BRAIN TUMORS

CONTEMPORARY NEUROLOGY SERIES AVAILABLE:

19 THE DIAGNOSIS OF STUPOR AND COMA, EDITION 3
Fred Plum, M.D., and Jerome B. Posner, M.D.

26 PRINCIPLES OF BEHAVIORAL NEUROLOGY
M-Marsel Mesulam, M.D., *Editor*

32 CLINICAL NEUROPHYSIOLOGY OF THE VESTIBULAR SYSTEM, EDITION 2
Robert W. Baloh, M.D., and Vincente Honrubia, M.D.

36 DISORDERS OF PERIPHERAL NERVES, EDITION 2
Herbert H. Schaumburg, M.D., Alan R. Berger, M.D., and P.K. Thomas, C.B.E., M.D., D.Sc., F.R.C.P., F.R.C.Path.

38 PRINCIPLES OF GERIATRIC NEUROLOGY
Robert Katzman, M.D., and John W. Rowe, M.D., *Editors*

42 MIGRAINE: MANIFESTATIONS, PATHOGENESIS, AND MANAGEMENT
Robert A. Davidoff, M.D.

43 NEUROLOGY OF CRITICAL ILLNESS
Eelco F. M. Wijdicks, M.D., Ph.D., F.A.C.P.

44 EVALUATION AND TREATMENT OF MYOPATHIES
Robert C. Griggs, M.D., Jerry R. Mendell, M.D., and Robert G. Miller, M.D.

45 NEUROLOGIC COMPLICATIONS OF CANCER
Jerome B. Posner, M.D.

46 CLINICAL NEUROPHYSIOLOGY
Jasper R. Daube, M.D., *Editor*

47 NEUROLOGIC REHABILITATION
Bruce H. Dobkin, M.D.

48 PAIN MANAGEMENT: THEORY AND PRACTICE
Russell K. Portenoy, M.D., and Ronald M. Kanner, M.D., *Editor*

49 AMYOTROPHIC LATERAL SCLEROSIS
Hiroshi Mitsumoto, M.D., D.Sc., David A. Chad, M.D., F.R.C.P., and Eric P. Pioro, M.D., D.Phil., F.R.C.P.

50 MULTIPLE SCLEROSIS
Donald W. Paty, M.D., F.R.C.P.C., and George C. Ebers, M.D., F.R.C.P.C.

51 NEUROLOGY AND THE LAW: PRIVATE LITIGATION AND PUBLIC POLICY
H. Richard Beresford, M.D., J.D.

52 SUBARACHNOID HEMORRHAGE: CAUSES AND CURES
Bryce Weir, M.D.

53 SLEEP MEDICINE
Michael S. Aldrich, M.D.

55 THE NEUROLOGY OF EYE MOVEMENTS, Edition 3
R. John Leigh, M.D., and David S. Zee, M.D.
(book and CD-ROM versions available)

BRAIN TUMORS

HARRY S. GREENBERG, M.D.
Professor of Neurology and Surgery
University of Michigan Medical School
Director, Neuro-Oncology Program
University of Michigan Medical Center
Ann Arbor, Michigan

WILLIAM F. CHANDLER, M.D.
Professor of Surgery
University of Michigan Medical School
Ann Arbor, Michigan

HOWARD M. SANDLER, M.D.
Associate Professor of Radiation Oncology
Associate Chair for Clinical Research
University of Michigan Medical School
Ann Arbor, Michigan

New York Oxford
OXFORD UNIVERSITY PRESS
1999

Oxford University Press

Oxford New York
Athens Auckland Bangkok Bogotá Buenos Aires Calcutta
Cape Town Chennai Dar es Salaam Delhi Florence Hong Kong Istanbul
Karachi Kuala Lumpur Madrid Melbourne Mexico City Mumbai
Nairobi Paris São Paulo Singapore Taipei Tokyo Toronto Warsaw

and associated companies in
Berlin Ibadan

Published by Oxford University Press Inc.,
198 Madison Avenue, New York, New York 10016
http://www.oup-usa.org

Library of Congress Cataloging-in-Publication Data

Greenberg, Harry, 1946-
Brain tumors / Harry S. Greenberg, William F. Chandler, Howard M. Sandler.
p. cm. — (Contemporary neurology series ; 54)
Includes bibliographical references and index.
ISBN 0-19-512958-X
1. Brain—Tumors. I. Chandler, William F. II. Sandler, Howard M. (Howard Mark), 1956- . III. Title. IV. Series.
[DNLM: 1. Brain Neoplasms. WL 358G798b 1999]
RC280.B7G74 1999
616.99'281—dc21
DNLM/DLC
for Library of Congress 98-27811
CIP

The science of medicine is a rapidly changing field. As new research and clinical experience broaden our knowledge, changes in treatment and drug therapy do occur. The author and the publisher of this work have checked with sources believed to be reliable in their efforts to provide information that is accurate and complete, and in accordance with the standards accepted at the time of publication. However, in light of the possibility of human error or changes in the practice of medicine, neither the author, nor the publisher, nor any other party who has been involved in the preparation or publication of this work warrants that the information contained herein is in every respect accurate or complete. Readers are encouraged to confirm the information contained herein with other reliable sources, and are strongly advised to check the product information sheet provided by the pharmaceutical company for each drug they plan to administer.

9 8 7 6 5 4 3 2 1

Printed in the United States of America
on acid-free paper.

This book is dedicated to my mother, Bea,
to my wife, Anne,
and my two stepsons, Ted and Will.

PREFACE

This monograph is written for neurologists and other physicians who participate in the diagnosis and treatment of patients with brain tumors. The authors, a neuro-oncologist, a neurosurgeon, and a radiation oncologist, based the book on their individual clinical experience, as well as on their experiences as members of a multidisciplinary treatment team of neurologists, neurosurgeons, radiation oncologists, neuropathologists, neuroradiologists, and basic scientists.

The text is practical. The first seven chapters provide a foundation for tumor pathology, biology, radiology, and the treatment modalities of surgery, radiation therapy, and chemotherapy. The chapter on biology presents an up-to-date summary of the recent advances in brain tumor biology that can be used as a springboard for comprehension of translational research and the development of clinical trials. Each of the tumor-specific chapters has a common format and reviews the history, epidemiology, biology, pathology, clinical symptoms, differential diagnosis, treatment, and prognosis and complications. There is particular emphasis on treatment in each of these chapters.

Many people helped in the writing of this work. Carol Cribbins typed many drafts of the manuscript, proofread all the chapters, and clarified the grammar, syntax, punctuation, and sometimes the thoughts and concepts. She prepared the figures and bibliography, and provided a kind, steering force through the detailed requirements of the text.

Several colleagues read chapters of the monograph and made valuable suggestions. Mila Blaivas, M.D., Ph.D., reviewed Chapter 1 on the pathology of brain tumors and provided almost all of the neuropathological figures. The comments of Al Yung, M.D., who reviewed Chapter 2, Stephen Gebarski, M.D., who reviewed Chapter 3, and Steven Telian, M.D., who reviewed Chapter 14, were helpful. Nicholas Vick, M.D. provided Figure 2–3 and Paul Kileny, Ph.D., Figure 14–1a,b.

Important collaboration came from my two co-authors, William Chandler, M.D., who wrote Chapters 4 and 13, and Howard Sandler, M.D., who wrote Chapters 5 and 6. They also contributed to many other chapters in this text. Without their collaboration and support, the book could not have been written.

I also want to thank Sid Gilman, M.D., Chairman of the Department of Neurology and Editor of the Contemporary Neurology Series, for inviting me to write this book. I am also indebted to the University of Michigan Medical School, which approved six months' sabbatical time for the book to germinate and grow toward completion.

I would also like to thank Jerome Posner, M.D., who has been a role model for me and for many other neuro-oncologists. Dr. Posner is the consummate physician–scientist who provided understanding and guidance during the critical years of my development.

Finally, a special thanks goes to my wife, Anne, who allowed me to spend four months writing this text in the mountains of Colorado while a construction project was taking place on the farm. Her love, strength, and support were truly appreciated.

Ann Arbor, Mich.
July 1998

H. S. G.

CONTENTS

Chapter 1

BRAIN TUMOR CLASSIFICATION, GRADING, AND EPIDEMIOLOGY

CLASSIFICATION AND GRADING
Historical Origins
Neuroepithelial Tumors
Tumors of Cranial and Peripheral Nerves
Mesenchymal Tumors
Lymphomas
Germ Cell Tumors
Sellar Region Tumors
Cysts and Other Benign Tumorlike Lesions
Brain Extension of Neighboring Regional Tumors
Metastatic Tumors
EPIDEMIOLOGY
Incidence
Environmental Exposure
Genetics

Brain tumors grow within a rigid, inelastic bony skull. Benign, slowly growing, and malignant brain tumors may produce significant neurological symptoms and signs prior to treatment or cure. Although brain tumors rarely metastasize outside the central nervous system (CNS), disability and death occur with brain tumors when the intracranial contents exceed the intracranial space, causing herniation and compression of respiratory centers. In this chapter, the classification and grading of brain tumors are discussed. The anatomic location of a brain tumor relative to surrounding structures is important in determining surgical therapy options; histologically identical tumors in different anatomic locations require radically different surgical and subsequent medical treatments. Histologically identical tumor types may occur in different locations within the CNS, and histologically diverse tumors are often common to the same location. The section on brain tumor epidemiology that completes the chapter discusses the different tumor incidences occurring in different age groups.

CLASSIFICATION AND GRADING

Historical Origins

The histological classification of most brain tumors is based on the normal CNS cell of origin, with the tumor named by the predominant cell type.[1,2] Despite progress in histological techniques and immunohistochemistry, the cell of origin of certain neoplasms has remained a mystery. Malignancy or anaplasia is determined by the histopathological features and is discussed under tumor type. Tumors are frequently an admixture of different neoplastic cell types, but a tumor is considered a mixed tumor only when a significant component of each neoplastic cell exists. The earliest classifications of brain tumors were those by Bailey and Cushing[2] (Fig. 1–1) and Kernohan and Sayre[3], with important contributions to classification made by Russell and Rubinstein.[4] The present system of classification of brain tumors was developed by neuropathologists under the auspices of the World Health Organization (WHO) in

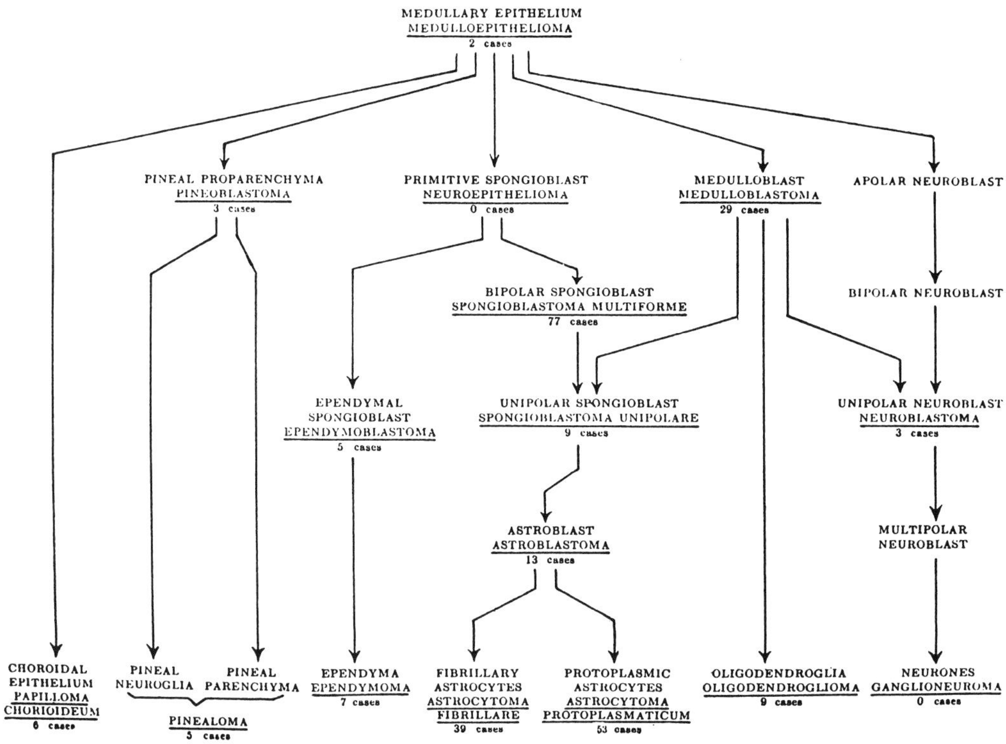

Figure 1–1. The Percival Bailey-Cushing classification, as given in the 1926 monograph (Schema IV, P 103). (From Bailey and Cushing,[2] p 103, with permission.)

1979 and revised in 1993.[5,6] It will be used for all classification in this chapter.

The initial major classification system was published in 1926 by Percival Bailey, a neuropathologist working with neurosurgeon Harvey Cushing, who published the work before Bailey had completed his studies.[1] This classification divided tumor types into 14 groups, with medulloepithelioma, arising from medullary epithelium, giving rise to all other malignant neoplasms (see Fig. 1–1). In this hierarchical classification system, medulloepithelioma differentiated into pineoblastoma, ependymoblastoma, spongioblastoma multiforme (glioblastoma multiforme), medulloblastoma, and neuroblastoma. The most differentiated neoplasms—pinealoma, ependymoma, astrocytoma fibrillare and astrocytoma protoplasmaticum, oligodendroglioma and ganglioglioma, and choroid plexus papilloma—were at the base of the chart, with choroid plexus papilloma arising directly from medulloepithelioma. Bailey and Cushing also established an expected clinical outcome for each tumor type in their classification scheme (Table 1–1).[2]

Oligodendroglioma was initially considered a differentiated form of medulloblastoma. The classification system was simplified in the next few years when Bailey and Bucy,[7] using the histological staining technique developed by del Rio-Hortega, proved the presence of oligodendroglia in oligodendrogliomas and reclassified these tumors of glial cell lineage. Bailey[8] made further changes, combining the two astrocytic tumors, eliminating the categories of medulloepithelioma, pineoblastoma, ependymoblastoma, and neuroblastoma, and noting that choroid plexus papilloma was not usually considered a glioma.

Kernohan and Sayre[3] classified tumors into five subtypes—astrocytoma, oligodendroglioma, ependymoma, gangliocytoma and medulloblastoma—and more importantly, added a grading system. Russell and Rubinstein[4] considered Kernohan's

Table 1–1. **Bailey and Cushing's Major Neurogenic Tumors and Their Clinical Outcomes**

Type of Tumor	Average Survival Period (mo)
Medulloepithelioma	8
Pineoblastoma	12
Spongioblastoma multiforme	12
Medulloblastoma	17
Pinealoma	18
Ependymoblastoma	19
Neuroblastoma	25
Astroblastoma	28
Ependymoma	32
Spongioblastoma unipolare	46
Oligodendroglioma	66
Astrocytoma protoplasmaticum	67
Astrocytoma fibrillare	86

Adapted from Bailey and Cushing,[2] p 108.

system oversimplified because of the omission of certain rare but real tumor types such as neuroepithelioma and polar spongioblastoma. They also believed tumors should be graded based on postmortem examination, when large samples could be analyzed.

Under the auspices of the WHO, neuropathologists met twice in the 1970s and developed a new classification and grading system for brain tumors, which Zülch published in 1979.[5] The classification system was to be comprehensive, clarify existing controversies in tumor typing, provide a histological grading system across a variety of intracranial neoplasms, and provide a means of communication between neuropathologists, neurosurgeons, neuro-oncologists, radiation oncologists, and other health professionals involved in the treatment of brain tumors.[5] The system was revised in 1993 by Kleihues, Burger, and Scheithauer[6] after two international working group meetings in 1988 and 1990. This new classification eliminated the separate entity of monstrocellular astrocytoma, which histological studies suggest is an astrocytoma. The major areas of controversy at the meetings were the use of grading systems to describe the degree of malignancy of tumors and the distinction between medulloblastoma and primitive neuroectodermal tumor.[9] Whereas one group of neuropathologists, led by Rubinstein, was initially opposed to all forms of grading, Zülch supported a grading system.[10] The introduction of the second edition of the WHO[6] classification system takes the compromise position that grading is not necessary for tumor typing, but if a grading system is used, it should be identified. Clearly, clinicians delivering care to patients with brain tumors feel a need for a grading system and understand the risk of sampling error with inaccurate prediction of biologic outcome.

This chapter covers nine major histological tumor types. Discussion of other aspects of these histologic tumor types is found in chapters or sections of chapters relating to specific tumors (Chapters 8–15)

Neuroepithelial Tumors

ASTROCYTOMA

The most common neuroepithelial tumors (Table 1–2) are astrocytic, composed predominantly of neoplastic astrocytes. Anaplasia or malignancy summarizes the histological features associated with a poor biologic outcome, as listed on Table 1–3.[6] An *astrocytoma* is a well-differentiated tumor that infiltrates the surrounding brain, spreading along white matter tracts (Fig. 1–2). These grade II astrocytomas are yellow-white, ill-defined, and expand the cortex, with tough rubbery fibrillary tumors and softer gelatinous protoplasmic astrocytomas. Microscopically, they infiltrate the surrounding brain diffusely. The astrocytes are neoplastic and vary with respect to cell processes and number of cytoplasmic glial filaments within these cell processes.[6] The histological classification of astrocytomas as fibrillary or protoplasmic has little prognostic significance because the same criteria of anaplasia are used in both types.[6]

Glial fibrillary acidic protein (GFAP) immunohistochemical staining is common in

Table 1–2. **Neuroepithelial Tumors**

Astrocytoma
Anaplastic astrocytoma
Glioblastoma multiforme
Gliosarcoma
Pilocytic astrocytoma
Pleomorphic xanthoastrocytoma
Subependymal giant-cell astrocytoma
Oligodendroglioma
Anaplastic oligodendroglioma
Oligo-astrocytoma
Anaplastic oligo-astrocytoma
Ependymoma
Anaplastic ependymoma
Myxopapillary ependymoma
Subependymoma
Choroid plexus tumors
Unclassified tumors
Astroblastoma
Polar spongioblastoma
Gliomatosis cerebri

fibrillary and gemistocytic astrocytoma, but much less marked in protoplasmic astrocytes without intracellular fibrils.[6,11] In the 1993 WHO classification, if mitoses are present, the tumor is a grade III astrocytoma. In the original WHO classification system from 1979, mitoses were included in the definition of grade II astrocytoma.[5,6] Pilocytic astrocytoma (grade I astrocytoma) is a surgically curable benign neoplasm. The differentiation of pilocytic astrocytoma from grade II astrocytoma is of critical importance because of the major differences in biologic behavior between these two types of astrocytomas.

Table 1–3. **Features of Increasing Malignancy in Neuroepithelial Tumor Grading**

Nuclear atypia
Cellular pleomorphism
Mitoses
Vascular proliferation
Necrosis

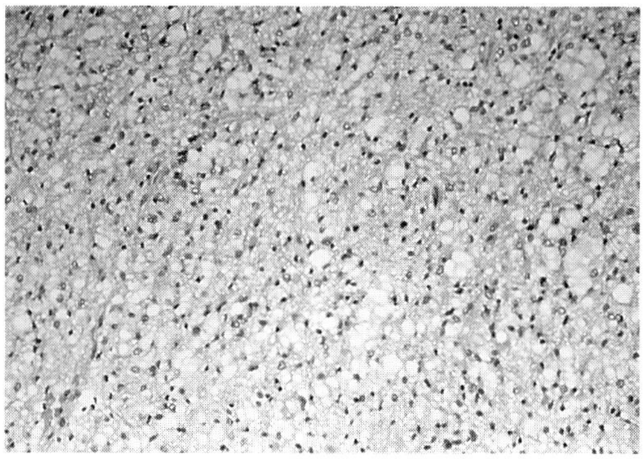

Figure 1–2. Grade II astrocytoma. Moderately pleomorphic astrocytic nuclei with little or no cytoplasm form fibillary microcystic matrix. Mitotic figures and vascular/endothelial proliferation are not present. H&E stain. Mag. ×200. (Courtesy of Mila Blaivas, MD, PhD, Department of Pathology, University of Michigan Medical School, Ann Arbor, MI.)

Anaplastic astrocytoma (malignant, grade III) has mitotic activity, increased nuclear atypia, cellular pleomorphism, and increased cellularity (Fig. 1–3A). This type of tumor often progresses rapidly and may transform into a glioblastoma. Vascular proliferation and necrosis are absent in an anaplastic astrocytoma. This differs from the 1979 WHO classification,[5] in which the presence of vascular proliferation classified the tumor as grade III. A cellular variant of the anaplastic astrocytoma is the gemistocytic anaplastic astrocytoma, which has a large amount of pink cytoplasm and small, frequently eccentric, nuclei (Fig. 1–3B). Patients with astrocytomas, with a gemistocytic cellular component of 20% or greater, have a median survival that is less than in patients with anaplastic astrocytomas.[12]

Glioblastoma is the most malignant tumor of the astrocytoma series. In addition to mitoses and nuclear pleomorphism, glioblastoma has either vascular proliferation or necrosis (Fig. 1–4). The descriptor "multiforme" indicates a variety of cytological features and patterns.To the surgeon, the affected brain regions appear macroscopically swollen and expanded. The tumor surfaces are mottled, with pinkish-gray peripheral tissue, most often surrounding a rim of yellow necrosis.[6]

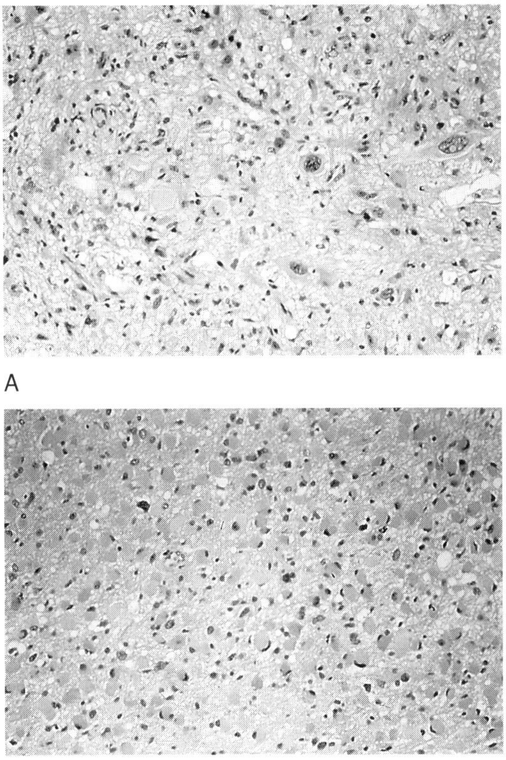

A

B

Figure 1–3. *(A.)* Grade III anaplastic astrocytoma. Markedly pleomorphic, hyperchromatic nuclei are frequently surrounded by a large amount of cytoplasm. Mitotic figures and multinucleated cells are easily found. Vascular and endothelial proliferation is not present. H&E stain. Mag. ×200. *(B)* Gemistocytic astrocytoma. Pink gemistocytic astrocytes exhibit large amounts of cytoplasm and relatively small, frequently eccentric nuclei. Multinucleated cells as well as nuclei with no surrounding cytoplasm, or large, pleomorphic, hyperchromatic nuclei are mixed within. The matrix is finely fibrillar. Mitotic figures are present. H&E stain. Mag. ×200. (Courtesy of Mila Blaivas, MD, PhD, Department of Pathology, University of Michigan Medical School, Ann Arbor, MI.)

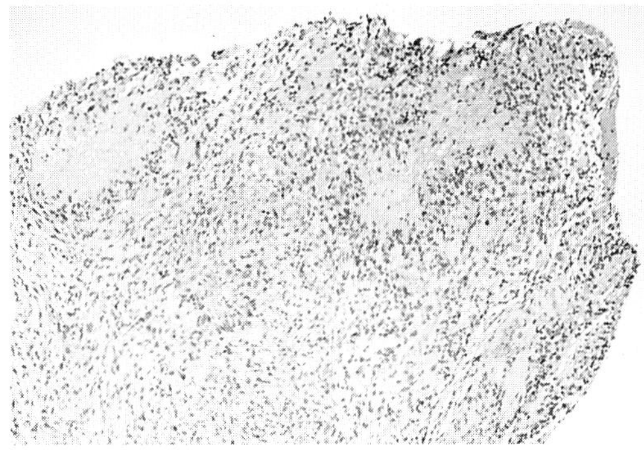

Figure 1–4. Glioblastoma multiforme. Hypercellular, pleomorphic neoplasm with visible mitotic figures and vascular/endothelial proliferation. The tumor contains several easily identified regions of geographic necrosis surrounded by palisades of neoplastic cells. H&E stain. Mag. ×100. (Courtesy of Mila Blaivas, MD, PhD, Department of Pathology, University of Michigan Medical School, Ann Arbor, MI.)

Hemorrhage is often present, and the tumor may invade the leptomeninges and attach to the dura or grow through the ependyma and seed cerebrospinal fluid (CSF).[6] The dura most often acts as a barrier to the glioma cell invasion.

Microscopically, glioblastoma is often composed of pleomorphic, poorly differentiated fusiform or round cells. Giant cells are occasionally present. These tumors frequently have large areas that are GFAP negative, consistent with progressive dedifferentiation. If bizarre multinucleated giant cells with eosinophilic cytoplasm predominate, the tumor is called a *giant-cell glioblastoma.* The giant-cell variant is associated with a slightly better prognosis than is the usual small-cell glioblastoma multiforme.[13]

Gliosarcoma has a malignant sarcomatous component, usually a malignant fibrous histiocytoma or fibrosarcoma. Gliosarcoma occurs in less than 5% of patients with glioblastoma multiforme, and the prognosis is similar to that of glioblastoma multiforme.[13,14]

On pathological examination, glial neoplasms show significant regional variability or heterogeneity.[6,15–18] Foci of high cellularity, nuclear pleomorphism, frequent mitosis with necrosis, and vascular proliferation may adjoin sheets of fibrillary astrocytes without anaplastic features. The tumor is graded pathologically by its most anaplastic component, which is most predictive of its biologic behavior. Anaplastic regions may represent dedifferentiated regions of less aggressive tumor or may arise de novo.

Daumas-Duport[18] has added a structural organization to tumor characterization, describing the relationship of tumor to brain. Type I tumors are solid and do not infiltrate surrounding brain. Type II tumors have solid portions; in addition, individual tumor cells infiltrate the surrounding brain and are not in contact with each other. Type III tumors are composed only of individual tumor cells that infiltrate normal brain, without a solid tumor mass. Astrocytoma, anaplastic astrocytoma, and glioblastoma most often have a type II structure.

Other grading systems have been frequently used in describing astrocytomas. The Kernohan system, introduced in 1950 by Kernohan and Sayre,[3] divided astrocytomas into grades I to IV, with increasing malignancy. Grade III and IV astrocytomas were both called *glioblastomas* and both contained mitoses, endothelial proliferation, and necrosis. A sharp distinction did not exist between using these grades and grading on a subjective evaluation by a pathologist.[3,19] In 1950, Ringertz[20] developed a three-tiered system of astrocytoma, anaplastic astrocytoma, and glioblastoma multiforme, using increasing cellular atypia, nuclear pleomorphism, vascular proliferation, and necrosis as criteria for increasing malignancy. The Ringertz system was also applied to oligodendroglioma and ependymoma, with the final category of anaplasia being glioblastoma.[21,22] In 1979, the first WHO classification was developed.[5] Because of opposition from pathologists, the WHO did not embrace grading, preferring instead to discuss tumors in terms of degree of malignancy. In 1989, the University of California-San Francisco introduced its grading system.[23] To develop a reproducible grading system, Daumas-Duport and colleagues (Mayo St. Anne, Paris)[18,24] proposed a discrete grading system based on the presence or absence of nuclear atypia, mitosis, endothelial proliferation, or necrosis in the pathological specimen. If no criteria are present, the tumor is classified as grade I; if one criterion, grade II; if two criteria, grade III; and if three or four criteria, grade IV. In summary, whereas Kernohan, Ringertz, and the WHO used a grading system with continuous variables, Daumas-Duport developed a discrete-variable classification system. A comparison of the pathological grading systems is shown in Table 1–4. The biologic behavior from the revised WHO classification system for major tumor types is summarized in Table 1–5.

Pilocytic astrocytoma (grade I astrocytomas) is most often a well-circumscribed astrocytoma (type I structure by Daumas-Duport) composed of bipolar piloid or fusiform cells that often form compact bundles (Fig. 1–5). The tumor contains microcysts that join together to form the larger cysts seen on computed tomography (CT) and magnetic resonance imaging (MRI). Glomeruloid capillary or endothelial proliferation may be responsible for contrast enhancement visualized on imaging studies.[6,25,26] Rosenthal fibers (elongated eosinophilic, club-shaped structures) and intracytoplasmic protein droplets (granular bodies) are histological markers of pilocytic astrocytoma in a circumscribed astrocytoma. Although tumor cell nuclei are often bizarre and endothelial proliferation or even necrosis is present, these features do not carry the same biologic significance as they do in an anaplastic astrocytoma. An anaplastic variant is characterized by multiple mitoses. Many pathologists believe that because of their benign biologic behavior, pilocytic astrocytomas should not be graded (with other astrocytomas) using the WHO, Kernohan, or Dumas-Duport systems; their histological features would classify them as higher-grade astrocytomas.[27]

Pleomorphic xanthoastrocytoma is a rare astrocytoma variant occurring in children and young adults. The tumor is most frequently located superficially in the temporal lobe and has areas of meningeal involvement, showing a dense intracellular reticulum network (Fig. 1–6A). Mitoses are rare, and endothelial proliferation and necrosis are absent. The pleomorphic cells vary from fibrillary astrocytes to giant, multinucleated, lipid-laden cells that raise the specter of aggressive behavior. Generally, the biologic behavior is grade II, with a minority of tumors progressing to more malignant astrocytic tumors (Fig 1–6B).[8]

Subependymal giant-cell astrocytoma occurs in young patients with tuberous sclerosis. The tumor is located in the walls of the lateral ventricle and is composed of astrocytes that appear to stream from vessel

Table 1–4. **A Comparison of Pathologic Grading Systems Commonly Used in Astrocytomas**

Kernohan[3] (1950)*	Ringertz [BMW[39]][20] (1950)	WHO[5] (1979)	UCSF[23] (1989)	Mayo/St Anne[24] (1993)**	WHO[6] (1993)
Grade IV astrocytoma	Glioblastoma	Glioblastoma	Glioblastoma	Grade IV astrocytoma	Glioblastoma
Grade III astrocytoma	Anaplastic astrocytoma	Anaplastic astrocytoma	Moderately anaplastic Astrocytoma	Grade III astrocytoma	*Glioblastoma*
Grade II astrocytoma	Astrocytoma	Astrocytoma	Mildly anaplastic astrocytoma	Grade II astrocytoma	Astrocytoma or Anaplastic astrocytoma
Grade I astrocytoma			Mildly anaplastic astrocytoma	Grade I astrocytoma	

*Grade III and IV both contain glioblastoma.
**Each number based on presence of four categories (nuclear atypia, mitoses, endothelial proliferation, necrosis); no categories, grade I; 3 or 4 categories, grade IV.

Table 1–5. **Biologic Behavior of Primary CNS Tumors**

Tumors	Grade I Benign	Grade II Semibenign	Grade III Relatively Malignant	Grade IV Highly Malignant
Astrocytoma		+		
Astrocytoma, anaplastic			+	
Glioblastoma				+
Gliosarcoma				+
Pilocytic astrocytoma	+			
Pilocytic astrocytoma, anaplastic			+	
Oligodendroglioma		+		
Oligodendroglioma, anaplastic			+	
Oligo-astrocytoma		+		
Oligo-astrocytoma, anaplastic			+	
Ependymoma	+	+		
Ependymoma, anaplastic			+	+
Myxopapillary ependymoma	+			
Subependymoma	+			
Choroid plexus papilloma	+			
Choroid plexus carcinoma			+	+
Gangliocytoma	+			
Ganglioglioma		+		
Central neurocytoma	+			
Desmoplastic infantile ganglioglioma	+			
Dysembryoplastic neuroepithelial tumor	+			

Continued on following page

walls. Tumor cells often cluster and palisade around blood vessels (Fig. 1–7). This type of tumor grows very slowly and can be surgically removed, resulting in cure. The histology of subependymal giant-cell astrocytoma and that of subependymal nodules are identical, with clinical convention calling the tumor a *subependymal giant-cell astrocytoma,* the appropriate nomenclature when symptomatic.[28] It is a grade I neoplasm.

OLIGODENDROGLIOMA AND OLIGOASTROCYTOMA

Oligodendroglial tumors are the second major type of astrocytic neoplasm. They may be solid and distinct from surrounding brain (i.e., Daumas-Duport type I structure), or at the opposite extreme, diffuse, with single infiltrating cells (i.e., type III structure). The *oligodendroglioma* is composed of neoplastic oligodendro-

Table 1–5.—*continued*

Tumors	Grade I Benign	Grade II Semibenign	Grade III Relatively Malignant	Grade IV Highly Malignant
Medulloblastoma				+
Neurofibroma	+			
Schwannoma	+			
Malignant nerve sheath tumor (Neurofibrosarcoma)				+
Meningioma	+			
Meningioma, atypical		+		
Meningioma, anaplastic			+	
Lymphoma			+	
Mesenchymal sarcoma				+
Pineocytoma		+		
Pineoblastoma				+
Germinoma		+		
Nongerminomatous germ cell			+	
Pituitary adenoma	+			
Pituitary carcinoma			+	
Craniopharyngioma	+			

cytes. On microscopic examination, a well-defined plasma membrane and a clear cytoplasm, swollen by fixation artifact, produce a fried-egg appearance. Focal calcifications are frequently seen in the marginal zones of tumor infiltration. Histologically, the neoplasms are moderately cellular with enlarged hyperchromatic nuclei. Mitoses are infrequent, and the extracellular matrix (ECM) contains small capillary blood vessels forming a lattice framework (Fig. 1–8). Currently, there is no reliable marker for oligodendroglial cells. A significant proportion of these tumors stain with GFAP when they become anaplastic.[6]

Anaplastic oligodendroglioma contains numerous mitoses, nuclear pleomorphism, and cellular atypia; it corresponds to the

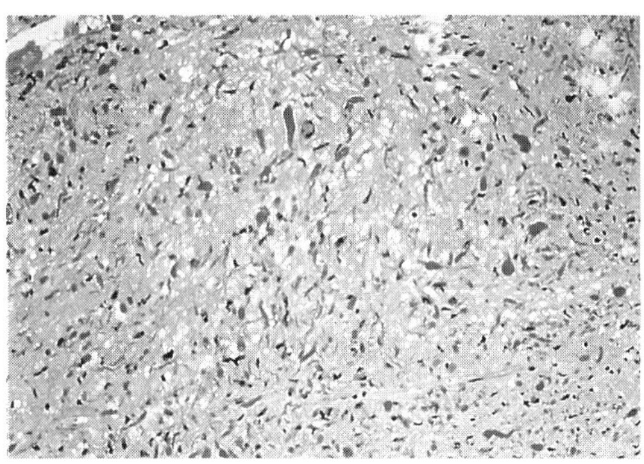

Figure 1–5. Pilocytic astrocytoma. Relatively hypocellular neoplasm with coarsely fibrillar matrix, slight nuclear pleomorphism and frequent Rosenthal fibers. Mitotic figures are inconspicuous. Vascular and endothelial proliferation is absent in this field. H&E stain. Mag. ×200. (Courtesy of Mila Blaivas, MD, PhD, Department of Pathology, University of Michigan Medical School, Ann Arbor, MI.)

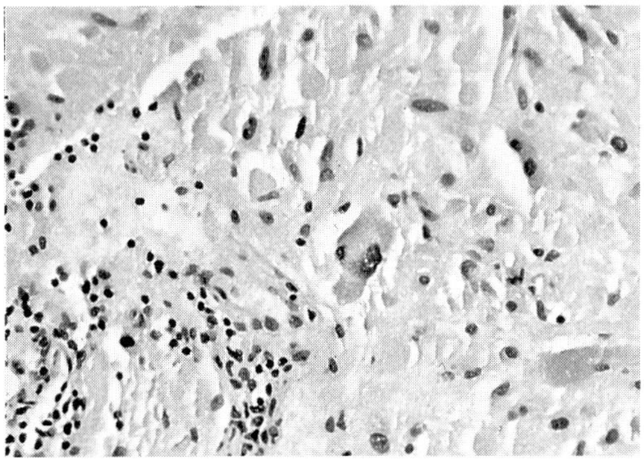

A

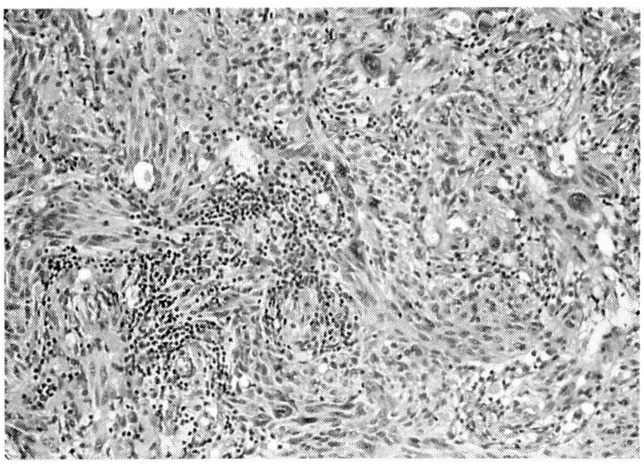

B

Figure 1–6. *(A)* Pleomorphic xanthoastrocytoma. This neoplasm is characterized by marked cellular pleomorphism, occasional multinucleated giant cells with lipidized (xanthochromatous) cytoplasm. Perivascular lymphocytic infiltrate is common. Mitotic figures and endothelial proliferation are absent. H&E stain. Mag. ×400. *(B)* Malignant pleomorphic xanthoastrocytoma. Much more cellular and even more pleomorphic than the benign variant, this neoplasm retains similar cytological features and perivascular lymphocytic inflammation. However, mitotic figures and endothelial proliferation are prominent and regions of tumor necrosis exist. H&E stain. Mag. ×200. (Courtesy of Mila Blaivas, MD, PhD, Department of Pathology, University of Michigan Medical School, Ann Arbor, MI.)

anaplastic or grade III astrocytoma. Endothelial proliferation and necrosis may be features of further anaplasia in an oligodendroglioma, and may be morphologically indistinguishable from a glioblastoma.

Oligo-astrocytomas are mixed tumors containing both malignant astrocytes and oligodendrocytes; the two individual cell types may occur in distinct areas or be intermingled (Fig. 1–9). Although oligo-astrocytoma, oligodendroglioma, and astrocytoma all have grade II biologic behavior, it is generally thought that tumors with an oligodendroglial component behave less aggressively. Whereas Glass and colleagues[29] concluded that oligodendroglioma and oligo-astrocytoma have the same biologic behavior, Shaw and colleagues[30] found that oligo-astrocytoma is slightly more aggressive than oligodendroglioma but more benign than astrocytoma in terms of biologic behavior. The bi-

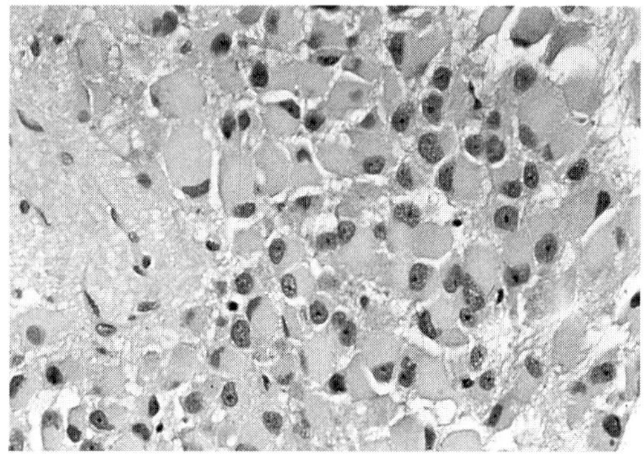

Figure 1–7. Subependymal giant-cell astrocytoma. Clusters of large rounded cells with large, frequently eccentric nuclei and prominent nucleoli are embedded within finely fibrillar matrix. The cells resemble both large astrocytes and neurons. Endothelial proliferation and necrosis and mitotic figures are rare or absent. H&E stain. Mag. ×400. (Courtesy of Mila Blaivas, MD, PhD, Department of Pathology, University of Michigan Medical School, Ann Arbor, MI.)

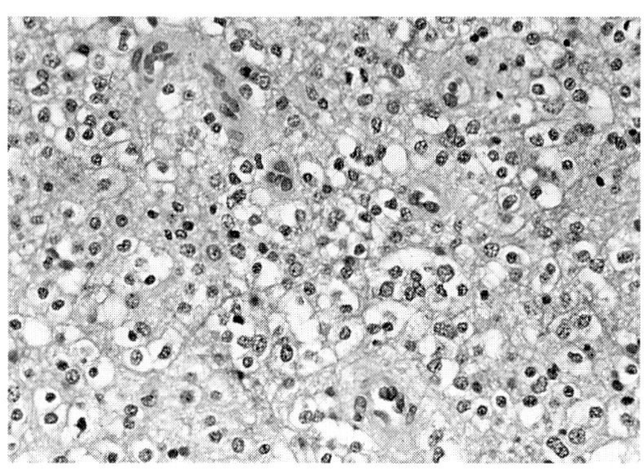

Figure 1–8. Grade II oligodendroglioma. Rounded cells with central or slightly eccentric round nuclei and clear perinuclear halos are gathered in small clusters or rows. Mitotic figures are rare, and the vessels are thin walled and lack endothelial proliferation. H&E stain. Mag. ×400. (Courtesy of Mila Blaivas, MD, PhD, Department of Pathology, University of Michigan Medical School, Ann Arbor, MI.)

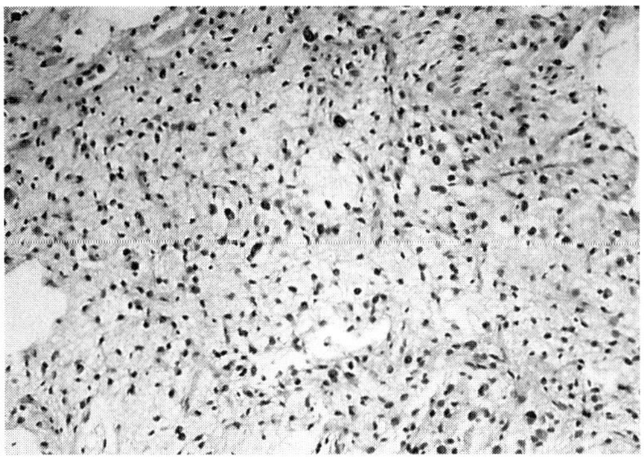

Figure 1–9. Grade II oligoastrocytoma. A mixture of rounded oligodendroglial and elongated or irregular astrocytic nuclei, with little or no cytoplasm, is situated in a microcystic fibrillary background. The vessels crossing the field are thin walled and long. Mitotic figures and endothelial proliferation are absent. H&E stain. Mag. ×200. (Courtesy of Mila Blaivas, MD, PhD, Department of Pathology, University of Michigan Medical School, Ann Arbor, MI.)

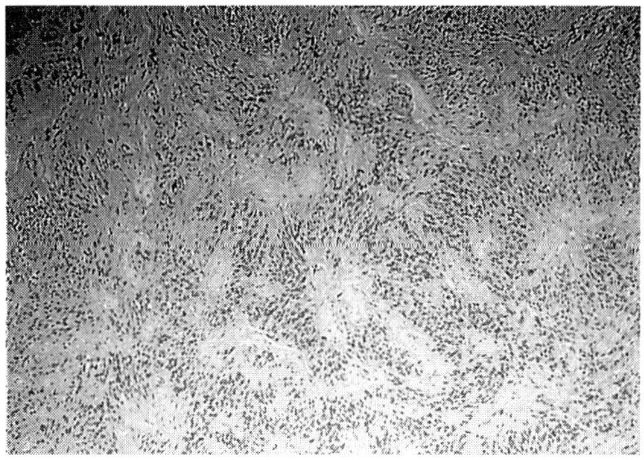

Figure 1–10. Ependymoma. Rather monotonously sized and shaped nuclei with "salt-and-pepper" chromatin are arranged around vessels forming perivascular pseudorosettes. The cells send their long processes toward the vessel walls, which are hypocellular and frequently hyalinized. Mitotic figures are rare, endothelial proliferation and necrosis are absent. H&E stain. Mag. ×100. (Courtesy of Mila Blaivas, MD, PhD, Department of Pathology, University of Michigan Medical School, Ann Arbor, MI.)

ologic behavior of the anaplastic variant is similar to that of both anaplastic oligodendroglioma and astrocytoma.

EPENDYMOMA

Ependymoma is a moderately cellular tumor composed of neoplastic ependymal cells. It originates from ependyma lining the ventricular walls, the central canal of the spinal cord, or the filum terminale. On microscopic examination, ependymal rosettes and perivascular pseudorosettes, occasional mitoses, nuclear atypia, and even necrosis are present. These histological features are not necessarily indicative of malignant biologic behavior (Fig. 1–10). In children and adolescents, ependymoma is most often located in the fourth ventricle and remains well demarcated from the surrounding brain. Whereas ependymomas in the cerebellum tend to be firm, those projecting into the fourth ventricle or foramen of Luschka may be soft and papillary.[6] In adults, ependymoma is most frequently found in the lumbosacral region. The three cellular variants of ependymoma are clear cell, cellular, and papillary (i.e., resembling a choroid plexus papilloma)

In terms of biologic behavior, ependymoma is a grade II tumor. It frequently has a type III structural organization, according to the Daumas-Duport classification. Until recently, it has been difficult to determine what histological changes predict more aggressive behavior. Two recent studies, one of supratentorial and the other of infratentorial ependymoma, find that marked mitotic activity, nuclear atypia, and prominent endothelial proliferation predict poor outcome and correspond to a

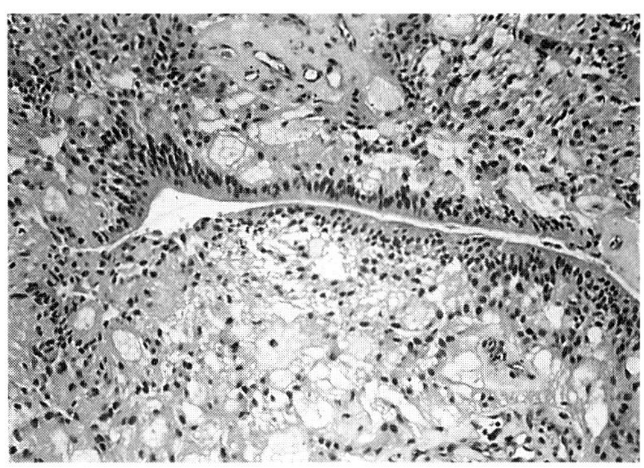

Figure 1–11. Myxopapillary ependymoma. The neoplasm forms ependymal lining in the center of the field. Pools of mucin separated by small clusters of elongated nuclei and thick-walled hyalinized vessels are important features of the tumor. Mitotic figures are not conspicuous. H&E stain. Mag. ×200. (Courtesy of Mila Blaivas, MD, PhD, Department of Pathology, University of Michigan Medical School, Ann Arbor, MI.)

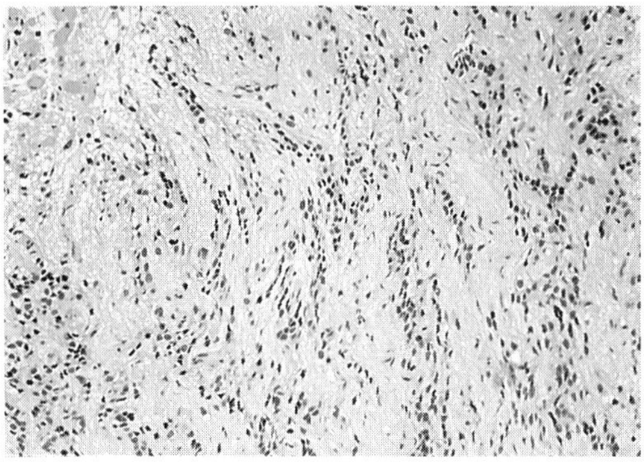

Figure 1–12. Subependymoma. Clusters of small rounded or elongated nuclei with salt-and-pepper chromatin pattern are separated by wide bands of fibrillary matrix. Mitotic figures are absent and vessels are not conspicuous. H&E stain. Mag. ×200. (Courtesy of Mila Blaivas, MD, PhD, Department of Pathology, University of Michigan Medical School, Ann Arbor, MI.)

grade III anaplastic tumor.[31] Rarely, the tumor evolves into a glioblastoma.

Myxopapillary ependymoma is an ependymoma variant that occurs only in the lumbosacral region, originating from ependymal nests in the filum terminale and growing in the cauda equina, with occasional invasion of the conus medullaris. Mucin-containing cysts or hyalinized vessels are surrounded by neoplastic ependymal cells, which are often cuboidal and papillary (Fig. 1–11). The tumor cells often are positive for GFAP on immunohistochemistry. This benign tumor can be resected completely when encapsulated; its biologic behavior is benign or grade I.

Subependymoma is a nest of round ependymal cells with glial fibrillary processes forming a dense network with frequent microcysts (Fig. 1–12). It occurs as single or multiple nodules in the fourth and lateral ventricles and has a benign biologic behavior (i.e., it is a grade I tumor).

CHOROID PLEXUS TUMORS

Choroid plexus papilloma is a benign (i.e., grade I) epithelial tumor, developing from choroid plexus in the cerebral ventricles.[6] Gross examination shows that the tumor is an irregular, mottled, pinkish-gray, jelly-like mass that expands the ventricle locally. It consists of columnar or cuboidal cells resting on basement membrane, which surround papilla of connective tissue containing blood vessels. Anaplastic features may be present without a change in biologic behavior. Histologically, it may be difficult to distinguish papillary ependymoma and normal choroid plexus from papilloma, particularly on small biopsy specimens. Its malignant form, *choroid plexus carcinoma,* is a rare entity characterized by loss of papillae, leaving a diffuse expanse of columnar and cuboidal cells with significant mitotic activity and nuclear atypia. These tumors may seed through the neuraxis and are biologically aggressive grade III tumors.

UNCLASSIFIED NEUROEPITHELIAL TUMORS

According to the most recent WHO classification, three other neuroepithelial tumors are probably ordinary gliomas, but their cell of origin remains unclear. They are astroblastoma, polar spongioblastoma, and gliomatosis cerebri. *Astroblastoma,* a tumor of young adults, is composed of neoplastic astrocytes that radiate to a blood vessel. Astroblastoma may have pseudorosettes that resemble an ependymoma.[6] Astroblastoma covers the spectrum of anaplasia, with higher-grade tumors having the usual features of malignancy.[32]

Polar spongioblastoma is composed of sheets of bipolar astrocytic tumor cells stacked with parallel nuclei. It occurs in children and has varying biologic behavior. The polar spongioblastoma may contain regions with pilocytic or oligodendroglial differentiation. The developers of the recent WHO classification[6] were unsure whether this tumor occurred as a separate entity or was more commonly observed focally in other glial neoplasms.

Gliomatosis cerebri is the last of the unclassified glial tumors and is a diffuse glial cell infiltration in multiple lobes of the brain. In its classic form, there is no solid tumor nodule and it corresponds to a type III structure of Daumas-Duport. In addition to histology, the diagnosis requires CT or MRI scan that demonstrates involvement of several lobes of the brain.

MIXED NEURONAL AND GLIAL TUMORS

Mixed neuronal and glial tumors (Table 1–6) are composed of a varying admixture of neuronal and glial cells. The first of these is *gangliocytoma* (Fig. 1–13A), a tumor with neoplastic ganglion cells and a supporting network of normal glial cells. These tumors tend to occur in the temporal lobe in children and young adults and are a benign neoplasm with a grade I biologic behavior. The tumor is composed of neoplastic ganglion cells, which are occasionally binucleate. The presence of Nissl substance and neurofibrils, identified by special staining techniques, conclusively identify neuronal populations. On immunohistochemistry, these tumors often stain with the neuronal markers for synaptophysin or neurofilament protein.[6,12] Whether these neuronal populations are a tumor or a hamartoma is often difficult to distinguish. Dysplastic gangliocytoma of cerebellum (Lhermitte-Duclos), a variant of gangliocytoma, occurs in the cerebellum and consists of unusual granular neurons that may resemble Purkinje cells.

Ganglioglioma (Fig. 1–13B) is a benign tumor with grade II biologic behavior, composed of both neoplastic astrocytes and ganglion cells. In contrast to gangliocytoma, this tumor possesses a neoplastic glial cell component and immunostains for both neuronal and glial markers. Blood vessels are often surrounded by lymphocytes. In the anaplastic variant, the glial component has anaplastic features.

Central neurocytoma is another newly recognized entity, described initially in 1992. It consists of round cells, often with clear cytoplasm, closely resembling oligodendroglia within a fibrillar matrix. This tumor usually occurs in the walls of the lateral ventricle, near the foramen of Monro, and has a grade I biologic behavior. Recently, a malignant variant has been described (Fig. 1–14A).[33] Central neurocytoma routinely stains with neuronal markers (Fig. 1–14B).

Desmoplastic infantile ganglioglioma (DIG), a mixed neuronal and glial neoplasm of infancy, has neoplastic ganglion cells and astrocytes in varying percentages. The neuronal component may react with neurofilament protein or synaptophysin; the

Table 1–6. **Neuronal or Mixed Neuronal-Glial Tumors**

Gangliocytoma
Ganglioglioma
Central neurocytoma
Desmoplastic infantile ganglioglioma
Dysembryoplastic neuroepithelial tumor
Olfactory neuroblastoma

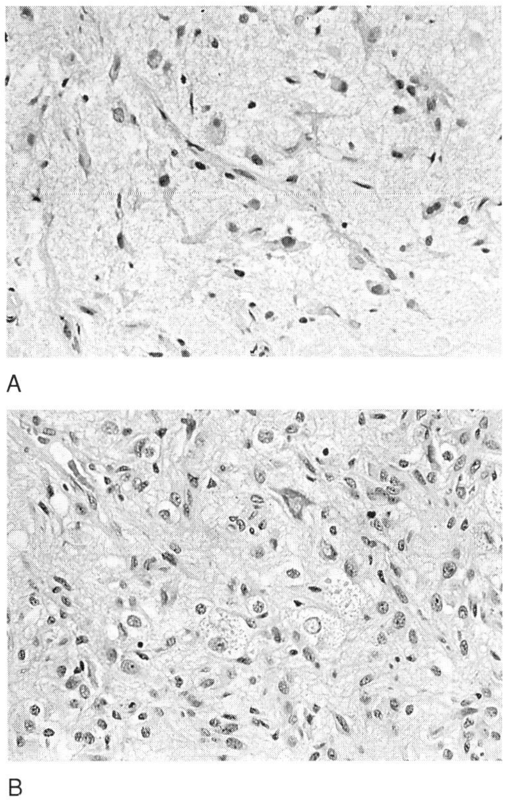

Figure 1–13. *(A)* Gangliocytoma. Various size and shape neurons, some binucleated, are haphazardly arranged within the vaguely fibrillar matrix that contains rare glial nuclei. There are no mitotic figures and the vessels crossing the section are very thin. H&E stain. Mag. ×400. *(B)* Gangliocytoma. Fibrillary microcystic matrix contains haphazardly arranged small and large misshapen neurons and rounded or elongated glial nuclei. No mitotic figures are present, and the vessels are thin walled with no endothelial proliferation. H&E stain. Mag. ×400. (Courtesy of Mila Blaivas, MD, PhD, Department of Pathology, University of Michigan Medical School, Ann Arbor, MI.)

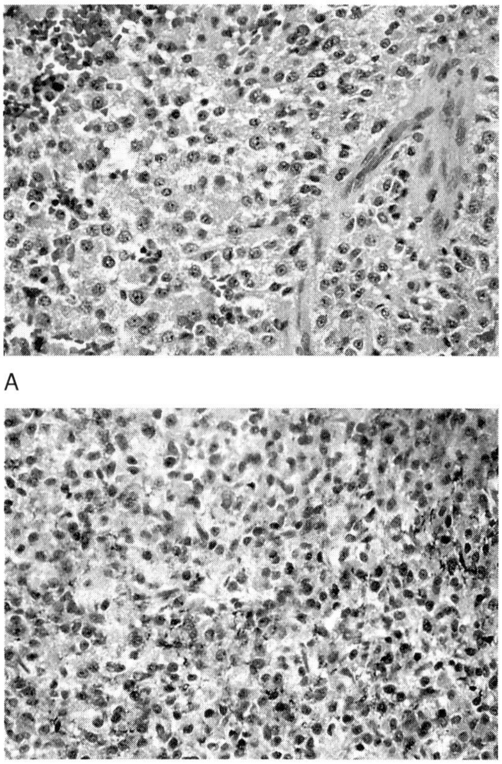

A

B

Figure 1–14. Central neurocytoma *(A)* Small rounded nuclei with prominent nucleoli and frequent perinuclear halos reminiscent of oligodendroglioma form this neoplasm. The vessels are usually thin walled and are reminiscent of those in oligodendroglioma. The mitotic figures are not conspicuous. H&E stain. Mag ×400. *(B)* The neoplastic cells stain positively for synaptophysin. Immunoperoxidase stain with antisynaptophysin antibody. Mag. ×400. (Courtesy of Mila Blaivas, MD, PhD, Department of Pathology, University of Michigan Medical School, Ann Arbor, MI.)

astrocytes express GFAP. This tumor is located close to the surface in the cerebral hemispheres and may be associated with a large cyst. The solid component is often a large fibrous mass, and the tumor displays a benign grade I biologic behavior.

A recently recognized neuropathological entity, *Dysembryoplastic neuroepithelial tumor* (DNET), is seen in children and young adults, particularly in those with medically intractable partial complex seizures. It is not associated with mental retardation or skin lesions and behaves as a benign tumor that does not recur after surgical resection. It is composed of neoplastic neurons, oligodendroglia, and astrocytes. The tumor is often cystic, with neurons eccentrically placed within the cyst (Fig. 1–15). The cortex surrounding the tumor is often dysplastic.[6,21]

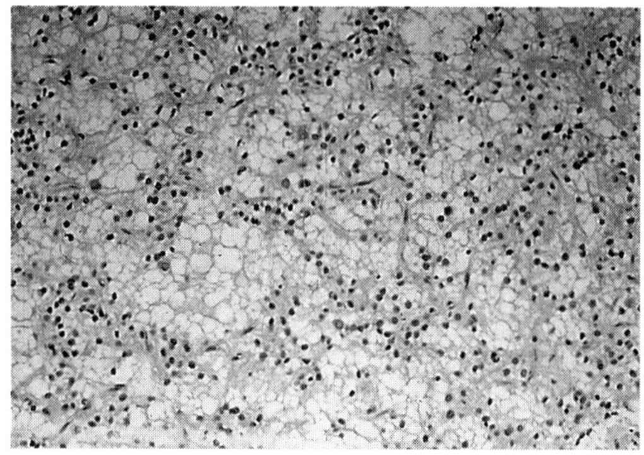

Figure 1–15. Dysembryoplastic neuroepithelial tumor. Clusters of small, rounded nuclei are present; some of these belong to small, young neurons and others to oligodendroglia. The clusters are arranged in groups among criss-crossing thin-walled vessels on the microcystic background. Some of the nuclei are larger, with prominent nucleoli and small amounts of cytoplasm, proclaiming them better-differentiated neurons. No mitotic figures are present. H&E stain. Mag. ×200. (Courtesy of Mila Blaivas, MD, PhD, Department of Pathology, University of Michigan Medical School, Ann Arbor, MI.)

Olfactory neuroblastoma is a neuronal malignant tumor arising from precursor cells of the nasal neuroepithelium.

From its origin in the vault of the nose, this tumor invades the sinuses, orbit, and brain. Histologically, the tumor is composed of neuroblasts located within a richly vascularized stroma. It behaves biologically as a grade III tumor.

PINEAL TUMORS

The pineal region of the brain is the site of many different tumor types, including pineocytoma, pineoblastoma, astrocytoma, dysgerminoma, non-germ-cell embryonal tumors, and teratoma. The astrocytoma was discussed previously. Dysgerminoma and non-germ-cell embryonal tumors are discussed with germ-cell tumors.

Pineocytoma is a moderately cellular, rare tumor that forms rosettes around blood vessels. These tumors grow slowly, exhibiting a grade II biologic behavior. They become symptomatic by producing hydrocephalus through compression of the aqueduct of Sylvius. The malignant variant is called a *pineoblastoma*. A continuous spectrum of malignancy is seen from pineocytoma to pineoblastoma; individual tumors often have components of both neoplasms. Pineocytoma most often occurs in children and young adults. The pineoblastoma has also been called a *primitive neuroectodermal tumor* by Rorke.[34] It has a grade IV biologic behavior.

PRIMITIVE NEUROECTODERMAL TUMOR OR EMBRYONAL TUMOR

Lucy Rorke introduced the name "primitive neuroectodermal tumor" (PNET) for a group of tumors that share a common progenitor cell. These tumors are believed to derive from the subependymal matrix level. PNET has variably been called *medulloblastoma, ependymoblastoma, neuroblastoma,* and *pineoblastoma*. Rorke's theory is that subependymal cells occur in various locations in the CNS and, depending on locale, a specific type of embryonal tumor occurs.[34] In its most recent classification, the WHO failed to embrace this theory and instead kept these tumors as separate diagnostic entities. One question was the origin of the medulloblastoma, generally believed to arise from the granular layer, a matrix zone for neurons but not for glial cells. Medulloblastomas display neuronal differentiation more often than glial differentiation.

Medulloblastoma is a cerebellar embryonal childhood tumor that is highly cellular with round, carrot-shaped, or oval nuclei and sparse cytoplasm. Mitoses are frequent, and the cells may form Homer Wright rosettes (Fig. 1–16). Neuronal differentiation is frequent, and most of these tumors express synaptophysin and neurofilament protein. Less frequently, the cells have astrocytic differentiation; ependymal features are rare. There may be GFAP staining without apparent histological evidence of astrocytic differentiation. These tumors grow aggressively from their site of origin in the vermis, filling the fourth ventricle, blocking CSF egress, invading the cerebellum and brainstem, and seeding the CSF.[6,35] Their biologic behavior is grade IV. A desmoplastic variant, with similar biologic behavior, has a network of reticulin fibers interspersed with areas of

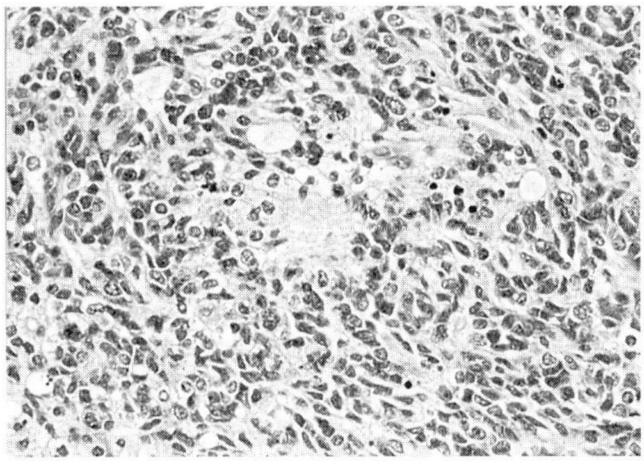

Figure 1–16. Medulloblastoma. Cellular neoplasm formed by small, angular, rounded, or oval hyperchromatic nuclei circling vessels or fibrillary cores and making rosettes. Mitotic figures and pyknotic degenerative nuclei of necrotic tumor cells are frequently observed. H&E stain. Mag. ×400. (Courtesy of Mila Blaivas, MD, PhD, Department of Pathology, University of Michigan Medical School, Ann Arbor, MI.)

typical neuronally differentiated medulloblastoma cells. Melanotic and rhabdomyoblastic variants occur rarely.

Medulloepithelioma is a rare childhood neoplasm similar in biologic behavior to medulloblastoma. It is formed by columnar cells arranged in glandular structures sitting on a basement membrane. The term "medulloepithelioma" was originally used by Bailey and Cushing[1,2] to describe the progenitor cell of all neuroepithelial neoplasms. The authors discarded the term shortly thereafter, but recent evidence suggests the existence of a rare primitive childhood tumor composed of undifferentiated ependymal-type cells forming true rosettes around a lumen.

Neuroblastoma is a rare primitive tumor of children, most often well circumscribed when found in the cerebral hemispheres. There is a high cellular density of neuroblasts, which are small and round or oval, in which rosettes may be seen. Maturation to ganglion cells may occur. Their biologic behavior is grade IV.

Tumors of Cranial and Peripheral Nerves

The two principal tumors in this class, neurofibroma and schwannoma, occur along cranial, spinal, and peripheral nerves. Both occur as solitary lesions in patients without neurofibromatosis and may be solitary or multiple in neurofibromatosis. *Neurofibromas* are often multiple and occur most commonly in the context of neurofibromatosis type I (NF1). A hyperplastic proliferation of all elements of nerve, including fibroblasts, glia, and Schwann cells, occurs, producing a swollen, distorted nerve with the axon bundles coursing through the nerve (Fig. 1–17). Neurofibroma is of grade I biologic behavior and immunostains positively for S-100.

In contrast, *schwannoma* is a proliferation of neoplastic Schwann cells that exhibits two histological patterns: Antoni A, consisting of compact, elongated cells (Fig. 1–18A) and Antoni B (Fig. 1–18B), consisting of less compact, pleomorphic cells, which grow to produce microcysts (in a bubbly pattern). Schwannoma also has a tendency to undergo xanthomatous change. Both patterns show immunoreactivity for S-100. The axons of the parent nerve are generally found draped over the tumor. Schwannoma occurs in plexiform, cellular, and melanotic variants. It is grade I in biologic behavior. A malignant variant, usually arising from the neurofibroma, is called a *malignant peripheral nerve sheath tumor* (neurofibrosarcoma, malignant schwannoma). The transformation is sarcomatous, and the tumor has a grade III or IV biologic behavior. It can occur in the setting of neurofibromatosis, particularly with plexiform neurofibromas.

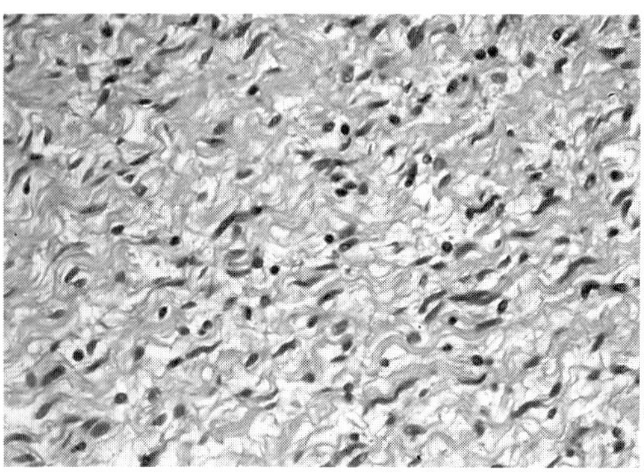

Figure 1–17. Neurofibroma. This neoplasm is formed by wavy connective tissue with elongated or round Schwann cell nuclei embedded within the bubbly myxomatous matrix. Some of the bubbly material belongs to myelinated axons traversing the neoplasm. Mitotic figures are not found. Nuclear pleomorphism is absent or minimal. H&E stain. Mag. ×400. (Courtesy of Mila Blaivas, MD, PhD, Department of Pathology, University of Michigan Medical School, Ann Arbor, MI.)

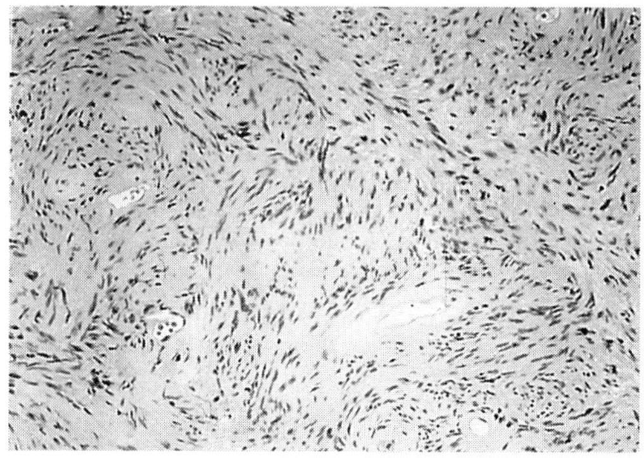

A

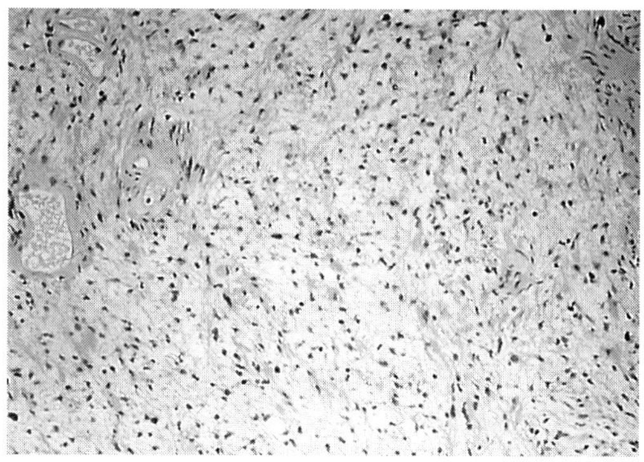

B

Figure 1–18. Schwannoma. *(A)* Antoni A region. Cellular portion of the neoplasm with fusiform, spindle-shaped, or small, rounded nuclei that are occasionally arranged in palisades of Verocay bodies. The vessels are characteristically hypocellular, thick walled, and hyalinized. H&E stain. Mag. ×200. *(B)* Antoni B region. This less cellular, cystic region of schwannoma is made of similar nuclei with the bubbly cytoplasm and cystic spaces that vary from microcystic to sizable cysts. Thick-walled hyalinized vessels are included within. H&E stain. Mag. ×200. (Courtesy of Mila Blaivas, MD, PhD, Department of Pathology, University of Michigan Medical School, Ann Arbor, MI.)

Mesenchymal Tumors

Meningiomas (Table 1–7) may be found attached to any of the three layers of the meninges, but most are thought to

Table 1–7. **Mesenchymal Tumors**

Meningioma
Osteocartilaginous tumor
Lipoma
Fibrous histiocytoma
Hemangiopericytoma
Rhabdomyosarcoma
Meningeal sarcoma
Melanoma

arise where arachnoidal villi are numerous. They are composed of neoplastic arachnoidal cells and have a grade I biologic behavior. Meningioma is most often cured by surgical resection. Located both intracranially and intraspinally, meningioma is a typically spherical tumor firmly attached to the dura. It does not invade the brain or spinal cord, but displaces it. Meningioma also occurs intraventricularly or "en plaque," spreading along one of the deeper dural surfaces. Immunohistochemically, it stains with the intermediate filament vimentin, epithelial membrane antigen, and desmoplakin. Histologically, the numerous variants—meningothelial, fibrous, transitional, psammomatous, angiomatous, microcystic, secretory, clear-cell, choroid, lymphoplasmacyte-rich, and metaplastic—all have the same basic biologic behavior (Fig. 1–19A to C). All tend to recur.

Atypical meningiomas are meningiomas with frequent mitoses, increased cellularity, high nuclear cytoplasmic ratios, uninterrupted sheetlike growth, and necrosis. They behave more aggressively than meningiomas, with a grade II biologic behavior. Anaplastic meningioma, with a grade III biologic behavior, shows a high mitotic index, malignant cytology, and

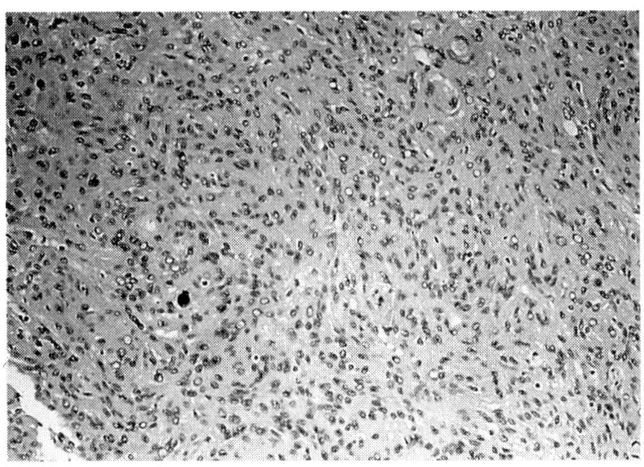

A

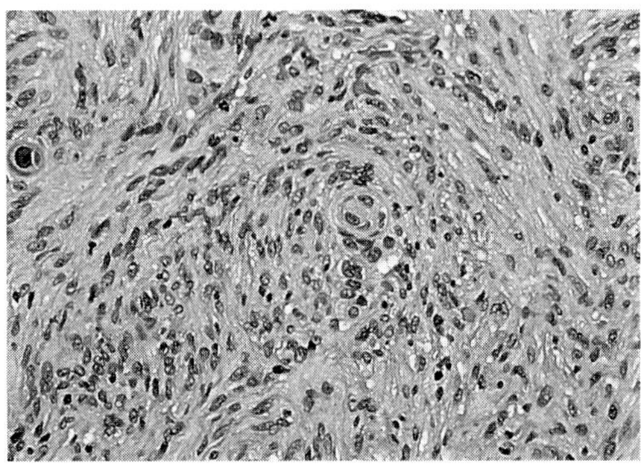

B

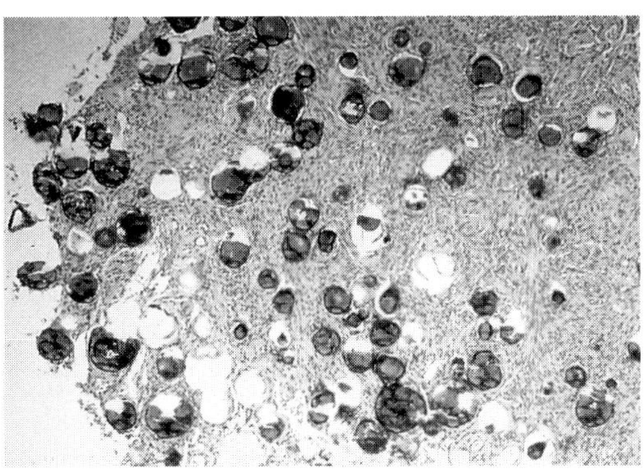

C

Figure 1–19. *(A)* Meningothelial meningioma. Meningioma cells have syncytial appearance with no clear-cut borders and frequent intranuclear cytoplasmic inclusions. A typical whorl on the left lower corner of the section and a psammoma body on the right-hand side. No mitotic figures or necrosis are present. H&E stain. Mag. ×200. *(B)* Fibroblastic meningioma. This neoplasm is composed of predominantly spindle-shaped cells arranged in bundles along with collagen fibers. Well-formed whorls and psammoma bodies are rare or absent. H&E stain. Mag. ×400. *(C)* Psammomatous meningioma. Numerous psammoma bodies are included within a cellular island of the neoplasm formed by mostly syncytial meningioma mixed with some transitional regions. No mitotic figures or tumor necrosis are present. H&E stain. Mag. ×100. (Courtesy of Mila Blaivas, MD, PhD, Department of Pathology, University of Michigan Medical School, Ann Arbor, MI.)

widespread necrosis. Some pathologists think gross brain invasion is necessary for the "anaplastic" designation.

Papillary meningioma is an aggressive histological variant with frequent recurrence, brain invasion, and metastases. It is a highly cellular tumor, with cell processes ending on vessels, producing pseudorosettes.

Tumors arising from mesenchymal structures other than the meninges include osteocartilaginous tumors, lipoma, fibrous histiocytoma, and hemangiopericytoma.[6] *Osteocartilaginous tumors* are composed of bone and cartilage, are most often durally based, and are known as *chondroma, osteoma,* and *osteochondroma. Chondrosarcoma* is a malignant variant found in the dura. *Lipoma* usually occurs in the midline but may also occur in the posterior fossa, in the cerebellopontine angle, and in the Sylvian fissure. It is thought to arise from the meninx primitiva, a mesenchymal derivative of the neural crest.[36] Macroscopically, lipoma looks like fat; microscopically, like histologically normal adipose tissue. It frequently occurs with dysraphic states. The *fibrous histiocytoma* is composed of fibroblasts and histiocytes. A malignant variant has significant mitoses and occasionally necrosis. The malignant fibrous histiocytoma may also arise intraparenchymally and contain spindle cells, including fibroblasts and giant lipid-laden cells. This tumor is similar to the sarcomatous element of the gliosarcoma. *Hemangiopericytoma* is composed of polygonal tumor cells with varying amounts of reticulin intracellular matrix interspersed (Fig. 1–20). The tumor-cell differentiation may be fibroblastic, myoid, or pericytic. Mitoses are frequent. This tumor is thought to be a malignant neoplasm with a propensity to metastasize and recur locally. Melanomas also arise in the meninges and range from benign to malignant. Other rare sarcomatous lesions that occur intracranially include the *rhabdomyosarcoma* and the *meningeal sarcoma*. These are not discussed in the text because of their rarity.

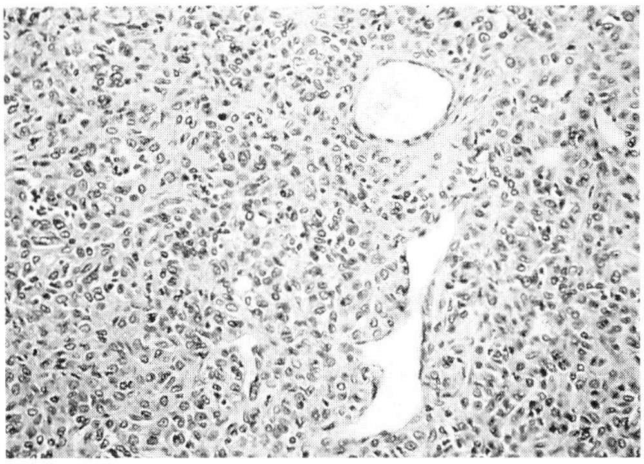

Figure 1–20. Hemangiopericytoma. Plump, polygonal tumor cells with increased mitotic activity in a dense fibrous stroma. Note the typical stag horn vasculature. (From Kleihues,[6] p 97, with permission.)

Lymphomas

Primary central nervous system lymphoma (PCNSL) occurs spontaneously in the CNS in otherwise healthy individuals. There is an increased incidence in patients who are immunodeficient, particularly those with AIDS. Previously, the tumor has been called a *reticulum cell sarcoma, histiocytic sarcoma,* and *microglioma*. Modern immunologic techniques have shown that these tumors are similar to systemic lymphomas of the non-Hodgkin's type, most often from a monoclonal B-cell population, where the cells are immunoblastic or large-cell in type (Fig. 1–21). Rarely, these neoplasms

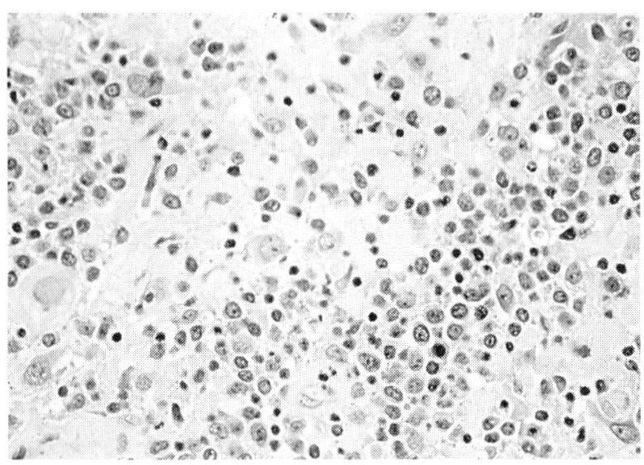

Figure 1–21. Primary CNS lymphoma. Gray matter with large neurons and small glial cells is infiltrated by rounded lymphoma cells with a narrow rim of cytoplasm that lacks processes. Mitotic figures and pyknotic or fragmented neoplastic nuclei are frequent. Prominent reactive astrocytes with large gemistocytic bodies and virtually invisible nuclei are scattered among lymphoma cells. H&E stain. Mag. ×400. (Courtesy of Mila Blaivas, MD, PhD, Department of Pathology, University of Michigan Medical School, Ann Arbor, MI.)

have a T-cell origin. Their biologic behavior is grade III. *Plasmacytoma* also occurs intracranially in the skull or dura and is composed of sheets of plasma cells.

Germ Cell Tumors

Germ cell tumors occur primarily in the suprasellar and pineal regions of the brain but may arise in the hypothalamus, thalamus, and basal ganglia, and they may infiltrate the brain. Pineal-region tumors are identical histologically to tumors that occur in the male testes.[6] *Germinoma* is the most frequent pineal tumor, representing about 65% of germ cell tumors. Histologically, the cells are identical to the testicular seminoma, with monotonous round cells that have large nuclei and prominent nucleoli. Lymphocytes are a regular component of the neoplasm and are often positioned along vascular connective tissue. Occasionally, the germinoma has granulomatous areas or multinucleated giant cells. This tumor immunostains positively for placental alkaline phosphatase and usually negatively for human chorionic gonadotropin (hCG) and alphafetoprotein (AFP). These tumors occur in early childhood, adolescence, and young adulthood, generally with a grade II biologic behavior.

Nongerminomatous germ cell tumors include choriocarcinoma, embryonal carcinoma, yolk sac tumor, and teratoma. Mixed germ cell tumors are composed of combinations of these four tumor types. Nongerminomatous germ cell tumors have a more aggressive biologic behavior (grade III) than do germinomas and frequently stain positively for hCG and AFP.

Sellar Region Tumors

The most common tumor of the sellar region is the *pituitary adenoma,* which represents about 10% of all intracranial neoplasms and has a grade I biologic behavior. This tumor is endocrinologically active, may form large cysts, and is composed of normal adenohypophyseal cells that have lost their glandular pattern (Fig. 1–22). It secretes prolactin, adrenocorticotropic hormone, growth hormone, thyrotropic hormone, or gonadotropic hormones.[6,37] It may be nonsecretory and is then called *null cell adenoma.* Secretory tumors are identified by immunostains and by molecular biologic in situ hybridization of messenger RNAs.[38]

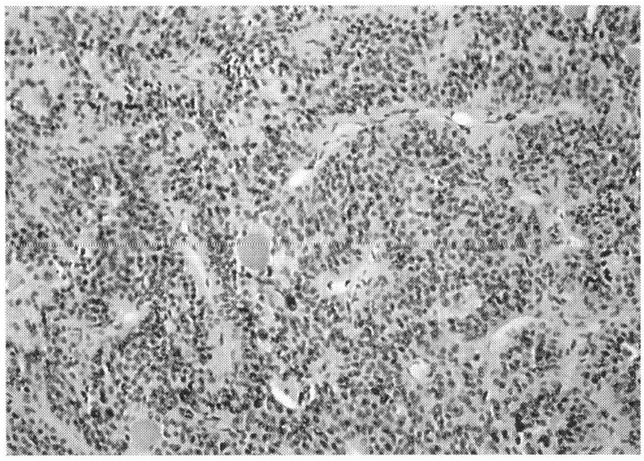

Figure 1–22. Pituitary adenoma. The neoplasm is formed by a sinusoidal arrangement of small, monotonous size and shape nuclei without significant hyperchromasia or prominent nucleoli. Occasional larger nuclei and droplets of colloid are seen in this section. No mitotic figures are present. H&E stain. Mag. ×200. (Courtesy of Mila Blaivas, MD, PhD, Department of Pathology, University of Michigan Medical School, Ann Arbor, MI.)

Pituitary carcinoma is an extremely rare tumor with the capacity to invade brain and metastasize systemically (i.e., grade III biologic behavior). It most frequently is anaplastic histologically, with mitoses and cellular atypia. It may not show the cellular features of malignancy or be functional.

Craniopharyngioma also occurs in the suprasellar region. These tumors are typically suprasellar but may be solely intrasellar. Craniopharyngioma is a dysontogenetic tumor that, although histologically benign, invades surrounding structures locally.[39] It ranges from small, well-circumscribed nodes to multilobular cysts. The two common histological types are adamantinomatous and papillary.

Adamantinomatous craniopharyngioma consists of epithelial masses with peripheral palisading and keratin nodules. These form large cysts filled with turbid fluid that contains cholesterol crystals (Fig. 1–23). Papillary craniopharyngioma, which is rarer histologically, is formed by sheets of squamous epithelium in the shape of papillae. It is seen more frequently in

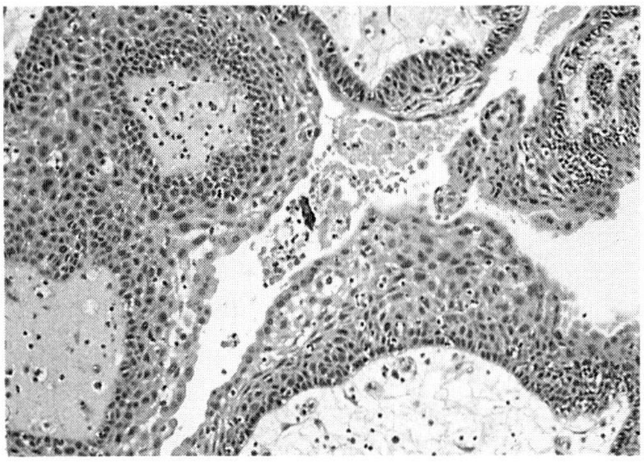

Figure 1–23. Craniopharyngioma. Ribbons of adamantinomatous epithelium with peripheral palisading demonstrate disintegration of the epithelial integrity and degeneration of the epithelial cells as well as the elements of reticulate center beneath the palisading layer. The debris produced by this process, together with inflammatory cells, cholesterol clefts, macrophages, and calcium, forms thick oily cystic content. H&E stain. Mag. ×200. (Courtesy of Mila Blaivas, MD, PhD, Department of Pathology, University of Michigan Medical School, Ann Arbor, MI.)

adults than in children and lacks cellular palisading and cholesterol crystals. Craniopharyngioma has a grade I to II biologic behavior but invades locally.

Cysts and Other Benign Tumorlike Lesions

Rathke's cleft cyst is similar to the cystic component of craniopharyngioma but is lined with a cuboidal or columnar epithelium, which is often ciliated in places. Rathke's pouch cyst closes in late embryonic life, except for the apical portion, which may persist into postnatal life and fill with gelatinous material. The epithelium is the same as that lining the normal small cysts and glands between the anterior and posterior lobes of the pituitary.[6] Epidermoid and dermoid cysts are caused by a neural tube closure defect early in embryogenesis, when neural ectoderm does not cleave from cutaneous ectoderm.[40] *Epidermoid cysts* occur laterally when embryonic cell rests are carried to the cerebellopontine angle with the developing otic vesicles. Epidermoid cysts are thin-walled and "pearly," with cheesy contents. They are lined by flattened, differentiated squamous epithelium resting on connective tissue. The epithelium contains keratohyaline granules and produces keratin. Also called *cholesteatomas,* these "pearly" tumors can also occur in the temporal lobe, bone, and throughout the neuraxis.

Dermoid cysts are more frequently situated in the midline, are thicker-walled than epidermoid cysts, and contain not only squamous epithelium but also dermal outgrowths (i.e., in hair follicles, adnexae, and, less commonly, bone). They are also lined by squamous epithelium but contain dermal adnexae underneath. Malignant transformation is rare in both dermoids and epidermoids, which both react immunologically with cytokeratins and epithelial membrane antigen (EMA).

Colloid cysts are smooth, spherical lesions arising in the anterior roof of the third ventricle, adjacent to the foramen of Monro. They sometimes obstruct CSF outflow through the foramen of Monro.[41] Histologically, the lining is composed of columnar, ciliated epithelial cells that are reactive for EMA and sit on a fibrous stroma (Fig. 1–24). Other rare tumorlike brain lesions include the *granular cell tumor,* an astrocyte-derived tumor of the pituitary; the *hypothalamic neuronal hamartoma,* a clustered mass of neurons and glia that most often occurs at the base of the brain; and the *plasma cell granuloma,* an inflammatory pseudotumor composed of

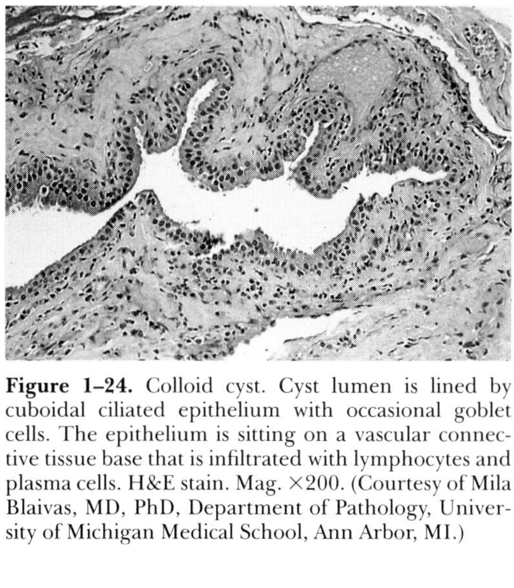

Figure 1–24. Colloid cyst. Cyst lumen is lined by cuboidal ciliated epithelium with occasional goblet cells. The epithelium is sitting on a vascular connective tissue base that is infiltrated with lymphocytes and plasma cells. H&E stain. Mag. ×200. (Courtesy of Mila Blaivas, MD, PhD, Department of Pathology, University of Michigan Medical School, Ann Arbor, MI.)

plasma cells that is usually attached to the meninges.

Brain Extension of Neighboring Regional Tumors

Paraganglioma is a tumor of the middle ear, glomus jugulare and carotid body, and cauda equina region. Through growth, this tumor compresses, but does not invade, neural structures. It may secrete catecholamines and is composed of "chief cells." *Chordoma* arises from notochordal remnants in the clivus or the sacrum. The tumor consists of lobular masses of highly vacuolated cells in a myxoid matrix. The vacuolated physaliphorous, or bubbly, cells have few mitoses and little cytoplasm. They immunostain with cytokeratin and EMA, unlike chondromas or chondrosarcomas, with which they are often confused (Fig. 1–25). Other tumors that grow through the skull include nasopharyngeal carcinoma and adenocystic carcinoma, both of which extend along nerves.

Metastatic Tumors

Metastatic brain tumors spread to the brain from a primary site elsewhere in the body.

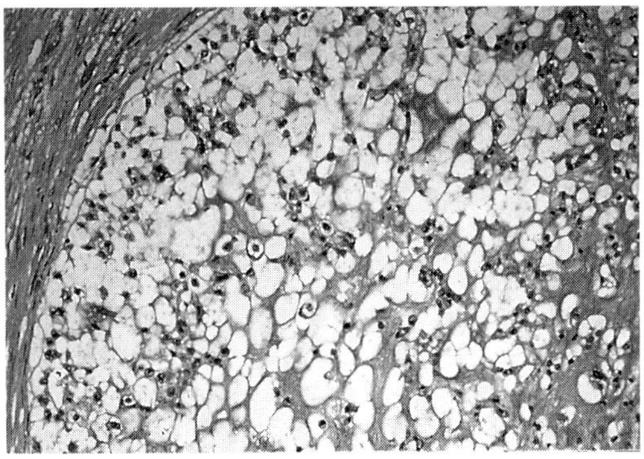

Figure 1–25. Chordoma. One of the chordoma lobules that is separated from other lobules by a band of collagenous connective tissue is composed of markedly vacuolated physaliphorous cells in a myxoid matrix. Mitotic figures are not present. Interlobular bands of connective tissue are frequently infiltrated by lymphocytes. H&E stain. Mag. ×200. (Courtesy of Mila Blaivas, MD, PhD, Department of Pathology, University of Michigan Medical School, Ann Arbor, MI.)

Most tumors reach the brain by hematogenous spread through arterial circulation. The brain metastasis most often originates from a primary lung malignancy or a metastasis to the lung. The pathology reflects the primary site of origin. Management depends on their location and on whether there are single or multiple metastases.

EPIDEMIOLOGY

Incidence

In the United States in 1991, primary malignant brain tumors were diagnosed in approximately 16,000 people; there were 11,000 deaths in patients with brain tumors.[42] Age-specific rates for symptomatic malignant astrocytoma and glioma increase from rates one and two per 100,000 annually, respectively, at ages 35 to 44, and reach a maximum of approximately 17 and 19 per 100,000 annually, in the 75- to 84-year-old age group (Fig. 1–26).

The incidence of primary intracranial malignant brain tumors appears to have increased dramatically in the past two decades, particularly in the elderly in developed countries.[44–46] Between the 1960s and 1985, the reported incidence of malignant brain tumors increased in the population by 40%. In elderly people, older than age 65 years, the reported incidence increased 100% in both the United States and Canada.[44–47] It is debatable whether the increased reported incidence is due to improved diagnostic tumor imaging with

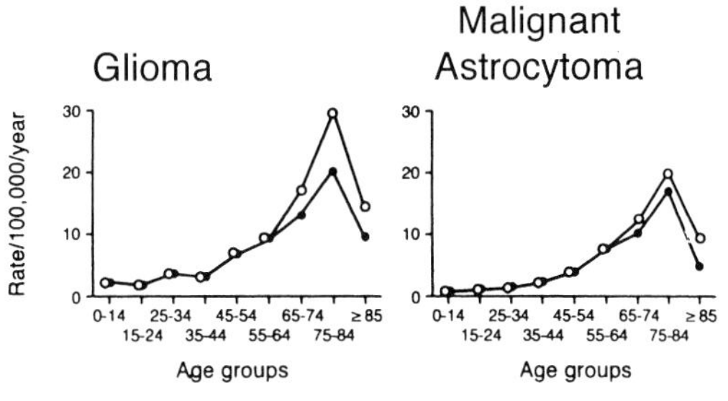

Figure 1–26. Age-specific incidence rates of primary glioma and malignant astrocytoma in Rochester, Minnesota, 1950–1989, by including all tumors (open circles) and excluding tumors diagnosed incidentally at autopsy and neuroimaging (closed circles). (From Radhakrishnan,[43] p 70, with permission.)

CT and MRI or reflects an actual increased incidence of malignant brain tumors.[47] In a retrospective chart review of 215 patients diagnosed with malignant brain tumor between 1985 and 1989, Desmeules, Mikkelsen, and Mao[48] eliminated CT and MRI information from patients' medical records and speculated that the diagnosis of malignant brain tumor would have been made in 80% of cases. They concluded that CT and MRI scans were partly but not solely responsible for the reported increase in brain tumor incidence.

A recent population study of malignant and nonmalignant symptomatic brain tumors in Rochester, Minnesota, found the incidence increased from 9.5 per 100,000 population annually from 1950 to 1969, to 12.5 per 100,000 annually in 1970 to 1989 (x^2 trend, 1.89; P = .17). During this period, the incidence of glioma, malignant astrocytoma, and meningioma showed no change for those younger or older than age 65 years.[43] The incidence of pituitary adenomas increased significantly, from 0.73 per 100,000 annually in 1950 to 1969, to 3.55 per l00,000 annually in 1970 to 1989.[43] The authors believed that the increase in pituitary adenomas was principally responsible for the nonsignificant increase in symptomatic malignant and nonmalignant brain tumors in the Rochester population. They attributed the increased incidence to improved endocrinologic function testing and pituitary imaging.

PCNSL incidence has been rising dramatically in both immunocompetent and immunocompromised patients.[49–51] The incidence of PCNSL increased by approximately 300% in the immunocompetent population between 1974 and 1988, with no increase in non-Hodgkin's lymphoma, the systemic histological counterpart.[49] In the immunocompromised AIDS population, patients are living longer because of more effective treatment of opportunistic infections, with resultant increased incidence of PCNSL.[50,51]

Environmental Exposure

A causal relationship has not been established between any environmental exposure and the development of brain tumors.[52] Numerous reports in the scientific and lay literature and in legal cases have attempted to establish a causal relationship, although an association only may exist. Associations have been suggested for occupations[53–56] (e.g., petrochemical, farming, rubber), chemical exposure (e.g., polycyclic hydrocarbons, nitroso compounds, vinyl chloride),[53–56] electromagnetic fields of low frequency, and even cellular telephones.[52] A convincing causal relationship has been established between therapeutic ionizing radiation and the development of brain tumors. When the analysis was confined to malignant head and neck tumors, there was a risk ratio of observed to expected of 4.5; for gliomas, 2.6; meningiomas, 9.5; and nerve sheath tumors, 18.8. A study of 10,800 Israeli children who underwent radiation therapy for tinea capitis[51] showed a relative risk of 6.9 (95% C.I.: 4.1–ll.6) of developing neural tumors when the children were compared with their sibling controls (who had not undergone radiation therapy). A striking dose-response relation was present, with the relative risk near 20 after doses of approximately 2500 cGy.[57] In Los Angeles County, risk factors for the development of meningiomas and neuromas include radiation treatment to the head or frequent full-mouth dental radiographs.[58] Following cranial radiation, lymphoblastic leukemia has occasionally been associated with the secondary development of malignant gliomas.[59] Trauma has not been established as a risk factor for the development of brain tumors.

Petrochemical workers in Texas were found to have greater brain tumor mortality than expected (22 observed versus 10.7 expected), with the majority of workers dying of brain tumor 15 or more years following the beginning of employment.[53] However, a subsequent meta-analysis concluded the petroleum industry had no excess risk of brain tumor mortality.[54] In workers involved with rubber and tire building, industry cohort studies[53–56] show a generally nonsignificant increase in the risk ratio of l.5 or less. In occupational exposures, causal relationships are often difficult to delineate because a specific chemical cannot be implicated, the time between exposure and disease is often long, and the affected individuals often have multiple exposures. In animals, gliomas have been caused by the direct implantation of polycyclic aromatic hydrocarbons and nitroso compounds. Nitroso compounds can also be infused intravenously and produce brain tumors. Nitrosoureas have been used extensively in the treatment of gliomas and do not appear to be associated with the development of second neoplasms in humans.

Farmers who are frequently exposed to pesticides have been reported to have an increased relative risk of brain tumors. In a case control study in Italy in 1980,[53] brain tumor patients were five times more likely to be farmers than were age-matched controls with non-neoplastic degenerative diseases. A similar follow-up study in 1984[56] found a 3.6 relative risk in farmers. A prospective study is ongoing in rural counties of four midwestern states to assess pesticide and other environmental risks in farmers compared with age-matched controls. In summary, the causal relationship between ionizing radiation and brain tumors is the only definite one.

Genetics

Fewer than 5% of patients with brain tumors have a predisposing genetic syndrome. The most common of these are the phakomatoses: von Recklinghausen's types I and II neurofibromatosis, tuberous sclerosis, von Hippel-Lindau disease, and the epidermal nevus syndrome. These dominantly inherited neurocutaneous syndromes are associated with an increased incidence of specific tumors.

Neurofibromatosis I (NF1) is due to a mutation of a gene locus on chromosome 17. In NF1, the number of optic nerve gliomas is increased, with a prevalence of 1.5% in one study.[60] Meningiomas and other gliomas do not appear to be increased in NF1.[61] Neurofibromas, neurofibrosarcomas, and malignant schwannomas of the peripheral nervous system occur with increased frequency in NF1.[62] *Neurofibromatosis II* (NF2) is due to a chromosomal defect on the long arm of chromosome 22 in an area thought to code for cytoskeletal proteins. In NF2, the incidence of bilateral acoustic schwannomas and single or multiple schwannomas on other cranial and spinal nerve roots is increased.[63] Meningiomas and brain and spine glial tumors, including pilocytic astrocytoma and ependymoma, occur more often in individuals with NF2.[63,64]

In *tuberous sclerosis*, 30% to 40% of families are chromosome-9 linked, with at least one other tuberous sclerosis gene elsewhere in the genome.[62] Tuberous sclerosis is associated with an increased incidence of subependymal glial nodules and, when symptomatic, these are classified as subependymal giant-cell astrocytomas.[65]

Von Hippel-Lindau disease is an inherited syndrome associated with hemangioblastomas in multiple organ systems, including the cerebellum, retina, and spinal cord. It is also associated with pheochromocytoma and renal cell carcinoma. Von Hippel-Lindau disease is due to a defective gene on chromosome 3.66

The *epidermal nevus syndrome* is associated with linear skin nevi and an increased incidence of malignant gliomas.

The *Li-Fraumeni syndrome* is characterized clinically by closely related family members who develop cancer between ages 25 and 35. The common cancers are breast, lung, colon, and osteogenic sarcoma. These individuals are at increased risk to develop second malignancies, and the syndrome may be associated with choroid plexus papilloma and anaplastic astrocytoma. Families with the Li-Fraumeni syndrome have p53 germline mutation, in which the individual is heterozygous for the allele and a missense mutation produces a faulty protein. When patients with multifocal glioma, unifocal glioma with an additional primary malignancy, or unifocal glioma with a family history of cancer were examined for germline p53 mutations, 12% of these patients had germline mutations. If two factors were present, 43% had germline mutations; if all three factors were present, there was a 67% rate of germline mutation.[67]

A very small subset of glioma patients have a family history of these tumors. The largest number of families have been compiled in the Johns Hopkins National Brain

Tumor Registry,[68,69] which has identified 59 families with 127 cases of primary brain tumors. There have been 20 parent-child cases, 27 sibling-sibling cases, and nine husband-wife pairs. Multiple generations were not affected. In 47% of the parent-child cases, the child was diagnosed before the parent. In 20% of the families, the second case was diagnosed within 2 years of the index case. The authors concluded that the findings were most consistent with a common toxic or infectious exposure, particularly in the husband-wife pairs; in 33% of these cases, both spouses, after decades of living together, were diagnosed within 1 year of each other.[69]

CHAPTER SUMMARY

This chapter has discussed the pathological classification and grading systems for brain tumors. Neuroepithelial tumors are the most common and feared tumors of adult life and occur most frequently as astrocytoma, oligodendroglioma, and ependymoma. Neuroepithelial tumors are frequently heterogeneous morphologically and immunohistochemically. Histological features of increasing neuroepithelial tumor malignancy that usually have a poor biologic outcome are nuclear atypia, cellular pleomorphism, mitoses, vascular proliferation, and necrosis. Meningiomas are mesenchymal tumors that arise from the meninges of the brain or spinal cord. They are cured surgically but may occur in more aggressive, noncurable atypical and anaplastic variants.

The incidence of astrocytic tumors has increased in the elderly, but this increase is probably the result of improved imaging techniques. Lymphomas are increasing in incidence in immunocompetent and immunocompromised hosts. Radiation is the only exposure known to produce an increased risk of brain tumors.

REFERENCES

1. Bailey, OT: Genesis of the Percival Bailey-Cushing classification of gliomas. Pediatr Neurosci 12: 261–265, 1985–1986.
2. Bailey, P and Cushing, H: A Classification of the Tumors of the Glioma Group on a Histogenetic Basis with a Correlated Study of Prognosis. JB Lippincott Company, Philadelphia, 1926.
3. Kernohan, JW and Sayre, GP: Atlas of Tumor Pathology: Tumors of the Central Nervous System. Armed Forces Institute of Pathology, Washington, 1950.
4. Russell, DS and Rubinstein, LJ: Pathology of Tumours of the Nervous System, Ed 4. The Williams and Wilkins Company, Baltimore, 1977.
5. Zülch, KJ: Histological Typing of Tumours of the Central Nervous System. World Health Organization, Geneva, 1979.
6. Kleihues, P, Burger, PC, and Scheithauer, BW: Histological Typing of Tumours of the Central Nervous System, Ed 2. World Health Organization, Springer-Verlag, Berlin, 1993.
7. Bailey, P and Bucy, PC: Oligodendrogliomas of the brain. J Path 32:735–751, 1929.
8. Bailey, P: Further remarks concerning tumors of the glioma group. Bull Johns Hopkins Hosp 40: 354–389, 1927.
9. Fields, WS: Brain tumours: Morphological aspects and classification. Brain Pathol 3:251–253, 1993.
10. Burger, PC: Revising the world health organization (WHO) blue book — 'Histological Typing of Tumours of the Central Nervous System'. J Neurooncol 24:3–7, 1995.
11. Wechsler, W and Reifenberger, G: Immunohistochemistry in brain tumor classification. In Paoletti, P. Takakura, K, Walker, MD et al (eds): Neuro-Oncology. Kluwer Academic Publishers, Netherlands, 1991, pp 11–19.
12. Krouwer, HGJ, Davis ,RL, Silver, P, and Prados, M: Gemistocytic astrocytomas: A reappraisal. J Neurosurg 74:399–406, 1991.
13. Margetts, JC and Kalyan-Raman, UP: Giant-celled glioblastoma of brain. A clinico-pathological and radiological study of ten cases (including immunohistochemistry and ultrastructure). Cancer 63:524–531, 1989.
14. Meis, JM, Martz, KL, and Nelson, JS: Mixed glioblastoma multiforme and sarcoma. A clinicopathologic study of 26 Radiation Therapy Oncology Group cases. Cancer 67:2342–2349, 1991.
15. Giangaspero, F and Burger, PC: Correlations between cytologic composition and biologic behavior in the glioblastoma multiforme. A postmortem study of 50 cases. Cancer 52:2320–2333, 1983.
16. Burger, PC: Malignant astrocytic neoplasms: Classification, pathologic anatomy, and response to treatment. Semin Oncol 13(1):16–26, 1986.
17. Bruner, J: Neuropathology of malignant gliomas. Semin Oncol 21(2):126–138, 1994.
18. Daumas-Duport, C: Histoprognosis of gliomas. Advances and Technical Standards in Neurosurgery 21:43–76, 1994.
19. VandenBerg, SR: Current diagnostic concepts of astrocytic tumors. J Neuropathol Exp Neurol 51(6):644–657, 1992.
20. Ringertz, N: Grading of gliomas. Acta Pathol Microbiol Scand 27:51–64, 1950.

21. Kleihues, P, Burger, PC, and Scheithauer, BW: The new WHO classification of brain tumours. Brain Pathol 3:255–268, 1993.
22. Mennel, H-D: Grading of intracranial tumors following the WHO classification. Neurosurg Rev 14:249–260, 1991.
23. Davis, RL: Grading of gliomas. In Fields, WS (ed): Primary Brain Tumors: A Review of Histologic Classification. Springer-Verlag, New York, 1989, pp 150–158.
24. Daumas-Duport, C, Scheithauer, B, O'Fallon, J, and Kelly, P: Grading of astrocytomas. A simple and reproducible method. Cancer 62:2152–2165, 1988.
25. Forsyth, PA, Shaw, EG, Scheithauer BW, et al: Supratentorial pilocytic astrocytomas. A clinicopathologic, prognostic, and flow cytometric study of 51 patients. Cancer 72:1335–1342, 1993.
26. Garcia, DM and Fulling, KH: Juvenile pilocytic astrocytoma of the cerebrum in adults. A distinctive neoplasm with favorable prognosis. J Neurosurg 63:382–386, 1985.
27. Newton, H: Pilocytic astrocytomas. In Gilman, S, Goldstein, G, and Waxman, S (eds): Neurobase. Arbor Publishing Corporation, San Diego, 1995.
28. Shepherd, CW, Scheithauer, BW, Gomez, MR, et al: Subependymal giant cell astrocytoma: A clinical, pathological, and flow cytometric study. Neurosurgery 28:864–868, 1991.
29. Glass, J, Hochberg, FH, Gruber, ML, et al: The treatment of oligodendrogliomas and mixed oligodendroglioma-astrocytomas with PCV chemotherapy. J Neurosurg 76:741–745, 1992.
30. Shaw, EG, Scheithauer, BW, O'Fallon, JR, and Davis, DH: Mixed oligoastrocytomas: A survival and prognostic factor analysis. Neurosurgery 34:577–582, 1994.
31. Burger, PC, and Fuller, GN: Pathology: Trends and pitfalls in histologic diagnosis, immunopathology, and applications of oncogene research. Neurologic Clinics 9(2):249–271, 1991.
32. Bonnin, JM and Rubinstein, LJ: Astroblastomas: A pathological study of 23 tumors, with a postoperative follow-up in 13 patients. Neurosurgery 25:6–13, 1989.
33. Yasargil, MG, von Ammon, K, von Deimling, A, et al: Central neurocytoma: histopathological variants and therapeutic approaches. J Neurosurg 76:32–37, 1992.
34. Rorke, LB: The cerebellar medulloblastoma and its relationship to primitive neuroectodermal tumors. J Neuropathol Exp Neurol 42:1–15, 1983.
35. Packer, RJ: Medulloblastoma. In Gilman, S, Goldstein, G, and Waxman, S (eds): Neurobase. Arbor Publishing Corporation, San Diego, 1995.
36. O'Rahilly, R and Mullen, F: The meninges in human development. J Neuropathol Exp Neurol 45:588–608, 1986.
37. Chandler, WF: Pituitary tumors. In Gilman, S, Goldstein, G, and Waxman, S (eds): Neurobase. Arbor Publishing Corporation, San Diego, 1995.
38. Lloyd, RV: Molecular biologic analysis of pituitary disorder. In Lloyd, RV (ed): Surgical Pathology of the Pituitary Gland. WB Saunders, Philadelphia, 1993, pp 85–93.
39. Recht, LW: Craniopharyngiomas. In Gilman, S, Goldstein, G, and Waxman S (eds): Neurobase. Arbor Publishing Corporation, San Diego, 1995.
40. Grant, R: Dermoid and epidermoid cysts. In Gilman, S, Goldstein, G, and Waxman, S (eds): Neurobase. Arbor Publishing Corporation, San Diego, 1995.
41. Recht, LW: Colloid cysts. In Gilman, S, Goldstein, G, and Waxman, S (eds): Neurobase. Arbor Publishing Corporation, San Diego, 1995.
42. Wrensch, M, Bondy, ML, Wiencke, J, and Yost, M: Environmental risk factors for primary malignant brain tumors: A review. J Neurooncol 17: 47–64, 1993.
43. Radhakrishnan, K, Mokri, B, Parisi, JE, et al: The trends in incidence of primary brain tumors in the population of Rochester, Minnesota. Ann Neurol 37:67–73, 1995.
44. Greig, NH, Ries, LG, Yancik, R, and Rapoport, SI: Increasing annual incidence of primary malignant brain tumors in the elderly. J Natl Cancer Inst 82:1621–1624, 1990.
45. Mao, Y, Desmeules, M, Semenciw, RM, et al: Increasing brain cancer rates in Canada. Can Med Assoc J 145:1583–1591, 1991.
46. Davis, DL, Lilienfeld, AD, Gittelsohn, A, and Scheckenbach, ME: Increasing trends in some cancers in older Americans: Fact or artifact? Toxicol Ind Health 2:127–144, 1986.
47. Davis, DL, Hoel, D, Fox, J, and Lopez, A: International trends in cancer mortality in France, West Germany, Italy, Japan, England and Wales, and the USA. Lancet 336:474–481, 1990.
48. Desmeules, M, Mikkelsen, T, and Mao, Y: Increasing incidence of primary malignant brain tumors: Influence of diagnostic methods. J Natl Cancer Inst 84:442–445, 1992.
49. Devesa, SS, and Fears, T: Non-Hodgkin's lymphoma time trends: United States and international data. Cancer Res 52(19 Suppl):5432s–5440s, 1992.
50. Gail, MH, Pluda, JM, Rabkin, CS, et al: Projections of the incidence of non-Hodgkin's lymphoma related to acquired immunodeficiency syndrome. J Natl Cancer Inst 83:695–701, 1991.
51. Pluda, JM, Yarchoan, R, Jaffe, ES, et al: Development of non-Hodgkin's lymphoma in a cohort of patients with severe human immunodeficiency virus (HIV) infection on long-term antiretroviral therapy. Ann Intern Med 113:276–282, 1990.
52. Brem, S, Rozental, JM, and Moskal, JR: What is the etiology of human brain tumors? A report of the first Lebow conference. Cancer 76(4):709–713, 1995.
53. Waxweiler, RJ, Alexander, V, Leffingwell, SS, et al: Mortality from brain tumor and other causes in a cohort of petrochemical workers. JNCI 70:75–81, 1983.
54. Wong, O, and Raabe, GK: Critical review of cancer epidemiology in petroleum industry employees with a quantitative meta-analysis by cancer site. Am J Indust Med 15:283–310, 1989.
55. Musicco, M, Filippini, G, Bordo, BM, et al: Gliomas and occupational exposure to carcinogens: Case-control study. Am J Epidemiol 116: 782–790, 1982.

56. Musicco, M, Sant, M, Molinari, S, et al: A case-control study of brain gliomas and occupational exposure to chemical carcinogens: The risk to farmers. Am J Epidemiol 128:778–785, 1988.
57. Ron, E, Modan, B, Boice, JD Jr, et al: Tumors of the brain and nervous system after radiotherapy in childhood. N Engl J Med 319:1033–1039, 1988.
58. Preston-Martin, S, Thomas, DC, Wright, WE, and Henderson, BE: Noise trauma in the etiology of acoustic neuromas in men in Los Angeles County. Br J Cancer 59:783–786, 1989.
59. Salvati, M, Artico, M, Caruso, R, et al: A report on radiation-induced gliomas. Cancer 67:392–397, 1991.
60. Purvin, VA, and Dunn, DW: Ophthalmological manifestations of neurofibromatosis 1 and 2. In Huson, SM and Hughes, RAC (eds): The Neurofibromatoses. A Pathogenetic and Clinical Overview. Chapman & Hall Medical, London, 1994, pp 253–274.
61. Hughes, RAC: Neurological complications of neurofibromatosis 1. In Huson, SM and Hughes, RAC (eds): The Neurofibromatoses. A Pathogenetic and Clinical Overview. Chapman & Hall Medical, London, 1994, pp 204–232.
62. Huson, SM and Upadhyaya, M: Neurofibromatosis 1. Clinical management and genetic counselling. In Huson, SM and Hughes, RAC (eds): The Neurofibromatoses. A Pathogenetic and Clinical Overview. Chapman & Hall Medical, London, 1994, pp 355–381.
63. Riccardi, VM: Neurofibromatosis: Clinical heterogeneity. Curr Probl Cancer 7:1–34, 1982.
64. Short, PM, Martuza, RL, and Huson, SM: Neurofibromatosis 2: Clinical features, genetic counselling and management issues. In Huson, SM and Hughes, RAC (eds): Neurofibromatoses. A Pathogenetic and Clinical Overview. Chapman and Hall, London, 1994, pp 414–444.
65. Haines, JL and Short, P: Tuberous sclerosis: Hamartomas, subependymal giant cell astrocytomas, and other central nervous system tumors. In Levine, AJ and Schmidek HH (eds): Molecular Genetics of Nervous System Tumors. Wiley-Liss, Inc, New York, 1993, pp 303–310.
66. Seizinger, BR: Tumor suppressor genes and hereditary tumor syndromes of the human nervous system: Isolation of a primary genetic defect in von Hippel-Lindau disease. In Levine, AJ and Schmidek, HH (eds): Molecular Genetics of Nervous System Tumors. Wiley-Liss, Inc, New York, 1993, pp 311–318.
67. Kyritsis, AP, Bondy, ML, Xiao, M, et al: Germline p53 gene mutations in subsets of glioma patients. J Natl Cancer Inst 86:344–349, 1994.
68. Lossignol, D, Grossman, SA, Sheidler, VR, et al: Familial clustering of malignant astrocytomas. J Neurooncol 9:139–145, 1990.
69. Grossman, SA, Osman, M, Hruban, RH, and Piantadosi, S: Familial gliomas: The potential role of environmental exposures. Proc Am Soc Clin Oncol 14:149, 1995.

Chapter 2

BRAIN TUMOR BIOLOGY

Basic research in malignant brain tumors is progressing at a rapid pace. Glial differentiation is the process by which astrocytic and oligodendroglial precursors differentiate into mature glial cells. Differentiation is under coordinated genetic control and includes sequential activation and deactivation of genes and the production of growth factors. Gene activation and deactivation produces a series of antigenic cell surface changes and eventually a mature astrocyte or oligodendroglial cell.[1]

Angiogenesis, or capillary sprouting from blood venules, is important during embryonic development, is quiescent during normal adult life, and becomes active during tumor growth. Angiogenic growth factors secreted by malignant glioma cells activate endothelial cells through tyrosine kinase receptors. [2] Normal brain endothelial cells have a tight blood-brain barrier (BBB). In malignant brain tumor cells, the BBB varies from normal to markedly abnormal, with endothelial gaps and clefts.[3] The BBB remains a formidable obstacle to drug transport into brain, particularly at the advancing edge of the tumor. Bradykinin analogs may offer selective means of opening the blood-tumor barrier (BTB) only.[4] Glial oncogenesis probably results from a series of chromosomal changes, which lead to inactivation of tumor-suppressor genes and the amplification of proto-oncogenes. Glial tumors have multiple chromosomal abnormalities, discovered initially by karyotypic analysis and analyzed now with molecular biologic techniques of restriction fragment length polymorphisms (RFLP), polymerase chain reaction (PCR), or fluorescence in situ hybridization (FISH).[5–9] No one chromosomal abnormality is the cause of, or specific for, all malignant gliomas. Astrocytic malignancy progression involves the accumulation of a series of allelic changes, with chromosomal loss of tumor-suppressor genes and amplification of proto-oncogenes.[6–9] These changes often occur in sequence, with certain genomic changes occurring early in astrocytoma development and other chromosomal changes occurring only with anaplastic change to a glioblastoma multiforme.[8,9] The chromosomal abnormalities among patients with malignant astrocytomas, among tumor regions in the same patient, and on serial analysis over time in the same patient vary significantly.[5–9] Chromosomal abnormalities have also been found in medulloblastomas involving the 17p region,[6–9] and in meningiomas on chromosome 22.[8,9] Results of recent studies have shown how chromosomal changes perturb cell cycle kinetics leading to uncontrolled tumor growth.[10,11] Malignant brain tumor growth is influenced by growth factors, both in an autocrine and a paracrine manner.[12,13] The invasion of malignant glial cells into normal brain is an interaction between receptors on the glial cell surface and extracellular matrix (ECM) proteins surrounding them.[14] Halopyrimidine monoclonal antibody(labeling techniques have been developed that enable neuro-oncologists to measure tumor growth fraction and doubling time.[15] These and other scientific discoveries—radiolabeled antibodies to growth factors, antisense oligonucleotides to transcription factors, differentiating agents, and gene therapy to correct allelic loss or to produce cell cytotoxicity—offer many avenues for future therapy.

GLIAL DIFFERENTIATION

An understanding of normal glial cell differentiation may provide insights into the development of brain tumors that may arise by dedifferentiation or an arrest of differentiation. In rat optic nerve and in other parts of the rat central nervous system (CNS), all glia are derived from two precursor cells, the T1A precursor, and the O2A progenitor cell.[1] T1A precursors are identified first on prenatal day 10, with mature forms on day l6 or l7. In the course of normal rat optic nerve differentiation, O2A progenitor cells first appear prenatally at day 16 of a 21-day gestational period. T2A mature astrocytes first appear on postnatal day 7 and increase into adulthood.[1] Growth factors, neighboring cells, and growth medium may influence the differentiation of precursor cells.

T1A Precursor Differentiation

The T1A precursor cell differentiates only into a T1A astrocyte (Fig. 2–1). The T1A precursor cell is rat cell surface protein RAN-2 positive and polysialoganglioside A2B5 negative, the reverse antigenicity of the O2A precursor cell. It acquires glial fibrillary acidic protein (GFAP) antigenicity as it differentiates into a mature T1A astrocyte.[1]

O2A Precursor Differentiation

The O2A progenitor cell can differentiate into either a mature oligodendrocyte or a T2A astrocyte. The O2A precursor cells' antigenic phenotype is polysialoganglioside A2B5 positive, and RAN-2 negative. If the O2A progenitor differentiates into an immature oligodendrocyte, it stains positively for the O4 cell surface sulfatide and negatively for the galactocerebroside, Gc. On further differentiation into a mature oligodendrocyte, the immature oligodendrocyte becomes Gc positive and then, quickly, antigenically A2B5 negative. Immature oligodendrocytes are bipotential; they are able to differentiate into mature oligodendrocytes or T2A astrocytes. However, when they express Gc, they are committed to become an oligodendroglial cell. If an O2A progenitor cell expresses GFAP, it differentiates into a T2A astrocyte. O2A progenitor cells are inhibited from differentiation into T2A astrocytes when placed in a culture with T1A astrocytes. They are stimulated to differentiate by platelet-derived growth factor (PDGF) and have been found to have PDGF receptors on their surface.[13] When O2A cells are placed in fetal calf serum (FCS), they differentiate into T2A astrocytes and permanently express GFAP; however, if they are grown in T1A-conditioned

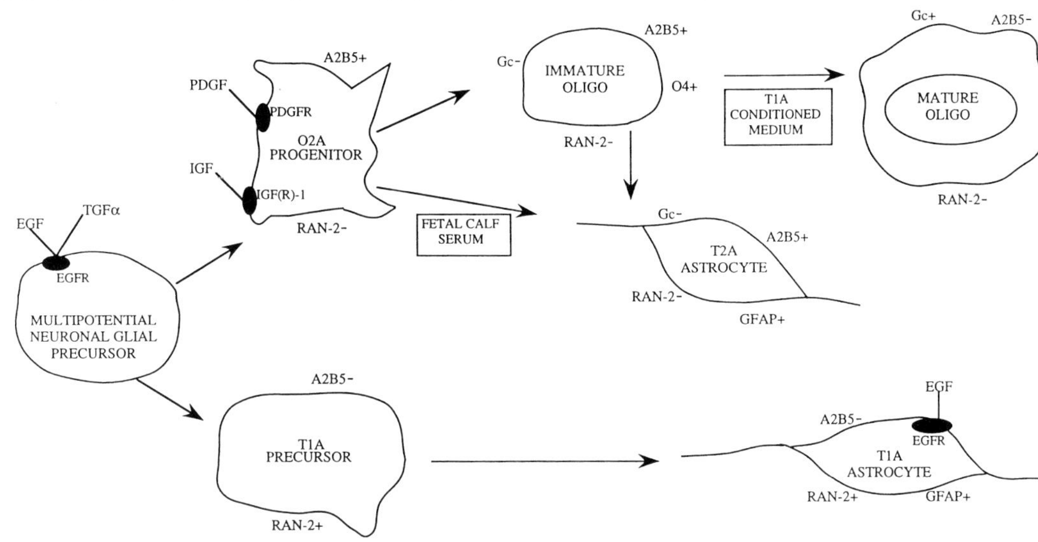

A2B5	POLYSIALOGANGLIOSIDE A2B5	PDGF(R)	PLATELET DERIVED GROWTH FACTOR (RECEPTOR)
RAN-2	RAT CELL SURFACE PROTEIN	IGF(R)-1	INSULIN GROWTH FACTOR (RECEPTOR)-1
GC	GALACTOCEREBROSIDE	+	ANTIGENICALLY POSITIVE
O4	O4 CELL SURFACE SULFATIDE	-	ANTIGENICALLY NEGATIVE
GFAP	GLIAL FIBRILLARY ACIDIC PROTEIN	▭	MEDIA THAT FACILITATE DIFFERENTIATION
EGF(R)	EPIDERMAL GROWTH FACTOR (RECEPTOR)	⬬	RECEPTOR
TGFα	TRANSFORMING GROWTH FACTOR α		

Figure 2–1. Glial cell differentiation of rat optic nerve. Cell surface antigenicity of glial progenitor cells, stimulatory growth factors and their receptors. (Adapted from Linskey and Gilbert,[1] p 3, with permission.)

medium with less than 0.5% FCS, they differentiate into mature oligodendrocytes.

Gene Activation

Glial differentiation involves the coordinated sequential activation of multiple genes with subsequent deactivation. The exact order of gene activation and the control and timing of the process remain to be delineated. For transcription to proceed, DNA, which is tightly packaged as chromatin, must unfold in response to a transcription factor binding to a promoter region. When DNA is methylated, transcription is repressed. DNA methyltransferase is necessary for the unfolding of DNA and for the process of transcription. Gene activation involves transcription of DNA beginning at the 5' end with the binding of RNA polymerase and other protein transcription factors. RNA polymerase has the ability to read and correct errors in transcription. Transcription may fail if a point mutation involves a single nucleotide substitution or if addition or deletion of base pairs produces a reading-frame shift.[1,16] Antisense DNA and mRNA are synthetic oligodeoxynucleotides that inhibit transcription or translation from their respective nucleic acid. When GFAP-positive astrocytoma cells are transfected with a murine complementary DNA for GFAP in an antisense orientation, the transfected cells lose their glial processes and become epithelioid. They also develop an enhanced proliferative potential with larger colonies than those present in nontransfected control cells.[17] The ability to modify glial antigenicity in tissue culture provides hope for future progress in glial differentiation research.

Glial Oncogenesis

Glial oncogenesis most likely results from a series of chromosomal changes that lead to the inactivation of tumor-suppressor genes or the amplification of proto-oncogenes. Stimulants for genetic dedifferentiation of mature cells or the arrest of stem cell development are largely unknown. Inherited phakomatoses, germline p53 mutations, and radiation are associated with increased risk of malignancy.

ANGIOGENESIS

Angiogenesis is the sprouting of capillaries from pre-existing small venules.[2] Venule-sprouting occurs through degradation of the venular basement membrane, followed by the proliferation, alignment, and migration of endothelial cells to the angiogenic stimulus.[18] In embryonic development, angiogenesis is the major process by which the brain and other organs become vascularized.[2] Angiogenesis is absent during adulthood, except for transient bursts during wound healing and in the female menstrual and reproductive process.[2] The growth of tumors requires blood vessel maintenance and growth and proliferation of capillaries to provide nutrients to the tumor.[19] The secretion of angiogenic factors by tumors was first proposed by Folkman and Klagsburn in 1987.[20] The angiogenic stimulus in malignant gliomas is the expression of tumor genes coding for the angiogenic growth factors—fibroblast growth factor (FGF), PDGF, and vascular endothelial growth factor (VEGF). Other possible sources of growth factors include the ECM and macrophages.[2] Angiogenic growth factors activate endothelial cells through receptor mechanisms (Fig. 2–2).[2,19] These receptors all belong to the transmembrane class of tyrosine kinases.[2]

Growth Factors and Angiogenesis

FGF has been cloned in eight different isoforms, and there are at least four high-affinity FGF receptors. FGF-1 and -2 are potent angiogenic factors present during chick brain development. FGF isoforms are not downregulated during adult life and are strongly mitogenic.[2] FGF messenger RNA has been found in tumor cells but not in vascular cells in tumors. These findings question the role of FGF in angiogenesis.

PDGF is a dimeric molecule formed by two polypeptide chains. It exists in three different dimers, PDGF-AA, -AB, and -BB, with two different receptors, and , that bind the PDGF dimers with different affinities. PDGF is a potent growth factor for both glial and mesenchymal cells. PDGF receptors (e.g., PDGFR-B) have recently been found on endothelial cells.[21] PDGFR-B is not expressed in normal brain, is present on low-grade glioma cells, and its expression is further increased on the endothelium of glioblastoma (see Fig. 2–2).[22]

VEGF is an endothelial cell mitogen expressed in glioma cells abutting areas of necrosis, with its receptor (e.g., VEGF-receptor 1, or flt-1) expressed in endothelial cells. Recently, a second VEGF receptor, KDR (or flk-1), has been described.[2,23] Flt-1 and KDR messages are not expressed on endothelial cells in normal brain, are expressed to a minor degree in some low-grade gliomas, and are highly co-expressed in glioblastoma.[23,24] Receptor activity of Flt-1 is greatest on the endothelial cells of glioblastoma, where it can be increased 20- to 50-fold in comparison with that in low-grade glioma. This suggests that VEGF is secreted from glioblastoma cells and that it acts to stimulate endothelial cells through paracrine mechanisms. VEGF and its receptor are also expressed in meningioma. [24] In glioma cell lines, VEGF secretion may be induced by epidermal growth factor (EGF) alone, by PDGF-BB or by bFGF, but not by PDGF-AA.[17]

Inhibition of Angiogenesis

The inhibition of angiogenesis is a possible avenue for control of malignant glioma growth. Minocycline, a semisynthetic tetracycline, inhibits 9L gliosarcoma growth when compared with controls.[25] AGM-1470 (or TNP-470), a fungal derived inhibitor of angiogenesis, inhibits the growth of nerve-sheath tumors.[26] TNP-470 also inhibits tumor vascularization in nonmalignant and malignant meningiomas, implanted under the renal cap-

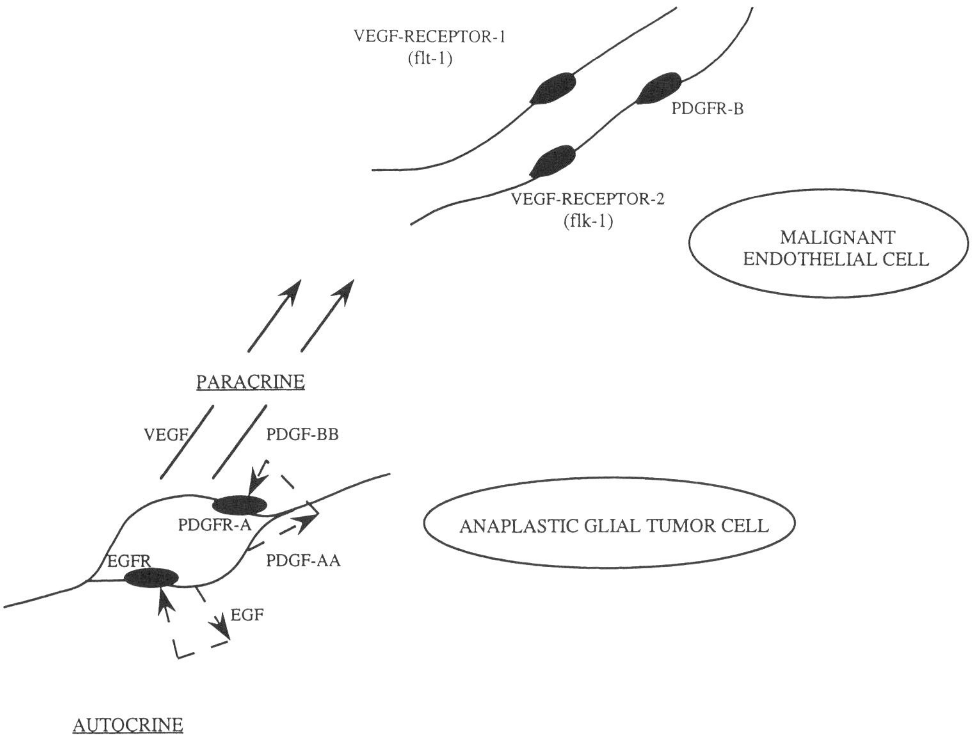

VEGF	VASCULAR ENDOTHELIAL GROWTH FACTOR
VEGF-RECEPTOR-1 (flt-1)	VASCULAR ENDOTHELIAL GROWTH FACTOR-RECEPTOR-1
VEGF-RECEPTOR-2 (flk-1)	VASCULAR ENDOTHELIAL GROWTH FACTOR-RECEPTOR-2
PDGF-AA or BB	PLATELET DERIVED GROWTH FACTOR-AA or BB
PDGFR-A or B	PLATELET DERIVED GROWTH FACTOR RECEPTOR-A or B
EGF	EPIDERMAL GROWTH FACTOR
EGFR	EPIDERMAL GROWTH FACTOR RECEPTOR
	RECEPTOR

Figure 2–2. Anaplastic glial tumor cell and endothelial cell growth factors and their receptors. Note autocrine glial tumor stimulation by EGF and PDGF-AA, and paracrine stimulation of endothelial cell by astrocyte produced PDGF-BB and VEGF.

sule in nude mice.[27] TNP-470 is undergoing clinical trials.

In the p53-deficient human glioblastoma cell line, LN-Z308, there is strong angiogenic activity, which is suppressed when the cell is transfected with wild type p53.[18] In tissue culture, U-251 glioma cells had their VEGF mRNA secretion downregulated by a ribosome molecule (i.e., vrZmI) packaged in a episomal plasmid vector. VrZmI acts by cutting all isoforms of VEGF mRNA.[28] Antisense oligodeoxynucleotides targeting VEGF inhibited glioma cells in tissue culture and in subcutaneously implanted D54 gliomas.[29] As the understanding of angiogenesis has increased markedly in the past decade, so has the potential for successful antiangiogenic therapy.

BLOOD-BRAIN BARRIER

Structure

Normal brain endothelial cells have tight junctions, lacking fenestrations, gaps, and clefts.[3] The tight junctions between normal brain endothelial cells make the cells functionally continuous and are responsible for the BBB. In brain tumors, a blood-tumor barrier (BTB) protects tumor cells from water-soluble substances. The endothelium of virally induced tumors in animals and human brain tumors is discontinuous (Fig. 2–3). Vick and colleague[30] found that clefts exist in the endothelium in brain tissue adjacent to tumor. On microscopic examination, they found the number of junctional clefts varied directly with the density of infiltrating tumor cells. Junctional clefts were present even when the tumor cell was not in direct contact with the blood vessel.[31] Brain tumor capillaries varied from normal to markedly abnormal in thickness of capillary walls and basement membranes, surface projections, pinocytotic vesicles, and endothelial gaps or defects.[32]

Function

In intracerebrally implanted tumor models, the transit of biologic tracers both into tumor and brain adjacent to tumor varies.[33] In RG-2 tumors implanted intracerebrally, the permeability of tumor was approximately 25 times greater than in tumor-free cortex.[34] Therefore, water-soluble drugs may pass into the brain tumor without passing through the BBB. The most active proliferation of tumor is at the advancing edge into normal brain. The permeability of the BBB in this advancing edge varies, as does water-soluble drug delivery to tumor. Whereas lipid-soluble drugs with a high octanol/-water partition coefficient (e.g., 1,3-bis-(2-chloroethyl)-1-nitrosourea [BCNU]) are highly permeable, the water soluble drugs (e.g., methotrexate [MTX], 5-fluorouracil, thymidine) are minimally permeable.[35]

Dexamethasone has been shown to decrease the permeability of rat brain capillary endothelium alone and when cocultured with glial cells.[36] In rats bearing unilateral hemispheric C6 gliomas, dexamethasone 10 mg/kg intraperitoneally decreased the permeability of the BBB marker, 14C-α-aminoisobutyric acid, into tumor and brain adjacent to tumor. One hour following infusion there was approximately a one-third decrease in tumor capillary permeability; at 12 hours the permeability was 25% of the untreated value. In

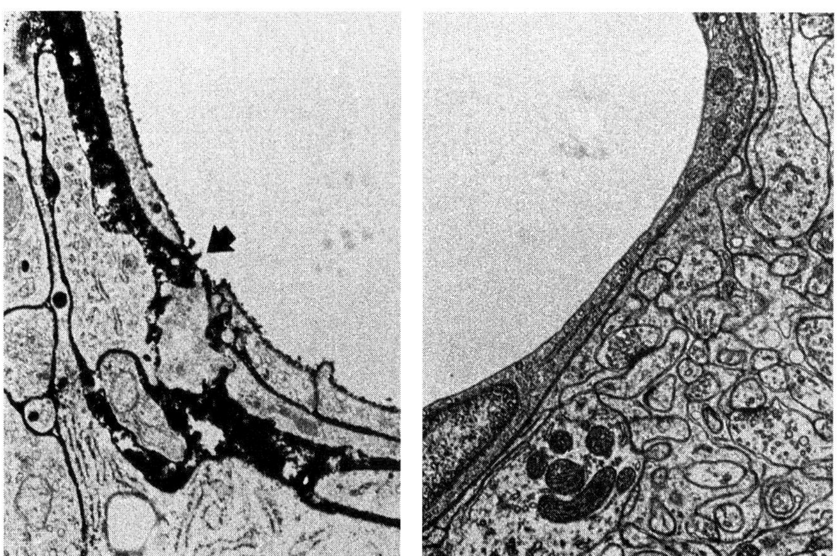

Figure 2–3. Endothelial cell with normal tight *(right)* and open *(left)* capillary junctions. Electron-dense reaction product fills intercellular spaces between processes in a virally induced rat glioma. Arrow at left indicates endothelial gap through which intravenously administered horseradish peroxidase has free access to brain. (From Vick, Khandekar, and Bigner[30], pp 524–525, with permission).

brain adjacent to tumor, permeability fell to 29% of its control value at 12 hours.[37] The decrease in permeability produced by dexamethasone may be mediated by the inhibition of vascular permeability factor secretion by malignant astrocytic cells.[38] Dexamethasone may decrease chemotherapy access to tumor, and its dose should be kept to a minimum. It is often needed for its anti-edema effect, decreasing transudation of fluid into the interstitial space of brain.

A glucose transporter (GLUT1) is expressed on differentiated brain vessels with an intact BBB. GLUT1 is necessary to transport glucose through tight junctions into the brain. In contrast, malignant tumor vessels with a permeable BBB often lose GLUT1 expression.[39,40] Dexamethasone treatment of 9L rat malignant gliomas produced a marked decrease in the leakage of vascular permeability marker, Evans blue, a 100% increase in GLUT1 expression, and a significantly smaller tumor size.[40] GLUT3 mRNA expression is increased when a tumor becomes more malignant and probably relates to the neovascularization that accompanies glioblastoma multiforme.[41]

Rats radiated with single large doses of 20 to 60 Gy had BBB breakdown, measured by Evans blue leakage, with the time to BBB breakdown inversely proportional to dose.[42] Following high-dose external-beam radiation therapy, or interstitial brachytherapy for treatment of malignant gliomas, transient contrast enhancement (BBB breakdown) may appear in the tumor or in the immediate surrounding area. After weeks to months, the area of contrast enhancement may evolve into an edematous mass, requiring surgical removal, or recede to an area of low density.

Drug Delivery to Tumor

Drug delivery to tumor depends not only on permeability but also on luminal surface area of capillaries.[31] Plasma protein binding limits drug entry into tissue, through either a closed or partially open BBB. Blood flow plays a role in drug delivery when a large capillary surface area exists and permeability is great. Blood flow to tumor is less critical with water-soluble drugs, in which permeability is small.[31] Adenosine, a potent vasodilator, increased blood flow more than twofold to avian sarcoma-induced rat tumors but did not affect blood flow to normal brain.[43]

Disruption

Osmotic blood-brain barrier disruption (BBBD) has been used to increase drug delivery to tumors prior to both IV and IA chemotherapy infusion. Although the BBB is partially open in most anaplastic brain tumors, the delivery of water-soluble chemotherapeutic agents to tumor and brain adjacent to tumor is limited. Osmotic BBBD is a reversible means of disrupting tight junctions in tumor, brain adjacent to tumor, and normal brain. In animals, tracers that mark the BBB opening include Evans blue staining and 14C-α-aminoisobutyric acid autoradiography. In humans, computed tomography (CT) contrast enhancement can be used to assess BBBD. Osmotic BBBD enables nonselective delivery of chemotherapeutic agents and monoclonal antibodies to human brain tissue.[44–47] A shortcoming of osmotic BBBD is that because the opening of the BBB is greater in normal brain than in tumor or brain adjacent to tumor, increased drug delivery to tumor produces a larger percentage increase in drug exposure of normal brain, with the potential for toxicity.[48] Osmotic BBBD has been used with apparent benefit in clinical lymphoma trials (see Chapter 12).[49]

New agents have been discovered that selectively open the BBB in tumor and have no effect in normal brain. Leukotriene C4, infused intra-arterially in rats with RG-2 tumors, produced a twofold increase in the permeability of 14C-α-aminoisobutyric acid in tumor, but had no effect in normal brain.[50] More recently, intracarotid infusion of the bradykinin analog RMP-7 in glioma-bearing rats increased the transport of [14C] carboplatin to tumors 2.7-fold, with no increase in normal brain. RMP-7 treated animals survived longer than untreated control animals, particularly if combined treatment was used at the time of tumor implantation.

Clinical trials with IA infusion of RMP-7, followed by intravenous (IV) carboplatin infusion, are in progress.[4,50]

CHROMOSOMAL CHANGES

Chromosomal abnormalities in brain tumors can be divided into three categories: (1) gain or loss of specific chromosome, (2) changes in ploidy, and (3) structural changes of specific loci on a chromosome.[5–9] Gain or loss of a chromosome and changes in ploidy in brain tumors were initially discovered using karyotypic analysis.[6,7] Karyotypic analysis can only detect large losses of genetic material of three to five megabases and involves tumor cell culture, which may introduce changes in the genome.[8,9] Karyotypic analysis has largely been replaced by molecular biologic techniques in the detection of chromosomal abnormalities. These new techniques enable the investigator to find smaller structural changes of specific loci on a chromosome, whether there is a deletion, insertion, point mutation, or duplication of genetic material.[51,52] Comparative genomic hybridization (CGH) is a recent cytologic method that detects losses or gains across the entire tumor genome.[53] Cytologic studies and molecular biologic techniques have not found a single chromosomal abnormality present in all malignant gliomas.[6–9] Chromosomal variability or heterogeneity occurs in different regions of a tumor. In addition, no chromosome abnormality is specific for gliomas. In contrast, most children with retinoblastoma have a specific abnormality of the retinoblastoma-susceptibility gene (Rb) on 13q14.[54]

Mutations or chromosomal changes may give rise to loss of function of a gene or an increase in function. Genetic mutations of tumor-suppressor genes result in a loss or markedly decreased expression of an inhibitory protein, resulting in uncontrolled growth. The loss of a small portion of chromosome 13, the retinoblastoma-susceptibility gene, is responsible for the absence of a gene product and the development of retinoblastomas.[8] Such mutations typically require the inactivation of both gene copies. Retinoblastoma gene abnormalities are also seen in high-grade astrocytomas. An analogy can be made to an automobile that suddenly loses its brakes and continues to accelerate going downhill. The reintroduction of normal, transcriptionally active sequences in these tumor cells is associated with a return to a more normal phenotype.[55] An increase in gene function by gene amplification or copy number may be associated with an increase in a protein product, stimulating cell growth. It is usually a dominant genetic change and can be compared to stepping on a car's accelerator.

Astrocytoma

Astrocytoma, like most other solid tumors, acquires a series of sequential allelic changes, with both the amplification and deletion of genetic material in their development and malignant evolution (Fig. 2–4).[6–9,55–63] The earliest changes involve the loss of genetic material on chromosomes 6,13,17gp (short arm), and 22, probably associated with the change from normal glia to low-grade glioma (LGA).[8,9,55,56,64] The p53 gene, a known tumor-suppressor gene located on chromosome 17, is mutated in up to 75% of glial tumors, with loss of one 17p allele.[60] The p53 protein is thought to be a regulator of the cell cycle, with its presence producing G1 arrest or apoptosis. Cells expressing a dominant-negative mutation had less G1 arrest and increased survival at all therapeutic radiation doses compared with cells with wild type p53.[11]

Allelic changes involving losses of chromosome 9p and 19q (long arm) are associated with progression from astrocytoma to anaplastic astrocytoma. These changes are not commonly seen in grade II astrocytoma but do appear in grade III, or anaplastic, astrocytoma.[8,55,59,60] The 9p21 region controls for a cyclin-dependent kinase (CDK4) that inhibits cell proliferation.[65] The protein is undetectable in greater than 50% of high-grade tumors. $P16^{INK4}$ is a cell cycle regulator that binds to and inactivates CDK4. It is absent in 50% of high-grade tumors. Hypermethylation of the CpG island in the 5' region of the p16/*CDKN2* gene may produce loss of

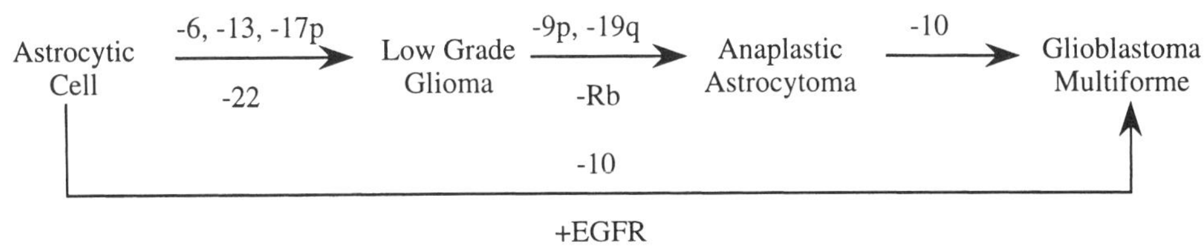

Figure 2–4. Chromosomal gain (+) or loss (−) associated with the evolution of the malignant process in astrocytic tumors. Glioblastoma may develop through two pathways: 1) Progression from low grade to anaplastic astrocytoma to glioblastoma where p 53 mutations are common, or 2) de novo from an astrocytic cell where EGFR amplification is common.

p16 expression without gene deletion. The transfection of the p16/*CDKN2* gene, in glioma cell lines with a homozygous gene deletion, suppresses U-373MG cell-line growth, suggesting the gene is a tumor suppressor.[66] When CDK4 is over-expressed in high-grade gliomas, P16^{INK4} is also over-expressed.[65] Deletions are also noted in the region of the 9p type 1 interferon locus, which suggests a loss of interferon function. Interferon normally inhibits cell growth.[9,67] Loss of part of chromosome 19q is seen in 46% of grade III tumors but in only 11% of grade II tumors.[59] In human high-grade astrocytoma, abnormalities of the retinoblastoma gene are present in 30% of tumors. CDKN2, CDK4 and Rb abnormalities are usually independent and do not overlap, possibly suggesting the existence of anaplastic astrocytoma biologic subsets.[68]

The most common chromosomal abnormality, occurring in almost all cases of glioblastoma, is a loss of chromosome 10.[8,9,55–57,59,69,70] Deletions of chromosome 10 occur in 93% of glioblastomas, 64% of anaplastic astrocytomas, and 32% of astrocytomas. In glioblastomas, the vast majority lost one entire chromosome 10; in astrocytomas, most lost only 10p.[71] The exact region that functions as a tumor-suppressor gene is on chromosome 10q23–24. This region was thought to contain a tumor-suppressor gene. Identification of homozygous deletions in four glioma cell lines further localized the region. A gene, *MMAC1* (PTEN), spans these deletions and encodes a widely expressed 5.5-kb mRNA. The predicted MMAC1 protein contains sequence motifs with significant homology to the catalytic domain of protein phosphatases and to the cytoskeletal proteins tensin and auxilin. MMAC1 coding-region mutations were observed in other tumors, including prostate, kidney, and breast carcinoma cell lines and tumor specimens.[72,72a] A considerable percentage of glioblastomas have no MMAC1 mutation despite a loss of heterogeneity, supporting the hypothesis that there is a least one other tumor suppressor gene on 10q.[72b] Amplification or rearrangement of the *EGFR* gene occurs primarily in glioblastoma. The *EGFR* or c-*erbB* gene is the most consistently amplified gene in gliomas; it is amplified in up to 50% of glioblastoma specimens from tissue culture, biopsy, and resection.[73–79] Amplification of the *EGFR* gene can occur from extra copies of chromosome 7 or a duplication of the *EFGR* gene region on chromosome 7.[75]

Watanabe and colleagues[80] found EGF over-expression was common in glioblastoma with a clinical history of less than 3 months and no previous history of low-grade astrocytoma. In this population, they found a low incidence of p53 mutations. In glioblastomas seen initially as low-grade astrocytoma or anaplastic astrocytoma, there was a high incidence of p53 mutations and frequent overexpression of EGF receptors.[80] This suggests two genetic pathways for the development of glioblastoma: a multistep sequential pathway and a second de novo pathway (see Fig. 2–4). Other genes amplified in glioblastoma include the *MDM2*, *N-myc*, and *gli* genes.[76,78,81]

MDM2 codes for a cellular protein that complexcs thc p53 tumor-suppressor gene and inhibits its function. The *MDM2* gene is amplified and overexpressed in 8% to 10% of anaplastic glioma and glioblastoma. No p53 abnormalities have been found in these cases when examined with RFLP analysis.[81]

Reduced or absent expression of the deleted colorectal carcinoma gene, a potential tumor-suppressor gene on 18q, is seen frequently in glioblastoma and less frequently but commonly in oligodendroglioma and oligo-astrocytoma.[82] Loss of regions of chromosome 22 has also been seen in glioblastoma.[56,58,59] The presence or absence of chromosomal abnormalities within a tumor grade has not been prognostically correlated with survival in astrocytic malignancy. Pediatric and juvenile astrocytic tumors have only rarely been found to have chromosomal abnormalities on chromosomes 10 or 17, or p53 gene alterations, suggesting a different pathway for oncogenesis in pediatric astrocytoma.[83]

Oligodendroglioma

Oligodendroglioma has an early loss of chromosomal material on 1p and 19q, with loss of CDKN2 (p16) and MTS2 (p15) on 9p, or amplification of CDK4 on 12q associated with the progression to anaplastic oligodendroglioma (Fig. 2–5).[84] The response of anaplastic oligodendroglioma to procarbazine, CCNU, and vincristine chemotherapy and survival has been positively correlated with the loss of chromosomal material on 1p, with or without 19q loss, and inversely correlated with CDKN2 loss.[84a]

Primitive Neuroectodermal Tumor

In primitive neuroectodermal tumor (PNET) chromosomal loss is predominantly on chromosome 17, but loss on chromosomes 12 and 22 also occurs.[8,9]

Meningioma

Meningioma is characterized by monosomy 22, or deletion of the long arm of chromosome 22, and by the increase in expression of the *sis* and c-*myc* oncogenes.[8,85]

The development of glial tumors and malignant transformation is due to the loss of tumor-suppressor genes and the gain and amplification of proto-oncogenes. These changes offer many targets for future gene therapy, with gene replacement and antisense oligonucleotides. The next section examines how growth factors and cytokines influence cell growth.

GROWTH FACTORS, RECEPTORS, AND CYTOKINES

Growth Factors and Receptors

Growth factors and their inhibitors are peptides involved in the normal development, proliferation, and differentiation of tissues in the CNS (Table 2–1). Growth-factor activity is normally under the control of proto-oncogenes and tumor-suppressor genes.[86]

The amplification and activation of the *EGFR* gene on chromosome 7 is at least partly responsible for the development

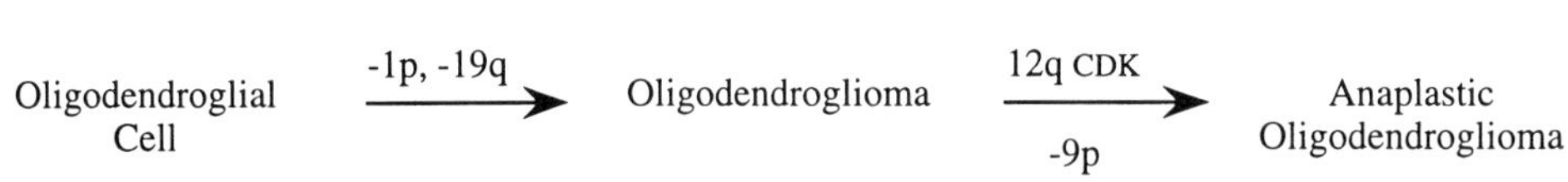

Figure 2–5. Chromosomal gain (+) or loss (−) associated with the evolution of the malignant process in oligodendroglial tumors.

Table 2–1. **Growth Factors**

Growth Factors	Present On and Secretion By	Probable Function
Epidermal growth factor	Astrocytoma	Stimulates astrocytoma cell growth (autocrinc)
Fibroblast growth factor	Astrocytoma, meningioma	Stimulates astrocytoma, growth, migration, and invasion (autocrine)
Insulin-like growth factor	IGF-I: Normal brain, meninges, choroid plexus, meningiomas	Growth regulation of meningiomas (autocrine)
	IGF-II: Meningiomas, astrocytomas	
Nerve growth factor	Neuroectodermal tumors	Stimulates neuroectodermal cell growth (autocrine)
Platelet-derived growth factor	PDGF-AA: Astrocytoma	Stimulates astrocytoma cell growth (autocrine)
	PDGF-BB: Astrocytoma Astrocytoma	Stimulates endothelial proliferation (paracrine)
Transforming growth factor	TGF-α Astrocytoma, meningioma	Phenotypic transformation of normal cells
	TGF-β Astrocytoma Astrocytoma	Inhibition of growth of astrocytoma cells in culture
Vascular endothelial growth factor	Astrocytoma	Stimulates endothelial cell proliferation (paracrine)

of glioblastoma.[87] The *EGFR* gene is amplified in up to 50% of cases of glioblastoma and is over-expressed in the majority.[73,79,88]

Growth factors may also act reciprocally to control the activity or expression of specific oncogenes and tumor-suppressor genes.[86] Malignant brain tumor cells generally lose their requirement for exogenous growth factors to maintain their cellular proliferation. They develop the machinery to synthesize and respond to endogenously produced growth factors. Brain tumor-generated growth factors act through autocrine, paracrine, and intracrine mechanisms to stimulate themselves and their neighbors, which also produce receptors for these and other peptides.[86]

EPIDERMAL GROWTH FACTOR AND RECEPTOR

In almost all cases, EGF has stimulated growth in human primary glioma biopsy specimens and in glioma cell lines grown both in tissue culture and as spheroids.[89,90] In addition, tumor-cell invasion into normal fetal rat brain aggregates was measured and found to be increased by EGF, in both primary biopsies and cultured glial cells. PDGF-BB—and FGF-stimulated glioma cell growth less consistently, with FGF only occasionally stimulating spheroid invasion into normal rat brain.[89,90]

The amplified or over-expressed *EGFR* gene did not appear to mediate the growth-promoting effect of EGF in glioblastoma. The level of expression of *EGFR* in glioblastoma cell lines did not predict the response to EGF, although cells with greater expression of *EGFR* were more resistant to the differentiating effect of retinoic acid.[88,91] *EGFR* was found to mediate EGF effects on GFAP and glial-process extension.[91]

Optimistically, we might hope that amplification of the *EGFR* gene would provide a target for effective treatment of gliomas.[92] Monoclonal antibodies to the *EGFR* expressed on human gliomas and in tumors of other tissue origin, but not in normal brain, have been developed.[93] Recurrent malignant glioma has been treated with an iodine-131 (^{131}I)–labeled monoclonal antibody to normal EGFR protein, delivered intra-arterially through the internal carotid artery.[94,95] CT scans showed occasional tumor regression, although the durability of response was not long. A new antibody has been developed to an aberrant form of the EGFR protein, seen in approximately 20% of glioblastomas. It is tumor specific and does not exist on any other cell. This antibody and others may be linked to toxins, radiation sources, or genetically engineered material to provide an effective treatment for a subset of malignant astrocytoma.[92]

FIBROBLAST GROWTH FACTOR (FGF) AND RECEPTOR

Glioma cells express FGF in at least two of the eight isoforms, aFGF and bFGF.[2,96] Human glioma cells have FGF proteins and receptors,[97] and meningiomas express message transcripts of fibroblast receptor genes and FGF receptors by immunohistochemistry.[98,99] The fibroblast growth factor receptor 1 (FGFR1) mRNA levels were significantly higher in glioblastoma, than in normal brain, brain adjacent to tumor, or on endothelial cells within the tumor.[2,96] Although FGF does not play a major role in angiogenesis (see angiogenesis section), it is thought to stimulate glioma cells in an autocrine manner.[2,96] The expression of bFGF increased proportionate to the degree of glial malignancy.[100] If bFGF is transfected into fibroblasts with a signal sequence for bFGF, the fibroblasts assume a malignant phenotype, with migration and invasion into surrounding neurophil. The transformed fibroblasts also secrete a proteolytic gelatinase and form branching networks.[101] If the signal peptide is absent when bFGF is transfected into the fibroblasts, the cells form a pseudocapsule with little secretion of gelatinase and minimal invasion of the ECM. Suppression of FGF expression with antisense oligodeoxynucleotides inhibits the in vitro growth of transformed astrocytes.[102,103]

INSULIN-LIKE GROWTH FACTOR AND RECEPTOR

In culture, human glioma cells express a high level of insulin-like growth factor-I (IGF-I) mRNA transcripts. There is no tumor growth when C6 glioma cells are transfected in vitro subcutaneously in rats with an antisense IGF-I expression construct in an Epstein-Barr virus expression vector. The antisense IGF-I expression construct also requires the presence of a $ZnSO_4$ promotor. In the absence of the $ZnSO_4$ promotor, C6 transfectants continue to express high levels of IGF-I mRNA.[104] Insulin-like growth factor-II (IGF-II) is present in normal human adult brain, in the meninges and the choroid plexus.[105] IGF-II message transcripts are found in most meningiomas but inconsistently in tumors of astrocytic lineage. IGF-I and IGF-II receptors are described in both in vitro normal brain and glial tumor cell lines.[106,107]

NERVE GROWTH FACTOR AND RECEPTOR

Nerve growth factor (NGF) mRNA has been found in a primitive neuroectodermal tumor (PNET) cell line. In l3 of 35 human PNET and the above cell line,[108] NGF receptors were localized to the cell surface. In C6 glioma cells, NGF receptors have been found to be upregulated by both NGF and brain-derived neurotrophic factor.[109]

PLATELET-DERIVED GROWTH FACTOR AND RECEPTOR

PDGF is formed by two polypeptide chains and exists in three isoforms, PDGF-AA, -AB, and -BB.[21] Whereas the PDGF A chain is expressed in almost all astrocytic tumors, the PDGF B chain is expressed in only 50% of anaplastic astrocytomas, and in much fewer low-grade gliomas.[22,110–112] PDGF-α and PDGF-β receptors are present on glioma cells, with the PDGF-β receptor also present on endothelial cells.[22,112] This suggests an autocrine receptor mechanism for PDGF-AA in glioma cells, and a paracrine receptor mechanism for PDGF-BB on endothelial cells.[22,112]

The PDGF B chain is identical in amino acid sequence and structural properties to the simian sarcoma virus sis oncogene that encodes for a protein, p28^{sis}.[113] The human homologue, c-*sis*, of the simian sarcoma virus oncogene *sis*, was used for a template for the synthesis of an 18-base antisense oligodeoxynucleotide. When the 5'-antisense c-*sis*-3' was transfected into A172 glioma cells in vitro, proliferation was inhibited in a dose-dependent fashion. Whereas the antisense primers inhibited the de novo synthesis of c-*sis* intracellular protein, cells transfected with sense primers had no effect on cell proliferation or c-*sis* protein synthesis.[113] This is a very exciting application of antisense technology; however, c-sis is expressed in only a minority of gliomas and, therefore, this is not likely to be a clinical target for human glioma trials.

Suramin, a growth factor scavenger, which binds to PDGF-BB, EGF, and IGF-I, significantly inhibited the growth of meningioma cells, but not glioma cells in culture.[114,115] In meningioma cells, EGF, IGF-I and PDGF-BB cell proliferation was abolished, and intracellular PDGF-BB was reduced.[114]

TRANSFORMING GROWTH FACTOR AND RECEPTOR

Transforming growth factors (TGFs) cause phenotypic transformation of normal cells. The phenotype transformation is accompanied by a loss of density-dependent inhibition of monolayer cell growth and the gain of anchorage-independent cell growth.[116] TGF-α has been found in both meningioma and glial tumors, with increased levels in recurrent meningioma and the more anaplastic gliomas.[117,118] TGF-β and its receptors, TBR-I and TBR-II, are expressed in gliomas; there is increased expression of TGF-β with increasing malignancy.[119,120] TGF-α produces a dose-dependent growth inhibitory effect on normal brain and glioma cells in culture. TGF-β_1 stimulates glioma cells in vitro to migrate and invade.[121] Further understanding TGF-β_1 antiproliferative and invasive mechanisms may allow scientists to develop more effective glioma therapy.[120,121] TGF-β_2 has been shown to mediate suppression of T lymphocyte activation within malignant gliomas and may be classified with the cytokines listed later. This suppression of lymphocyte activation can be abolished by preincubation of two glioblastoma cell lines with a TGF-β_2-specific phosphorothioate antisense oligodeoxynucleotide.[122]

Kinase Receptors

Tyrosine kinase receptors bind naturally occurring ligands on their extracellular domain. Ligand binding results in the phosphorylation of tyrosine on cytoplasmic proteins. EGF may be a ligand both for tyrosine and serine receptor kinases.[123] Protein tyrosine kinase signals are amplified in cellular proliferation, and inhibition of these signals with benzodiazepin-2-one produces apoptosis in glioma cell lines.[124]

Protein kinase C (PKC) is a serine kinase. PKC is part of a signal transduction system and acts through second messengers. When an extracellular ligand binds to its receptor, an activated complex is formed that associates with a G protein and activates the enzyme phospholipase C. Phospholipase C catalyzes the hydrolysis of phosphatidylinositol-1,4-diphosphate into inositol 1,4,5-triphosphate (IP3) and diacylglycerol. IP3 mobilizes calcium, and the calcium facilitates the activation of pyruvate kinase, the second messenger. PKC exerts its regulatory influence through phosphorylation of the transcriptional control elements, c-*fos* and c-*jun*.[125] All human glioma cell lines examined showed high levels of PKC activity.[126] Further studies demonstrated higher PKC expression in low-grade gliomas than in anaplastic astrocytoma and glioblastoma.[127] When PKC was activated by phorbol esters, there was a dose-dependent inhibition of human glioma cell-line growth, as measured by the incorporation of tritiated thymidine uptake.[127,128] The growth factors EGF and FGF stimulate PKC activity, and this can be reversed with staurosporine, a PKC inhibitor.[126] The PKC inhibitor tamoxifen inhibits glioma DNA synthesis and cell proliferation in vitro in a dose-dependent manner. These gliomas are estrogen-receptor negative; therefore, inhibition is not mediated through the estrogen receptor.[129] Clinical trials of recurrent glioma treated with tamoxifen have produced significant tumor responses in a small percentage of patients.[130]

The estrogen receptor–related antigen has been expressed in embryonal and germ cell tumors.[131] Meningiomas are rich in progestin receptor. RU-486, an antiprogestational agent, is currently being evaluated for the treatment of recurrent meningiomas that have failed radiation therapy.[132,133] Glucocorticoid receptors have been found on some glioma cell lines (e.g., HU197, D384, LW5). They respond to dexamethasone with cell growth.[134,135] In the clinical management of patients, there may be a tradeoff between the antiedema effect and tumor-growth stimulation. Other receptors expressed in brain tumors include the grade-related expression of the vitamin D receptor in astrocytic tumors;[136] the endothelin receptor in astrocytoma and glioblastoma;[137] the diazepam-binding inhibitor polypeptide;[138] kappa opiate receptors in glioblastoma; sigma opiate receptors in neuroblastoma;[139] and the folate receptor in ependymoma.[140]

Cytokines

Cytokines are soluble factors controlling a wide variety of leukocyte functions, including activation, growth, differentiation, and functional inhibition (Table 2–2).[141] Cytokine effects are mediated through high-affinity cell surface receptors, which may stimulate other cytokines. Tumors produce cytokines, and some such as TGF-β_2, are functionally inhibitory.[122,141] TGF-$\beta_2$may be partially responsible for the impaired leukocyte function of gliomas.

TUMOR NECROSIS FACTOR

Tumor necrosis factor-α (TNF-α), a cytokine, plays a key role as a immunoregulatory molecule in various neurologic diseases, such as multiple sclerosis (MS), Alzheimer's disease, and AIDS. TNF-α mRNA is expressed and protein is present in all grades of astrocytic malignancy and is correlated with lymphocyte infiltration of glial tumor tissue.[142] TNF-α exerts a marked antiproliferative and anti-invasive effect on human glioblastoma.[143] Twenty patients with glioblastoma were treated with TNF-α the initial five were treated intravenously, and the others were treated intra-arterially, all at a dose of 1 x 10^5 U/m^2 per day. Ten patients were evaluable, with one complete response and one partial response in the IA group.[144]

INTERLEUKINS AND INTERFERONS

Interleukins 1, 6, 8 and 10 are all found on astrocytomas, often with an increase in activity when stimulated with other cy-

Table 2–2. **Cytokines**

Cytokines	Present On and Secretion By	Probable Function
Tumor necrosis factor-α	Astrocytoma	Anti-invasive and antiproliferative effect on astrocytoma cells
Interleukins • IL-1 • IL-6 • IL-8 • IL-10	Astrocytoma	Neutrophil mediated inflammation accompanying malignancy
Interferons • A and B	Astrocytoma	Inhibition of growth and loss of colony-forming ability

tokines, such as TNF-α or another interleukin.[144–146] Their exact role in tumor growth and invasion is not yet elucidated. Fourteen of 28 glioblastomas stained with a monoclonal antibody to IL-1α.[147] Whereas IL-10 is expressed more frequently in invasive tumors, IL-6 and granulocyte macrophage-colony stimulating factor (GM-CSF) are more common in localized tumors.[148] Glioblastoma cell lines have receptors for IL-1α, interferon β, and GM-CSF, suggesting autocrine loop function.[149]

Interferon α and β genes are detectable in a high percentage of malignant gliomas, but the presence or absence of the gene is unrelated to the growth inhibitory effect of either interferon α or β in these cell lines.[150]

Table 2–3. **Extracellular Matrix Structures and Their Components**

Glial limitans externa basement membrane
Fibrillar type I and III collagen
Nonfibrillar type IV collagen
Fibronectin
Laminin
Heparan sulfate
Vascular basement membrane
Type IV collagen
Laminin
Vitronectin
Entactin
Heparan sulfate
Brain parenchyma
Hyaluronic acid
Chondroitin sulfate
Glycoproteins

INVASION

Brain tumor invasion into brain adjacent to tumor is mediated by the interaction of the ECM, with adhesion molecules expressed and secreted by tumor cells and their transmembrane receptors. Proteases are secreted by tumor cells through adhesion molecule interaction with protease receptors and degrade the ECM.

Extracellular Matrix

The ECM of brain is a poorly understood structure. The function and identity are largely unknown. The ECM of brain is composed of at least three structures: (1) the glial limitans externa basement membrane, (2) the vascular basement membrane, and (3) brain parenchyma. These structures are composed of collagen, proteoglycans, glycoproteins, and binding proteins (Table 2–3).[151]

The ability of cells to infiltrate into the ECM, spread and establish themselves in distant organs is a property of both nonmalignant and malignant cells. Nonmalignant hematopoietic cells, such as polymorphonuclear cells and lymphocytes, are produced in the bone marrow, enter into blood vessels, and migrate into tissues to perform their many functions.[151] Angiogenesis involves the proliferation and then migration of endothelial cells to the angiogenic stimulus.[2,18,151] A difference between the invasion of normal and malignant cells is the control of the process in normal cells by the ECM.[152] Tumor invasion involves changes in tumor cell attachment to the ECM, mediated by adhesion molecules and their transmembrane receptors.

Adhesion Molecules and Receptors

The adhesion molecules are expressed on the extracellular surface of brain tumor cells, and expression is produced by a complex interaction between the tumor cell and the glial limitans externa, the vascular basement membrane, and the brain parenchyma. Glioma cell adhesion is important for tumor anchorage and to facilitate growth and migration through the white matter of brain.[151,152] In malignant transformation, there is alteration in adhesion molecule transmembrane receptor type, number, and function. Adhesion molecules are classified by their chemical structure and fall into three major categories: (1) the integrins, (2) the immunoglobulin superfamily, and (3) the selectins and CD44 (Table 2–4).[151] Typically, in normal cells, the ECM receptors are collected at the cell membrane into adhesion plaques with the adhesion molecules. The plaques serve as a transmembrane link for

Table 2–4. **Types of Adhesion Molecules**

Type	Cell Type Expression	Ligand
Integrins		
Lymphocyte function-associated antigen-1 (LFA-1)	Hematopoietic cells	ICAM-1
Very late antigen (VLA-4)	Hematopoietic cells, gliomas, neural crest derivatives	VCAM-1, fibronectin
Immunoglobulin Superfamily		
Neural cell adhesion molecule (NCAM)	Gliomas, medulloblastomas, neuroblastomas, and ependymomas	NCAM, types I-VI collagen
Lymphocyte function-associated antigen-3 (LFA-3)	Gliomas, leukocytes	CD2
Intercellular adhesion molecule (ICAM-1)	Gliomas, endothelial cells, leukocytes	LFA-1
Vascular cell adhesion molecule (VCAM-1)	Astrocytes, gliomas, endothelial cells	VLA-4
Selectins		
Endothelial leukocyte adhesion molecule-1 (ELAM-1)	Endothelial cells	Sialyl-lex
Other		
CD44	Normal brain, gliomas, primitive neuroectodermal tumors	Types I-VI collagen, fibronectin, hyaluronic acid

Adapted from Couldwell et al[151], p 783, with permission.

communication between the ECM and the cell cytoskeleton. In avian sarcoma virus transformed cells, an abnormally tyrosine-phophorylated integrin is present, which may serve as a substrate for growth factors in producing disordered growth.[153]

Vascular cell adhesion molecule-1 (VCAM-1), an adhesion molecule that belongs to the immunoglobulin superfamily, is expressed by astrocytes and astrocytoma cell lines and is a ligand for very late antigen (VLA-4). In astrocytoma cell lines, VCAM-1 expression is upregulated by the cytokines TNF-α, INF-γ, and IL-1β.[154] CD44H is expressed in normal brain, glial tumors, and PNET and is an adhesion molecule with a cell surface receptor for hyaluronic acid, the major component of the ECM.[155] CD44 exists in other isoforms in colon carcinoma. The interaction with the ECM may be responsible for the invasive potential of glioma and the metastatic potential of colon carcinoma.[154] CD44 expression appears to be highest at the margins of infiltrating glial tumors and is absent in the proliferating cells in the tumor's mass.[156]

Proteases and Their Natural Inhibitors

Transmembrane receptors for adhesion molecules also play an important role in modulating the production and secretion of proteases, essential for the breakdown of the ECM. Several classes of proteases exist: matrix metalloproteinases (MMPs), serine proteases, cysteine proteases, aspartic proteinases, and endoglycosidases

Table 2–5. **Types of Proteases**

Proteases	Substrates	Natural Inhibitors
Matrix metalloproteases		
Type IV collagenase	Fibrillar collagens	TIMP-1, TIMP-2, TIMP-3
Gelatinase A & B	Gelatins, collagens (IV, V), elastin	TIMP-1, TIMP-2, TIMP-3
Matrilysin	Proteoglycans, elastin, fibronectin, laminin	TIMP-1, TIMP-2, TIMP-3
Serine proteases		
Urokinase plasminogen activator (uPA), tissue plasminogen activator (TPA)	Glycoproteins and collagens	PAI-1, PAI-2, protease nexin 1
Elastase	Elastin	—
Cysteine proteases		
Cathepsin B and L	Glycoproteins, collagens (telopeptide)	Cystatin, stefin
Aspartic proteases		
Cathepsin D	Glycoproteins, collagens (telopeptide)	—
Endoglycosidases		
Hyaluronidase	Hyaluronic acid	—
Heparanase	Heparan sulfate	—

Adapted from De Clerck et al[152], p 113, with permission.

(Table 2–5). Natural inhibitors of MMPs, serine and cysteine proteases, have now been recognized.[152]

MATRIX METALLOPROTEINASES

The MMPs degrade major components of the ECM. High levels of type IV collagenase, an MMP, have been found in malignant gliomas and on endothelial cells. The MMPs are regulated by the tissue inhibitors of MMPs (TIMPs), and invasion is a balance between MMPs and TIMPs.[157]

Tissue inhibitor metalloproteinases are negative regulators of MMPs and play an important role in modulating the activity of MMPs.[157–59] Northern blot analysis of TIMP-1 and TIMP-2 transcripts showed lower levels of these transcripts in anaplastic astrocytoma and glioblastoma multiforme than in meningioma or normal brain.[157] In addition, in malignant glioma, the over-expression of the MMPs gelatinase A, gelatinase B, and matrilysin genes was accompanied by the over-expression of the TIMP-1 gene. TIMP-1 suppressed the invasion of glioma cells through a growth medium.[158,159]

SERINE PROTEASES

Tissue plasminogen activator (tPA) and urokinase (uPA) are serine proteases that activate plasminogen through a single peptide bond cleavage to plasmin, which degrades various glycoproteins and collagens in extracellular matrix. The serine proteases are regulated by the plasminogen activator inhibitors. Pro-uPA is released by a tumor cell, with subsequent binding to its cell surface receptor. It is activated by plasmin and has proteolytic activity for the ECM components fibronectin, laminin, and type IV collagenase.[160–162] Upregulation of uPA mRNA and receptors was significant in anaplastic astrocytoma and particularly in glioblastoma when compared with normal brain and LGA.[163] An anti-uPA receptor monoclonal antibody blocked glioma invasion into a growth medium.[164]

CYSTEINE PROTEASES

Cathepsin B is one of a series of cysteine proteases expressed in astrocytoma. Expression increases with anaplasia and is present on peripheral infiltrating cells.[163,165,166] An inhibitor of cathepsin B, peptidyl methyl ketone, inhibits invasion of tumor cells in a dose-dependent fashion.[166] The understanding of brain tumor invasion, the interactions of adhesion molecules and their ECM receptors, and proteases and their inhibitors is evolving. I suspect there will be great heterogeneity in interaction of adhesion molecules and receptors within a histologic type of tumor and between tumors of different histology. The goal will be a search for a common thread that can be use for treatment.

CELL KINETICS AND PROLIFERATIVE INDICES

Cell Kinetics

Brain tumor growth is a balance between cell proliferation and cell death. Four different basic pathways can be followed by a brain tumor cell: it can rest, proliferate, differentiate, or die.[167] When a brain tumor is diagnosed clinically with CT or magnetic resonance imaging, it usually weighs 30 to 60 g, corresponding to a cellular burden of 3 to 6 x 10^{10} cells. The smallest brain tumors diagnosed clinically weigh slightly more than 1 g (10^9 cells), with 100 g (10^{11} cells) of tumor fatal because of the inelastic skull.[168]

The tumor contains proliferating cells, referred to as the *growth fraction,* and nonproliferating cells, which are quiescent.[169,170] The latter cells may revert to a proliferative state or may have lost the ability to proliferate through differentiation. Alternatively, they may be in the process of dying.[169] The proliferating cell cycle is divided into four discrete phases: (1) postmitotic or presynthetic (G1), (2) deoxyribonucleic acid synthesis (S), (3) postsynthetic or premitotic (G2), and (4) mitotic (M) (Fig. 2–6).[169,170] During the S-phase, the cell DNA is doubled in preparation for mitosis.

In untreated glioblastoma, necrosis is spontaneous cell death. Tumor cell death can be passive, with the morphologic changes of cell membrane disruption and pyknosis, or active, through apoptosis. Apoptosis, or "programmed" cell death, is characterized morphologically by chromatin condensation with an intact cell membrane and cytoplasmic granules.[167] In apoptosis, the cell actively provides substances for the process to proceed. Apoptosis can be stimulated by growth factors, by substances such as endonuclease, or by the action of oncogenes (*bcl*-2). It may be inhibited by other oncogenes (c-*myc*) or viral transfection.[167] Fas ligand is a transmembrane glycoprotein in the tumor necrosis factor family that, when placed in the supernatant of T98G glioma cells, produces apoptosis.[171] E2F-1 is a gene product transcription factor that is regulated by its interaction with the retinoblastoma protein. It is involved in promoting apoptosis and suppressing proliferation. Mice deficient in E2F-1 develop tumors in many organs. In glioma cell lines, transfection of E2F-1 with a replication deficient adenoviral vector produced a massive entry of glioma cells into the S phase and then triggered apoptosis. The induction of apoptosis was independent of p53, p16, or Rb gene status.[172]

Radiation-induced neuronal damage may be mediated by apoptotic cell death. Following radiation of cultured postmitotic fetal rodent neurons and astrocytes, radiation-induced apoptotic changes are seen only in the neurons. In the future, radiation neuronal damage may be treated with antisense oligonucleotides or apoptosis oncogenes.[173] Although the molecular basis of apoptosis is a "work in

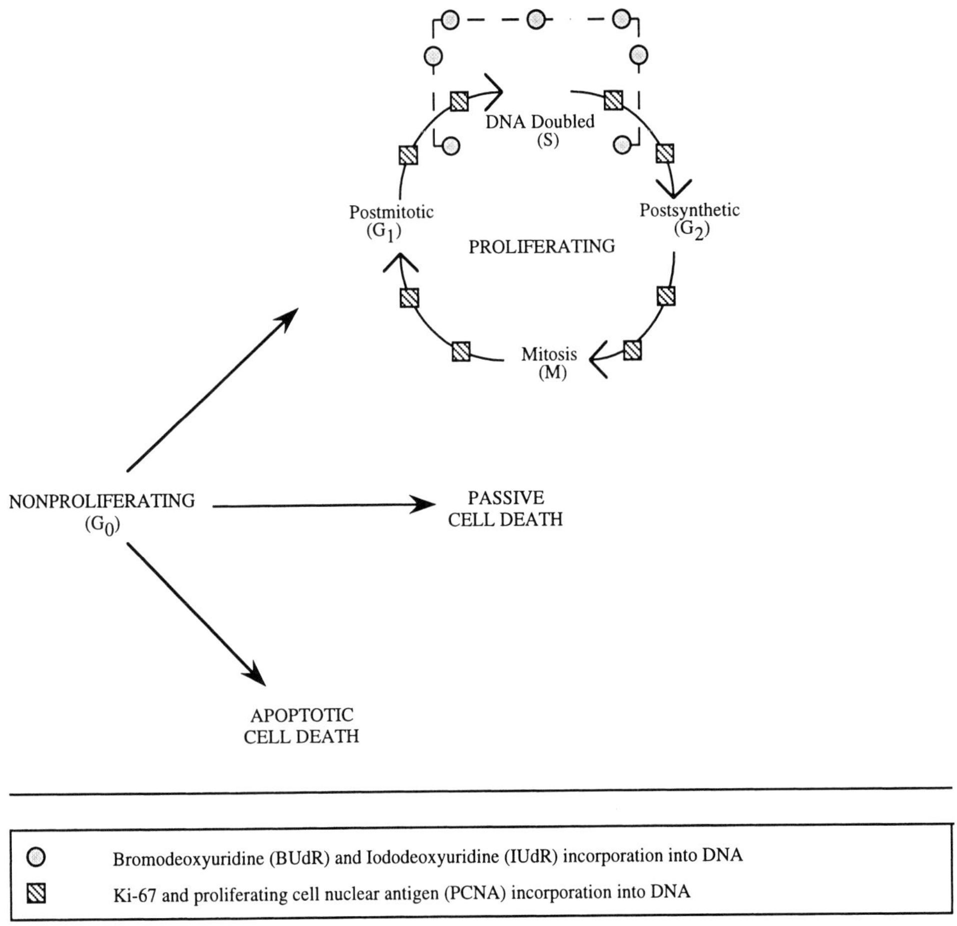

Figure 2–6. In the proliferating phase of the cell cycle, thymidline analogs (BUdR, IUdR) and antigens (Ki-67, PCNA) are labeled by specific monoclonal antibodies. Nonproliferating tumor cells and the pathways they can follow.

progress," the proliferative phase of the glioma cell cycle is better understood.

Proliferative Indices

THYMIDINE

In the 1970s, Hoshino and colleagues[170] infused ^{3}H-thymidine, a pyrimidine nucleotide necessary for DNA synthesis, into patients intravenously immediately prior to tumor resection. After tumor removal, histologic sections were fixed for autoradiography and counted for incorporation of ^{3}H-thymidine. The percentage of cells incorporating the tritiated nucleoside is the growth fraction. A second portion of tumor was minced and then immediately exposed to ^{14}C-thymidine for a second time period.[170] This tissue was partly labeled with both ^{3}H-thymidine and ^{14}C-thymidine, with a percentage of cells having a single label of either ^{3}H-thymidine or ^{14}C-thymidine. Assuming a constant rate of cell division and no cell death, the single-labeled cells are the cells entering or leaving S-phase. A tumor's S-phase duration can be calculated if the interval between isotope administration is known. A doubling, or turnover, time is obtained by dividing the growth fraction by the S-phase duration (see Fig. 2–6). In glioblastoma, the labeling varied from near 0% in necrotic areas to 20% in the most actively growing regions of the tumor. The tumor range for five glioblastomas was 4.4% to 11.4%; for anaplastic astrocytoma, it was 2.3% to 8.2%; and for astrocytoma, it was less than 1%. The duration of DNA synthesis was 7 to 10 hours regardless of tumor grade, with tumor doubling time of 58 to 203 hours in glioblastoma, 154 to 316 hours in anaplastic astrocytoma, and 1154 hours in the one astrocytoma studied.

BROMODEOXYURIDINE

In the 1980s, growth fraction estimation techniques evolved with the IV infusion of the thymidine analog bromodeoxyuridine (BUdR) prior to surgery. Surgical tumor specimens were stained with a monoclonal antibody to BUdR in paraffin-fixed sections, with the percentage of BudR-labeled cells called the *growth fraction*. This technique ended the need for infusion of radioactive tracers (thymidine) and time-consuming autoradiography.[15,174–176] Growth fractions (or labeling index) ranged from 9.1% to 46.5% in malignant glioma to 2.0% to 6.7% in low-grade glioma.[167] Medulloblastoma had an average labeling index of 14%; meningioma, 3.5%; ependymoma, 4.5%; pituitary tumor, 1.4%; and metastatic tumor, 13.7%.[176] These values were similar to tritiated thymidine determinations. There was also significant regional heterogeneity in BUdR labeling in different regions of an individual tumor.

Hoshino and coworkers[174,176] believed that the labeling index correlated with the histology in predicting biologic behavior. In two separate studies, Bookwalter[175] and Ritter[177] and their associates found the BudR-labeling index not predictive of survival, with the latter study examining specimens from both initial surgery and reoperation. Ritter and colleagues[177] cited the following reasons for a lack of correlation of BudR-labeling index with survival:(1) following surgery, the ratio of proliferating to nonproliferating cells may change; (2) cell death may be decreased by decreasing tumor burden; (3) tumor bulk removal may allow better access to nutrients; or (4) alternatively, a greater number of slowly proliferating cells may be present. An in vitro technique for determination of the BUdR- labeling index on postsurgical specimens was developed, and its correlation with survival was reported.[178,179]

Double-labeling techniques were developed to determine tumor doubling time measurements. BUdR and iododeoxyuridine (IUdR) are infused at 2- to 3-h intervals prior to tumor resection.[180] After tumor resection, pathological specimens are stained with two antibodies, one that recognizes BUdR alone and a second that recognizes both BUdR and IUdR.[180,181] In glioblastoma, the range of S-phase duration was 6 to 10 hours, with doubling time ranging from 2 days to more than 1 month. Actual in vivo tumor doubling will be slower because of cell loss.[181] Although most studies suggest BUdR is safe for IV clinical use, there is evidence in some experimental systems that it may be a carcinogen or mutagen. The in vitro BUdR-labeling technique does not have this risk.[178,179] A search for a better measure of proliferative index continues. It is necessary to find one that has a stronger correlation to biological outcome.[182]

KI-67

Ki-67 is a reactive antigen expressed on proliferating glioma cells in all four phases of the cell cycle; G1, S, G2, and M. The monoclonal antibody to Ki-67 can be used in vitro for staining frozen sections or fresh tissue. Ki-67 labeling has been correlated with survival, with a Ki-67—labeling index of greater than 3% correlating with a shorter survival.[183] Ki-67 monoclonal antibody labeling generally parallels BUdR labeling but tends to be somewhat higher because the antigen is expressed in all parts of the proliferating cell cycle.[184] A newer method uses fixed microwave-heated paraffin-embedded tumor sections. The heating activates an epitope of the Ki-67 antigen, recognized by the MIB-1 monoclonal antibody. MIB-1 labeling correlates with the BUdR labeling index.[185] The immunostaining technique is superior in quality to Ki-67 labeling and is quantitatively 2.5 times greater than the BUdR-labeling index.[185]

PROLIFERATIVE CELL NUCLEAR ANTIGEN

Proliferating cell nuclear antigen (PCNA), or cyclin, is a nuclear protein expressed in all phases of the proliferating cell cycle.[186] Antibodies to PCNA have been successfully used to measure a proliferative index.[186,187] The labeling of glioblastoma was greater than that of anaplastic astrocytoma, which was greater than that of astrocytoma.[186] The labeling index was greater in CT regions of contrast enhancement than in hypodense CT regions.[187] In addition, PCNA labeling was greater at the solid tumor–parenchyma interface than in the solid tumor or more distally infiltrated brain.

NUCLEOLAR ORGANIZER REGIONS

Nucleolar organizer regions are portions of DNA that code for ribosomal RNA with the transcription enzyme RNA polymerase.[188,189] These regions, located on the short arms of chromosomes 13, 14, 15, 21, and 22, are stained with a silver colloid–staining technique.[189,190] Nucleolar organizer regions are greater in LGA than in gliosis[191] and increase in number, with increasing anaplasia from astrocytoma to glioblastoma multiforme.[189,190] Malignant neoplasms, including metastatic brain tumor, meningeal sarcoma, and recurrent meningioma, have increased nucleolar organizer regions compared with those in pituitary adenoma, ependymoma, and LGA.[191]

All proliferative index measures report increased labeling with increasing anaplasia, both within and across tumor types. The ability of these measures to predict biologic outcome and be a useful additive prognostic tool to histopathology is uncertain. The decision will determine whether proliferative index measures are used clinically or remain for research investigation only.

FLOW CYTOMETRY

Flow cytometry has been used to show abnormalities in glial tumor cellular DNA content with diploid, aneuploid, uniploid, and multiploid populations. Ploidy differences have been found between tumors and within different regions of the same tumor.[192,193] Whether flow cytometry is a reliable prognostic indicator has been in dispute. Independent recent studies have found the percentage of S-phase DNA a negative predictor of survival.[194] A large aneuploid population has been found to be a positive predictor of outcome in anaplastic astrocytoma.[195] And finally, a hypertriploid DNA histogram has been found to be a positive predictor of survival.[196] Other investigations [192,193] found no correlation between outcome and DNA distribution. When flow cytometry study results were positive,[194–196] different outcome measures were predictive in different studies, which shows that flow cytometry may not be a reliable prognostic indicator.

DRUG SENSITIVITY AND RESISTANCE

Sensitivity

A goal of neuro-oncologists is to predict malignant brain tumor response to chemotherapeutic agents, with the hope of selecting the optimal treatment for each patient. Drug sensitivity assays have been developed in vitro in cell culture to test astrocytic tumor response to chemotherapeutic agents. Various tissue culture techniques are used to determine tumor drug sensitivity; two of the most common are the colony-forming assay and the microcytotoxicity assay.[197] The colony-forming assay involves the separation of a tumor into a single cell suspension, which is treated with a drug. The cells are then plated into a growth medium as a monolayer. Two to 4 weeks later, the number and size of colonies are compared with control cells, and sensitivity is determined by qualitative criteria. In the microcytotoxicity assay, cells are treated with drug plated in wells and then counted at a set time interval and compared with control specimens.

In 1981, Kornblith and colleagues,[198] using a microcytotoxicity assay, showed that six of nine patients who had a positive in vitro response to BCNU had a decrease in tumor size after treatment with BCNU. Five patients with a negative response to BCNU had tumor progression when treated with BCNU. In general, the assays predicted a positive clinical response in 50% to 70% of patients and drug resistance in 100% of patients.[197]

These assays have not received wide acceptance because of their poor ability to predict a positive response. A single cell assay cannot duplicate the complex environment of a tumor in vivo. In vivo, the tumor cell has numerous cell-cell interactions that present the cell with nutrients, growth factors, cytokines, and ECM proteins. In situ, the tumor may be heterogeneous, and certain cell types may be in a nonproliferating pool. After treatment, a tumor cell may undergo a chromosomal change, or a gene may be upregulated to return a cell to the proliferating pool or to promote migration. In conclusion, in vitro assays are less effective in predicting drug sensitivity than drug resistance.

Resistance

Drug resistance may be an intrinsic property of tumor cells, or it can be acquired after treatment.[199] Drug resistance can be divided into factors extrinsic or intrinsic to the cell (Table 2–6). Extrinsic factors include drug pharmacokinetics and delivery of adequate drug concentrations through the BBB. Drug metabolism governs the conversion of drug into its active or inactive form. The more rapidly a drug or its metabolite is cleared from the body, the shorter its duration of action. The delivery of adequate drug concentrations to the brain depends on the protein binding of drug in the vascular compartment, the lipid solubility of the drug, the surface area of the tumor capillaries, and the state of the BBB.[31] Intrinsic factors include the BTB and the ability of tumor to transport and retain drug; the change in drug concentration in tissue produced by the presence of or activation of metabolic processes; and the ability of tumor to repair drug-induced DNA damage.[199] Drug resistance mechanisms are discussed in this chapter for astrocytoma and PNET and for the most common chemotherapy drugs (i.e., nitrosoureas, platinum compounds, and cyclophosphamide), as well as drugs in which resistance is mediated by the multidrug-resistance gene (MDR1), such as vincristine, doxorubicin, and etoposide. More than one mechanism of resistance may be operational in a particular tumor. Mechanisms of drug resistance may vary in tumors of different histology or among different tumors of identical histology.

Table 2–6. **Factors in Drug Resistance**

Extrinsic factors
Drug pharmacokinetics
Drug delivery to tumor
Intrinsic factors
Tumor transport and retention of drug
Tumor drug metabolism
Tumor DNA damage repair

Nitrosoureas (i.e., ACNU, BCNU, and CCNU) and procarbazine are the most active single agents for treatment of malignant astrocytoma. However, less than 50% of patients with malignant astrocytoma have a useful clinical response to BCNU or procarbazine. Nitrosourea and procarbazine cytotoxicity are mediated by DNA alkylation at the O^6 position of guanine, followed by crosslink formation between DNA strands, or between DNA and protein. Resistance is mediated by the tumors' quantity of the enzyme O^6-methylguanine-DNA methyl transferase (MGMT). MGMT removes drug alkyl groups from the O6 position on DNA.[199–203] Schold and coworkers[200] found that procarbazine-treated brain tumor cells lines with MGMT levels higher than 100 had growth delays of less than 20 days; those with undetectable MGMT levels had growth delays of more than 30 days. Similar results are obtained with nitrosoureas.[201–203] MGMT is also present in oligodendroglioma, ependymoma, and medulloblastoma.[204,205] MGMT levels in normal brain and tumor are inversely correlated with age.[205] This supports the clinical observation of a shorter time to progression and shorter survival for nitrosourea-treated patients age 60 years and older than for those younger than age 60 years.[206]

Streptozotocin, methylnitrosourea, O^6-methylguanine, and O^6-benzylguanine are all used in tissue culture to deplete tumor MGMT before chloroethylnitrosourea exposure, with increase in cytotoxicity.[207–210] Early phase I and II clinical trials with O^6-benzylguanine are in progress.

Reduced glutathione (GSH) is important in the protection of cells from free radical damage and from radiation- and nitrosourea-induced cytoxicity. High levels of glioma GSH cause decreased BCNU crosslinking and decreased nitrosourea cytotoxicity.[211] Glioblastoma has lower levels of GSH than do anaplastic astrocytoma and astrocytoma. GSH levels were greater in normal brain and meningiomas than in astrocytomas.[212] Radiosensitive tumors such as myeloma and small cell lung cancer had low levels of GSH. In addition, glutathione-S-transferase- (GST-π), an enzyme that catalyzes the conjugation of glutathione to electrophilic species, was increased with increasing grade of glial anaplasia.[199,211,213] Nontoxic substrates for GST-π and buthionine sulfoximine, a glutathione depletor, are being evaluated for their ability to potentiate nitrosourea-induced cytotoxicity.[199] Buthionine sulfoximine acts by inhibiting an enzyme in the synthesis of glutathione. In rare glioma cell lines, multidrug resistance (see following) has been found without amplification of the MDR1 gene.[214]

PNET drug resistance was examined using the medulloblastoma cell line (DAOY). Cell lines were made resistant to actinomycin D through exposure to increasing concentrations of drug. The inhibitory concentration of actinomycin D was 10 times greater in the resistant line, and the *MDR1* gene was expressed in the resistant and not the parental line.[215] Fifteen de novo and recurrent medulloblastoma cell lines were examined for *MDR1* gene amplification, and no amplification was found. Six of 12 patients had MDR message on polymerase chain reaction (PCR) and Northern blotting, and two of 15 patients had detectable P-glycoprotein on Western blotting.[216] Resistance to actinomycin D is mediated by the MDR1 gene and its protein product, P-glycoprotein. P-glycoprotein is adenosine triphosphate (ATP) energy–dependent and provides drug efflux from the cell.[198,216] The degree of MDR resistance is proportional to the amount of P-glycoprotein present.[216]

Platinum compounds develop drug resistance by three primary mechanisms: decreased intracellular drug uptake and accumulation, increased inactivation by the protein metallothionen, and increased DNA repair.[199] Cyclophosphamide, an alkylating agent, is an inactive prodrug that undergoes activation in the liver. It has activity in recurrent high-grade brain tumors. Resistance to cyclophosphamide is at least partly due to increased inactivation by elevated concentrations of aldehyde dehydrogenase. Other mechanisms include increased levels of GSH and GST.[199] Resistance to vincristine, etoposide, and doxorubicin is mediated by the *MDR1* gene and involves P-glycoprotein.[199,217] New therapeutic possibilities to treat drug resistance include gene transfection of both alkyltransferases and antisense oligodeoxynucleotides to the *MDR1* gene.

CHAPTER SUMMARY

Mature astrocytes can develop from an O2A progenitor cell or a T1A astrocyte. The O2A progenitor cell is bipotential and may also differentiate into an oligodendroglial cell. Glial differentiation involves the coordinated sequential activation of multiple genes, with subsequent deactivation. Glial dedifferentiation occurs when antisense DNA, complementary to glial fibrillary acidic protein, is transfected into cultured astrocytoma cells; they lose their glial processes and become epithelioid. Glial oncogenesis probably results from a series of sequential chromosomal changes. These chromosomal changes lead to the inactivation of tumor-suppressor genes and the amplification of proto-oncogenes and may lead to the uncontrolled growth of malignancy. The growth of tumors requires the maintenance, growth, and proliferation of capillaries. Angiogenic growth factors are secreted from glioma cells. They stimulate glioma cells through autocrine mechanisms and endothelial cells through paracrine mechanisms.

Growth factors, peptides involved in the development, proliferation, and differentiation of tissues, are controlled by tumor-suppressor genes and proto-oncogenes. Growth factors themselves may also control the activity of tumor-suppressor genes or proto-oncogenes. Malignant tumor cells often lose their requirement for exogenously produced growth factors and stimulate themselves through endogenously produced growth factors. Cytokines, such as TNF-α, interleukins, and interferons, control a wide variety of leukocyte functions and may stimulate other cytokines or growth factors to influence glioma cell growth.

Malignant glial tumor cells invade the brain by infiltrating the ECM, which is composed of glial and vascular basement membrane and brain parenchyma. The glial cells express adhesion molecules and proteases on their surface. The adhesion molecules bind to ECM proteins, such as hyaluronic acid or fibronectin or their transmembrane protein receptors. The transmembrane receptor proteins work predominantly through second messenger systems. Proteases degrade the ECM. The interaction between the glioma cell and the ECM plays an important role in tumor invasion.

Brain tumor growth is a balance between cell proliferation and cell death. A brain tumor cell can rest, proliferate, differentiate, or die. The proliferating portion of the cell cycle is divided into four phases: G1, S, G2, and M. Labeling techniques have been developed to measure S-phase growth fraction, S-phase duration, and tumor-doubling time. Sequential chromosomal changes may lead to abrogation of normal cell cycle checkpoints, such as G1/S, that produce uncontrolled growth.

Astrocytomas may have intrinsic resistance to chemotherapeutic agents, or the resistance may be acquired after treatment. Drug resistance can be caused by factors that are intrinsic or extrinsic to the cell. Intrinsic factors are the ability of the tumor to retain drug, to metabolize drug, and to repair DNA damage. Extrinsic factors include the BBB and drug pharmacokinetics.

REFERENCES

1. Linskey, ME, Gilbert, MR: Glial differentiation: a review with implications for new directions in neuro-oncology. Neurosurgery 36:1–21, 1995.
2. Plate, KH, Breier, G, Risau, W: Molecular mechanisms of developmental and tumor angiogenesis. Brain Pathol 4:207–218, 1994.
3. Reese, TS, Karnovsky, MJ: Fine structural localization of a blood-brain barrier to exogenous peroxidase. J Cell Biol 34:207–217, 1967.
4. Matsukado, K, Inamura, T, Nakano, S, Black, KL: Enhanced tumor uptake of carboplatin and survival in glioma-bearing rats by intracarotid infusion of bradykinin analog, RMP-7. J Neurooncol 28:50, 1996.
5. Bigner, SH, Mark, J, Bullard, DE, et al: Chromosomal evolution in malignant human gliomas starts with specific and usually numerical deviations. Cancer Genet Cytogenet 22:121–135, 1986.
6. Shapiro, JR: Biology of gliomas: Heterogeneity, oncogenes and growth factors. Semin Oncol 13: 4–15,1986.
7. Bigner, SS, Mark, J, and Bigner, DD: Cytogenetics of human brain tumors. Cancer Genet Cytogenet 47:141–154, 1990.
8. Collins, VP, and James, CD: Molecular genetics of primary intracranial tumors. Curr Opin Oncol 2:666–672, 1990.
9. James, CD, and Collins, VP: Molecular genetic characterization of CNS tumor oncogenesis. Adv Cancer Res 58:121–142, 1992.
10. James, CD, Ekstrand, AJ, and He, J: Gene alterations and disruption of cell cycle regulation in glial tumors. J Neurooncol 28:57, 1996.
11. Gupta, N, Vij, R, Haas-Kogan, DA, et al: Cytogenetic damage and the radiation-induced p53-dependent G1 checkpoint. J Neurooncol 28:52, 1996.
12. Westphal, M, and Herrmann, HD: Growth factor biology and oncogene activation in human gliomas and their implications for specific therapeutic concepts. Neurosurgery 25:681–694, 1989.
13. Eppenberger, U, and Mueller, H: Growth factors and their ligands. J Neurooncol 22:249–254, 1994.
14. Rutka, JT: Effects of extracellular matrix proteins on the growth and differentiation of an

anaplastic glioma cell line. Can J Neurol Sci 13: 301–306, 1986.
15. Hoshino, T: Cell kinetics of glial tumors. Rev Neurol (Paris) 148:396–401, 1992.
16. Harding, AE: Clinical and molecular genetics in neurosurgery. Adv Tech Stand Neurosurg 20: 81–104, 1993.
17. Rutka, JT, Hubbard, SL, Fukuyama, K, et al: Effects of antisense glial fibrillary acidic protein complementary DNA on the growth, invasion, and adhesion of human astrocytoma cells. Cancer Res 54:3267–3272, 1994.
18. Van Meir, EG, Polverini, PJ, Chazin, VR, et al: Release of an inhibitor of angiogenesis upon induction of wild type p53 expression in glioblastoma cells. Nature Genet 8:171–176, 1994.
19. Tsai, J-C, Goldman, CK, and Gillespie, GY: Vascular endotheial growth factor in human glioma cell lines: Induced secretion by EGF, PDGF-BB, and bFGF. J Neurosurg 82:864–873, 1995.
20. Folkman, J, and Klagsburn, M: Angiogenic factors. Science 235:442–447, 1987.
21. Beitz, JG, Kim, IS, Calabresi, P, and Frackelton, AR Jr: Human microvascular endothelial cells express receptors for platelet-derived growth factor. Proc Natl Acad Sci USA 88: 2021–2025, 1991.
22. Hermanson, M, Funa, K, Hartman, M, et al: Platelet-derived growth factor and it receptors in human glioma tissue: Expression of messenger RNA and protein suggests the presence of autocrine and paracrine loops. Cancer Res 52: 3213–3219, 1992.
23. Plate, KH, Breier, G, Weich, HA, et al: Vascular endothelial growth factor and glioma angiogenesis: Coordinate induction of VEGF receptors, distribution of VEGF protein and possible in vivo regulatory mechanisms. Int J Cancer 59: 520–529, 1994.
24. Weindel, K, Moringlane, JR, Marmé, D, and Weich, HA: Detection and quantification of vascular endothelial growth factor/vascular permeability factor in brain tumor tissue and cyst fluid: The key to angiogenesis? Neurosurgery 35:439–448, 1994.
25. Weingart, J, Tamargo, R, and Brem, H: Minocycline, an angiogenesis inhibitor, inhibits brain tumor growth. Proc Annu Meet Am Assoc Cancer Res 33:A450, 1992.
26. Takamiya, Y, Friedlander, RM, Brem, H, et al: Inhibition of angiogensis and growth of human nerve-sheath tumors by AGM-1470. J Neurosurg 78:470–476, 1993.
27. Yazaki, T, Takamiya, Y, Costello, PC, et al: Inhibition of angiogenesis and growth of human non-malignant and malignant meningiomas by TNP-470. J Neurooncol 23:23–29, 1995.
28. Ke, LD, Chen, XS, Steck, PA, and Yung, WKA: Molecular modulation of vascular endothelial growth factor (VEGF) expression in glioma cells by a ribozyme. J Neurooncol 28:62, 1996.
29. Schlageter, K, Vick, N, and Groothuis, D: bFGF and VEGF antisense oligonucleotide therapy of malignant gliomas. J Neurooncol 35 (Suppl 1): S40, 1997.
30. Vick, N, Khandekar, JD, and Bigner, DD: Chemotherapy of brain tumors. The "blood-brain barrier" is not a factor. Arch Neurol 34: 523–526, 1977.
31. Stewart, PA, Hayakawa, K, Farrell, CL, and Del Maestro, RF: Quantitative study of microvessel ultrastructure in human peritumoral brain tissue. Evidence for a blood-brain barrier defect. J Neurosurg 67:697–705, 1987.
32. Blasberg, RG, and Groothuis, DR: Chemotherapy of brain tumors: physiological and pharmacokinetic considerations. Semin Oncol 13:70–82, 1986.
33. Groothuis,, DR, Fischer JM, Vick, NA, and Bigner, DD: Comparative permeability of different glioma models to horseradish peroxidase. Cancer Treat Rep 65(Suppl 2):13–18, 1981.
34. Groothius, DR, Fischer, JM, Pasternak, JF, et al: Regional measurements of blood-to-tissue transport in experimental RG-2 rat gliomas. Cancer Res 43:3368–3373, 1983.
35. Groothuis, DR, and Blasberg, RG: Rational brain tumor chemotherapy: The interaction of drug and tumor. Neurol Clin 3:801–816, 1985.
36. Grabb, PA, and Gilbert, MR: Neoplastic and pharmacological influence on the permeability of an in vitro blood-brain barrier. J Neurosurg 82:1053–1058, 1995.
37. Shapiro, WR, Hiesiger, EM, Cooney, GA, et al: Temporal effects of dexamethasone on blood-to-brain and blood-to-tumor transport of 14C-alpha-aminoisobutyric acid in rat C6 glioma. J Neurooncol 8:197–204, 1990.
38. Bruce, JN, Criscuolo, GR, Merrill, MJ, et al: Vascular permeability induced by protein product of malignant brain tumors: Inhibition by dexamethasone. J Neurosurg 67:880–884, 1987.
39. Harik, SI, and Roessmann, U: The erythrocyte-type glucose transporter in blood vessels of primary and metastatic brain tumors. Ann Neurol 29:487–491, 1991.
40. Guerin, A, Wolff, JEA, Laterra, J, et al: Vascular differentiation and glucose transporter expression in rat gliomas: Effects of steroids. Ann Neurol 31:481–487, 1992.
41. Nishioka, T, Oda Y, Seino, Y, et al: Distribution of the glucose transporters in human brain tumors. Cancer Res 52:3972–3979, 1992.
42. Remler, MP, Marcussen, WH, and Tiller-Borsich, J: The late effects of radiation on the blood brain barrier. Int J Radiat Oncol Biol Phys 12:1965–1969, 1986.
43. Panther, LA, Baumbach, GL, Bigner, DD, et al: Vasoactive drugs produce selective changes in flow to experimental brain tumors. Ann Neurol 18:712–715, 1985.
44. Neuwelt, EA, Frenkel, EP, Rapoport, S, and Barnett, P: Effect of osmotic blood-brain barrier disruption on methotrexate pharmacokinetics in the dog. Neurosurgery 7:36–43, 1980.
45. Neuwelt, EA, Frenkel, EP, Diehl, J, et al: Reversible osmotic blood-brain barrier disruption in humans: Implications for the chemotherapy of malignant brain tumors. Neurosurgery 7:44–52, 1980.

46. Neuwelt, EA, Maravilla, KR, Frenkel,EP, et al: Osmotic blood-brain barrier disruption. Computerized tomographic monitoring of chemotherapeutic agent delivery. J Clin Invest 64: 684–688, 1979.
47. Neuwelt, EA, and Rapoport, SI: Modification of the blood-brain barrier in the chemotherapy of malignant brain tumors. Fed Proc 43:214–219, 1984.
48. Hiesiger, EM, Voorhies, RM, Basler, GA, et al: Opening the blood-brain and blood-tumor barriers in experimental rat brain tumors: The effect of intracarotid hyperosmolar mannitol on capillary permeability and blood flow. Ann Neurol 19:50–59, 1986.
49. Neuwelt, EA, Goldman, DL, Dahlborg, SA, et al: Primary CNS lymphoma treated with osmotic blood-brain disruption: Prolonged survival and preservation of cognitive function. J Clin Oncol 9:1580–1590, 1991.
50. Inamura, T, Nomura, T, Bartus, RT, Black, KL: Intracarotid infusion of RMP-7, a bradykinin analog: a method for selective drug delivery to brain tumors. J Neurosurg 81:752–758, 1994.
51. Korf, B: Molecular medicine: Molecular diagnosis. (first of two parts). N Engl J Med 332(18): 1218–1220, 1995.
52. Korf, B: Molecular medicine: Molecular diagnosis. (second of two parts). N Engl J Med 332–22):1499–1502, 1995.
53. Kim, DH, Mohapatr,a G, Bollen, A, et al: Chromosomal abnormalities in glioblastoma multiforme tumors and glioma cell lines detected by comparative genomic hybridization. Int J Cancer 60:812–819, 1995.
54. Mulligan, LM, and Mole, SE: Strategies for isolating genes in hereditary and sporadic tumors. In Levine AJ, Schmidek HH (eds): Molecular Genetics of Nervous System Tumors. Wiley-Liss Inc, New York, 1993, pp 195–208.
55. James, CD, Mikkelsen, T, Cavenee, WK, and Collins, VP: Molecular genetic aspects of glial tumour evolution. Cancer Surveys 9(4):631–644, 1990.
56. James, CD, Carlbom, E, Dumanski ,JP, et al: Clonal genomic alterations in glioma malignancy stages. Cancer Res 48:5546–5551, 1988.
57. Fults, D, Brockmeyer, D, Tullous, MW, et al: p53 mutation and loss of heterozygosity on chromosomes 17 and 10 during human astrocytoma progression. Cancer Res 52:674–679, 1992.
58. Westphal, M, Hänsel, M, Hamel, W, et al: Karyotype analyses of 20 human glioma cell lines. Acta Neurochir (Wien) 126:17–26, 1994.
59. von Deimling, A, Bender, B, Jahnke, R, et al: Loci associated with malignant progression in astrocytomas: A candidate on chromosome 19q. Cancer Res 54:1397–1401, 1994.
60. Lang, FF, Miller, DC, Koslow, M, and Newcomb, EW: Pathways leading to glioblastoma multiforme: A molecular analysis of genetic alterations in 65 astrocytic tumors. J Neurosurg 81:427–436, 1994.
61. Henson, JW, Schnitker, BL, Correa, KM, et al: The retinoblastoma gene is involved in malignant progression of astrocytomas. Ann Neurol 36:714–721, 1994.
62. Schlegel, U: Molekulare Entstehungsmechanismen menschlicher gliome (Molecular genetics of human gliomas). Nervenarzt 64:485–493, 1993.
63. Steck, PA, and Saya, H: Pathways of oncogenesis in primary brain tumors. Curr Opin Oncol 3:476–484, 1991.
64. Liang, BC, Ross, DA, Greenberg ,HS, et al: Evidence of allelic imbalance of chromosome 6 in human astrocytomas. Neurology 44:533–536, 1994.
65. Nishikawa, R, Furnari, FB, Lin, H, et al: Loss of P16^{INK4} expression is frequent in high grade gliomas. Cancer Res 55:1941–1945, 1995.
66. Arap, W, Nishikawa, R, Furnari ,FB, et al: Replacement of the p16/CDKN2 gene suppresses human glioma cell growth. Cancer Res 55: 1351–1354, 1995.
67. Ichimura, K, Schmidt, EE, Yamaguchi, N, et al: A common region of homozygous deletion in malignant human gliomas lies between the *IFN/* gene cluster and the *D9S171* locus. Cancer Res 54:3127–3130, 1994.
68. Louis, DN: Molecular genetic classification of glioblastoma: An update. J Neurooncol 35(Suppl 1):S53, 1997.
69. Dalrymple, SJ, Herath, JF, Ritland ,SR, et al: Use of fluorescence *in situ* hybridization to detect loss of chromosome 10 in astrocytomas. J Neurosurg 83:316–323, 1995.
70. Leenstra, S, Bijlsma, EK, Troost, D, et al: Allele loss on chromosomes 10 and 17p and epidermal growth factor receptor gene amplification in human malignant astrocytoma related to prognosis. Br J Cancer 70:684, 1994.
71. Ichimura, K, Schmidt, EE, and Collins ,VP: Deletion mapping of chromosome 10 in astrocytic gliomas. J Neurooncol 35(Suppl 1):S21, 1997.
72. Steck, PA, Pershouse, MA, Jasser, SA, et al: Identification of a candidate tumour suppressor gene, MMAC1, at chromosome 10q23.3 that is mutated in multiple advanced cancers. Nature Genetics 15(4):356–362, 1997.
72a. Li, J, Yen, C, Liaw, D, et al: PTEN, a putative protein tyrosine phosphatase gene mutated in human brain, breast, and prostate cancer. Science 275:1943–1947, 1997.
72b. Bostrom, J, Cobbers, JM, Wolter, M, et al: Mutation of the PTEN (MMAC1) tumor suppressor gene in a subset of glioblastomas but not in meningiomas with loss of chromosome 10q. Cancer Res 58:29–33, 1998.
73. Yamazaki, H, Fukui, Y, Ueyama, Y, et al: Amplification of the structurally and functionally altered epidermal growth factor receptor gene (c-*erbB*) in human brain tumors. Molecular Cellular Biology 8(4):1816–1820, 1988.
74. Sang, U H, Kelley, PY, Hatton, JD, and Shew, JY: Proto-oncogene abnormalities and their relationship to tumorigenicity in some human glioblastomas. J Neurosurg 71:83–90, 1989.
75. Humphrey, PA, Wong, AJ, Vogelstein, B, et al: Amplification and expression of the epidermal

growth factor receptor gene in human glioma xenografts. Cancer Res 48:2231–2238, 1988.
76. Bigner, SH, Burger, PC, Wong, AJ, et al: Gene amplification in malignant human gliomas: Clinical and histopathologic aspects. J Neuropathol Exp Neurol 47:191–205, 1988.
77. Huritt, MR, Moossy, J, Donovan-Peluso, M, and Locker, J: Amplification of epidermal growth factor receptor gene in glomas: Histopathology and prognosis. J Neuropathol Exp Neurol 51: 84–90, 1992.
78. Fuller, GN, and Bigner, SH: Amplified cellular oncogenes in neoplasms of the human central nervous system. Mutation Research 276:299–306, 1992.
79. Olson, JJ, James, CD, Krisht, A, et al: Analysis of epidermal growth factor receptor gene amplification and alteration in stereotactic biopsies of brain tumors. Neurosurgery 36:740–748, 1995.
80. Watanabe, K, Tachibana, O, Sato, K, et al: Overexpression of the EGF receptor and p53 mutations are mutually exclusive in the evolution of primary and secondary glioblastomas. Brain Pathol 6:217–224, 1996.
81. Reifenberger, G, Liu, L, Ichimura, K, et al: Amplification and overexpression of the *MDM2* gene in a subset of human malignant gliomas without *p53* mutations. Cancer Res 53:2736–2739, 1993.
82. Scheck, AC, and Coons, SW: Expression of the tumor suppressor gene *DCC* in human gliomas. Cancer Res 53:5605–5609, 1993.
83. Rasheed, BKA, McLendon, RE, Herndon, JE, et al: Alterations of the TP53 gene in human gliomas. Cancer Res 54:1324–1330, 1994.
84. Collins, VP: Molecular basis of glial oncogenesis. J Neurooncol 28:53, 1996.
84a. Cairncross, JG, Ueki, K, Zlatescu, MC, et al: Specific genetic predictors of chemotherapeutic response and survival in patients with anaplastic oligodendrogliomas. J Natl Cancer Inst 90: 1473–1479, 1998.
85. Kazumoto, K, Tamura, M, Hoshino, H, and Yuasa, Y: Enhanced expression of the sis and c-myc oncogenes in human meningiomas. J Neurosurg 72:786–791, 1990.
86. Salomon, DS, Brandt, R, Ciardiello, F, and Normanno, N: Epidermal growth factor-related peptides and their receptors in human malignancies. Crit Rev Oncol Hematol 19:183–232, 1995.
87. Eppenberger, U, and Mueller, H: Growth factor receptors and their ligands. J Neurooncol 22: 249–254, 1994.
88. Hoi Sang, U, Espiritu, OD, Kelley, PY, et al: The role of the epidermal growth factor receptor in human gliomas: I. The control of cell growth. J Neurosurg 82:841–846, 1995.
89. Engebraaten, O, Bjerkvig, R, Pedersen ,P-H, and Laerum, OD: Effects of EGF, bFGF, NGF and PDGF(bb) on cell proliferative, migratory and invasive capacities of human brain-tumour biopsies in vitro. Int J Cancer 53:209–214, 1993.
90. Pedersen, P-H, Ness, GO, Engebraaten, O, et al: Heterogeneous response to the growth factors [EGF, PDGF (bb), TGF-, bFGF, IL-2] on glioma spheroid growth, migration and invasion. Int J Cancer 56:255–261, 1994.
91. Hoi Sang, U, Espiritu, OD, Kelley, PY, et al: The role of the epidermal growth factor receptor in human gliomas: II. The control of glial process extension and the expression of glial fibrillary acidic protein. J Neurosurg 82:847–857, 1995.
92. Collins, VP: Epidermal growth factor receptor gene and its transcripts in glioblastomas. Recent Results Cancer Res 135:17–24, 1994.
93. Takahashi, H, Herlyn, D, Atkinson, B, et al: Radioimmunodetection of human glioma xenografts by monoclonal antibody to epidermal growth factor rceptor. Cancer Res 47:3847–3850, 1987.
94. Epenetos, AA, Courtenay-Luck, N, Pickering, D, et al: Antibody guided irradiation of brain glioma by arterial infusion of radioactive monoclonal antibody against epidermal growh factor receptor and blood group A antigen. Br Med J 290:1463–1466, 1985.
95. Kalofonos, HP, Pawlikowska, TR, Hemingway, A, et al: Antibody guided diagnosis and therapy of brain gliomas using radiolabeled monoclonal antibodies against epidermal growth factor receptor and placental alkaline phosphatase. J Nucl Med 30:1636–1645, 1989.
96. Morrison, RS, Yamaguchi, F, Bruner, JM, et al: Fibroblast growth factor receptor gene expression and immunoreactivity are elevated in human glioblastoma multiforme. Cancer Res 54: 2794–2799, 1994.
97. Morrison, RS, Gross, JL, Herblin, WF, et al: Basic fibroblast growth factor-like acitvity and receptors are expressed in a human glioma cell line. Cancer Res 50:2524–2529, 1990.
98. Takahashi, JA, Suzui, H, Yasuda, Y, et al: Gene expression of fibroblast growth factor receptors in the tissues of human gliomas and meningiomas. Biochem Biophys Res Comm 177(1): 1–7, 1991.
99. Ueba, T, Takahashi, JA, Fukumoto, M, et al: Expression of fibroblast growth factor receptor-1 in human glioma and meningioma tissues. Neurosurgery 34:221–226, 1994.
100. Takahashi, JA, Fukumoto, M, Igarashi, K, et al: Correlation of basic fibroblast growth factor expression levels with the degree of malignancy and vascularity in human gliomas. J Neurosurg 76:792–798, 1992.
101. Gately, S, Tsanaclis, AMC, Takano, S, et al: Cells transfected with the basic fibroblast growth factor gene fused to a signal sequence are invasive in vitro and in situ in the brain. Neurosurgery 36:780–788, 1995.
102. Morrison, RS: Suppression of basic fibroblast growth factor expression by antisense oligodeoxynucleotides inhibits the growth of transformed human astrocytes. J Biol Chem 266:728–734, 1991.
103. Redekop, GJ, and Naus, CCG: Transfection with bFGF sense and antisense cDNA resulting in modification of malignant gioma growth. J Neurosurg 82:83–90, 1995.

104. Trojan, J, Blossey, BK, Johnson, TR, et al: Loss of tumorigenicity of rat glioblastoma directed by episome-based antisense cDNA transcription of insulin-like growth factor I. Proc Natl Acad Sci USA 89:4874–4878, 1992.
105. Hultberg, BM, Haselbacher, G, Nielsen FC, et al: Gene expression of insulin-like growth factor II in human intracranial meningioma. Cancer 72:3282–3286, 1993.
106. Merrill, MJ, and Edwards, NA: Insulin-like growth factor-I receptors in human glial tumors. J Clin Endocrinol Metab 71:199–209, 1990.
107. Sara, VR, Prisell, P, Sjögren, B, et al: Enhancement of insulin-like growth factor 2 receptors in glioblastoma. Cancer Letters 32:229–234, 1986.
108. Baker, DL, Reddy, UR, Pleasure, S, et al: Human central nervous system primitive neuroectodermal tumor expressing nerve growth factor receptors: CHP707m. Ann Neurol 28:136–145, 1990.
109. Spoerri, PE, Romanello, S, Petrelli, L, et al: Nerve growth factor (NGF) receptors in a central nervous system glial cell line: Upregulation by NGF and brain-derived neurotrophic factor. J Neurosci Res 33:82–90, 1992.
110. Mapstone, T, McMichael, M, and Goldthwait, D: Expression of platelet-derived growth factors, transforming growth factors, and the *ros* gene in a variety of primary human brain tumors. Neurosurgery 28:216–222, 1991.
111. Mapstone, TB: Expression of platelet-derived growth factor and transforming growth factor and their correlation with cellular morphology in glial tumors. J Neurosurg 75:447–451, 1991.
112. Mauro, A, Bulfone, A, Turco, E, and Schiffer, D: Coexpression of platelet-derived growth factor (PDGF) B chain and PDGF B-type receptor in human gliomas. Child Nerv Syst 7:432–436, 1991.
113. Nitta, T, and Sato, K: Specific inhibition of c-sis protein synthesis and cell proliferation with antisense oligodeoxynucleotides in human glioma cells. Neurosurgery 34:309–315, 1994.
114. Schrell, UMH, Gauer, S, Kiesewetter, F, et al: Inhibition of proliferation of human cerebral meningioma cells by suramin: effects on cell growth, cell cycle phases, extracellular growth factors, and PDGF-BB autocrine growth loop. J Neurosurg 82:600–607, 1995.
115. Westphal ,M, Ackermann, E, Hoppe, J, and Herrmann, H-D: Receptors for platelet derived growth factor in human glioma cell lines and influence of suramin on cell proliferation. J Neurooncol 11:207–213, 1991.
116. Rutka, JT, Rosenblum, ML, Stern, R, et al: Isolation and partial purification of growth factors with TGF-like activity from human malignant gliomas. J Neurosurg 71:875–883, 1989.
117. Linggood, RM, Hsu, DW, Efird, JT, and Pardo, FS: TGF expression in meningioma: Tumor progression and therapeutic response. J Neurooncol 26:45–51, 1995.
118. Schlegel, U, Moots, PL, Rosenblum, MK, et al: Expression of transforming growth factor alpha in human gliomas. Oncogene 5:1839–1842, 1990.
119. Maxwell, M, Galanopoulos, T, Neville-Golden, J, and Antoniades, HN: Effect of the expression of transforming growth factor-2 in primary human glioblastomas on immunosuppression and loss of immune surveillance. J Neurosurg 76: 799–804, 1992.
120. Yamada, N, Kato, M, Yamashita, H, et al: Enhanced expression of transforming growth factor- and its type-I and type-II receptors in human glioblastoma. Int J Cancer 62:386–392, 1995.
121. Merzak, A, McCrea, S, Koocheckpour, S, and Pilkington, GJ: Control of human glioma cell growth, migration and invasion *in vitro* by transforming growth factor . Br J Cancer 70:199–203, 1994.
122. Jachimaczak, P, Bogdahn, U, Schneider, J, et al: The effect of transforming growth factor-2-specific phosphorothioate-anti-sense oligodeoxynucleotides in reversing cellular immunosuppression in malignant glioma. J Neurosurg 78:944–951, 1993.
123. Kristt, DA, Reedy, E, and Yarden, Y: Receptor tyrosine kinase expression in astrocytic lesions: Similar features in gliosis and glioma. Neurosurgery 33:106–115, 1993.
124. Wong, ET, Yung, WKA, Fueyo, J, et al: Induction of apoptosis in glioma cells by a benzodiazepin-2-one. J Neurooncol 35(Suppl 1):S49, 1997.
125. Vertosick, FT Jr : The role of protein kinase C in the growth of human gliomas: implications for therapy. Cancer Journal 5:328–331, 1992.
126. Couldwell, WT, Antel, JP, and Yong, VW: Protein kinase C activity correlates with the growth rate of malignant gliomas: Part II. Effects of glioma mitogens and modulators of protein kinase C. Neurosurgery 31:717–724, 1992.
127. Benzil, DL, Finkelstein, SD, Epstein, MH, and Finch, PW: Expression pattern of -protein kinase C in human astrocytomas indicates a role in malignant progression. Cancer Res 52:2951–2956, 1992.
128. Couldwell, WT, Antel, JP, Apuzzo, MLJ, and Yong, VW: Inhibition of growth of established human glioma cell lines by modulators of the protein kinase-C system. J Neurosurg 73:594–600, 1990.
129. Pollack, IF, Randall, MS, Kristofik, MP, et al: Effect of tamoxifen on DNA synthesis and proliferation of human malignant glioma lines *in vitro*. Cancer Res 50:7134–7138, 1990.
130. Couldwell, WT, Weiss, MH, DeGiorgio, CM, et al: Clinical and radiographic response in a minority of patients with recurrent malignant gliomas treated with high-dose tamoxifen. Neurosurgery 32:485–490, 1993.
131. Khalid, H, Yasunaga, A, Kishikawa, M, and Shibata, S: Immunohistochemical expression of the estrogen receptor-related antigen –ER-D5) in human intracranial tumors. Cancer 75:2571–2578, 1995.
132. Blakenstein, MA, Koehorst, SGA, van der Kallen, CJH, et al: Oestrogen receptor inde-

pendent expression of progestin receptors in human meningioma - a review. J Steroid Biochem Molec Biol 53(1–6):361–365, 1995.

133. Grunberg, SM, Weiss, MH, Spitz, IM, et al: Treatment of unresectable meningiomas with the antiprogesterone agent mifepristone. J Neurosurg 74:861–866, 1991.

134. Zibera, C, Gibelli, N, Butti, G, et al: Proliferative effect of dexamethasone on a human glioblastoma cell line (HU 197) is mediated by glucocorticoid receptors. Anticancer Research 12:1571–1574, 1992.

135. Langeveld, CH, van Wass, MP, Stoof, JC, et al: Implication of glucocorticoid receptors in the stimulation of human glioma cell proliferation by dexamethasone. J Neurosci Res 31:524–531, 1992.

136. Magrassi, L, Bono, F, Milanesi, G, and Butti, G: Vitamin D receptor expression in human brain tumors. J Neurosurg Sci 36:27–30, 1992.

137. Kurihara, M, Ochi, A, Kawaguchi, T, et al: Localization and characterization of endothelin receptors in human gliomas: a growth factor? Neurosurgery 27:275–281, 1990.

138. Alho, H, Kolmer, M, Harjuntausta, T, and Helén P: Increased expression of diazepam binding inhibitor in human brain tumors. Cell Growth Differ 6:309–314, 1995.

139. Thomas, GE, Mamone, JY, Coscia, CJ, and Johnson, FE: Sigma and opioid receptors in human brain tumors. Proc Am Soc Clin Oncol 9:92, 1990.

140. Weitman, SD, Frazier, KM, and Kamen, BA: The folate receptor in central nervous system malignancies of childhood. J Neurooncol 21: 107–112, 1994.

141. Merlo, A, Juretic, A, Zuber, M, et al: Cytokine gene expression in pimary brain tumours, metastases and meningiomas suggests specific transcription patterns. Eur J Cancer 29A(15): 2118–2125, 1993.

142. Roessler, K, Suchanek, G, Breitschopf, H, et al: Detection of tumor necrosis factor- protein and messenger RNA in human glial brain tumors: comparison of immunohistochemistry with *in situ* hybridization using molecular probes. J Neurosurg 83:291–297, 1995.

143. Iwasaki, K, Rogers, LR, Barnett, GHet al: Effect of recombinant tumor necrosis factor- on three-dimensional growth, morphology, and invasiveness of human glioblastoma cells *in vitro*. J Neurosurg 78:952–958, 1993.

144. Yoshida, J, Wakabayashi, T, Mizuno, M, et al: Clinical effect of intra-arterial tumor necrosis factor- for malignant glioma. J Neurosurg 77:78–83, 1992.

145. Barnum, SR, Jones, JL, and Benveniste, EN: Interleukin-1 and tumor necrosis factor-mediated regulation of C3 gene expression in human astroglioma cells. GLIA 7:225–236, 1993.

146. Gauthier, T, Hamou, M-F, Monod, L, et al: Expression and release of interleukin-1 by human glioblastoma cells in vitro and in vivo. Acta Neurochir (Wien) 121:199–205, 1993.

147. Nitta, T, Allegretta, M, Okumura, K, et al: Neoplastic and reactive human astrocytes express interleukin-8 gene. Neurosurg Rev 15:203–207, 1992.

148. Nitta, T, Hishii, M, Sato, K, and Okumura, K: Selective expression of interleukin-10 gene within glioblastoma multiforme. Brain Research 649:122–128, 1994.

149. Tada, M, Diserens, A-C, Desbaillets, I, and de Tribolet, N: Analysis of cytokine receptor messenger RNA expression in human glioblastoma cells and normal astrocytes by reverse-transcription polymerase chain reaction. J Neurosurg 80:1063–1073, 1994.

150. Miyakoshi, J, Dobler, KD, Allalunis-Turner, J, et al: Absence of *IFNA* and *IFNB* genes from human malignant glioma cell lines and lack of correlation with cellular sensitivity to interferons. Cancer Res 50:278–283, 1990.

151. Couldwell, WT, de Tribolet, N, Antel, JP, et al: Adhesion molecules and malignant gliomas: implications for tumorigenesis. J Neurosurg 76: 782–791, 1992.

152. De Clerck, YA, Shimada, H, Gonzalez-Gomez, I, and Raffel, C: Tumoral invasion in the central nervous system. J Neurooncol 18:111–121, 1994.

153. Berens, ME, Rutka,, JT, and Rosenblum ML: Brain tumor epidemiology, growth, and invasion. Neurosurg Clin N Am 1(1):1–18, 1990.

154. Rosenman, SJ, Shrikant, P, Dubb, L, et al: Cytokine-induced expression of vascular cell adhesion molecule-1 (VCAM-1) by astrocytes and astrocytoma cell lines. J Immunology 154:1888–1899, 1995.

155. Nagasaka, S, Tanabe, KK, Bruner, JM, et al: Alternative RNA splicing of the hyaluronic acid receptor CD44 in the normal human brain and in brain tumors. J Neurosurg 82:858–863, 1995.

156. O'Neill, K, Martin, K, King, A, et al: CD44 immunocytochemistry of sequential biopsies taken across the margins of human gliomas. J Neurooncol 35(Suppl 1):S33, 1997.

157. Mohanam, S, Wang, SW, Rayford, A, et al: Expression of tissue inhibitors of metalloproteinases: negative regulators of human glioblastomas invasion *in vivo*. Clin Exp Metastasis 13:57–62, 1995.

158. Nakano, A, Tani, E, Miyazaki, K, et al: Matrix metalloproteinases and tissue inhibitors of metalloproteinases in human gliomas. J Neurosurg 83:298–307, 1995.

159. Nakagawa, T, Kubota, T, Kabuto, M, et al: Production of matrix metalloproteinases and tissue inhibitor of metalloproteinases-1 by human brain tumors. J Neurosurg 81:69–77, 1994.

160. Reith, A, and Rucklidge, GJ: Invasion of brain tissue by primary glioma: evidence for the involvement of urokinase-type plasminogen activator as an activator of type IV collagenase. Biochem Biophys Res Comm 186:348–354, 1992.

161. Yamamoto, M, Sawaya, R, Mohanam, S, et al: Expression and localization of urokinase-type plasminogen activator in human astrocytomas *in vivo*. Cancer Res 54:3656–3661, 1994.

162. Yamamoto, M, Sawaya, R, Mohanam, S, et al: Expression and localization of urokinase-type

plasminogen activator receptor in human gliomas. Cancer Res 54:5016–5020, 1994.
163. Gladson, CL, Pijuan-Thompson, V, Olman, MA, et al: Up-regulation of urokinase and urokinase receptor genes in malignant astrocytoma. Am J Pathol 146(5):1150–1160, 1995.
164. Mohanam, S, Sawaya, R, McCutcheon, I, et al: Modulation of *in vitro* invasion of human glioblastoma cells by urokinase-type plasminogen activator receptor antibody. Cancer Res 53: 4143–4147, 1993.
165. Sivaparvathi, M, Sawaya, R, Wang, SW, et al: Overexpression and localization of cathepsin B during the progression of human gliomas. Clin Exp Metastasis 13:49–56, 1995.
166. Rosenblum, ML, Spencer, D, Nelson, K, et al: Novel cystein protease inhibitors in the control of glioma cell migration. J Neurooncol 28:58, 1996.
167. Green, DR, Bissonnette, RP, and Cotter, TG: In: Rosenberg, SA (ed): Apoptosis and Cancer, Principles and Practice of Oncology PPO Updates. JB Lippincott, Philadelphia, Number 1, 1994.
168. Shapiro, WR: Treatment of neuroectodermal brain tumors. Ann Neurol 12:231–237, 1982.
169. Tannock, IF: Principles of cell proliferation: Cell kinetics. In DeVita, VT, Hellman, S, and Rosenberg, SA (eds): Principles and Practice of Oncology. JB Lippincott, Philadelphia, 1989, pp 3–13,.
170. Hoshino, T, Barker, M, Wilson, CB, et al: Cell kinetics of human gliomas. J Neurosurg 37:15–26, 1972.
171. Tabuchi, K, Shiraishi, T, Kawaguchi, S, and Mineta, T: Induction of apoptosis in glioma cells by recombinant fas ligand. J Neurooncol 35(Suppl 1):S43, 1997.
172. Fueyo, J, Gomez-Manzano, C, Liu, TJ, et al: E2F-1-mediated apoptosis in glioma cells. J Neurooncol 35(Suppl 1):S17, 1997.
173. Gobbel, GT, Bellinzona, M, Vogt, AR, et al: Radiation induces apoptosis in post-mitotic neurons. J Neurooncol 28:53, 1996.
174. Yoshii, Y, Maki, Y, Tsuboi, K, et al: Estimation of growth fraction with bromodeoxyuridine in human central nervous system tumors. J Neurosurg 65:659–663, 1986.
175. Bookwalter, JW III, Selker, RG, Schiffer, L, et al: Brain-tumor cell kinetics correlated with survival. J Neurosurg 65:795–798, 1986.
176. Hoshino, T, Nagashima, T, Cho, KG, et al: S-phase fraction of human brain tumors in situ measured by uptake of bromodeoxyuridine. Int J Cancer 38:369–374, 1986.
177. Ritter, AM, Sawaya, R, Hess, KR, et al: Prognostic significance of bromodeoxyuridine labeling in primary and recurrent glioblastoma multiforme. Neurosurgery 35:192–198, 1994.
178. Nishizaki, T, Orita, T, Saiki ,M, et al: Cell kinetics of human brain tumors by in vitro labeling using anti-BUdR monoclonal antibody. J Neurosurg 69:371–374, 1988.
179. Nishizaki, T, Orita, T, Kajiwara, K, et al: Correlation of in vitro bromodeoxyuridine labeling index and DNA aneuploidy with survival or recurrence in brain-tumor patients. J Neurosurg 73:396–400, 1990.
180. Asai, A, Shibui, S, Barker, M, et al: Cell kinetics of rat 9L brain tumors determined by double labeling with iodo- and bromodeoxyuridine. J Neurosurg 73:254–258, 1990.
181. Hoshino, T, Ito, S, Asai, A, et al: Cell kinetic analysis of human brain tumors by in situ double labeling with bromodeoxyuridine and iododeoxyuridine. Int J Cancer 50:1–5, 1992.
182. Freese, A, O'Rourke, D, Judy, K, and O'Connor, MJ: The application of 5-bromodeoxyuridine in the management of CNS tumors. J Neurooncol 20:81–95, 1994.
183. Montine, TJ, Vandersteenhoven, JJ, Aguzzi, A, et al: Prognostic significance of Ki-67 proliferation index in supratentorial fibrillary astrocytic neoplasms. Neurosurgery 34:674–679, 1994.
184. Sasaki, K, Matsumura, K, Tsuji, T, et al: Relationship between labeling indices of Ki-67 and BrdUrd in human malignant tumors. Cancer 62:989–993, 1988.
185. Onda, K, Davis, RL, Shibuya, M, et al: Correlation between the bromodeoxyuridine labeling index and the MIB-1 and Ki-67 proliferating indices in cerebral gliomas. Cancer 74:1921–1926, 1994.
186. Kim, DK, Hoyt, J, Bacchi, C, et al: Detection of proliferating cell nuclear antigen in gliomas and adjacent resections margin. Neurosurgery 33:619–626, 1993.
187. Dalrymple, SJ, Parisi, JE, Roche, PC, et al: Changes in proliferating cell nuclear antigen expression in glioblastoma multiforme cells along a stereotactic biopsy trajectory. Neurosurgery 35:1036–1045, 1994.
188. Louis, DN, Meehan, SM, Ferrante, RJ, et al: Use of the silver nucleolar organizer region (AgNOR) technique in the differential diagnosis of central nervous system neoplasia. J Neuropathol Exp Neurol 51–2):150–157, 1992.
189. Shiraishi, T, Tabuchi, K, Mineta, T, et al: Nucleolar organizer regions in various human brain tumors. J Neurosurg 74:979–984, 1991.
190. Kajiwara, K, Nishizaki, T, Orita, T, et al: Silver colloid staining technique for analysis of glioma malignancy. J Neurosurg 73:113–117, 1990.
191. Hara, A, Sakai, N, Yamada, H, et al: Rapid detection of proliferating potential in human brain tumors by nucleolar organizer region staining on squash preparations. J Cancer Res Clin Oncol 117:510–514, 1991.
192. Cho, KG, Nagashima, T, Barnwell, S, and Hoshino, T: Flow cytometric determination of modal DNA population and relation to proliferative potential of human intracranial neoplasms. J Neurosurg 69:588–592, 1988.
193. Coons, SW, and Johnson, PC: Regional heterogeneity in the DNA content of human gliomas. Cancer 72:3052–3060, 1993.
194. Mckeever, PE, Feldnezer, JA, McCoy, JP, et al: Nuclear parameters as prognostic indicators in glioblastoma patients. J Neuropath Exp Neurol 49:71–78, 1990.

195. Salmon, I, Dewitte, O, Pasteels, J-L, et al: Prognostic scoring in adult astrocytic tumors using patient age, histopathological grade, and DNA histogram type. J Neurosurg 80:877–883, 1994.
196. Ganju, V, Jenkins, RB, Scheithauer, B, et al: Prognostic factors in gliomas: multivariate analysis of cytogenetic, flow cytometry, and clinical parameters. Proc Annu Meet Am Assoc Cancer Res 33:A1558, 1992.
197. Kimmel, DW, Shapiro, JR, and Shapiro, WR: *In vitro* drug sensitivity testing in human gliomas. J Neurosurg 66:161–171, 1987.
198. Kornblith, PL, Smith, BH, and Leonard, LA: Response of cultured human brain tumors to nitrosoureas: correlation with clinical data. Cancer 47:255–265, 1981.
199. Phillips. PC: Antineoplastic drug resistance in brain tumors. Neurologic Clin 9(2):383–404, 1991.
200. Schold, SC Jr, Brent, TP, von Hofe, E, et al: O^6-alkylguanine-DNA alkyltransferase and sensitivity to procarbazine in human brain-tumor xenografts. J Neurosurg 70:573–577, 1989.
201. Hotta, T, Saito, Y, Fujita, H, et al: O^6-alkylguanine-DNA alkyltransferase activity of human malignant glioma and its clinical implications. J Neurooncol 21:135–140, 1994.
202. Citron, M, Decker, R, Chen, S, et al: O^6-methylguanine-DNA methyltransferase in human normal and tumor tissue from brain, lung, and ovary. Cancer Res 51:4131–4134, 1991.
203. Mineura, K, Izumi, I, Watanabe, K, and Kowada, M: Influence of O^6-methylguanine-DNA methyltransferase activity on chloroethylnitrosourea chemotherapy in brain tumors. Int J Cancer 55:76–81, 1993.
204. Mineura, K, Izumi, I, Watanabe, K, and Kowada, M: O^6-methylguanine-DNA methyltransferase activity in cerebral gliomas. A guidance for nitrosourea treatment? Acta Oncologica 33(1):29–32, 1994.
205. Silber, JR, Mueller, BA, Ewers, TG, and Berger, MS: Comparison of O^6-methylguanine-DNA methyltransferase activity in brain tumors and adjacent normal brain. Cancer Res 53:3416–3420, 1993.
206. Grant, R, Liang, BC, Page, MA, et al: Age influences chemotherapy response in astrocytomas. Neurology 45:929–933, 1995.
207. Zhao, K-M, Chen, J-M, Zuo, H-Z, et al: Modulation of O^6-methylguanine-DNA methyltransferase-mediated nimustine resistance in recurent malignant gliomas by streptozotocin: A preliminary report. Anticancer Res 15:645–648, 1995.
208. Marathi, UK, Kroes, RA, Dolan, ME, and Erickson, LC: Prolonged depletion of O^6-methylguanine DNA methyltransferase activity following exposure to O^6-benzylguanine with or without streptozotocin enhances 1,3-bis(2-chloroethyl)-1-nitrosourea sensitivity *in vitro*. Cancer Res 53: 4281–4286, 1993.
209. Baer, JC, Freeman, AA, Newlands, ES, et al: Depletion of O^6-alkylguanine-DNA alkyltransferase correlates with potentiation of temozolomide and CCNU toxicity in human tumour cells. Br J Cancer 67:1299–1302, 1993.
210. Chen, J-M, Zhang, Y-P, Moschel, RC, and Ikenaga, M: Depletion of O^6-methylguanine-DNA methyltransferase and potentiation of 1,3-bis(2-chloroethyl)-1-nitrosourea antitumor activity by O^6-benzylguanine *in vitro*. Carcinogenesis 14(5): 1057–1060, 1993.
211. Ali-Osman, F, Stein, DE, and Renwick, A: Glutathione content and glutathione-S-transferase expression in 1,3-bis(2-chloroethyl)-1-nitrosourea-resistant human malignant astrocytoma cell lines. Cancer Res 50:6976–6980, 1990.
212. Kudo, H, Mio, T, Kokunai, T, et al: Quantitative analysis of glutathione in human brain tumors. J Neurosurg 72:610–615, 1990.
213. Hara, A, Yamada, H, Sakai, N, et al: Immunohistochemical demonstration of the placental form of glutathione S-transferase, a detoxifying enzyme in human gliomas. Cancer 66:2563–2568, 1990.
214. Matsumoto, T, Tani, E, Kaba, K, et al: Amplification and expression of a multidrug resistance gene in human glioma cell lines. J Neurosurg 72:96–101, 1990.
215. Tishler, DM, and Raffel, C: Development of multidrug resistance in a primitive neuroectodermal tumor cell line. J Neurosurg 76:502–506, 1992.
216. Tishler, DM, Weinberg, KI, Sender, LS, et al: Multidrug resistance gene expression in pediatric primitive neuroectodermal tumors of the central nervous system. J Neurosurg 76:507–512, 1992.
217. Rothenberg, M, and Ling, V: Multidrug resistance: Molecular biology and clinical relevance. J Natl Cancer Inst 81(12):907–910, 1989.

Chapter 3

TUMOR IMAGING AND RESPONSE

TUMOR IMAGING

Tumor imaging has changed dramatically since 1970 (Table 3–1). The modern era of central nervous system imaging began in 1973 with the introduction of computed tomography (CT). In 1975, Oldendorf and Hounsfeld received the Lasker award for their contribution to early CT imaging theory. In 1979, Hounsfeld and Cormack were awarded the Nobel Prize for their discovery. Magnetic resonance imaging (MRI), the static imaging procedure of choice for brain tumors, was developed in the mid-1980s. The development of MRI fostered a clinical partnership among neurologist, neurosurgeon, neuroradiologist, and radiation oncologist for the interpretation of scans. The myriad different pulse sequences—spin-echo (SE), gradient-echo, and inversion recovery—combined with different repetition (TR) and echo (TE) times, required the specialization of a neuroradiologist or, less commonly, a neurologist.

In the early 1980s, dynamic functional imaging with positron emission tomography (PET) was developed, initially measuring regional glucose utilization with (^{18}F)-2-fluoro-2-deoxyglucose (FDG) in tissue, including tumors. PET required a cyclotron for the generation of short half-life photon emitting isotopes and a special camera for the recording of photon emissions. Since then, other cyclotron-generated photon-emitting isotopes have been developed to measure blood flow, oxygen consumption, blood-brain barrier (BBB) function, protein synthesis, nucleic acid precursor uptake, neurotransmitter uptake, and drug uptake. In clinical neuro-oncology, the main use of FDG-PET has been in the differentiation of tumor recurrence from radiation necrosis. Early reports[1–3] that glial tumor FDG uptake is predictive of survival have not withstood the test of time.[4,5] Single photon emission tomography (SPECT) with thallium tracers is a less sensitive means of acquiring physiologic information about brain tumors.[6–8] SPECT and FDG-PET are used preoperatively to supplement static imaging with localization of the highest metabolic area in tumor for biopsy.[9–12] SPECT tracers do not require a cyclotron for generation, and SPECT scanners are more readily available and less expensive. PET is the best available nonsurgical means of differentiating between radiation necrosis and tumor recurrence. In patients heavily treated with radiation or chemotherapy, PET is less reliable.[13]

Angiography, the oldest of the imaging techniques currently in use, is an invasive procedure associated with significant risk (see section on angiography farther on). It is used less frequently in presurgical treatment planning but is still the best technique for visualizing small penetrating

Table 3–1. **Tumor Imaging Techniques**

Static
Magnetic resonance imaging (MRI)
Computed tomography (CT)
Dynamic
Angiography
MRI angiography
Positron emission tomography (PET) and activated PET
Single photon emission tomography (SPECT)
Magnetic resonance spectroscopy (MRS)
Functional MRI (echo-planar MR)
Co-registration of Images and Treatment Planning

blood vessels, aneurysms, and arteriovenous malformations. MRI angiography and echo-planar MR with faster scan times of 0.1 second per image are developing techniques to visualize major tumor vasculature. Echo-planar MR and PET activation studies monitor task-related increases in blood flow and provides more information about brain physiology. Brain tumor localization is aided by cortical mapping of changes in blood flow to eloquent areas of brain adjacent to tumor. MRI spectroscopy noninvasively and repetitively monitors metabolic changes in tumor and adjacent tissue and provides metabolic parameters for early tumor response.

Co-registration techniques, combining three-dimensional (3-D) anatomic imaging information from CT, MRI, and PET scans, have been developed and applied in 3-D radiation therapy (RT) treatment planning.[14] The transposition of this information to the reference stereotactic frame has produced great advances in stereotactic biopsy and is responsible for sophisticated interstitial radiotherapy and laser-guided stereotactic resection.

The advent of new static imaging techniques has allowed for the more precise definition of tumor margins, the development of criteria for response determination, and the determination of tumor recurrence. However, survival is the major endpoint of most randomized clinical trials.

Static Imaging Techniques

MAGNETIC RESONANCE IMAGING

MRI, with and without gadolinium, is the procedure of choice for initial diagnostic imaging of patients suspected of having an intracranial primary brain neoplasm or other malignancy.[15–17] Compared with CT, MRI is a more sensitive imaging modality for lesion identification,[18,19] and the margin of the T_2-weighted abnormality is a more accurate marker of the primary glioma boundary.[20] The anatomic detail obtained with MRI thin slices and the ability to obtain multiplanar images without reformatting provide superior detail with less artifact than those found in static or functional imaging. There is no radiation exposure. The intravenous (IV) paramagnetic contrast material, gadolinium, crosses into the brain at discontinuities in the BBB. It interacts with tissue to increase the T_1-weighted signal and provide an imaging separation between enhancing tumor, with a disrupted BBB and edema or normal brain.

The scientific basis of MRI is based on the excitation of tissue protons with a radiofrequency pulse sequence, and measuring tissue proton parameters, such as tissue T_1- and T_2-relaxation times, proton density, magnetic susceptibility and chemical shift, to obtain imaging differences in adjacent tissues. The Spin-echo (SE) technique is the most widely used pulse sequence for the imaging of brain tumors.[21] In this technique, a 90-degree radiofrequency pulse is followed, after a delay, by a second 180-degree pulse. Whereas the initial pulse causes a 90-degree change in the orientation of the body's protons, the second pulse maintains that change and prevents internal field distortion. When the protons return to more stable energy levels, radiowave signals are emitted and the location of the protons in the brain are encoded in the signal wavelength. Magnetic gradients in three dimensions can provide a point location in space, and an image is produced using Fourier transformation. Every tissue has a speed of magnetization and signal decay that are related to the T_1 and T_2 relaxation times of tissue. The disadvantage of SE pulse sequences is the time required for patient imaging. Gradient-echo imaging is being used increasingly in uncooperative and pediatric patients because there is only a single pulse, which requires less time. Gradient-echo imaging can also visualize moving blood and is used in MRI angiography.[21]

T_1-weighted SE images with a short TR and TE produce excellent anatomic detail in normal brain. T_1-weighted SE images often fail to identify tumors in brain because of the small imaging differences between tumor and brain when short TR and TE are employed. T_2-weighted SE images with long TRs and TEs delineate differences in signal intensity between normal brain and tumor. However, both tumor tissue and edematous brain parenchyma have prolonged relaxation times and cannot be distinguished on T_2-weighted images.[22] The combined volume of tumor plus brain edema is imaged with T_2-weighted SE sequences. Mass effect is seen with both T_1- and T_2-weighted images. IV infusion of gadolinium with SE pulse sequences and T_1-weighted images increases the relaxation of protons, shortening T_1- and lengthening T_2-relaxation times (Fig. 3–1). This allows distinction between tumor and edema, not possible on T_2-weighted sequences. On T_1-weighted images, the tumor appears very bright, similar to the image obtained with infused iodinated contrast in CT. However, in CT the iodinated contrast electron density is measured in tissue; in MRI, an interaction between the tissue and gadolinium is measured.[21]

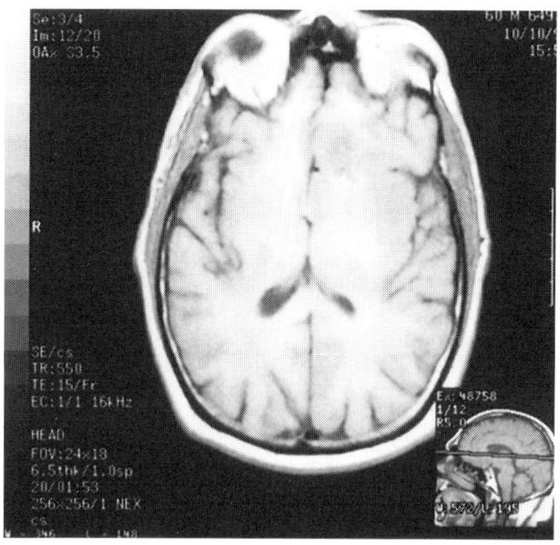

A

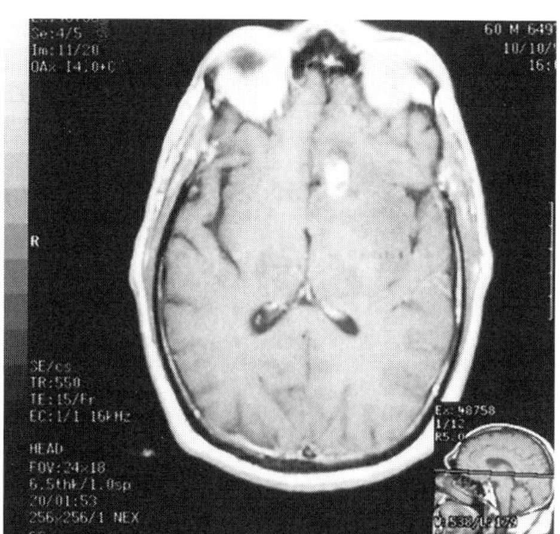

B

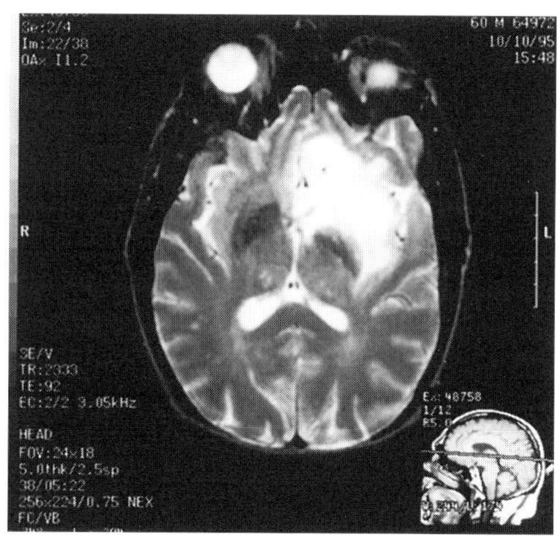

C

Figure 3–1. Tumor edema *(A)* T_1-weighted MRI precontrast, small left low frontal hypointense area of biopsy proven glioblastoma multiforme that *(B)* enhances with gadolinium. *(C)* T_2-weighted MRI shows extensive area of hyperintense signal including both enhancing tumor and edema surrounding tumor. The edema involves predominantly white matter. On stereotactic biopsy studies tumor cells may extend beyond T_2 abnormality.

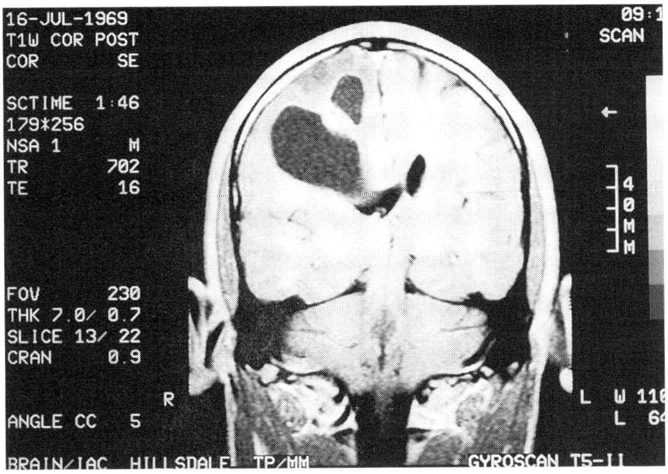

Figure 3–2. Tumor cyst. T_1-weighted MRI with contrast infusion of anaplastic astrocytoma with multicystic hypointense area with rim enhancement of the cyst walls and the area between cysts.

Tumor cysts are identified on T_1-weighted SE sequences as homogeneous low-signal areas. The TR and TE values are slightly higher than the levels of cerebrospinal fluid because of the cyst protein content (Fig. 3–2). The cyst may also be seen on T_2-weighted sequences when it has a long TR and TE. Acute hemorrhage is seen as high signal on T_1-weighted images (Fig. 3–3). Tumor hemorrhage often evolves more slowly than nontumoral hemorrhage with a greater time delay before the development of decreased signal on T_1-weighted images. The development of a low-intensity peripheral ring signal on T_2-weighted images, characteristic of nontumoral hemorrhage, is rarely seen in chronic tumoral hemorrhage. Most importantly, tumoral hemorrhage has marked signal heterogeneity, pronounced or marked edema, and often, but not always, nonhemorrhagic tumor tissue.[23] MRI cannot visualize calcification reliably.[24] Fat has a very high signal on T_1-weighted images and a very low signal on T_2-weighted images.

Kelly and colleagues[20] correlated abnormalities on preoperative CT and MRI, with serial fresh surgical stereotactic bi-

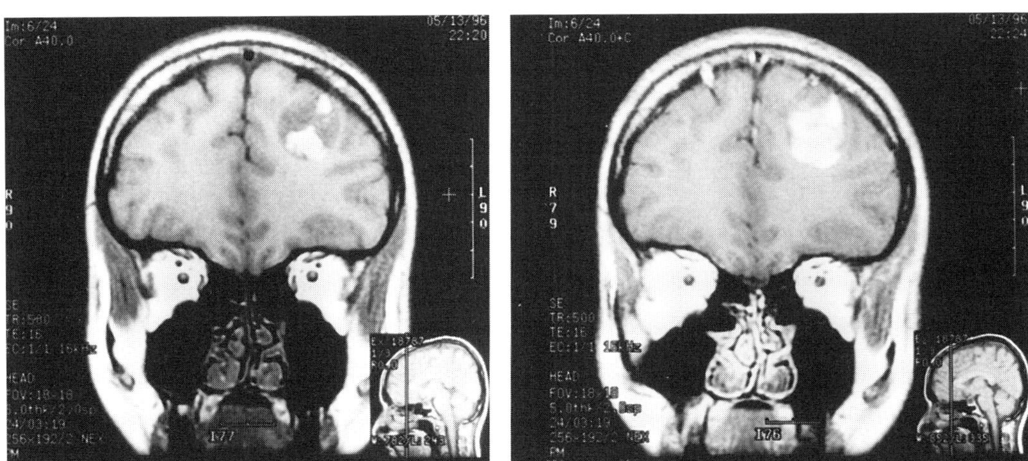

A B

Figure 3–3. Tumor hemorrhage. *(A)* T_1-weighted MRI precontrast of glioblastoma multiforme shows hypointense circular area, with two areas of hyperintense signal of acute hemorrhage. *(B)* On T_1-weighted MRI postcontrast there is heterogeneous contrast enhancement.

opsy specimens.[25] In this study, tumors were grouped anatomically according to the Daumas-Duport classification of structural organization (see Chapter 1). In high-grade lesions, CT and MRI areas of contrast enhancement accurately depicted the volume of solid tumor. In malignant gliomas, areas of CT low attenuation corresponded to pathological tumor necrosis. Low-grade gliomas were usually hypodense on T_1-weighted MRI scans but could be isodense. In low-grade gliomas, the T_2-weighted area of MRI abnormality matched more accurately the histological distribution of tumor cells than the area of CT hypodensity. However, in gliomas, tumor cells frequently extended beyond the area of T_2-weighted abnormality, particularly in low-grade gliomas (Fig. 3–4).[20] Tumor infiltration into host brain beyond the imaging abnormalities makes planned surgical resection and cure unlikely, without unacceptable toxicity to normal brain. Effective postoperative treatment techniques must be able to selectively destroy infiltrating tumor cells.[26]

Not all high-grade astrocytomas enhance with gadolinium. In these cases, the increased T_2-weighted MRI signal may mimic imaging abnormalities seen in low-grade glioma (LGA) or nonmalignant conditions, such as multiple sclerosis, radiation or chemotherapy toxicity, or edema from vascular or infectious disease.[27–29] Radiation oncologists have extended focal conformal radiation fields to include a margin around the T_2-weighted abnormality to encompass the extent of tumor infiltration.[20]

Because MRI cannot accurately predict the type or grade of malignancy, surgical histologic diagnosis is imperative if the surgical morbidity and mortality are acceptable. A static imaging technique cannot predict tumor biologic behavior as measured by such parameters as growth fraction, doubling time, rate of cell death, invasiveness, spread, or sensitivity or resistance to therapy. Preoperative MRI has been assessed for prognostic variables in a selected series of 48 patients who underwent gross total resection and adjuvant RT and chemotherapy. Multivariate analysis revealed that quantitative tumor necrosis, the intensity of enhancement, and the extent of edema were independently, and negatively, associated with survival.[30]

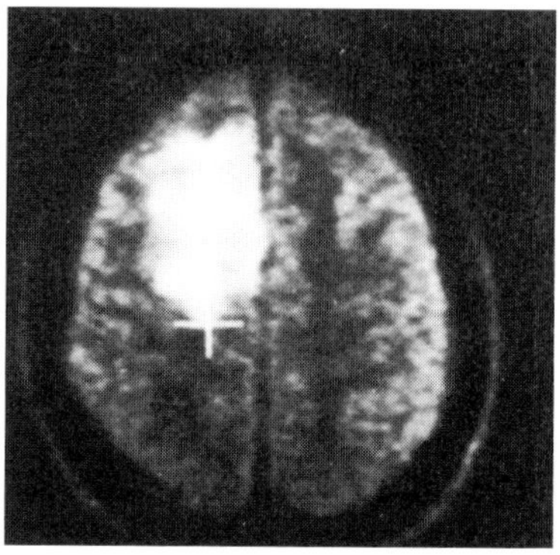

A

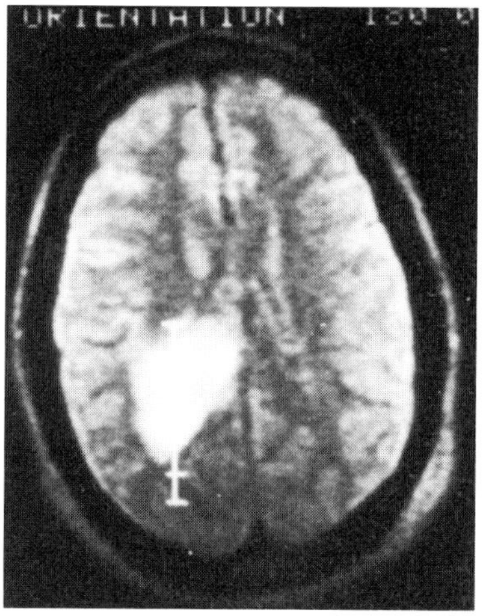

B

Figure 3–4. Low grade oligodendroglioma. Serial biopsies taken along *(A)* anterior-posterior trajectory and *(B)* posterior-anterior trajectory. Tumor cells are found in the uninvolved white matter surrounding the T_2 abnormality. The hash marks correspond to stereotactic position of each biopsy section and are separated by 1 cm. (From Kelly et al[20], p453, with permission).

Diffusion MRI measures the diffusion of intracellular and extracellular water. Water diffusion varies in different tissues and is restricted by cell membranes and tissue macromolecules. Diffusion measures are different from T_1 and T_2 relaxation times and are obtained with varying amplitude SE sequences, delivered from three orthogonal directions. Diffusion MRI has measured different diffusion coefficients in areas of solid tumor, cyst formation, edema, necrosis, and normal white matter.[31] Conventional MRI, with T_1 and T_2

relaxation times, sometimes cannot differentiate among cyst formation, necrosis, and solid tumor. Diffusion MRI may help the surgeon plan surgical biopsy and resection preoperatively.[31]

Ideally, MRI is ordered by a clinician in consultation with a neuroradiologist and monitored by a neuroradiologist during scan performance. MRI cannot be performed if the patient has a pacemaker, paramagnetic aneurysm clips, metallic foreign bodies, or other magnetic devices in the orbits or cranium. MRI is difficult to perform for claustrophobic patients. IV sedation with 1.0 to 1.5 mg of lorazepam, or 3 to 5 mg of diazepam can be used. Often an oral dose of 10 mg diazepam, given 45 minutes prior to the scan, is effective in relieving anxiety and the majority of the claustrophobia.[32] If MRI is unobtainable, CT is a good alternative. MRI is not performed during the first trimester of pregnancy, although the risks are not well defined and MRI is probably safer than CT with its radiation exposure.[32]

COMPUTED TOMOGRAPHY

CT was the first brain imaging method to determine tumor size. Radionuclide scanning depended on BBB breakdown for visualization of tumor. CT depends upon the varying electron density of tissues and their attenuation of photon energy. The photon energy is measured by a detector after traversing the patient. Intravenously infused iodinated and noniodinated contrast dyes cross the BBB where it is discontinuous, are taken into malignant tumor, and increase the electron density. Approximately 4% of patients with supratentorial glioblastoma multiforme do not have tumoral contrast enhancement.[33] Contrast CT is not as sensitive as gadolinium MRI in diagnosing tumors and defining their margins.[18–20] Calcification within tumors is most accurately seen with CT (Fig. 3–5).[16,17] CT is more useful than MRI in detecting lytic bony change in the cranium but is not as effective in imaging any associated soft-tissue mass. CT is excellent for the diagnosis of acute parenchymal and subarachnoid hemorrhage.[32]

Dynamic Imaging Techniques

ANGIOGRAPHY

Angiography is an invasive procedure involving transfemoral catheterization of the femoral artery. After catheterization, a guidewire is passed through the catheterization trochar, and then the catheter is threaded over the guidewire and positioned in the intracranial vessel to be imaged. An iodinated contrast dye is injected by an automated injector, and then

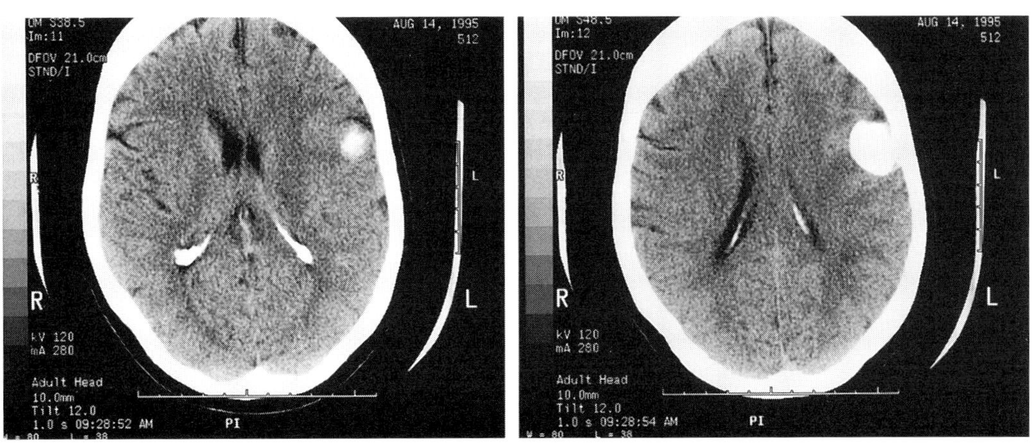

A B

Figure 3–5. Tumor calcification. *(A)* CT without contrast showing densely calcified right frontal meningioma. No brain invasion or edema is seen. *(B)* CT with contrast shows a larger area of enhancement surrounding calcified area.

a series of rapid sequence radiographs are taken. The rapid-sequence radiographs show the great vessels leading to the brain, the small penetrating blood vessels, a capillary phase, and, finally, a venous phase. The major arterial vessels and tumor blood vessels, supplying meningiomas or other vascular tumors—hemangioblastoma or glioma—are frequently visualized with selective arterial contrast injections. The endothelial proliferation of malignant gliomas is imaged as a vascular blush because of the vascular retention of contrast. Angiography can also show mass effect, imaged as distortion, and displacement of major arteries and veins. Angiograms are no longer routinely performed preoperatively on patients with brain tumors. MRI can delineate tumor and normal tissue anatomic relations to vessels, often obviating the need for angiography.

The major risks of angiography are thromboembolic complications, vessel rupture, and arterial dissection from catheter manipulation within a proximal artery. The vascular complication rate of angiography should be less than 2% when performed by experienced clinicians. Other significant complications include groin hematoma, femoral nerve injury, and anaphylactic shock secondary to contrast-dye allergy. Angiographic procedures are being performed less frequently because of advances in static imaging, ultrasound, and noninvasive MRI angiography.

MRI ANGIOGRAPHY

MRI angiography is noninvasive and utilizes gradient-echo pulse sequence to evaluate flowing blood. Gradient-echo imaging uses only a single non–90-degree pulse, and images can be obtained much more rapidly than with SE sequences. Blood flowing into the imaging volume will not have received a single pulse and will be fully magnetized; surrounding stationary tissue has received multiple pulses and has not remagnetized. On T_1-weighted gradient-echo sequences, the fully magnetized blood appears brighter than the partially magnetized surrounding area.[22] MRI angiography can be used to visualize major vessels and their branches but does not show small arterioles or capillaries. MRI angiography might be used preoperatively to visualize the vascular supply of a presumed meningioma but not the small vessel supply of a malignant astrocytoma. MRI angiography may be used to examine the patency of a vessel for IA chemotherapy infusion or arterial chemotherapy pump placement.

POSITRON EMISSION TOMOGRAPHY

PET is a functional imaging technique developed in the 1970s and applied to brain tumors in the early 1980s. PET requires a cyclotron for the generation of photon-emitting isotopes, with half-lives of minutes to hours. A special PET camera is needed to record the photon emissions, and it must be situated near the cyclotron because of the short isotope half-life. Positrons travel only very short distances in tissue before colliding with electrons of negative charge. The positrons and electrons are destroyed by the collision, and two photons are emitted, which travel in 180-degree opposite directions. The PET camera photomultipliers and detectors record oppositely directed simultaneously arriving photons and ignore out-of-phase photons. The resolution of the best PET cameras is approximately 3 to 4 mm.[3,34] Tracer distribution is counted three dimensionally and quantitatively, with computerized algorithms similar to those in static CT.[34] Kinetic models for the distribution and metabolism of tracer in tissue are critical to the interpretation of data, and can be found elsewhere.[34,35]

Positron emitting isotopes include:

- FDG for the study of glucose utilization in tumor[1–5,10–12,15,17,35–43]
- $^{15}O_2$ for oxygen utilization[44,45]
- $C^{15}O_2H_2{}^{15}O$ for blood flow[44,45]
- ^{11}C-methionine for amino acid uptake[37,46,47]
- ^{11}C-BCNU for drug uptake[48]
- ^{82}Rubidium (^{82}Rb) for BBB function[36]
- (^{18}F)-fluorodeoxyuridine[49] for nucleic acid uptake into DNA
- ^{11}C-PK11195 for tumor grading[50]

PET studies with FDG in gliomas, have attempted to (1) predict malignancy and prognosis,[1–5,38,40–43] (2) localize the highest metabolic region for stereotactic biopsy to maximize the likelihood of obtaining a sample of maximum anaplasia,[10–12] (3) quantitate residual tumor after surgical resection,[40,41] (4) distinguish between radiation necrosis and recurrent tumor,[13,36,40] and (5) evaluate malignant degeneration in low-grade gliomas.[38] An early report by Di Chiro and colleagues[1] found a positive correlation between the histologic grade of the malignancy and the glucose utilization. Subsequent reports of FDG-PET in recurrent gliomas, by Patronas and associates,[2] found that a PET-scan ratio of tumor frontal lobe glucose utilization to normal brain of greater than 1.4 was associated with a poor prognosis. In addition, PET glucose utilization more accurately predicted survival than pathology.[2,3] Initial surgical pathology was analyzed and followed by RT, and in approximately two-thirds of the patients, by chemotherapy. After RT or chemotherapy failure, a FDG-PET scan was obtained and was more predictive of survival than initial pathology.[2,3] Three additional FDG-PET studies in patients with recurrent glioma found a correlation among glucose utilization, survival, and histology.[38,42,43] None of these studies reported FDG-PET a better predictor of survival than histology, and in the only study using multivariate analysis,[43] histology was not a studied variable. In 16 patients with untreated cerebral glioma examined with FDG-PET, glucose utilization did not correlate with tumor size or grade.[4] Subsequent studies by Junck and colleagues[5] on more than 40 untreated cerebral gliomas found a correlation between glucose metabolism and tumor grade, but histology was more predictive of survival. In conclusion, the use of PET scanning in determining survival in patients with de novo, untreated glioma has not been established. For de novo and recurrent disease, there may be a correlation of glucose utilization with histological grade; in recurrent tumors, the FDG-PET scan may have prognostic value. Some practical questions need an answer, however: (1) Does the predictive value of PET in recurrent patients help in patient management (i.e., after surgery, radiation and chemotherapy failure)? (2) Is the management change going to produce a change in survival and outcome measures? and (3) Who will pay for the scan?

The second application of FDG-PET is preoperative imaging for the area of maximum glucose utilization to help the surgeon localize the tumor with worst biologic behavior for biopsy.[10–12] There are no studies comparing the accuracy of tumor tissue surgical diagnosis with both preoperative MRI and PET localization versus MRI localization alone.

After surgical resection, Glantz and colleagues[41] used FDG-PET to document residual tumor. Twenty patients had hypermetabolic abnormalities on their postoperative scan, and 19 had early recurrence of tumor. None of the 12 patients with FDG-PET hypometabolic abnormalities had recurrence at the initial postoperative evaluation. The clinical value of early postoperative FDG-PET is unclear because patients with malignant glioma are assumed to have residual tumor after maximal resection. Conformal external-beam RT is most often based on the preoperative T2-weighted MRI, with a margin added for infiltrating tumor cells.

After surgical resection, Glantz and colleagues[41] found tumor FDG-PET glucose utilization to be unaffected by steroid treatment. In previous CT studies of recurrent malignant glioma, steroids produced decreased contrast enhancement in six of eight patients, and reduction was greater than 50% after steroids in two patients.[51]

Clinicians have not been able to distinguish between tumor recurrence and radiation necrosis using MRI and CT scans. Increased glucose utilization in tumor recurrence and negligible glucose utilization in radiation necrosis were found on FDG-PET scans (Fig. 3–6). In seven patients, there was histologic confirmation of the PET findings.[36] In 50 patients examined with FDG-PET for tumor recurrence, five patients' glucose utilization values were the opposite of their surgical pathology. Two patients had negligible glucose utilization with tumor at surgery, and three patients had increased glucose utilization and benign histology. These five were

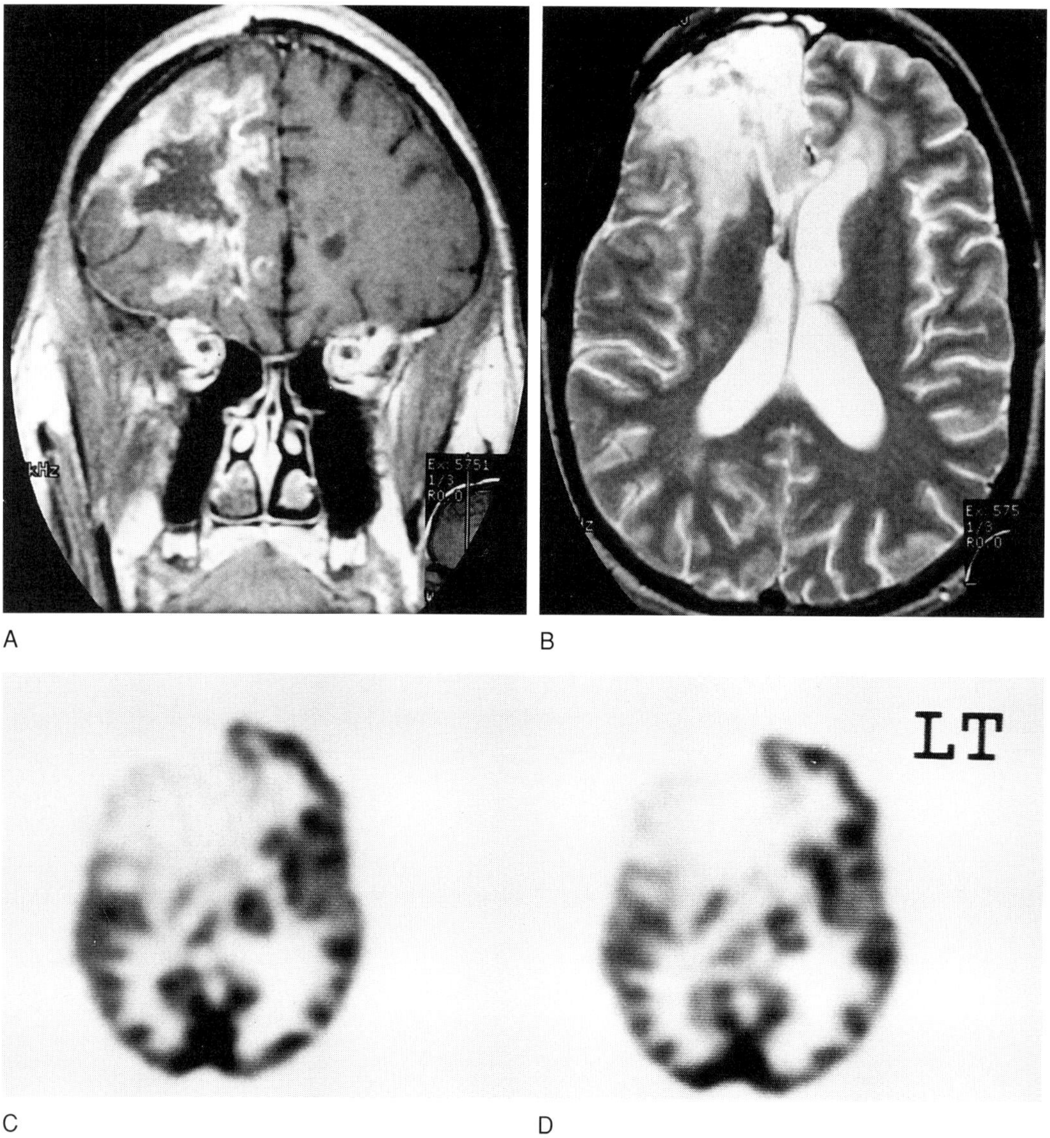

Figure 3–6. Radiation necrosis. 40-year-old man 9 months after gross total resection of a right frontal anaplastic astrocytoma and 8000 cGy focal conformal radiation therapy. Neurologic exam was normal. *(A)* MRI shows a large right frontal cystic mass with heterogeneous contrast enhancement with *(B)* extensive hyperintense T_2 signal extending into the opposite hemisphere. *(C and D)* ^{18}FDG-PET scan has no significant metabolism in the right frontal lobe.

among 17 patients heavily pretreated with accelerated fraction or interstitial radiation.[13] FDG-PET is the best noninvasive method for the determination of radiation necrosis versus recurrent tumor, but surgical resection may be needed in patients treated with high-dose experimental RT.

PET studies that included inhalation of $^{15}O_2$ for oxygen utilization found that the cerebral metabolic rate for oxygen and oxygen extraction ratio were low in all glial tumors. When $C^{15}O_2H_2^{15}O$ was used for blood flow studies, there was regional heterogeneity within tumors and variation between tumors.[34,44] Activated PET studies with blood flow tracers can be performed before and after a task. Areas with increased blood flow are presumably in-

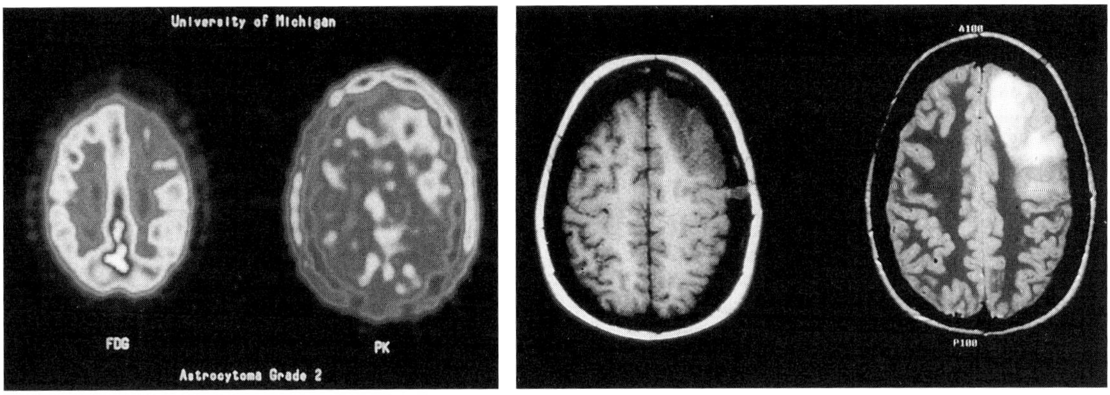

A B C D

Figure 3–7. PET ^{11}C-PK11195 binding of left frontal low grade astrocytoma. *(A)* [18]FDG-PET shows left frontal hypometabolism. *(B)* PET ^{11}C-PK11195 scan has increased binding in the left frontal lobe. *(C)* T_1-weighted MRI with left frontal hypointense signal. *(D)* T_2-weighted MRI, an area of hyerintense signal, greater in area than the T_1 hypointensity in *C*.

volved in task performance. Activation and localization of the motor or sensory cortex, or critical speech areas, using specifically designed tasks may permit greater tumor resection by localizing these critical cortical areas. Future studies should reveal whether this is additive to electrocorticographic stimulation or is a less invasive and less costly means of obtaining similar information.

L-methionine is an amino acid transported across the BBB by a specific amino acid transport system. After transport, it is rapidly incorporated into protein. ^{11}C-methionine is a positron emitting isotope, that has been studied in brain tumors. Uptake of this positron emitter was variable in LGA but increased with anaplasia.[46,47] Oligo-astrocytomas and meningiomas also showed increased uptake.[47]

PET ^{11}C-BCNU uptake distribution in gliomas and in normal brain is similar, as expected of a diffusible, highly lipophilic drug.[48] Another nitrosourea, sarcosinamide chloroethyl-nitrosourea, was PET labeled and found to be concentrated in gliomas and transported actively.[48] [82]Rb has been measured by PET and found to have increased brain extraction where CT contrast enhancement is present, and therefore is probably a BBB marker.[34] A positron-emitting halogenated pyrimidine, fluoro-2'-deoxyuridine, has been synthesized. In rats implanted with C6 glioma, there was a markedly increased incorporation in the tumor.[49] Halogenated pyrimidines are incorporated in cells in S-phase, so this would be a means of preoperatively obtaining a labeling index.

[11]C-PK11195 is a peripheral benzodiazepine receptor agonist that binds to glial cells and gliomas. Untreated gliomas have been found to have increased binding of ^{11}C-PK11195, which increases with anaplasia (Fig. 3–7). ^{11}C-PK11195 binding had stronger correlation with bromodeoxyuridine (BUdR) labeling index and histology than FDG-PET.[5,50] However, histology was a better predictor of survival than either ^{11}C-PK11195 or FDG-PET.

In untreated gliomas, none of the PET analogs is a better predictor of survival than histology. PET can be used to localize the area of maximum utilization of glucose, but it has not been determined if this increases the yield of stereotactic biopsy. PET is the noninvasive procedure of choice for the determination of tumor recurrence versus radiation necrosis, but in patients heavily pretreated with accelerated fraction or interstitial RT, significant false-positive and negative results occur.

SINGLE PHOTON EMISSION TOMOGRAPHY

SPECT is a functional imaging technique used to grade glioma malignancy and differentiate tumor necrosis from tumor recurrence. ^{201}thallium (^{201}Tl), infused intravenously, is localized in tumor and not necrotic tissue or normal brain.[6] Thallium is a potassium analog. Increased tumor uptake is probably due to increased potassium transport in tumor by a Na^+/K^+–ATPase pump mechanism in the cell membrane.[6] The physiologic role of thallium in SPECT is not as easily perceived and is more empirical than the role of ^{18}FDG in PET.[17] SPECT tracers have longer half-lives than PET tracers. SPECT radioisotopes for brain tumor studies besides ^{201}Tl are [^{99m}Tc] gluceptate,[67] gallium, DL-3–123I-iodo-α-methyltyrosine, and hexakis (methoxyisobutylisonitrile) technetium (I).[16,52,53] The spacial resolution is 7 to 8 mm with a 5-mm slice thickness and is inferior to PET and MRI.

Several ^{201}Tl SPECT studies have a found correlation between the ratio of tumor ^{201}Tl uptake to contralateral normal brain Tl uptake, and the tumor grade.[7,8,54,55] Black and colleagues[54] reported that Tl uptake was modified by surgical resection but not by steroids. CT contrast enhancement (barrier function) is modified by surgery and steroids, with surgery leading to an increase in CT contrast enhancement, and steroids, decreasing CT contrast enhancement in patients with recurrent gliomas.[51] Steroids are unable to repair the barrier abnormality responsible for ^{201}Tl passage, suggesting it is transported at a different location than CT contrast most likely by an active ATPase-mediated mechanism. Tl uptake ratio of tumor to opposite normal cortex has been correlated retrospectively with survival[8] and to locate the area of maximum malignancy for biopsy.[9] ^{201}Tl SPECT has been reported to be more effective than CT in documenting change in tumor burden.[56] It has not been compared with MRI.

^{201}Tl has been used to differentiate clinically radiation necrosis from tumor recurrence but does not appear nearly as effective as PET.[57] ^{201}Tl was infused, and a ratio of tumor to scalp uptake was used. If this ratio was greater than 3.5, recurrent tumor was found in 12 of 13 cases. If the ratio was less than 3.5, technetium-99m hexamethylpropylene amine oxime (^{99m}Tc HMPAO) blood flow studies were performed, with the rationale that blood flow is decreased in most regions of radiation necrosis. If blood flow was less than 0.5 and the thallium uptake ratio was less than 3.5, 11 of 12 patients had radiation necrosis. If blood flow was greater than 0.5, a diagnosis could not be made. Pathologically, rats and monkeys with radiation necrosis may have severely dilated capillaries and venules (telangiectasia), which may lead to increased blood flow and be a shortcoming of this technique.[58,59]

The exact role of thallium ^{201}Tl SPECT in clinical practice is uncertain. At present, it does not seem to have a significant role in differentiating tumor from necrosis. The preoperative use of tumor grading is unclear. SPECT may be able to consistently localize the highest metabolic area in a tumor. Unlike FDG-PET, ^{201}Tl SPECT uptake is influenced by surgical changes in BBB function.

MAGNETIC RESONANCE SPECTROSCOPY

Magnetic resonance spectroscopy (MRS) is a noninvasive imaging technique that measures the metabolism of brain tumors.[60] MRS tumor spectra are always different from normal brain, but no spectrum is diagnostic of any one tumor.[61] MRS tumor spectra vary widely in different locations within the same tumor. MRS is usually done concordantly with static MRI. Proton (1-H) and phosphorus 31 (P-31) spectra are measured in vivo using a high field strength magnet, in voxels of roughly 1.5 × 1.5 × 1.5 cm.[60–62] P-31 spectra brain tumor pH measurements have averaged 6.99, or significantly more alkaline than normal brain.[62] MRS pH measurements confirm previous studies with PET.[63]

1-H MRS has yielded three important metabolic findings. First is the presence of lactate in brain tumors. Lactate is only sporadically produced in normal brain.[64,65] In malignant gliomas, glycolytic activity is increased as measured by increased FDG-PET glucose utilization. Using both FDG-PET and 1-H MRS, Herholz and colleagues[65] examined patients with histologically confirmed malignant gliomas, and found good correlation of glucose metabolism with lactate production. High-grade astrocytomas had significant glucose uptake and lactate production (Fig. 3–8). However, in high-grade astrocytomas, high lactate production was not in the same areas as high glucose uptake. LGA often had no lactate production, and glucose utilization was below normal. Whereas the highest lactate production was in necrotic areas, tumor cysts, and abutting the ventricular system, the highest glucose uptake was in the tumor.[65]

Another finding has been the loss of *N*-acetyl aspartate (NAA) in gliomas and all other brain tumors, regardless of histologic type (see Fig. 3–8). NAA is a metabolite present predominantly in neuronal cell populations, and decreased NAA represents a loss of neurons in the tumor area.[64,66]

Finally, 1-H MRS has shown that choline is increased in all tumor types, when measured as choline-to-creatinine tumor ratios. The ratio increased with grade in astrocytoma, but the highest ratios were seen in meningioma and pituitary adenoma.[64,66] Choline levels decreased in areas of tumor necrosis and radiation necrosis.[18] Choline is a major component of cell membranes, and active cell membrane biosynthesis occurs in tumor. It is not known why benign pituitary adenomas tumors have the greatest choline-to-creatinine ratios.

MRS's clinical role is still developing, but findings from individual clinical studies offer little reason for optimism. In vitro studies with oxidants, with P-31 MRS monitoring used as a predictor of clinical response, are much more exciting. Rats were implanted with 9L glioma and treated with the enzyme glucose oxidase attached to polyethylene glycol for the generation of H_2O_2 and free radicals. The P-31 MRS energy state of the 9L tumors was dramatically impaired, with decreases in phosphocreatine, ratio of ATP to inorganic phosphorus, and pH value.[67] These changes correlated with decreased 9L tumor growth in cytotoxicity assays. In a similar study with 1-H MRS, rats were implanted with 9L brain tumors and treated with BCNU or adenoviral thymidine kinase gene therapy. Animals with a 9L tumor growth delay had a large increase in the 1-H MRS lipid/lactate peak.[68] These MRS studies are encouraging and provide hope for early prediction of tumor response. However, the animal experiments use hosts that are genetically similar and tumors that are identical.

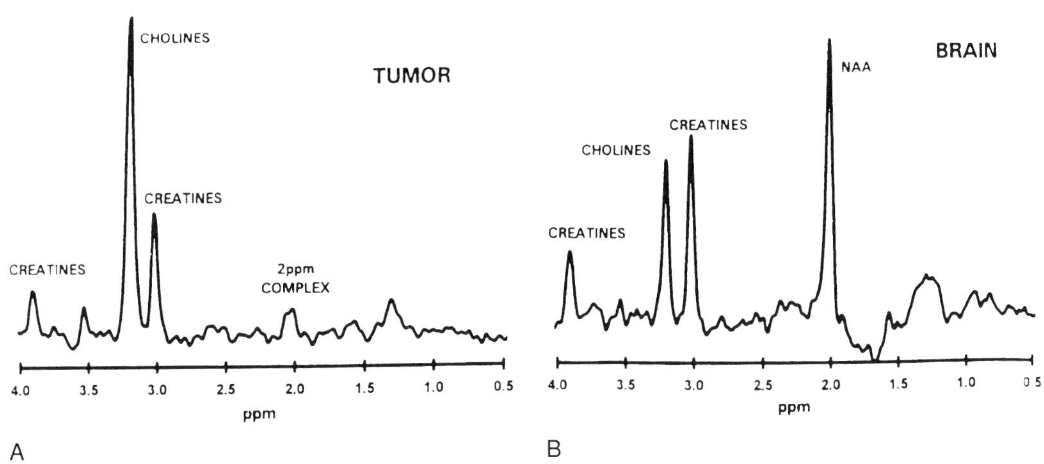

Figure 3–8. Magnetic resonance spectroscopy. *(A)* Malignant astrocytoma with increased choline and decreased N-acetyl aspartate peaks. *(B)* Normal brain spectroscopy from contralateral homologous brain. (From Negendank WG, Sauter R, Brown TR, et al: Proton magnetic resonance spectroscopy in patients with glial tumors: A multicenter study. J Neurosurg 84, 1996, p452, with permission).

FUNCTIONAL MRI (ECHO-PLANAR MR)

Echo-planar MR is performed on a conventional MRI scanner retrofitted with echo-planar technology. Echo-planar MR maps cerebral blood volume at the capillary level and can measure blood-brain transport of contrast dye past a disrupted BBB.[69] The region of interest analyzed is approximately 1.5 × 1.5 mm, with a 7-mm slice thickness, which is greater resolution than with PET blood flow. All patients have a conventional T_1- and T_2-weighted MRI. A single slice is selected to monitor with functional MRI. Patients are then injected with IV gadolinium, and a SE pulse sequence is given. Over 60 seconds, a series of 60 images is collected at the single selected level, with weighting of TR = 1000ms and TE = 100ms. Blood volume maps are mathematically obtained by integration of the first-pass tissue concentration through each region of interest.[69]

Eight patients with malignant astrocytoma were studied postoperatively with echo-planar MR and FDG-PET. Two patients had small areas of increased blood volume shown on echo-planar MR in their resection bed, indicating residual tumor. PET scans were hypometabolic in these two regions. The patients' radiation fields were adjusted to incorporate the blood flow (residual tumor) information. One had an excellent clinical outcome, and the other had tumor recurrence.[69]

It is hoped that echo-planar MR will be of use in differentiating radiation necrosis from tumor recurrence. However, because echo-planar MR may have the same potential problems as SPECT, relying on a rationale of decreased blood flow in radiation necrosis, we await future developments to determine its role.

Co-registration of Images and Treatment Planning

Modern computer technology has made it possible to wed CT, MRI, PET and SPECT images to develop 2- or 3-D reconstruction of identical planes or overlays in cranial space, from different tumor imaging modalities.[70,71] Image integration requires simultaneous display of imaging techniques in a single imaging system for stereotactic biopsy. This imaging system would be transferred to a stereotactic frame refer-

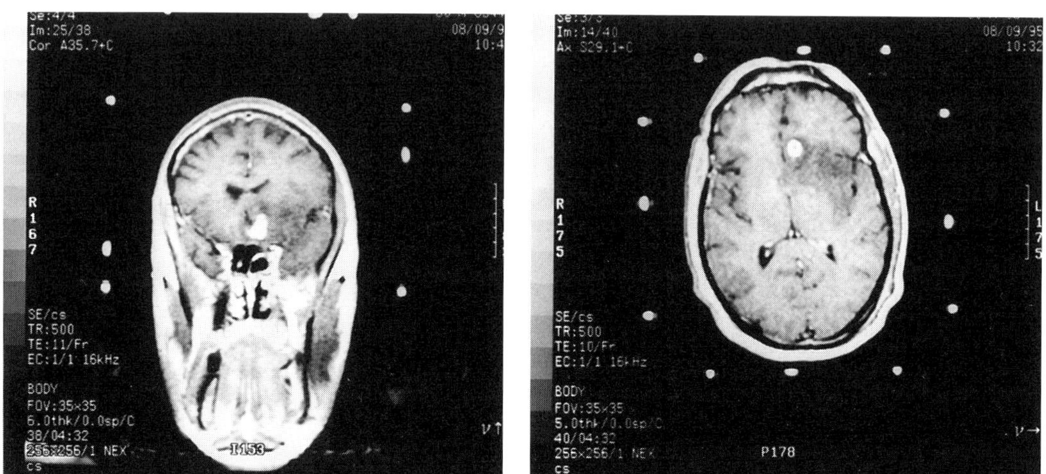

A B

Figure 3–9. Localization system for MRI in *(A)* coronal and *(B)* axial plane that creates a series of reference marks on each MRI image. Computer measurement of distance between reference marks of each image allows calculation of location of each slice from which stereotactic coordinates can be a calculated. Stereotactic biopsy revealed glioblastoma multiforme.

ence system, or the imaging procedures could be performed with a stereotactic frame in place (Fig. 3–9).[71–74] The transfer of MRI angiography or digital subtraction angiography images to a reference frame provides the neurosurgeon with information to select the best tract for a stereotactic biopsy or resection of a tumor. Ideally, these reference systems are interactive. The surgeon selects a target point for biopsy, and the computer calculates the mechanical adjustments of the stereotactic frame to place the target point for biopsy in the target area of the frame.[74] Next, the neurosurgeon selects the entry point, and the computer overlays the vascular study. An avascular entry point is selected. The computer then calculates the trajectory for biopsy to reach target point.[74]

Kelly and colleagues[75–78] have developed an innovative method for integrating preoperative imaging information into the operating microscope field for deep-laser stereotactic resection of low- and high-grade astrocytomas, oligodendroglioma, and metastatic lesions. In 34 grade IV astrocytomas treated with either stereotactic biopsy (n = 27), or stereotactic laser resection (n = 7) followed by RT, the mean survival was 21 weeks for the biopsy cohort and 62 weeks for the resection cohort.[78] This was an uncontrolled study, with procedure selection by the neurosurgeon. The resection group had more discrete lesions with less brain infiltration or edema.

Computerized 3-D reconstruction can also be used for RT treatment planning.[14,70,79,80] Information from one or more imaging modalities can be converted to three dimensions.[14,79,80] If CT and MRI data are being used, a margin around the data set would be added to treat infiltrating cells beyond the CT hypodensity or the T2-weighted MRI abnormalilty.[80] The computer would select conformal radiation fields to minimize radiation dose to normal brain and optimally radiate the tumor-volume selected.

Computer imaging advances in the past decade have been staggering, and their applications are exciting. The future should bring further translation of these techniques into clinical practice, with benefit for the patient.

TUMOR TREATMENT AND IMAGING

Determination of Tumor Margins

Clinical treatment planning for brain tumors requires an understanding of tumor margins in this predominantly focal disease process. Gliomas extend along white matter tracts peripherally into other lobes, deeply into the white matter and brainstem and across the corpus callosum to the opposite hemisphere.[81] CT and MRI have been rapidly assimilated into clinical practice because they enable clinicians to visualize tumor, necrosis, and edema, but they have given rise to a question: Does tumor visualized on CT and MRI scans accurately mirror histopathology from surgical specimens or time-locked autopsy material?

Burger and coworkers[82] compared clinical history with CT and matched whole-mount surgical or autopsy specimens in 20 patients with glioblastoma multiforme. They examined untreated, quiescent, and recurrent tumors. CT scans of the untreated lesions revealed a necrotic center, with a rim of contrast enhancement surrounded by low-density area. The whole-mount pathology showed necrotic areas corresponding to CT necrotic center, with a dense cellular rim of small anaplastic cells and significant vascular proliferation where CT contrast enhancement was seen. In untreated patients, the total imaging abnormality enhancement and low-density area contained the neoplasm, but tumor extended beyond the enhancing area, into the low-density area. Small anaplastic cells may have been present in more distant regions.[82]

Daumas-Duport and associates[83] compared diagnostic stereotactic biopsy specimens with preoperative CT in 100 patients with astrocytoma, oligo-astrocytoma, and oligodendrocytoma (oligodendroglioma). They found that solid tumor and microvascularity were observed only in the contrast-enhancing regions, confirming the CT findings in untreated gliomas of Burger and colleagues.[82] No correlation was found between contrast enhancement and malignancy, although contrast enhancement was a constant feature of grade IV gliomas. CT low attenuation corresponded to either edema or edematous parenchyma infiltrated by isolated tumor cells.[83]

Lesions in remission were localized necrotic masses with CT contrast enhancement in the most cellular areas and low-density regions, corresponding to pathologic edema. Vascular proliferation was absent or minor, and neoplastic cells were confined to the original tumor bed. Recurrent lesions were markedly different, with small anaplastic tumor cells extending far beyond the matched CT low-density area, and in two cases extending to the opposite hemisphere without radiologic abnormality.[83] In six patients, posterior fossa extension was seen pathologically but not on CT scan. CT was insensitive in documenting the invasiveness of recurrent gliomas.

Kelly and colleagues[20] extended the CT and stereotactic biopsy correlative pathology study of Daumas-Duport and associates[83] to include MRI. T_2-weighted high-signal MRI abnormalities extended significantly beyond the CT hypodensity. Stereotactic biopsies documented infiltrating tumor cells in areas of T_2-weighted high signal beyond CT hypodensity. Finally, and most importantly, tumor cells were found in "MRI normal brain," in both low- and high-grade astrocytomas. The frequency of tumor cell infiltration into "MRI normal brain" was greater in LGA. In a separate report,[84] the same group found MRI contrast enhancement corresponded to vascular proliferation, tumor extended beyond enhancement, and areas of decreased signal corresponded to necrosis. These results were similar to the CT stereotactic biopsy pathology study results of Daumas-Duport and colleagues.[83] The MRI area of contrast enhancement in this study was greater than on CT.

Chamberlain and coworkers[33] reported the absence of CT contrast enhancement in 4% of patients with glioblastoma and in 54% of patients with highly anaplastic astrocytoma.

In summary, in high-grade astrocytomas, the MRI area of enhancement and T_2-weighted increased signal is greater than the CT area of enhancement and hypodensity. In LGA, the MRI T_2-weighted area of increased signal is greater than the CT hypodensity. Low- and high-grade astrocytomas frequently have infiltrating tumor cells beyond the area of MRI T_2-weighted abnormality. CT and MRI abnormalities frequently do not accurately reflect the extent of solid or infiltrating tumor. Most randomized clinical trials continue to use survival as the primary endpoint, at least partly because of uncertainties in documenting accurately the extent of disease and response.

Timing of Scans

Surgical disruption of the BBB can cause increased CT or MRI contrast enhancement and increased ^{201}Tl uptake.[51,54] FDG-PET glucose utilization is unaffected by surgical procedures.[41] Cairncross and associates[85] performed serial CT scans in the postoperative period in 10 patients with gliomas or metastatic lesions and found that surgical contrast enhancement did not appear until the fifth postoperative day and was most intense at 2 weeks postoperatively. CT was recommended for the third or fourth postoperative day for the accurate assessment of residual tumor. After surgery, MRI enhancement may appear within the first 24 hours, both in the tumor bed and the meninges, clouding the interpretation of postoperative MRI.[86,87]

Steroids affect the degree of contrast enhancement on CT and MRI scans[51] but not ^{201}Tl uptake in SPECT[54] or FDG-PET scans.[44] After an increase in steroid dose, determining MRI or CT tumor treatment response is problematic. Serial response imaging with ^{201}Tl SPECT and FDG-PET is unaffected by steroids, but the anatomical definition is poorer. In addition, low-grade tumors may not image distinctly with these tracers. It is far easier to obtain a scan for treatment response before changing the steroid dose.

Definition of Response

Using a widely accepted simple set of standard response criteria for both phase II and III clinical trials is important. It helps clinicians to compare patients' therapeutic responses in studies by individual investigators with the same or different therapeutic agents. It also provides more meaningful data for meta-analyses of small phase II trials. Four response categories are recommended: complete response (CR), partial response (PR), stable disease (SD), and progressive disease (PD) (Table 3–2). Response is based on a change in tumor size on enhanced CT or MRI at an interval from the treatment. No steroid dose increase is permitted in the interval between baseline and treatment scans to document response assessment as CR, PR, or SD.[88] The response must last for 1 month.

PR is usually defined as a decrease in contrast enhancement equal to or greater than 50% on stable or decreased doses of steroids, documented on two CT or MRI scans performed at least 1 month apart.[88] In some trials, a 25% reduction in contrast-enhancing size is considered a PR; in yet others, a fifth category representing a 25% reduction is added and labeled a "minor response."

PD is usually defined as a 25% increase in tumor enhancement but may be defined as a 50% increase in some studies. In systemic tumors, an increase of 50% is used to define PD, but this is probably too great a percentage increase for brain tumor clinical trials because the rigid, inelastic skull does not often allow a tumor growth of 50% before quality of life is compromised.

Grant and colleagues[89] examined the predictive ability of the four response categories[88] in 136 patients with recurrent malignant astrocytoma treated with nitrosourea chemotherapy. None of the patients had complete responses. Patients with PD had significantly decreased survival compared with those with SD and PR. No significant difference existed between the PR and SD groups in time to progression or survival. No difference in survival was shown if PR was considered a 25%, rather than a 50%, tumor reduction. The value of a four-tiered system is not supported by this study;[89] in fact , the data support a two-tiered system of "PD" and "other."

Rozental and coworkers[91] measured FDG-PET glucose utilization shortly after treatment in two groups of patients: the first group, patients with malignant gliomas before and after chemotherapy;[90] and the second, patients with gliomas or metastases before and after stereotactic radiosurgery (SR). After chemotherapy, patients whose tumors had the greatest increase in glucose utilization (75% to 100%) had the shortest survival. The longest survival time occurred in patients who had a decrease in glucose uptake.[90] After SR, glucose utilization increased from 25% to 40% on day 1 postradiation and then de-

Table 3–2. **Treatment Response Critieria***

Category	Steroid Dose	Change in Enhancing Tumor**
Complete response (CR)	None	Complete resolution
Partial response (PR)	Stable or decreased	≥ 50% decrease
Stable disease (SD)	Stable or decreased	< 50% decrease, or < 25% increase
Progressive disease (PD)	Stable or increased	≥25% increase in existing tumor, any new tumor, or neurologically worse

* Table developed from Macdonald et al.[88]
** As documented on two CT or MRI scans at least 1 month apart.

creased to 10% below baseline to 10% above baseline at 7 days. No prognostic information was given.[91]

Pitfalls in Response Determination

Changes that may compromise determination of a patient's treatment response are important to recognize. Serial imaging studies may be performed with differing doses of contrast dye, or the timing between contrast injection and imaging may change. The patient may be positioned at a gantry angle different from that used in the original baseline scan. The CT windows, or the MRI T_1- and T_2-weighted TR and TE relaxation times, may change. Changes are much more likely to occur if the patient undergoes imaging in a new center, alternate machine, or with a different neuroradiologist prescribing the scan.

Quantitative examination of serial CT scans is also important. Serial quantitative CT enhancement volume measurements were compared with a quantitative visual "gestalt" change. Investigators found a significant change (± 20%) in 28% of quantitative comparisons when "gestalt" reading did not identify change.[92] The 20% change criteria used in this study is less than typical PR of 50% decrease, but significant 3-D changes may be missed when examining 2-D images. In clinical trials, the observer should be blinded to the identity of the individual, the treatment received, and the order of the scan. Careful attention must be paid by patient, resident, or colleague to changes in steroid dose.[51]

CHAPTER SUMMARY

CT and MRI have markedly increased neuro-oncologists' ability to:

1. visualize tumor and surrounding edema
2. define tumor margins
3. localize tumor for stereotactic biopsy and resection
4. plan and treat patients with focal external beam and interstitial RT
5. monitor treatment responses to therapeutic modalities
6. develop and implement criteria for tumor response
7. determine tumor recurrence

The development of CT and MRI has fostered a clinical partnership among neurologist, neurosurgeons, neuroradiologists, and radiation oncologist for the interpretation of scans, with the aims listed.

FDG-PET is the noninvasive procedure of choice for the determination of tumor recurrence versus radiation necrosis, but it is imperfect in patients heavily pretreated with high-dose RT. The exact role of SPECT in clinical practice is uncertain. SPECT can localize the tumor area of highest metabolism. In tumor-bearing animals, MRI spectroscopy serial imaging has shown early metabolic changes of energy depletion that correlate with tumor-cell cytotoxicity. It is premature to extrapolate predictive ability in a more heterogeneous human population. Echoplanar MR, a technique in development, will probably be able to measure regional cerebral blood flow changes and blood-to-brain transport of contrast agents.

Computer technology has allowed the co-registration of imaging techniques for surgical and RT treatment planning. MRI is the best method available for tumor margin determination. Tumor cells often extend beyond the area of T_2-weighted abnormality on SE sequences. Tumor response determination is made using MRI and CT scans and preset response criteria. The pitfalls of response determination involve the inadvertent use of different scanning techniques, with serial scan interpretation by different physicians and patients receiving different medications.

REFERENCES

1. Di Chiro, G, DeLaPaz, RL, Brooks, RA, et al: Glucose utilization of cerebral gliomas measured by 18F fluorodeoxyglucose and positron emission tomography. Neurology 32:1323–1329, 1982.
2. Patronas, NJ, Di Chiro, G, Kufta, C, et al: Prediction of survival in glioma patients by means of

positron emission tomography. J Neurosurg 62: 816–822, 1985.
3. Di Chiro, G: Positron emission tomography using [18F]fluorodeoxyglucose in brain tumors. A powerful diagnostic and prognostic tool. Invest Radiol 22:360–371, 1987.
4. Tyler, JL, Diksic, M, Villemure, J-G, et al: Metabolic and hemodynamic evaluation of gliomas using positron emission tomography. J Nucl Med 28:1123–1133, 1987.
5. Junck, L, Strawderman, M, Ross, DA, et al: Prognostic value of PET-FDG scans in untreated gliomas. Neurology 45(4):A387, 1995.
6. Mountz, JM, Raymond, PA, McKeever, PE, et al: Specific localization of thallium 201 in human high-grade astrocytoma by microautoradiography. Cancer Res 49:4053–4056, 1989.
7. Slizofski, WJ, Krishna, L, Katsetos, CD, et al: Thallium imaging for brain tumors with results measured by a semiquantitative index and correlated with histopathology. Cancer 74:3190–3197, 1994.
8. Vertosick, FT Jr, Selker, RG, Grossman, SJ, and Joyce, JM: Correlation of thallium-201 single photon emission computed tomography and survival after treatment failure in patients with glioblastoma multiforme. Neurosurgery 34:396–401, 1994.
9. Alexander, E III, Loeffler, JS, Schwartz, RB, et al: Thallium-201 technetium-99m HMPAO single-photon emission computed tomography (SPECT) imaging for guiding stereotactic craniotomies in heavily irradiated malignant glioma patients. Acta Neurochir (Wien) 122:215–217, 1993.
10. Hanson, MW, Glantz, MJ, Hoffman, JM, et al: FDG-PET in the selection of brain lesions for biopsy. J Comput Assist Tomogr 15(5):796–801, 1991.
11. Herholz, K, Pietrzyk, U, Voges, J, et al: Correlation of glucose consumption and tumor cell density in astrocytomas. J Neurosurg 79:853–858, 1993.
12. Levivier, M, Goldman, S, Pirotte, B, et al: Diagnostic yield of stereotactic brain biopsy guided by positron emission tomography with [18F]fluorodeoxyglucose. J Neurosurg 82:445–452, 1995.
13. Janus, TJ, Kim, EE, Tilbury, R, et al: Use of [18F]fluorodeoxyglucose positron emission tomography in patients with primary malignant brain tumors. Ann Neurol 33:540–548, 1993.
14. Glatstein, E, Lichter, AS, Fraass, BA, et al: The imaging revolution and radiation oncology: use of CT, ultrasound, and NMR for localization, treatment planning and treatment delivery. Int J Radiat Oncol Biol Phys 11:299–314, 1985.
15. Bragg, DG, and Osborn, AG: CNS imaging of neoplasms. Int J Radiat Oncol Biol Phys 21:841–845, 1991.
16. Jaeckle, KA: Neuroimaging for central nervous system tumors. Seminars in Oncology 18(2):150–157, 1991.
17. Byrne, TN: Imaging of gliomas. Semin Oncol 21(2):162–171, 1994.
18. Zimmerman, RA: Imaging of adult central nervous system primary malignant gliomas. Staging and follow-up. Cancer 67:1278–1283, 1991.
19. Price, AC, Runge, VM, Allen, JH, et al: Primary glioma: diagnosis with magnetic resonance imaging. J Comput Tomogr 10:325–334, 1986.
20. Kelly, PJ, Daumas-Duport, C, Scheithauer, BW, et al: Stereotactic histologic correlations of computed tomography- and magnetic resonance imaging-defined abnormalities in patients with glial neoplasms. Mayo Clin Proc 62:450–459, 1987.
21. Segall, HD, Destian, S, Nelson, MD, et al: CT and MR imaging in malignant gliomas. In Apuzzo, MLJ (ed): Malignant Cerebral Gliomas. American Association of Neurosurgeons, Park Ridge, Illinois, 1990, pp 63–77.
22. Jolesz, FA, Schwartz, RB, and Guttmann, CRG: Diagnostic imaging of gliomas. In Black, PM, Schoene, WC, Lampson, LA (eds): Astrocytomas: Diagnosis, Treatment, and Biology. Blackwell Scientific Publications, Boston, 1993, pp 37–49.
23. Atlas, SW, Grossman, RI, Gomori, JM, et al: Hemorrhagic intracranial malignant neoplasms: Spin-echo MR imaging. Radiology 164:71–77, 1987.
24. Holland, BA, Kucharcyzk, W, Brant-Zawadzki, M, et al: MR imaging of calcified intracranial lesions. Radiology 157:353–356, 1985.
25. Daumas-Duport, C, Scheithauer, BW, and Kelly, PJ: A histologic and cytologic method for the spatial definition of gliomas. Mayo Clin Proc 62: 435–449, 1987.
26. Burger, PC: The anatomy of astrocytomas. Mayo Clin Proc 62:527–529, 1987.
27. Rogers, LR, Weinstein, MA, Estes, ML, et al: Diffuse bilateral cerebral astrocytomas with atypical neuroimaging studies. J Neurosurg 81:817–821, 1994.
28. Dooms, GC, Hecht, S, Brant-Zawadzki, M, et al: Brain radiation lesions: MRI imaging. Radiology 158:149–155, 1986.
29. Frytak, S, Earnest F, IV, O'Neill, BP, et al: Magnetic resonance imaging for neurotoxicity in long-term survivors of carcinoma. Mayo Clin Proc 60:803–812, 1985.
30. Hammoud, MA, Sawaya, R, Shi, W, et al: Prognostic significance of preoperative MRI scans in glioblastoma multiforme. J Neurooncol 27:65–73, 1996.
31. Brunberg, JA, Chenevert, TL, McKeever, PE, et al: In vivo MRI determination of water diffusion coefficients and diffusion anisotropy: correlation with structural alteration in gliomas of the cerebral hemispheres. Am J Neuroradiol 16:361–371, 1995.
32. Leeds, NE, and Kumar, AJ: Diagnostic imaging: Magnetic resonance imaging and computed tomography. In Levin, VA (ed): Cancer in the Nervous System. Churchill Livingstone, New York, 1996, pp 13–49.
33. Chamberlain, MC, Murovic, JA, and Levin, VA: Absence of contrast enhancement on CT brain scans of patients with supratentorial malignant gliomas. Neurology 38:1371–1374, 1988.

34. Thomas, DGT, Gill, SS, and Wilson, C: Current and future utilization of PET scanning in the evaluation and management of malignant cerebral glioma. In Apuzzo, MLJ (ed): Malignant Cerebral Glioma. American Association of Neurosurgeons, Park Ridge, Illinois, 1990, pp 79–89.
35. Phelps, ME, Huang, SC, Hoffman, EJ, et al: Tomographic measurement of local cerebral glucose metabolic rate in humans with (F-18)2-fluoro-2-deoxy-D-glucose: Validation of method. Ann Neurol 6:371–388, 1979.
36. Doyle, WK, Budinger, TF, Valk, PE, et al: Differentiation of cerebral radiation necrosis from tumor recurrence by [^{18}F]FDG and ^{82}Rb positron emission tomography. J Comput Assist Tomogr 11(4):563–570, 1987.
37. Bergström, M, Collins, VP, Ehrin, E, et al: Discrepancies in brain tumor extent as shown by computed tomography and positron emission tomography using [^{68}Ga]EDTA, [^{11}C]glucose, and [^{11}C]methionine. J Comput Assist Tomogr 7(6): 1062–1066, 1983.
38. Alavi, JB, Alavi, A, Chawluk, J, et al: Positron emission tomography in patients with glioma: A predictor of prognosis. Cancer 62:1074–1078, 1988.
39. Francavilla, TL, Miletich, RS, Di Chiro, G, et al: Positron emission tomography in the detection of malignant degeneration of low-grade gliomas. Neurosurgery 24:1–5, 1989.
40. Coleman, RE, Hoffman, JM, Hanson, MW, et al: Clinical application of PET for the evaluation of brain tumors. J Nucl Med 32:616–622, 1991.
41. Glantz, MJ, Hoffman, JM, Coleman, RE, et al: Identification of early recurrence of primary central nervous system tumors by [^{18}F]fluorodeoxyglucose positron emission tomography. Ann Neurol 29:347–355, 1991.
42. Ishikawa, M, Kikuchi, H, Miyatake, S, et al: Glucose consumption in recurrent gliomas. Neurosurgery 33:28–33, 1993.
43. Chang, SM, Barker, FG, Pounds, TR, et al: 18-fluorodeoxyglucose uptake and survival in patients with suspected recurrent malignant glioma. J Neurooncol 28:85, 1996.
44. Mineura, K, Sasajima, T, Kowada, M, et al: Perfusion and metabolism in predicting the survival of patients with cerebral gliomas. Cancer 73: 2386–2394, 1994.
45. Ogawa, T, Uemura, K, Shishido, F, et al: Changes of cerebral blood flow, and oxygen and glucose metabolism following radiochemotherapy of gliomas: A PET study. J Comput Assist Tomogr 12(2):290–297, 1988.
46. Derlon, J-M, Bourdet, C, Bustany, P, et al: [^{11}C]L-methionine uptake in gliomas. Neurosurgery 25:720–728, 1989.
47. Ericson, K, Lilja, A, Bergström, M, et al: Positron emission tomography with ([^{11}C]methyl)-L-methionine, [^{11}C]D-glucose, and [^{68}Ga]EDTA in supratentorial tumors. J Comput Assist Tomogr 9(4):683–689, 1985.
48. Mitsuki, S, Diksic, M, Conway, T, et al: Pharmacokinetics of ^{11}C-labelled BCNU and SarCNU in gliomas studied by PET. J Neurooncol 10:47–55, 1991.
49. Tsurumi, Y, Kameyama, M, Ishiwata, K, et al: ^{18}F-fluoro-2'-deoxyuridine as a tracer of nucleic acid metabolism in brain tumors. J Neurosurg 72:110–113, 1990.
50. Junck, L, Olson, JMM, Ciliax, A, et al: PET imaging of human gliomas with ligands for the peripheral benzodiazepine binding site. Ann Neurol 26:752–758, 1989.
51. Cairncross, JG, Macdonald, DR, Pexman,, W, Iand ves FJ: Steroid-induced CT changes in patients with recurrent malignant glioma. Neurology 38:724–726, 1988.
52. Guth-Tougelidis, B, Muller, S, Mehdorn, MM, et al: Uptake of DL-3-123I-iodo-alpha-methyltyrosine in recurrent brain tumors. Nuklearmedizin 34(2):71–75, 1995.
53. O'Tuama, LA, Packard, AB, and Treves, ST: SPECT imaging of pediatric brain tumor with hexakis (methoxyisobutylisonitrile) technetium (I). J Nucl Med 31(12):2040–2041, 1990.
54. Black, KL, Hawkins, RA, Kim, KT, et al: Use of thallium-201 SPECT to quantitate malignancy grade of gliomas. J Neurosurg 71:342–346, 1989.
55. Kaplan, WD, Takvorian, T, Morris, J, et al: Thallium-201 brain tumor imaging: A comparative study with pathologic correlation. J Nucl Med 28:47–52, 1987.
56. Lorberboym, M, Baram, J, Feibel, M, et al: A prospective evaluation of thallium-201 single photon emission computerized tomography for brain tumor burden. Int J Radiat Oncol Biol Phys 32(1):249–254, 1995.
57. Carvalho, PA, Schwartz, RB, Alexander, E III, et al: Detection of recurrent gliomas with quantitative thallium-201/technetium-99m HMPAO single-photon emission computerized tomography. J Neurosurg 77:565–570, 1992.
58. Caveness, WF: Pathology of radiation damage to the normal brain of the monkey. Natl Cancer Inst Monogr 46:57–76, 1977.
59. Plotnikova, ED, Levitman, MK, Shaposhnikova, VV, et al: Protection of microvasculature in rat brain against late radiation injury by gammaphos. Int J Radiat Oncol Biol Phys 15: 1197–1201, 1988.
60. Ross, BD, Ben-Yoseph, O, and Chenevert, TL: In vivo magnetic resonance imaging and spectroscopy: Application to brain tumors. In Bachelard, HS (ed): Magnetic Resonance Spectroscopy and Imaging in Neurochemistry (Vol. 8 of Advances in Neurochemistry). Plenum Press, New York, 1997, pp 145–178.
61. Ott, D, Hennig, J, and Ernst, T: Human brain tumors: Asessment with in vivo proton MR spectroscopy. Radiology 186:745–752, 1993.
62. Hubesch, B, Sappey-Marinier, D, Roth, K, et al: P-31 MR spectroscopy of normal human brain and brain tumors. Radiology 174:401–409, 1990.
63. Rottenberg, DA, Ginos, JZ, Kearfott, KJ, et al: In vivo measurement of brain tumor pH using [^{11}C]DMO and positron emission tomography. Ann Neurol 17:70, 1985.
64. Heesters, MAAM, Kamman, RL, Mooyaart, EL, and Go, KG: Localized proton spectroscopy of inoperable brain gliomas. Response to radiation therapy. J Neurooncol 17:27–35, 1993.

65. Herholz, K, Heindel, W, Luyten, PR, et al: In vivo imaging of glucose consumption and lactate concentration in human gliomas. Ann Neurol 31:319–327, 1992.
66. Usenius, J-PR, Kauppinen, RA, Vainio, PA, et al: Quantitative metabolite patterns of human brain tumors: detection of 1H NMR spectroscopy in vivo and in vitro. J Comput Assist Tomogr 18(5): 705–713, 1994.
67. Ben-Yoseph, O, and Ross, BD: Oxidation therapy: The use of a reactive oxygen species-generating system for tumour treatment. Br J Cancer 70:1131–1135, 1994.
68. Ross, BD, Kim, B, and Davidson, BL: Assessment of ganciclovir toxicity to experimental intracranial gliomas following recombinant adenoviral-mediated transfer of the herpes simplex virus thymidine kinase gene by magnetic resonance imaging and proton magnetic resonance spectroscopy. Clin Cancer Res 1:651–657, 1995.
69. Pardo, FS, Aronen, HJ, Kennedy, D, et al: Functional cerebral imaging in the evaluation and radiotherapeutic treatment planning of patients with malignant glioma. Int J Radiat Oncol Biol Phys 30(3):663–669, 1994.
70. Fraass, BA, and McShan, DL: 3-D treatment planning: I Overview of a clinical planning system. In Bruinvis, IAD (ed): The Use of Computers in Radiation Therapy. Elsevier Science Publishers BV, Amsterdam, 1987, pp 273–276.
71. Kelly, PJ, Daumas-Duport, C, Kispert, DB, et al: Imaging-based stereotaxic serial biopsies in untreated intracranial glial neoplasms. J Neurosurg 66:865–874, 1987.
72. Jolesz, FA, Kikinis, R, Cline, HE, and Lorensen, WE: The use of computerized image processing for neurosurgical planning. In Black, PM, Schoene, WC, and Lampson, LA (eds): Astrocytomas: Diagnosis, Treatment, and Biology. Blackwell Scientific Publications, Boston, 1993, pp 50–56.
73. Zamorano, L, Katanick, D, Dujovny, M, et al: Tumour recurrence vs radionecrosis: An indication for multitrajectory serial stereotactic biopsies. Acta Neurochir 46(Suppl):90–93, 1989.
74. Kelly, PJ, Earnest, F IV, Kall, BA, et al: Surgical options for patients with deep-seated brain tumors: Computer-assisted stereotactic biopsy. Mayo Clin Proc 60:223–229, 1985.
75. Kelly, PJ, Kall, BA, Goerss, S, and Cascino, TL: Results of computer-assisted stereotactic laser resection of deep-seated intracranial lesions. Mayo Clin Proc 61:20–27, 1986.
76. Kelly, PJ, Kall, BA, Goerss, S, and Earnest, F IV: Computer-assisted stereotaxic laser resection of intra-axial brain neoplasms. J Neurosurg 64: 427–439, 1986.
77. Kelly, PJ: Volumetric stereotactic surgical resection on intra-axial brain mass lesions. Mayo Clin Proc 63:1186–1198, 1988.
78. Kelly, PJ: Stereotactic biopsy and resection of thalamic astrocytomas. Neurosurgery 25:185–195, 1989.
79. Thornton, AF Jr, Hegarty, TJ, Ten Haken, RK, et al: Three-dimensional treatment planning of astrocytomas: A dosimetric study of cerebral irradiation. Int J Radiat Oncol Biol Phys 20:1309–1315, 1991.
80. Ten Haken, RK, Thornton, AF Jr, Sandler, HM, et al: Quantitative assessment of the addition of MRI to CT-based 3-D treatment planning of brain tumors. Radiotherapy and Oncology 25: 121–133, 1992.
81. Salazar, OM, Rubin, P: The spread of glioblastoma multiforme as a determining factor in the radiation treated volume. Int J Radiat Oncol Biol Phys 1:627–637, 1976.
82. Burger, PC, Dubois, PJ, Schold, SC Jr, et al: Computerized tomographic and pathologic studies of the untreated, quiescent, and recurrent glioblastoma multiforme. J Neurosurg 58:159–169, 1983.
83. Daumas-Duport, C, Monsaigneon, V, Blond, S, et al: Serial stereotactic biopsies and CT scan in gliomas: correlative study in 100 astrocytomas, oligo-astrocytomas and oligodendrocytomas. J Neurooncol 4:317–328, 1987.
84. Earnest, F IV, Kelly, PJ, Scheithauer, BW, et al: Cerebral astrrocytomas: Histopathologic correlation of MR and CT contrast enhancement with stereotactic biopsy. Radiology 166:823–827, 1988.
85. Cairncross, JG, Pexman, JHW, Rathbone, MP, and DelMaestro, RF: Postoperative contrast enhancement in patients with brain tumor. Ann Neurol 17:570–572, 1985.
86. Burke, JW, Podrasky, AE, and Bradley ,WG Jr: Meninges: benign postoperative enhancement on MR images. Radiology 174:99–102, 1990.
87. Elster, AD, and DiPersio, DA: Cranial postoperative site: assessment with contrast-enhanced MR imaging. Radiology 174:93–98, 1990.
88. Macdonald, DR, Cascino, TL, Schold, SC Jr, and Cairncross, JG: Response criteria for phase II studies of supratentorial malignant glioma. J Clin Oncol 8(7):1277–1280, 1990.
89. Grant, R, Liang, B, Greenberg, HS, and Junck, L: Chemotherapy response criteria in malignant glioma. Neurology 46:A474, 1996.
90. Rozental, JM, Levine, RL, Nickles, RJ, and Dobkin, JA: Glucose uptake by gliomas after treatment. A positron emission tomographic study. Arch Neurol 46:1302–1307, 1989.
91. Rozental, JM, Levine, RL, Mehta, MP, et al: Early changes in tumor metabolism after treatment: The effects of stereotactic radiotherapy. Int J Radiat Oncol Biol Phys 20:1053–1060, 1991.
92. Mahaley, MS Jr, Gillespie, GY, and Hammett, R: Computerized tomography brain scan tumor volume determinations. J Neurosurg 72:872–878, 1990.

Chapter 4

SURGERY FOR BRAIN TUMORS

GENERAL PRINCIPLES
OPEN SURGERY
STEREOTACTIC SURGERY
ENDOSCOPIC SURGERY

Surgery for neoplasms within the brain and its surrounding structures has evolved over the past 100 years. The advent of the operating microscope in the 1970s and computerized imaging and guidance in the 1990s have provided significant technical advances in surgical technique. This chapter will outline the principal factors involved in neurosurgical procedures.

GENERAL PRINCIPLES

The main guiding principle of intracranial tumor surgery is maximum resection with minimal or no harm to neural or supporting structures. A wide range of surgical approaches designed to provide access to tumors and minimize damage to the brain has been developed and refined over the decades. Modern computer-driven imaging has provided an entirely new way of localizing lesions, both before and during surgical procedures.

Another principle guiding the surgeon is the importance of placing the role of surgery in an informed perspective with other methods of treatment. For example, although a large prolactin-producing pituitary tumor may be readily and safely reached with the transsphenoidal approach, simple treatment with oral bromocriptine is the preferred and definitive treatment.

It is also important to individualize every operation to the overall needs and prognosis of the patient involved. A situation may arise in which a given approach would allow access to a tumor, but the short life expectancy of the individual would not warrant the discomfort and hospitalization required by the procedure.

Surgeons and institutions should also know the limits of the surgical skills available and be willing to refer the patient to a location where the most appropriate procedure can be performed. Surgeons need to know when to solicit the assistance of colleagues in other surgical and medical specialties to assist with certain operative procedures.

Preoperatively, assessment of patients with brain tumors includes evaluation of general medical risks for surgery and evidence of neoplasm in other locations. Most patients are loaded with an anticonvulsant prior to surgery even if no history of seizures exists. Intraoperatively, mannitol is usually given intravenously to help shrink the surrounding brain to allow safer access to the region of the tumor. Steroids, usually decadron 4 mg every 6 hours, are given on the day of surgery and gradually tapered postoperatively. Hyperventilation to a CO_2 level of 25 mEq/L is generally used during open procedures to reduce brain volume.

Postoperatively, patients undergoing open surgery are watched in an intensive care unit for 24 hours. Patients who have undergone stereotactic procedures may go directly to a standard hospital room to be discharged the next day. Patients are watched for any sign of postoperative intracranial bleeding or seizures. Patients usually continue with prophylactice treatment with an anticonvulsant drug for 2 to 3 months postoperatively.

Patients who have hydrocephalus related to obstruction of cerebrospinal fluid (CSF) pathways may require a ventriculoperitoneal shunt prior to or after tumor removal. Tumor resection often alleviates the obstruction, thus eliminating the need for shunting.

Modern neurosurgery can approach lesions of the brain in a variety of different ways, which are described in the appropriate sections of this chapter: open, or traditional craniotomy; stereotactic; and endoscopic. As technology advances, the boundaries between even these categories begin to blur.

OPEN SURGERY

Traditionally, most intracranial tumors have been accessed by a sizable craniotomy flap and direct visualization of the lesion. Localization has been greatly enhanced by computed tomography (CT) and magnetic resonance imaging (MRI), but defining the lesion at the time of surgery has still largely been a matter of the surgeon's judgment and the availability of anatomic landmarks. Intraoperative ultrasound, introduced in the early 1980s, provided the first intraoperative localization of intracerebral tumors.[1] This technique is still used widely and provides the only true "real-time" look at the anatomic location of a tumor.

With the development of the link between computerized imaging and stereotactic equipment in the mid-1980s, surgeons began to perform craniotomies with patients in a stereotactic frame, thus providing accurate localization of deep brain lesions. In the mid-1990s, sophisticated "frameless stereotactic" devices have proliferated, providing even better and more continuous intraoperative localization.[2] These frameless stereotactic systems work by computerized three-dimensional linkage of the preoperative imaging of the tumor to the surface landmarks of the patient during surgery. This provides the surgeon with immediate and three-dimensional feedback, which shows precisely where an instrument is placed or is heading within the entire intracranial space. This allows much more accurate identification of the borders between tumor and brain, thus allowing safer and greater resection of tumor tissue.

Over the past decade, CT scanners have been occasionally used in the operating room for localization. The latest intraoperative imaging technique involves open tumor resection actually within an MRI scanner.[3] Specially designed MRI units have enough room on either side of the patient for a person to stand and perform surgery with newly designed nonmagnetic instruments. This allows real-time assessment of the degree of tumor resection. Use of this equipment is expensive and cumbersome but has the advantage over framed or frameless stereotaxy because it assesses the actual residual tumor in its current anatomic location rather than relying on preoperative data.

The operating microscope was brought into clinical use in the neurosurgical operating room in the 1970s, originally for vascular lesions. It has become a standard operating tool for many surgical approaches to tumors, including most tumors deep in the brain or attached to cranial nerves. Ultrasonic aspiration devices and lasers are other tools that are available to assist in tumor resection, usually in conjunction with the microscope.

Although most open procedures are performed under general anesthesia, an increasing number of operative procedures require the patient to be awake. In patients who are awake, brain mapping for speech and vital motor areas is performed to safely demarcate the borders between tumor and eloquent areas of brain. Intraoperative electroencephalographic (EEG) monitoring may also assist in the resection of epileptogenic brain surrounding certain neoplasms.

During the past 10 years, considerable advances have been made in "skull base" surgery. Working closely with oncologic otorhinolargyngologist surgeons, neurosurgeons have developed a variety of approaches to the base of the skull, allowing much safer and wider resection of invasive tumors. Tumors invading or surrounding the internal carotid artery can now be resected by vein-graft bypassing of the carotid artery. Resected areas of the skull base can be reconstructed using vascularized free flaps, thus preventing CSF leakage. Tumors involving the cavernous sinus region can be more aggressively resected with preservation of cranial nerves. These techniques allow greater resection of benign tumors such as meningiomas and schwannomas and also malignant skull base and sinus tumors. These procedures involve the active cooperation and skills of ENTs and plastic surgeons.

STEREOTACTIC SURGERY

Stereotactic concepts and techniques have been used to localize intracranial structures for decades. In the 1950s and 1960s, frames were attached to the skull and brain landmarks were identified by the installation of intraventricular air or contrast material. Structures (e.g., the thalamus for thalamotomies) were calculated in relation to the third ventrical and the anterior commissure based on the appearance of the structures defined in atlases of the brain. Surprising accuracy could be achieved with these relatively crude systems.[4]

With the advent of CT scanning, deep anatomic structures and pathologic lesions were seen for the first time in detail. These identifiable structures could also be placed in a mathematical relationship to markers attached to the skull. A variety of frames have been devised to take advantage of these measurable relationships, thus allowing accurate stereotactic localization in the operating room. The advent of MRI made it natural to incorporate this even more detailed imaging modality into stereotactic systems.

Most "framed" stereotactic systems involve attaching an MRI-compatible metal device to the patient's skull using local anesthesia, then scanning the area of interest in either the CT or MRI scanner. The patient is then taken to the operating room, and a procedure is performed, usually under local anesthesia. The most common stereotactic procedure performed is needle biopsy of a deep brain lesion, usually a suspected tumor. Modern stereotactic systems can provide accuracy of 1 mm within the intracranial space. Stereotactic devices are also used to drain tumor cysts and to install chemotherapy or radioactive material within tumor cysts. An example of this is the installation of radioactive P32 within craniopharyngioma cysts.[5] Stereotactic systems are also used to place deep EEG electrodes in the brain and radioactive brachytherapy elements in tumors.

ENDOSCOPIC SURGERY

Opportunities for the use of endoscopic techniques for intracranial tumors are limited because of the relatively small extracerebral space within the cranium. These techniques are gaining wider acceptance and use because of the development of smaller and more refined endoscopic instruments.[6]

Patients who have a component of their tumor within the ventricular system and who have hydrocephalus may be candidates for endoscopic biopsy through the ventricular system. At the time of the biopsy, the floor of the third ventricle may be fenestrated to relieve the obstructive hydrocephalus.[7] An example of this is a tumor of the posterior third ventricle causing obstructive hydrocephalus. The endoscope can also be used within large cystic tumors to biopsy the wall of the cyst or a mural nodule under direct visualization.

Endoscopic instruments are also being used in selected intrasellar lesions through the transsphenoidal route. Although this does not provide nearly the view that is provided by an open microscopic transsphenoidal procedure, this procedure may be adequate for drainage of a cyst or debulking of a large soft adenoma.

Overall, significant technical advances continue, making surgical procedures for brain tumors safer and more effective. Specific surgical approaches are discussed in subsequent chapters.

REFERENCES

1. Rubin, JM, and Chandler, WF: Ultrasound in Neurosurgery. Raven Press, New York, 1990.
2. Spetzger, U, Laborde, G, and Gilsbach, JM: Frameless neuronavigation in modern neurosurgery. Minim Invasive Neurosurg 38:163–166, 1995.
3. Black, PM, Moriarty, T, Alexander, E, et al: Development and implementation of intraoperative magnetic resonance imaging and its neurosurgical applications. Neurosurgery 41:831–845, 1997.
4. Guiot, G, and Derome, P: The principles of stereotaxic thalamotomy. In Schneider, RC, Kahn, EA, Crosby, EC, and Taren, JA (eds): Correlative Neurosurgery, Charles C Thomas, Springfield, IL, 1982.
5. Saaf, M, Thoren, M, Bergstrand, CG, et al: Treatment of craniopharyngiomas - the stereotactic approach in a ten to twenty-three years' perspective. I. Surgical, radiological and ophthalmological aspects. Acta Neurochir (Wien) 99: 11–19, 1989.
6. Lewis, AI, Keiper, GL, and Crone, KR: Endoscopic treatment of loculated hydrocephalus. J Neurosurg 82:780–785, 1995.
7. Heilman, CB, and Cohen, AR: Endoscopic ventricular fenestration using a "saline torch." J Neurosurg 74:224–229, 1991.

Chapter 5

RADIATION THERAPY FOR BRAIN TUMORS: CURRENT PRACTICE

Radiation therapy (RT) is used frequently as a component of brain tumor therapy along with surgical resection and chemotherapy. Most often radiation therapy is used to treat neoplastic cells that remain *in situ* after a neurosurgical procedure; this helps define the tumor types for which RT has a role. That is, RT is generally used for invasive lesions that are difficult if not impossible to resect completely microscopically (i.e, most astrocytomas) or for lesions that, when accessible, are surgically curable but are technically unresectable (i.e., certain skull-based meningiomas). This chapter introduces radiotherapeutic principles, including the mechanisms of radiotherapy, issues regarding treatment regimens, radiotherapy planning and fractionation, and the tolerance of the normal central nervous system (CNS) to radiotherapy.

MECHANISMS OF RADIOTHERAPY

Radiotherapy, commonly delivered using external-beam treatment, consists of energetic photons in the range of 4 to 20 MeV x-rays created using a linear accelerator. The technology that allowed the widespread development of machines that could reliably deliver therapeutic doses was developed in the late 1950s and early 1960s. In the 1940s, cobalt-60 therapy units were the most widespread sources of therapeutic irradiation. Both linear accelerators and cobalt-60 units were significant improvements over lower-energy devices that were extensions of diagnostic radiology machines and operated at much lower energies. The use of higher-energy machines revolutionized RT because photons in this higher-energy range deposit dose deep to the skin; this allowed higher therapeutic doses to tumors (that is the dose was not limited, as in the past, by skin tolerance).

From a physics viewpoint, the ionizing radiation used for RT accounts for its action in cellular systems. Although the physics of the effect of ionizing RT are well known, the biologic response to irradiation is a very active area for investigation. Events that occur between photons and atomic electrons are the most common interactions between therapy-energy photons and matter that result in a transfer of energy to the target structure. At therapeutic photon energies, the interaction is through the Compton process.[1] Electrons are produced within tissue with various amounts of energy nearly up to the energy of the incident photons. Electrons with enough kinetic energy to disrupt other electrons are generated, and this disruption leads to the ionization of many molecules in tissue. Of importance for therapy are both the direct effect of electrons on DNA and an indirect effect on DNA secondary to creation of reactive-free radicals from water molecules. The presence of molecular oxygen leads to irreversible chemical changes in the double helix and solidifies the effect of x-rays on cellular DNA. Radiation has been long known to create single-strand breaks and double-strand breaks in DNA. The primary target of cellular injury is nuclear DNA, not other cellular elements (e.g., proteins, membranes). This is known from studies that involve selective cellular irradiation to either the cytoplasm or the nucleus. However, membrane effects may be very important in the cellular recognition of radiation-induced oxidative injury and may have a large effect in initiating the cellular response to radiation injury.

A complete discussion of the cellular response to irradiation is beyond the scope of this chapter. However, an introduction is appropriate because it is likely that radiation resistance is somehow related to various cellular response pathways, and experimental strategies (discussed in Chapter 6) are related to the current understandings of some of these.

Free radical–induced DNA damage, as describe previously, is a model for cellular injury that occurs during exposure to ionizing radiation, although it is likely that other mechanisms are involved. Cells have complex mechanisms for detecting radiation lesions and DNA damage and then repairing the injury. The ability of cells to repair potentially lethal DNA injury has been recognized for some time. Alternatively, rather than DNA repair, cells may undergo active DNA destruction and cellular suicide after exposure to ionizing radiation (i.e., programmed cell death, or apoptosis).[2] Investigation of the molecular biology involved in post-radiation cellular events (i.e., DNA repair, induction of apoptosis, effects on cell cycle checkpoints) may provide prognostic information or therapeutic strategies.

For example, the irradiation of normal cycling cells may lead to a number of events. Cells may undergo lethal DNA damage and rapid unregulated death; alternatively, if the cell survives the immediate free-radical insult, an increase in cellular p53 and cell cycle arrest in G1 are induced. Cells can either repair DNA damage or undergo apoptosis. Naturally, these pathways are highly regulated. The *Bcl-2* gene product interacts with other members from its family of genes, including *Bax* or *Bc-*, to either promote or inhibit the induction of apoptosis.[3] Tumor cells, including glial cell lines with mutant p53 proteins that are unable to use this pathway to undergo apoptosis, may then be more resistant to the effects of irradiation[4,5] although these data are conflicting.[6] Thus, determining the status of CNS tumors with respect to gene functions, such as the p53 or *Bcl-2* family members, may allow information regarding prognosis and may help direct therapy.

The understanding of the cellular events that occur after irradiation has been assisted by the elucidation of some of the pathways used in the repair process. For example, nucleotide excision repair, required to repair damage occurring during exposure to ultraviolet radiation, is defective in cells that carry the xeroderma pigmentosum mutation and results in frequent dermal neoplasia. In addition, cell lines from patients with ataxia-telangiectasia, a recessive disorder with neurological abnormalities related to gradual loss of Purkinje cells and extreme sensitivity to ionizing radiation, have altered cell cycle kinetics and loss of the normal G1 arrest after irradiation. However, the relationship between these changes and the radiosensitivity is unclear. Alteration in the cells' response to p53-induced apoptosis may be responsible.[7]

PRINCIPLES OF RADIOTHERAPY

Radiation Fractionation

Fractionation concepts tend to be perplexing to non-radiation oncologists and thus deserve some discussion. The term *fractionation* refers to the number of individual treatments used to deliver a planned total course of radiation. For example, to give a dose of 40 Gy to a tumor, one could prescribe 40 Gy in one treatment (or one fraction) or 2 Gy/fraction given once a day over 20 treatment days, 1 Gy/fraction given twice a day over 20 days, and so on.

Early this century, it was discovered that late side effects, such as fibrosis or chronic ulcers, were increased with respect to early side effects and tumor control when RT was given in relatively large dose (i.e. greater than or equal to 2.5 Gy/fraction) per fraction regimens. Early and late times refer to the periods after RT that these effects are noted. The reason for this difference (favoring smaller doses per fraction) is that distinct cellular components are responsible for these effects. Acutely responding tissues (i.e., skin) and tumor cells are generally more rapidly growing, generally spending more time actively moving throughout the cell cycle. Therefore, they are more likely to be damaged by RT during a sensitive portion of the cycle (i.e., M and G2). In contrast, the cells that are responsible, when damaged, for late effects and chronic complications (i.e., subepithelial fibroblasts, glial tissue) are more likely to be in G0 and be relatively resistant. To quote Hall,[8] "Fraction size is the dominant factor in determining late effects, while overall treatment time has little influence. By contrast, fraction size and overall treatment time both determine the response of acutely responding tissues."

These principles, gathered empirically over decades, explain attempts to increase the efficacy of RT by altering the standard fractionation regimen of 1.8 to 2.0 Gy/d. Attempts to increase the effect on tumor (and incidentally on acutely responding normal tissue) while sparing the late responding tissues generally consist of two fractions per day, so-called *hyperfractionation*. The Radiation Therapy Oncology Group (RTOG) has performed a number of studies investigating hyperfractionation in the treatment of CNS neoplasms. The group has completed two randomized dose-escalation studies for malignant glioma patients. The first one randomized patients to one of four treatment arms ranging in total dose from 64.8 to 81.6 Gy using a 1.2 Gy/fraction, twice-daily regimen. The second study randomized patients to either 48.0 or 54.4 Gy using 1.6 Gy/fraction twice daily. All told, the treatment arm with the best overall survival was the 72-Gy arm, perhaps indicating that the higher-dose arms were associated with an increase in toxicity despite the lower dose/fraction employed.[9,10] Neither of these studies had a comparison one fraction per day treatment arm. Another group used a fraction scheme that consisted of three times per day (TID) fractionation at 1 Gy/fraction.[11] This study was a sequential dose-escalation trial, and the highest dose reached 80 Gy. These investigators found no significant difference in median survival or time to progression among the three doses used, and they did not observe an increase in radiation complications with the escalated dose. One hypothesis for the lack of beneficial effect with the escalation in this study may be that the dose per fraction was too low and there was some sparing of the malignant cells. It may be that malignant astrocytomas behave somewhat like late-responding tissues with respect to dose per fraction. Although the results for CNS neoplasms have been disappointing to date, the concept of hyperfractionation has received some validation in a large study[12] from Europe for the treatment of squamous cell carcinoma of the oropharynx. In this two-arm trial, patients received either 70 Gy in standard, once-daily fractionation or 80.5 Gy given twice a day using 1.15 Gy fractions. They discovered statistically superior local tumor control, which has been translated into a trend in overall survival improvement. Importantly, the study showed no difference in late morbidity between the two treatment arms.

Note that *hypofractionation,* such as the large single-fraction technique used during typical radiosurgery treatments, has an increased effect on late-responding mature tissues, such as CNS parenchyma.

Radiation Therapy Techniques

Radiotherapy should be delivered to tissues that contain malignant cells in a dose sufficiently high to have an acceptable probability that these cells will be completely eliminated, while at the same time avoiding irradiation exposure to tissues that do not harbor a malignant cohort of cells. This obvious statement represents an idealized, nonclinical extrapolation and, in some fashion, also describes the idealized surgical approach to CNS neoplasms. Among the three general anticancer modalities (i.e., surgery, radiotherapy, and chemotherapy), radiotherapy and surgery are conceptually more closely related in their approach to a particular malignant process. Unfortunately, it is not usually known with certainty exactly where all the malignant cells are located. Although it is usually known from modern imaging results where gross accumulations of CNS neoplasia are lodged, the location of microscopic tumor cells in any individual situation is generally a speculative matter. Thus, compromises are made when designing RT to include tissues that contain gross disease but also may contain microscopic amounts of tumor that are not visible using any imaging modality.

Since the dose required to eradicate any amount of cancer is related to the number of cells present, it has become a standard technique in radiation oncology to use a "cone-down" technique. That is, tissue that is considered to contain both gross and microscopic disease is irradiated comprehensively to a dose known to be effective in eradicating microscopic amounts of

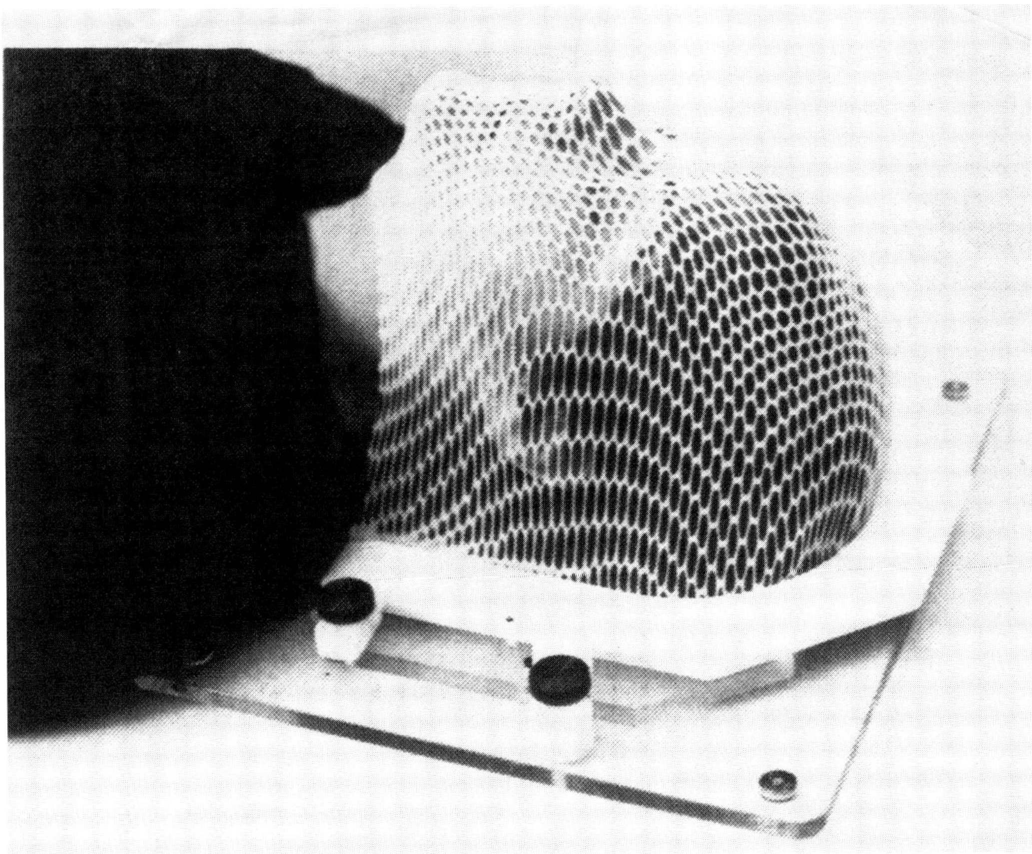

Figure 5–1. Patient immobilized in a thermoplastic mask for radiotherapy treatment of brain neoplasms. (Photograph courtesy of KGF Enterprise, Inc.)

Table 5–1. **Procedures Used During a Course of Radiotherapy**

Procedure	Purpose
Treatment simulation	Create custom immobilization
	Design treatment portals, unless additional treatment imaging required
Treatment imaging CT, MR	Additional imaging is often necessary to define the target volume, although sometimes previously acquired images may be used
Treatment planning	Tumor is defined on imaging datasets, critical normal structures are defined, and final treatment plan is created
First treatment day	Extra time is allotted to quality assure the entire treatment
Remainder of treatment	Usually Quality Assurance is weekly, additional planning for "cone down" may be required

tumor.[13] Then this larger treatment volume is reduced, and the therapy is directed only at the grossly identifiable disease. This accomplishes an improvement in risk/benefit ratio by tailoring the dose delivery to the density of tumor cells.

With the exception of single-dose radiosurgery treatments, RT is given in a fractionated manner; that is, the same treatment is given repeatedly over a course of therapy, with adjustments as necessary for cone-downs, as described. In order to ensure reproducible treatment for CNS neoplasms, patients must be placed in the treatment room, which contains a source of radiation, generally a linear accelerator, that rotates precisely about a fixed isocenter with minimal uncertainty (< 5 mm). In addition, since the treatment session may last approximately 15 minutes, the patient must be comfortably immobilized for treatment. This is usually accomplished by creating a customized mask-like device (Figure 5–1) marked with indelible lines by a laser light system in the room. This provides immobilization and reproducibility and does not interfere with the delivery of the radiation beam. The standard radiotherapy routine is outlined in Table 5–1.

Defining the target that is considered to be at risk for involvement by microscopic disease is a critical part of the design of RT plans. The current formalism in RT consists of three separate volumes that are helpful to consider for conceptual purposes (Table 5–2).

For example, when treating an infiltrating lesion such as a malignant astrocytoma, the gross tumor volume (GTV) consists of the enhancing lesion imaged on

Table 5–2. **Radiotherapy Tumor and Target Volumes**[40]

Volume	Definition
Gross tumor volume (GTV)	Gross palpable or visible/demonstrable extent of lesion
Clinical target volume (CTV)	Contains GTV and/or subclinical microscopic disease that has to be eliminated
Planning target volume (PTV)	Contains CTV and adds the net effect of all possible geometrical variations and inaccuracies in order to ensure that the prescribed dose is actually absorbed in the CTV

International Commission on Radiological Units definitions.

computed tomography (CT) or magnetic resonance imaging (MRI). The clinical target volume (CTV) adds 1 to 2 cm to account for subclinical infiltration, and 0.5 cm is added for uncertainties associated with treatment setup. For a non-infiltrating lesion such as a benign meningioma, the GTV consists of the enhancing lesion. The CTV may be the same as the GTV because no microscopic invasion is present, and 0.5 cm would be added to account for setup uncertainty. Thus, one adjusts the volume treated depending on the volume of tissue that may contain microscopic tumor infiltration.

TOLERANCE OF THE BRAIN TO RADIATION THERAPY

The tolerance of the normal brain to therapeutic doses of RT is a concept frequently discussed but not well understood. What is meant by "tolerance"? In general in RT literature, it is assumed that complications increase with dose according to a sigmoid-shaped, dose-response curve, a relationship that is derived from the statistically random nature inherent in the probability that irradiated cells will be inactivated.[14] Therefore, the tolerance is defined as the dose associated with a defined risk of complications, that is, the dose associated with a 5% risk of a certain complication, a 50% risk, and so on. However, this is a vast simplification. Generally, the dose-toxicity curves for humans are elucidated from limited retrospective data concerning whole-organ treatment.[15] Although most treatment is delivered to partial organs, even partial-organ therapy can result in vastly different clinical expressions of therapeutic complications. As an example involving the CNS, consider partial spinal cord irradiation: even if a small segment of the spinal cord is affected by RT, the clinical manifestations are severe. The entire organ can stop functioning in this situation. In analogy with electrical circuits, the spinal cord would be considered an organ arranged *in series:* any injury that interrupts the continuity of the organ results in functional deficits. In contrast, an organ such as the liver, which is constructed with many subunits arranged *in parallel,* can sustain a substantial loss of functional tissue before injury becomes clinically apparent.[14]

The risk that a patient will develop a clinically significant complication depends on many factors, including the volume irradiated, the dose of RT, the function of the tissue irradiated, the clinical effect of the loss of that function, the malignancy of the tumor, and the age of the patient. Elderly patients with malignant gliomas have a different chance of developing radiation-induced neoplasms than do young patients with more curable lesions. Risk should not necessarily be avoided at all times; that is, strict dose restrictions may be detrimental to patient outcome. Maintaining a dose of 60 Gy for patients with glioblastoma multiforme to avoid a risk of RT complications seems irrational in the face of an overwhelming probability of tumor recurrence; however, doses should be increased only as improved tumor control is evident. Outcome data for interstitial brachytherapy indicate that patients who developed radiation necrosis and required surgical management of this "complication" actually had a better outcome than did patients who did not develop this side effect. These data indicate that an event that may be considered adverse in the abstract had a net benefit for the individual.[16]

Radiation side effects are often discussed with respect to the time of occurrence because it relates to the cells affected by RT. Tissues may be (1) *rapidly proliferative* (as on most epithelial surfaces and in hair follicles) and respond to radiation quickly, usually during the course of RT; (2) *slowly proliferative* (as in endothelial and glial cells) and respond to radiation in a delayed manner months to years after a course of RT; or (3) *nonproliferative* (as in muscles and neurons) and only express injury indirectly due to damage of a proliferative component resulting in fibrosis, an obliterative vascular effect, or demyelinization, which in turn modifies the nonproliferative tissue.[17]

Based on these principles, early side effects, which are usually reversible, include cutaneous reactions; mucosal irritation; mild hematologic changes (primarily changes in lymphocyte numbers); and fatigue, a nonspecific effect of RT. Later manifestations include cognitive changes; frank radiation necrosis; and a number of other potential hazards, such as insufficiency of the hypothalamic-pituitary axis, optic nerve injury, and radiation-induced neoplasia.

RADIATION NECROSIS

Radiation necrosis is reaction that occurs in a region of relatively high radiation dose (i.e., it cannot occur at a distance from the high-dose volume). The primarily injured cells are the glial and vascular cellular compartments and not the postmitotic neuronal compartment. Radiation necrosis presents clinically as a contrast-enhancing mass lesion that is difficult to differentiate from a recurrent neoplasm; frequently, the two entities coexist. In experimental animal models, no pathognomonic pathological lesions are noted, although characteristic demyelinization and cell loss are noted in the white matter, where most RT-induced necrotic events occur.[18] Vascular lesions, including telangiectasias, thickening and hyalinization of vessel walls, and, frequently, fibroid necrosis (i.e., fibrin exudates surrounding necrotic small blood vessels) are also seen.[19] Burger and Boyko[19] note that a fibrin exudate in a layer of hypocellularity along the gray-white junction is a diagnostic pathological finding.

Radiation necrosis occurs usually between 6 to 24 months after a therapeutic course of conventional radiation, and 75% of cases occur within 3 years.[20] The time interval until the development of radiation necrosis is shortened after radiosurgery and interstitial therapy because of the intensity of the large dose per fraction scheme of radiosurgery and because of the very high doses delivered next to the radioactive sources during interstitial treatment. In addition, the time to necrosis is shortened when patients are re-treated with a second course of radiotherapy. The risk of RT necrosis is usually described in terms of the dose delivered, and it is clear that the dose per fraction is very important: when doses greater than 2 Gy/d are used to deliver high doses of therapy, the risk of RT necrosis increases.[21] However, for standard fractionation of 1.8 Gy/d, the risk is near 0 below 57.6 Gy, with 0 of 51 patients developing necrosis. For doses between 57.6 and 64.8 Gy, 2 of 60 patients developed necrosis, and among those who received 64.8 to 75.6 Gy, 5 of 28 developed necrosis.[22] Recall that necrosis may not be an absolute adverse event *per se,* especially if it results in longer tumor control. Modern imaging and RT techniques are treating much smaller volumes with high doses, and this will certainly influence the risk for necrosis and the morbidity of necrotic events, if they occur.

Therapy of radiation necrosis involves either corticosteroids alone, since some of these events are self-limited, or surgical removal of the necrotic foci.[23]

Diagnosis of radiation necrosis without surgical resection to provide tissue for pathological confirmation can be challenging. When confronted with a patient in the postradiation setting who has the typical features of an enlarging enhancing abnormality associated with adjacent edema and mass effect, clinical factors can be useful in contrasting the probability of necrosis with the probability of disease recurrence (Table 5–3).

(^{18}F)-2-fluoro-2-deoxyglucose positron emission tomography (FDG-PET) imaging can help distinguish between the two entities, although a hypometabolic PET image obviously cannot exclude a microscopic

Table 5–3. **Factors That Distinguish Radiation Necrosis from Recurrent Tumor**

Radiation Necrosis	Recurrent Tumor
6–24 months after RT	< 6 months,> 24 months
High-dose RT (> 65 Gy)	Low-dose RT (< 56 Gy)
Low-grade lesion	High-grade lesion
Lesion in high-dose volume	Lesion distant from high dose
^{18}F-FDG PET: Low uptake	^{18}F-FDG PET: High uptake

amount of active tumor. The basis for PET imaging as a useful test lies in the pathological characteristic of radiation necrosis as a hypovascular, necrotic, hypometabolic volume of brain versus the hypermetabolic behavior of recurrent neoplasm. In heavily pretreated patients (i.e., those treated with interstitial brachytherapy, hyperfractionation protocols, or radiosurgery), the risk of false-positive and false-negative PET scan results is higher.[24]

EFFECTS OF RADIOTHERAPY ON INTELLIGENCE

The intellectual changes that may occur as a consequence of RT are difficult to quantify and relate to patient and treatment factors. The variables that seem to be important in RT-induced injury include age at RT, volume irradiated, dose, and dose per fraction. However, other factors may be important in determining intellectual function after RT, including baseline function, chemotherapy and steroid use, direct tumor effect on sensorimotor function, loss of special sensory function (i.e., hearing deficits secondary to chemotherapy resulting in difficulty learning), and poorly controlled hydrocephalus.[25]

Radiographically diffuse, high-signal, T_2-weighted white matter changes are seen on MRI scans, and other analogous changes are imaged less well on CT in a proportion of patients irradiated. These changes are related to brain volume irradiated, dose, and dose per fraction. Discussing the relationship between volume irradiated and risk of MRI-detected white matter changes, Constine et al,[26] used a four-tier system to grade the white matter changes (Table 5–4), where grade 1 and 2 lesions may occur in some normal persons. They found that whereas treatment using localized RT fields produces grade 3 or 4 lesions in 15% of patients, whole brain RT, with or without a local RT boost, produces the same grade lesions in 50%. Despite similar total doses, there was a marked increase in incidence in grade 3 and 4 lesions with whole brain RT, confirming the relationship between brain volume irradiated and morbidity, at least as far as white matter changes are concerned.

Notably, assignment to either local or whole brain treatment was not random in this retrospective analysis. The white matter changes seen are presumably pathologically related to diffuse effects, such as widespread demyelinization, endothelial cell proliferation and loss, and vasogenic edema, with ultimate evolution occurring with loss of brain substance and atrophy. Burger and Boyko[19] note that necrotic foci are usually not seen in the white matter of diffusely affected patients; rather, there is global effacement of the white matter, with pallor and reactive astrocytosis.

The effect of RT on intelligence is often considered in two separate clinical situations: (1) as prophylaxis using relatively low doses to prevent clinical CNS failure in patients known to be at high risk for subclinical involvement (e.g., children with acute lymphoblastic leukemia [ALL] or adults with small cell lung cancer); and (2) as therapy, usually using higher doses, in patients with clinical CNS disease (e.g., primary CNS tumors). The reported data are perhaps best for children irradiated as CNS prophylaxis for ALL, although results of the many studies conflict even in this setting. Typical CNS prophylaxis

Table 5–4. **MRI Grading System for White Matter Changes Seen Following Radiotherapy**[26]

Grade 1	Discontinuous periventricular hyperintensity (PVH)
Grade 2	Continuous PVH surrounding the ventricles (thin line)
Grade 3	Periventricular halo (thicker line)
Grade 4	Diffuse white matter abnormality extending from ventricles to gray-white junction

doses are 18 Gy or 24 Gy given at 1.5 to 2.0 Gy/fraction. A recent review by Roman and Sperduto[27] summarizes the literature.

Using IQ as a measure of intelligence, a group at St. Jude Children's Hospital[28] followed up with patients with ALL who received three different CNS prophylaxis regimens: (1) intravenous (IV) methotrexate (MTX) and intrathecal (IT) MTX without RT; (2) IT MTX and 18 Gy of cranial RT; and (3) IT MTX and 24 Gy of cranial RT. The patients were prospectively evaluated with IQ and academic achievement testing. Groups 1 and 2 (as described) had their type of CNS prophylaxis assigned as part of a randomized trial, reducing the potential for selection bias. During 4 years of follow-up, there were no significant IQ differences between the three groups; however, approximately 20% of each group did experience an IQ decrease of 15 points or more.

In contrast, a retrospective report from the M.D. Anderson Cancer Center [29,30] comparing children who received cranial RT and IT chemotherapy for leukemia or lymphoma with children who received chemotherapy for other malignancies without cranial RT, found decreases in IQ in the group who received the cranial RT.

An additional report from Australia[31] compared three groups of patients: 100 with ALL who received chemotherapy and cranial RT, 50 with other malignancies who received chemotherapy without cranial RT, and 100 healthy control subjects. Overall, significant differences were seen in cognitive skills between the group who received cranial RT and the other groups. The cranial RT dose employed was either 18 Gy or 24 Gy and was not randomly assigned. This study also found significant differences between the two dose levels with respect to intelligence and academic achievement, with the higher dose level having a greater decline in intelligence. This difference with respect to dose was also seen by Halberg and associates,[32] although it was not seen in the randomized comparison mentioned earlier.

The Australian study[31] also found an age relationship. That is, patients irradiated when older than 5 years of age had no difference in intelligence or academic performance when compared with healthy controls or patients who received chemotherapy without cranial RT.

Other recent pediatric studies examining intelligence after a pilot study of low-dose craniospinal radiotherapy for medulloblastoma therapy[33] or during total body irradiation[34] show no loss of intellectual capacity.

The contrasts in the findings among the studies mentioned here, some of which show an effect of RT on intellectual function and some of which do not, seems to typify the state of this field.

For children irradiated with higher doses in the cranium for primary tumors such as medulloblastoma, the long-term outcome may be worse than for ALL patients. Hoppe-Hirsch and colleagues[35] compared patients with medulloblastoma who received cranial RT doses of 35 Gy with patients with posterior fossa ependymoma who received posterior fossa RT only. At 1 year after treatment, there was no difference. Beyond 1 year, ependymoma patients irradiated to the posterior fossa had maintained their IQ level. However, the medulloblastoma patients had progressive decline in IQ, with only 20% having an IQ of more than 90. Surgical postoperative complications also increased the morbidity, with only approximately 30% of patients having an IQ greater than 90 at 1 to 2 years after treatment. These complications, usually related to brainstem involvement, were more common in the medulloblastoma group.

It is reasonable to conclude that doses of 18 Gy or less in patients older than 5 years of age are associated with minimal intellectual changes. Younger patients and those treated to higher doses are particularly at risk, although many factors need to be considered as potentially contributory to intellectual deficits after treatment.

Finally, the use of alternative treatment modalities to decrease RT use and RT morbidity must be considered carefully. Complications associated with potential alternatives must be compared carefully with RT and the risks associated with RT. A recent study was performed in an effort to avoid the effects of cranial RT in 71 children treated with primary chemotherapy and no RT for CNS germ cell tumors (including germinomas, a subset often cured with RT alone). Seven patients died from the study chemotherapy; of the survivors, 60% eventually received RT as part of salvage therapy after recurrence or after an incomplete response.[36] Thus, although the effects of RT should not be diminished, the potential toxicity of alternatives needs to be considered as well.

The data for adults are less clear and more contradictory than those for children. Two articles from a single issue of the *Journal of Clinical Oncology*, with an accompanying editorial,[37] recently examined the issue of prophylactic cranial irradiation (PCI) during the management of patients with small cell lung cancer (SCC). One article[38] suggests that PCI for SCC is toxic to the CNS and should be avoided because of the morbidity associated with it and the other demonstrates the efficacy of PCI in decreasing the incidence of CNS metastases without causing important CNS toxicity.[39] The editorial suggests that the explanation for the different observations is the difference between the two studies in the timing of the systemic chemotherapy and the radiotherapy–: the study that revealed toxicity used concurrent chemotherapy and radiotherapy, and the study without resulting toxicity used PCI after the systemic treatment was complete. Turrisi[37] therefore recommends PCI following systemic chemotherapy in this type of setting.

REFERENCES

1. Khan, FM: The Physics of Radiation Therapy. Williams & Wilkins, Baltimore, 1984, pp 67–86.
2. Dewey, WC, Ling, CC, and Meyn, RE: Radiation-induced apoptosis: Relevance to radiotherapy. Int J Radiat Oncol Biol Phys 33:781–96, 1995.
3. Oltvai, ZN, Milliman, CL, and Korsmeyer, SJ: Bcl-2 heterodimerizes in vivo with a conserved homolog, Bax, that accelerates programmed cell death. Cell 74:609–19, 1993.
4. McIlwrath, AJ, Vasey, PA, Ross, GM, and Brown, R: Cell cycle arrests and radiosensitivity of human tumor cell lines: dependence on wild-type p53 for radiosensitivity. Cancer Res 54:3718–22, 1994.
5. Kanady, K, Su ,M, and Pardo, FS: Mutant p53 transfection of low grade astrocytic cells alters cell cycle control, tumorigenicity and intrinsic radiation resistance (Meeting abstract). Growth Control in Central Nervous System: Angiogenesis, Boston, 1995.
6. Slichenmyer, WJ, Nelson, WG, Slebos, RJ, and Kastan, MB: Loss of a p53-associated G1 checkpoint does not decrease cell survival following DNA damage. Cancer Res 53:4164–4168, 1993.
7. Jorgensen, TJ, and Shiloh, Y: The ATM gene and the radiobiology of ataxia-telangiectasia. Int J Radiat Biol 69:527–537, 1996.
8. Hall, EJ: Radiobiology for the Radiologist, Ed 4. J B Lippincott Co, Philadelphia, 1994, pp 211–229.
9. Murray, KJ, Nelson, DF, Scott, C, et al: Quality-adjusted survival analysis of malignant glioma. Patients treated with twice-daily radiation (RT) and carmustine: A report of Radiation Therapy Oncology Group (RTOG) 83–02. Int J Radiat Oncol Biol Phys 31:453–459, 1995.
10. Curran, WJ Jr, Scott, CB, Horton, J, et al: Recursive partitioning analysis of prognostic factors in three Radiation Therapy Oncology Group malignant glioma trials. J Natl Cancer Inst 85:704–710, 1993.
11. Fulton, DS, Urtasun, RC, Scott-Brown, I, et al: Increasing radiation dose intensity using hyperfractionation in patients with malignant glioma. Final report of a prospective phase I-II dose response study. J Neurooncol 14:63–72, 1992.
12. Horiot, JC, Le Fur, R, N'Guyen, T, et al: Hyperfractionation versus conventional fractionation in oropharyngeal carcinoma: Final analysis of a randomized trial of the EORTC cooperative group of radiotherapy. Radiother Oncol 25:231–241, 1992.
13. Fletcher, GH: Clinical dose-response curves of human malignant epithelial tumours. Br J Radiol 46:1–12, 1973.
14. Withers, HR: Biological basis of radiation therapy. In Perez, CA, and Brady, LW (eds): Principles and Practice of Radiation Oncology. J B Lippincott Co, Philadelphia, 1992, pp 64–96.
15. Emami, B, Lyman, J, Brown, A, et al: Tolerance of normal tissue to therapeutic irradiation. Int J Radiat Oncol Biol Phys 21:109–22, 1991.
16. Gutin, PH, Prados, MD, Phillips, TL, et al: External irradiation followed by an interstitial high activity iodine-125 implant "boost" in the initial treatment of malignant gliomas: NCOG study 6G-82–2. Int J Radiat Oncol Biol Phys 21:601–606, 1991.
17. Rubin, P: The Franz Buschke lecture: late effects of chemotherapy and radiation therapy: A new hypothesis. Int J Radiat Oncol Biol Phys 10:5–34, 1984.
18. Schultheiss, TE, Kun, LE, Ang, KK, and Stephens, LC: Radiation response of the central nervous system [published erratum appears in Int J Radiat Oncol Biol Phys 1995 Jul 15;32(4): 1269]. Int J Radiat Oncol Biol Phys 31:1093–1112, 1995.
19. Burger, PC, and Boyko, OB: The pathology of central nervous system radiation injury. In Gutin, PH, Leibel, SA, and Sheline, GE (eds): Radiation Injury to the Nervous System. Raven Press, Ltd, New York, 1991, pp 191–208.

20. Rubin, P, Constine, LS, and Nelson, DF: Late effects of cancer treatment: radiation and drug toxicity. In Perez, CA, and Brady, LW (eds): Principles and Practice of Radiation Oncology. J B Lippincott Co, Philadelphia, 1992, pp 124–161.
21. Sheline, G, Wara, W, and Smith, V: Therapeutic irradiation and brain injury. Int J Radiat Oncol Biol Phys 6:1215–1228, 1980.
22. Leibel, SA, and Sheline, GE: Radiation therapy for neoplasms of the brain. J Neurosurg 66:1–22, 1987.
23. Edwards, MS, and Wilson, CB: Treatment of radiation necrosis. In Gilbert, HA, and Kagan, AR (eds): Radiation Damage to the Nervous System: A Delayed Therapeutic Hazard. Raven Press, Ltd, New York, 1980, pp 129–143.
24. Janus, TJ, Kim, EE, Tilbury, R, et al: Use of [18F]fluorodeoxyglucose positron emission tomography in patients with primary malignant brain tumors. Ann Neurol 33:540–548, 1993.
25. Mulhern, RK, Ochs J, and Kun, LE: Changes in intellect associated with cranial radiation therapy. In Gutin, PH, Leibel, SA, and Sheline, GE (eds): Radiation Injury to the Nervous System. Raven Press, Ltd, New York, 1991, pp 325–340.
26. Constine, LS, Konski, A, Ekholm, S, et al: Adverse effects of brain irradiation correlated with MR and CT imaging. Int J Radiat Oncol Biol Phys 15:319–330, 1988.
27. Roman, DD, and Sperduto, PW: Neuropsychological effects of cranial radiation: current knowledge and future directions. Int J Radiat Oncol Biol Phys 31:983–998, 1995.
28. Mulhern, RK, Fairclough, D, and Ochs, J: A prospective comparison of neuropsychologic performance of children surviving leukemia who received 18-Gy, 24-Gy, or no cranial irradiation [published erratum appears in J Clin Oncol 1991 Oct;9(10):1922]. J Clin Oncol 9:1348–1356, 1991.
29. Copeland, DR, Fletcher, JM, Pfefferbaum-Levine, B, et al: Neuropsychological sequelae of childhood cancer in long-term survivors. Pediatrics 75:745–753, 1985.
30. Copeland, DR, Dowell, RE, Jr., Fletcher, JM, et al: Neuropsychological effects of childhood cancer treatment. J Child Neurol 3:53–62, 1988.
31. Smibert, E, Anderson, V, Godber, T, and Ekert, H: Risk factors for intellectual and educational sequelae of cranial irradiation in childhood acute lymphoblastic leukaemia. Br J Cancer 73:825–830, 1996.
32. Halberg, FE, Kramer, JH, Moore, IM, et al: Prophylactic cranial irradiation dose effects on late cognitive function in children treated for acute lymphoblastic leukemia. Int J Radiat Oncol Biol Phys 22:13–16, 1992.
33. Goldwein, JW, Radcliffe, J, Johnson, J, et al: Updated results of a pilot study of low dose craniospinal irradiation plus chemotherapy for children under five with cerebellar primitive neuroectodermal tumors (medulloblastoma). Int J Radiat Oncol Biol Phys 34:899–904, 1996.
34. Kramer, JH, Crittenden, MR, Halberg, FE, et al: A prospective study of cognitive functioning following low-dose cranial radiation for bone marrow transplantation. Pediatrics 90:447–50, 1992.
35. Hoppe-Hirsch, E, Brunet, L, Laroussinie, F, et al: Intellectual outcome in children with malignant tumors of the posterior fossa: influence of the field of irradiation and quality of surgery. Childs Nerv Syst 11:340–345; discussion 345–346, 1995.
36. Balmaceda, C, Heller G, Rosenblum, M, et al: Chemotherapy without irradiation: A novel approach for newly diagnosed CNS germ cell tumors: Results of an international cooperative trial. The First International Central Nervous System Germ Cell Tumor Study. J Clin Oncol 14:2908–2915, 1996.
37. Turrisi, AT: Brain irradiation and systemic chemotherapy for small-cell lung cancer: dangerous liaisons? J Clin Oncol 8:196–199, 1990.
38. Fleck, JF, Einhorn, LH, Lauer, RC, et al: Is prophylactic cranial irradiation indicated in small-cell lung cancer? J Clin Oncol 8:209–14, 1990.
39. Lishner, M, Feld, R, Payne, DG, et al: Late neurological complications after prophylactic cranial irradiation in patients with small-cell lung cancer: the Toronto experience. J Clin Oncol 8:215–221, 1990.
40. Measurements ICoRUa: ICRU Report 50: Prescribing, recording, and reporting photon beam therapy. Bethesda, Maryland, 1993.

Chapter 6

RADIATION THERAPY FOR BRAIN TUMORS: RECENT ADVANCES AND EXPERIMENTAL METHODS

CONFORMAL RADIOTHERAPY
RADIOSURGERY
INTERSTITIAL BRACHYTHERAPY
BORON NEUTRON CAPTURE THERAPY

Radiation oncology has had substantial technological development over the last decade. The application of new computerized planning in conjunction with modern imaging studies has markedly changed the radiotherapy of brain tumors. This chapter highlights some of these recent advances and describes their influence on brain tumor treatment.

CONFORMAL RADIOTHERAPY

The concept of three-dimensional conformal radiation therapy is not new. The principles involved were articulated in the late 1940s. Simply stated, three-dimensional radiotherapy involves an anatomic description of the tumor-bearing volume of the patient and a three-dimensional description of the uninvolved normal tissues for the delivery of radiotherapy to the tumor-bearing volume to the exclusion of the uninvolved regions of the patient. Delivering treatment to the tumor and sparing normal tissue is intuitive, but its implementation has been difficult. Crude attempts at performing therapy using these three-dimensional techniques were performed in the 1960s. These early technical efforts were hampered by a lack of three-dimensional imaging devices and the lack of a three-dimensional treatment planning system allowing for the complex calculations and graphical dose displays necessary to implement and describe three-dimensional radiotherapy dose distribution.

The modern development of three-dimensional treatment planning began in the late 1970s with the advent of cross-sectional imagers, such as the computed tomography (CT) scanner. With a parallel development of computer technology that allows practical reconstruction of three-dimensional images from stacked two-dimensional CT slices, three-dimensional conformal therapy became practical clinically. One of the primary graphical display tools necessary for the implementation of three-dimensional therapy is the beam's-eye view. This display allows a radiation oncologist to view along the axis of the treating machine and to create custom-designed shielding devices based on reconstructed CT anatomy. An additional benefit of computer technology in the treatment of brain tumors is the ability to integrate multiple imaging modalities into the treatment planning process. Magnetic resonance imaging (MRI) and CT are being widely used, not just for qualitative purposes but as fully fused database sets (Fig. 6–1). In addition, the use of positron emission tomography and functional MRI

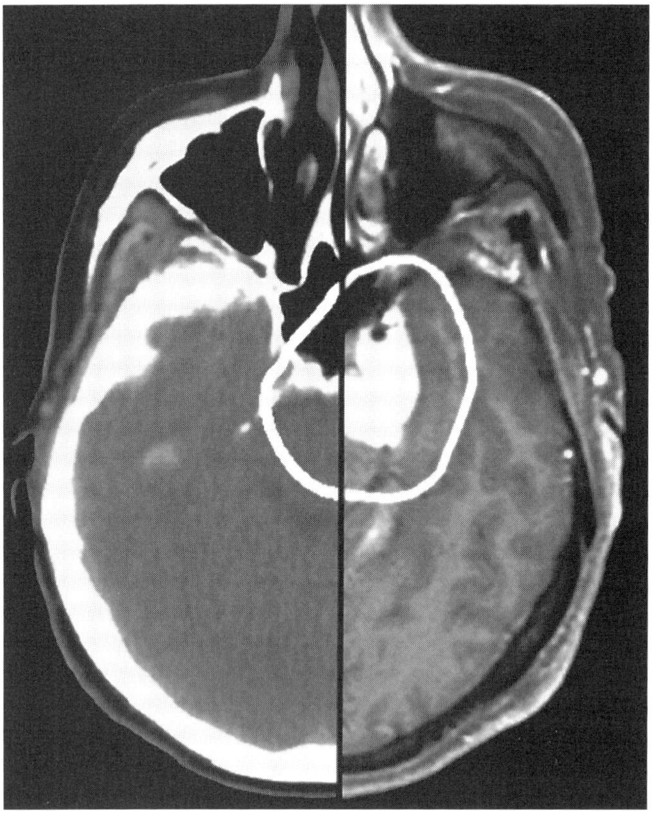

Figure 6–1. A patient with a skull-based meningioma who underwent fractionated radiotherapy to a dose of 55.8 Gy. The treatment was planned using both CT and MR. The MR and CT datasets were geometrically registered in the treatment planning system using anatomical landmarks. The white line represents the target volume and includes the enhancing tumor with a 1-cm additional margin. The additional margin provides for uncertainties in microscopic tumor location and daily patient set-up variation.

may allow the radiation oncologist to create dose distributions that exclude high doses of radiation from particular functional regions.[1]

Prior to the development of conformal radiotherapy, radiation oncologists treated patients with static or rotational therapy portals designed to encompass soft tissue and tumors based on bony landmarks, which were visible on treatment simulators. It was assumed that the tumor anatomy could be described in a reproducible way with respect to skeletal landmarks or other landmarks visible with fluoroscopy. Today three-dimensional technology is practical and becoming widely used for daily radiotherapy treatments and allows novel treatment techniques.[2–4] It is beginning to extend the upper limit on the maximum dose that can be delivered to the tumor while minimizing the dose given to the surrounding normal tissues. The University of Michigan is currently embarked on a trial using high doses of external beam therapy for malignant astrocytomas. These tumors have a propensity for local recurrence despite radiotherapy to conventional doses. The maximum tolerated dose achievable with fractionated external-beam therapy has not been reached and, in the current study, patients are treated to doses of 90 Gy, which far exceeds the conventional "safe" dose of near 60 Gy.

RADIOSURGERY

Although a complete discussion of radiosurgery is beyond the scope of this chapter, a short review with attention to newer issues is appropriate. Radiosurgery, as defined by Leksell in 1951 and quoted in a recent review,[5] refers to the destruction of a precisely defined intracranial target with a single high dose of ionizing radiation. Now commonly available, this procedure has had spectacular growth during the past 10 years. The three available types of units or methods for delivering radiosurgery treatments are cobalt (Co)-60 devices (i.e., Gamma Knife),[6] particle beams (i.e., proton therapy),[7,8] and modified linear accelerators.[9] The Co-60 units contain approximately 200 individual Co-60 sources arranged in a large hemisphere and surrounding the patient's head during the procedure. The sources have collimating apertures of various diameters that allow the gamma irradiation from the Co-60 sources to converge on a tumor or other target and create roughly spherical zones of high-dose irradiation. This type of procedure, as well as the others, uses stereotactic guidance to place the tumor at the desired location in the treatment device. Precise stereotactic localization of the radiosurgery beam to accurately treat the desired target with a minimal amount of dose delivered to uninvolved surrounding tissues generally requires the use of rigidly attached stereotactic head frames that are placed before target localization and removed after the treatment procedure. Many investigators are exploring the use of relocatable head frames that will facilitate fractionated stereotactic techniques. This procedure, known as *stereotactic radiotherapy,* may blend the radiobiologic advantage of fractionation with the spatial accuracy and favorable dose distribution associated with radiosurgery.[10]

Proton-beam radiotherapy uses particle beams that can provide for conventional fractionated radiotherapy or for single-fraction radiosurgery. Three facilities are currently in use in the United States: one in Loma Linda, CA, at Loma Linda University Medical Center: one in Cambridge, MA, at the Harvard Cyclotron Laboratory; and one in Bloomington, IN, at the Midwest Proton Radiation Institute. Proton-beam treatment, because of the physics of charged particle interactions, produces a low entry dose of radiation and no exit dose beyond the range of the proton in tissue. The vast majority of the proton energy is deposited in a well-defined manner at a depth that is dependent on the incident energy of the particle. The depth-dose curve has a peak deep in tissue that is called the *Bragg peak.* The Bragg peak phenomenon allows potentially superior dose distributions when compared with other radiosurgery devices. It is not known whether this improvement is clinically significant for radiosurgical treatment, and currently the limited availability of proton-beam units hampers additional study. New proton facilities cost about $60 million to construct.

Modified linear accelerators are also used in radiosurgical treatment.[11,12] Linear accelerators used for conventional therapy require only modest modification to be used for radiotherapy. The machines can provide conventional therapy throughout the day and can be quickly converted to use for radiosurgery. The technique uses a collimating device with a circular cross-section that attaches to the treatment gantry. The gantry rotates about a fixed point in space (i.e., the isocenter) while delivering radiation. This ensures that peripheral tissues receive only a low dose of radiation while an intense dose is delivered to the isocenter, which is generally where the center of the tumor, or target, is located. The diameter of the dose distribution is adjusted by choosing one of a series of circular collimators, up to about 4 cm in diameter.

Currently, radiosurgery is employed for both benign central nervous system conditions and benign and malignant tumors. The radiation dose is tightly confined and thus the role of radiosurgery for more infiltrative conditions remains poorly defined. The uses are summarized in Table 6–1. Radiosurgery with modified linear accelerators and with Gamma Knife units is widespread. Since the radiation that is emitted by each machine is essentially the same, the clinical outcomes should be the same regardless of the type of x-ray or gamma device used.

Recent advances in radiosurgery have been directed toward creating even more conformal dose distributions. Two advances include the creation of more conformal beam apertures using multileaf collimators[13,14] and intensity-modulated therapy using inverse planning.[15,16]

One of the main limitations in the use of conventional radiosurgery systems is their reliance on fixed, circular collimators to define the treatment beams. This results in excellent tumor coverage by the radia-

Table 6–1. **Indications for Radiosurgery**

Role for Radiosurgery	Indications
Radiosurgery well established	Arteriovenous malformations
	Acoustic neuromas
	Solitary brain metastases
Radiosurgery has a role	Meningiomas
	Recurrent malignant glial tumors
Radiosurgery is investigational	Trigeminal neuralgia
	Age-related macular degeneration
	Initial therapy for malignant gliomas
	Pituitary adenomas

tion isodose surfaces for spherical tumor volumes that do not exceed the diameter of the collimating system, typically 4 cm. When the tumor volumes are larger than the maximum tumor diameter or are irregularly shaped and nonspherical, conventional systems typically use multiple circular treatments added together to approximate the given tumor volume. Unfortunately, this method yields dose inhomogeneities within the brain and can contribute to complications.[17] In addition, multiple isocenter techniques add to treatment complexity and perhaps increase the likelihood of treatment error. As an alternative to fixed collimators, investigators are looking at multileaf collimators to customize the beam aperture to the projected profile of the tumor volume along the beam axis. This type of treatment, already in clinical use,[13] provides a benefit in target dose homogeneity and normal tissue sparing. Figure 6–2 demonstrates the conformal isodose distribution produced by radiosurgery with multileaf collimation.

Intensity-modulated radiosurgery involves intentional manipulation of the intensity or force of the radiation beam perpendicular to the axis of the treatment during a fixed treatment position in order to create complex dose distributions; it is exemplified by the Peacock system.[15] The treatment is delivered with a collimator of 2 × 20 cm that is modified by a small set of leaves. The collimator rotates about the patient and creates a 2-cm thick axial slab of conformal dose. During the axial rotation, at 5-degree intervals, the collimator stops, the set of leaves is adjusted, and the radiation beam is turned on. The leaves block the beam when critical structures would be exposed and are not inserted when the target volume is in view of the beam. The complex dose distributions

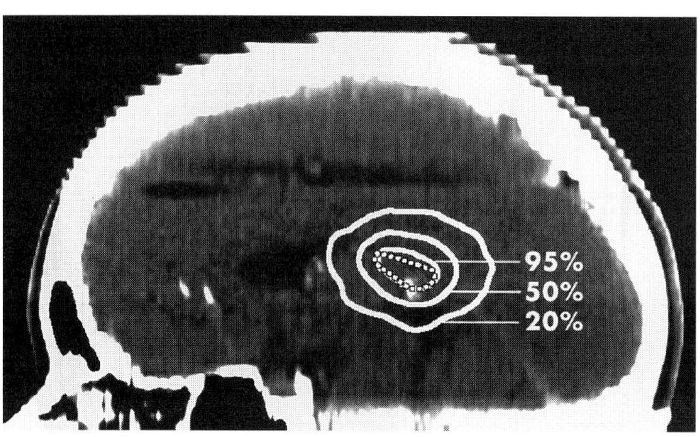

Figure 6–2. A sagittal reconstruction of the dose distribution of a patient with an irregular lesion (*dotted line*) who was treated with radiosurgery. The radiosurgery beams were shaped using a multileaf collimator. Despite the irregular contour of the abnormality, the dose distribution is conformal and homogeneous. The solid white lines represent the isodose contours. The 95%, 50%, and 20% lines are shown. The dose falls off rapidly from 95% to 20% over a distance of approximately 1 cm.

that are created in this way can be considered the inverse of the acquisition of CT radiographic images. Instead of the differential absorption of x-rays creating an axial density map (i.e., CT), the therapy x-rays created an axial dose distribution through computer control of the collimating leaves. Early clinical studies have shown that complex dose distributions are feasible, and a comparison between Peacock and conventional external-beam stereotactic radiosurgery suggests a dosimetric advantage, especially for large and irregularly shaped targets.[16]

INTERSTITIAL BRACHYTHERAPY

Brachytherapy, the treatment of tumors by placing radioactive sources close by or within lesions, has been used in the treatment of malignancies since the early 1900s. Iodine-125 (^{125}I), a radioactive isotope with a half-life of approximately 60 days, emits a low-energy spectrum of photons that are absorbed within a few centimeters of placement in tissue-density material.[125] It has been used in the past primarily as a temporary implant for the treatment of high-grade gliomas.[18,19] Gutin and coworkers[19] describe 107 patients with malignant gliomas treated on a nonrandomized protocol with brachytherapy after external-beam therapy. Patients with unifocal, well-defined malignant gliomas were initially treated with focal external-beam therapy to a dose of 60 Gy. A planned, temporary, brachytherapy procedure was performed afterwards unless tumor enlargement precluded the implant (if it did, patients received chemotherapy). A total of 63 of 101 evaluable patients underwent the brachytherapy procedure; the others could not because of tumor growth. The survival of the patients with implanted glioblastoma was felt to be encouraging and was measured at 88 weeks. The authors concluded that the non-glioblastoma patients did not benefit from the additional treatment.

For temporary implants such as those used by Gutin and associates,[19] the brachytherapy dose is usually given over a period of 1 week through surgically placed, transcranial catheters. The high-dose rate delivered by these implanted, ^{125}I-loaded catheters necessitates inpatient radiation safety restrictions. However, since ^{125}I emits radiation that is well absorbed by tissue, permanent low-dose rate ^{125}I implants are feasible and can deliver radiotherapy at low-dose rates for approximately 6 months (about three half-lives). The radioactive seeds are placed directly into the resection cavity, and no special radiation shielding is necessary.

Recent low-dose rate brachytherapy trials for recurrent gliomas,[20] upfront glioma therapy,[21] and cerebral metastases[22] indicate a high level of interest for permanent ^{125}I implantation. In the series of patients treated at the time of glioma recurrence, no patients underwent re-operation for radiation necrosis; however, in the patients treated adjuvantly at the time of original diagnosis, 20% underwent re-operation for necrotic lesions that developed after the implant, consistent with clinical radiation necrosis. The concept of maximal surgical debulking followed by placement of radioactive seeds in the periphery of the tumor cavity to help control the known remaining microscopic disease seems to have logical justification. Naturally, further studies and longer follow-up times are needed.

BORON NEUTRON CAPTURE THERAPY

For approximately 40 years, there have been clinical trials using boron neutron capture therapy (BNCT), and work continues on this modality. Investigators find BNCT compelling because the nuclear reaction: boron (B)-10 + neutron (thermal) $\rightarrow$ α–particle + lithium (Li)-7* releases substantial amounts of kinetic energy over short, biologically important distances. When B-10, a naturally occurring stable isotope, is irradiated by thermal neutrons, a reaction occurs that produces an α-particle and a Li-7* nucleus in an excited state, which rapidly decays by emitting a γ ray.

The α-particle and the Li-7 nucleus share significant kinetic energy, and the moving heavy particles cause tremendous local damage over their range, which is on the order of 1 cell diameter. The (B)-10 + neutron (thermal) reaction has a large cross section, and neutrons preferentially react in this fashion. Neutrons also react with hydrogen and nitrogen nuclei. Although these reactions are much less probable than the B-10 reaction, they become the dose-limiting events because of the large number of hydrogen and nitrogen nuclei in biological systems.[23]

If B-10 and thermal energy neutrons can be brought together in tumor cells, significant tumor cell death occurs. Barth and colleagues note that $\sim 10^9$ B-10 atoms/cell and neutron fluences of 10^{12} n·cm^2 are required.[23] The challenge facing investigators has been to create nontoxic boron compounds that are taken up preferentially by tumor cells and to construct useful neutron fluences from available nuclear reactors. Thermal neutrons are ideal for BNCT. Thermal neutrons are those that have an average kinetic energy equal to that of the ambient environment (i.e., $\sim$1/40 eV); therefore, their motion is somewhat hard to direct. Epithermal neutrons with slightly higher than thermal energies (0.4 to 10 keV) are also desirable because they can be directed at a tumor and become thermalized through nuclear collisions. The cross-section for the B-10 + neutron reaction, and the probability that the reaction will occur, decreases as the neutron energy increases; therefore, thermal energies are desirable at the tumor.

Although many laboratory studies evaluating the pharmacokinetics of various compounds are underway, and animal studies have been reported, few human in vivo data are available. In a report[24] of 120 patients treated in Japan between 1968 and 1992, 40 patients had intracranial grade 3 or 4 astrocytomas and were treated before 1985. Patients were treated with the borated compound[10] B-sodium-mercaptoundecahydrododecarborate. A 5-year survival rate of 19% versus 5% for conventionally treated nonrandomized controls was reported. Several patients were long-term survivors, and quality of life was reported to be good. However, some patients suffered from radiation toxicity, especially those who were treated previously with conventional radiotherapy and then had tumor recurrence before treatment with BNCT. In the United States, clinical work is underway at the MIT and Brookhaven, NY, reactors.

CHAPTER SUMMARY

Radiotherapy has been an important component in the therapy of brain tumors for most of this century. The past decade has witnessed significant improvements in the use of technological improvements to enhance the usefulness of radiotherapy delivery. Clearly, morbidity of therapy has dramatically improved for most patients with the use of more conformal therapy. Future challenges for radiation oncologists include developing strategies for dose intensification without sacrificing the gains made in morbidity reduction. After all, oncologists and patients alike are dissatisfied with current rates of tumor control. Applications of dose-escalation strategies are in their infancy. Using conformal therapy and intensity modulation in combination with improved imaging modalities that may highlight microscopic tumor cell aggregations may allow radiation dose distributions that precisely mirror the tumor cell distribution in each tumor. This would allow maximum therapeutic benefit by applying the therapy only when it is needed and allowing the most treatment for any individual.

REFERENCES

1. Hamilton, RJ, Sweeney, PJ, Pelizzari, CA, et al: Functional imaging in treatment planning of brain lesions. Int J Radiat Oncol Biol Phys 37: 181–188, 1997.
2. Fraass, BA: Investigating the potential of three-dimensional treatment planning. Med Prog Technol 18:227–238, 1992.
3. Ten Haken, RK, Thornton, A, Jr, Sandler, HM, et al: A quantitative assessment of the addition of MRI to CT-based, 3-D treatment planning of brain tumors. Radiother Oncol 25:121–133, 1992.
4. Thornton, A, Jr., Sandler, HM, Ten Haken, RK, et al: The clinical utility of magnetic resonance

imaging in 3-dimensional treatment planning of brain neoplasms. Int J Radiat Oncol Biol Phys 24:767–775, 1992.

5. Flickinger, JC, Loeffler, JS, and Larson, DA: Stereotactic radiosurgery for intracranial malignancies. Oncology (Huntingt) 8:81–86; discussion 86, 94, 97–88, 1994.
6. Wu, A: Physics and dosimetry of the gamma knife. Neurosurg Clin N Am 3:35–50, 1992.
7. Serago, CF, Thornton, AF, Urie, MM, et al: Comparison of proton and x-ray conformal dose distributions for radiosurgery applications. Med Phys 22:2111–2116, 1995.
8. Raju, MR: Proton radiobiology, radiosurgery and radiotherapy. Int J Radiat Biol 67:237–259, 1995.
9. Kooy, HM, Nedzi, LA, Loeffler, JS, et al: Treatment planning for stereotactic radiosurgery of intra-cranial lesions. Int J Radiat Oncol Biol Phys 21:683–693, 1991.
10. Shrieve, DC, Tarbell, NJ, Alexander, Er, et al: Stereotactic radiotherapy: A technique for dose optimization and escalation for intracranial tumors. Acta Neurochir Suppl (Wien) 62:118–123, 1994.
11. Winston, KR, and Lutz, W: Linear accelerator as a neurosurgical tool for stereotactic radiosurgery. Neurosurgery 22:454–464, 1988.
12. Loeffler, JS, Larson, DA, Shrieve, DC, and Flickinger, JC: Radiosurgery for the treatment of intracranial lesions. Important Adv Oncol 141–156, 1995.
13. Balter, JM, McShan, DL, Sandler, HM, et al: Segmental conformal radiosurgery using a multileaf collimator and computer controlled radiotherapy system: Clinical implementation. Int J Radiat Oncol Biol Phys 1997, in press.
14. Shiu, AS, Kooy, HM, Ewton, JR, et al: Comparison of miniature multileaf collimation (MMLC) with circular collimation for stereotactic treatment. Int J Radiat Oncol Biol Phys 37:679–688, 1997.
15. Carol, M, Grant, WH, Pavord, D, et al: Initial clinical experience with the Peacock intensity modulation of a 3-D conformal radiation therapy system. Stereotact Funct Neurosurg 66:30–34, 1996.
16. Woo, SY, Grant, WH, Bellezza, D, et al: A comparison of intensity modulated conformal therapy with a conventional external beam stereotactic radiosurgery system for the treatment of single and multiple intracranial lesions. Int J Radiat Oncol Biol Phys 35:593–597, 1996.
17. Nedzi, LA, Kooy, H, Alexander, E, et al: Variables associated with the development of complications from radiosurgery of intracranial tumors. Int J Radiat Oncol Biol Phys 21:591–599, 1991.
18. Green, SB, Shapiro, WR, Burger, PC, et al: A randomized trial of interstitial radiotherapy (RT) boost for newly diagnosed malignant glioma: Brain Tumor Cooperative Group (BTCG) trial 8701 (Meeting abstract). Proc Annu Meet Am Soc Clin Oncol 13:A486, 1994.
19. Gutin, PH, Prados, MD, Phillips, TL, et al: External irradiation followed by an interstitial high activity iodine-^{125} implant "boost" in the initial treatment of malignant gliomas: NCOG study 6G-82-2. Int J Radiat Oncol Biol Phys 21:601–606, 1991.
20. Halligan, JB, Stelzer, KJ, Rostomily, RC, et al: Operation and permanent low activity ^{125}I brachytherapy for recurrent high-grade astrocytomas. Int J Radiat Oncol Biol Phys 35:541–547, 1996.
21. Fernandez, PM, Zamorano, L, Yakar, D, et al: Permanent iodine-125 implants in the up-front treatment of malignant gliomas. Neurosurgery 36:467–473, 1995.
22. Schulder, M, Black, PM, Shrieve, DC, et al: Permanent low-activity iodine-125 implants for cerebral metastases. J Neurooncol 33:213–221, 1997.
23. Barth, RF, Soloway, AH, and Brugger, RM: Boron neutron capture therapy of brain tumors: Past history, current status, and future potential. Cancer Invest 14:534–550, 1996.
24. Hatanaka, H, and Nakagawa, Y: Clinical results of long-surviving brain tumor patients who underwent boron neutron capture therapy. Int J Radiat Oncol Biol Phys 28:1061–1066, 1994.

Chapter 7

BRAIN TUMOR CHEMOTHERAPY AND IMMUNOTHERAPY

Neurosurgery has had major technical advances in the past 20 years, with stereotactic biopsy and resection. Radiation oncology has developed focal conformal radiation therapy (RT), stereotactic radiosurgery (SR), and interstitial RT. Despite these major technical advances, the median survival for patients with glioblastoma multiforme has not changed significantly in the past 20 years. The neurosurgeon is limited by the infiltrating growth pattern of brain tumors and the regionally specialized normal brain. A neurosurgeon can only incompletely resect tumor to the margins of normal brain, and although RT does significantly prolong survival, it does not produce sufficient cytotoxicity to cure brain tumors. The goal of chemotherapy and immunotherapy has been to effect a cure or a prolonged response, with increased quality of life and decreased suffering. The effectiveness of chemotherapy and immunotherapy have been impaired by the blood-brain barrier (BBB)'s limiting access of water-soluble drugs and biologic response modifiers and reduced and variable tumor blood flow decreasing tumor exposure to lipid-soluble agents.

CHEMOTHERAPY

The development of rational therapy regimens for brain tumors depends on an understanding of the principles of chemotherapy: tumor cytoreduction, drug delivery to tumors, and tumor drug resistance (Table 7–1). Drug delivery to tumor is a function of the BBB and the blood-tumor barrier (BTB). Chemotherapy rests on the principle that the tumor is more susceptible to treatment than normal brain. Tumor resistance to chemotherapy or immunotherapy is intrinsic, or acquired through gene activation or mutation.[1–5]

Principles

TUMOR CYTOREDUCTION

At the time of diagnosis, intraparenchymal brain tumors range from 30 to 60 g, or 3 to 6 times 10^{10} cells, with 100 g or 10^{11} cells fatal (Table 7–2).[6–8] If a neurosurgeon removes 90% to 99% of the tumor, the cellular burden remaining will be 10^8 or 10^9 cells. Frequently, because of tumor location, the maximum tumor resection possible is less than 50%, or less than 1 log cell kill. After surgical resection, RT can be expected to produce an additional 2 log cell kill, leaving 10^6 to 10^7 cells. It is hoped

Table 7–1. **Principles of Chemotherapy**

Tumor cytoreduction
Early treatment
Maximize drug exposure (C × T)
Drug delivery to tumor
Blood-tumor barrier
Blood flow to tumor
Drug properties
Tumor drug resistance
Intrinsic
Acquired

that chemotherapy will produce an additional 2 log cell kill, leaving 10^4 or 10^5 cells. Immunotherapy or the body's natural cellular defenses may then produce a cure. The problem with this scenario is that surgery, RT, and chemotherapy rarely produce their maximum cytotoxicity (Table 7–3). The immunologic surveillance mechanisms of patients with brain tumors are decreased, and RT and chemotherapy may further impair them, so they are unable to destroy the remaining cellular burden.[9]

DRUG DELIVERY TO TUMOR

Drug delivery to tumor is a function of the BBB and BTB. In Chapter 2, normal brain endothelial cells were noted to be continuous, with tight junctions between the capillary endothelial cells. They lack gaps, clefts, and fenestrations.[10] Drug characteristics that enhance delivery across the tight BBB are high lipid solubility, weak protein binding, and low ionization (Table 7–4).[5] Malignant brain tumors have long been known to possess a BTB.[1,3,5] Angiography has shown a vascular tumor blush, and histologic examination reveals endothelial proliferation. Vick and colleagues[11] found that in brain adjacent to tumor, there were clefts in endothelial cells, and the number of clefts varied directly with the density of infiltrating tumor cells. Brain tumor capillaries vary from structurally normal to grossly abnormal, depending on tumor type and location within a tumor.[1,3,5] The structural abnormalities in human and experimental brain tumor capillaries include thickened capillary walls, surface projections, altered basement membranes, increased pinocytotic vessels, fenestrations, and endothelial gaps or defects.[3,5]

Drug delivery to tumor depends on the permeability and the surface area of the capillary endothelial cells.[1,3,5] The density of capillaries in brain and brain tumor regions is variable. Blood flow plays a major role in the delivery of lipid-soluble drugs, which pass readily through the BBB. Blood flow is less important with water-soluble drugs. The permeability and surface area of capillaries determines the rate of drug delivery.[1,3,5] Plasma protein binding and clearance of drug from the capillaries also influence drug delivery to tumor. The greater the clearance of drug

Table 7–2. **Tumor Cytoreduction and Therapy 1**

Scenario for Cure of Malignant Astrocytomas	Tumor Burden	
	Grams	Cell Number (log)
At diagnosis	30 to 60	3 to 6 × 10^{10}
After stereotactic biopsy	30 to 60	3 to 6 × 10^{10}
After subtotal resection	3 to 6	3 to 6 × 10^9
After "gross total resection" (GTR)	0.3 to 0.6	3 to 6 × 10^8
After GTR + RT	0.003 to 0.006	3 to 6 × 10^6
After GTR + RT + chemotherapy	0.00003 to 0.00006	3 to 6 × 10^4
After GTR + RT + chemotherapy + host response or immunotherapy		CURE

Table 7–3. **Tumor Cytoreduction and Therapy II**

Scenario for failure
Surgery often removes less than 50% of tumor
Radiation produces less than a 2-log cell kill
Chemotherapy frequently produces less than a 2-log cell kill
Immunotherapy is ineffective
The host's immunological response is compromised
Radiation therapy is often damaging to normal brain

from capillaries (shorter plasma half-life), through excretion or metabolism, the less drug will be present in the capillaries.[1,3,5] Assuming the capillaries of a tumor have a fixed permeability and surface area and two drugs have the same molecular weight, lipid solubility, ionization, and protein binding, the drug with the shorter plasma half-life will have decreased tumor exposure. In rat microvessels, the endothelial cells participate in drug metabolism.[12] Tumor cells distant from capillaries may not receive sufficiently cytotoxic drug concentrations. The cytotoxic drug may be metabolized during its journey in the extracellular space.[13,14]

A goal of chemotherapy is to maximize tumor drug exposure, which is the product of drug concentration at the tumor cell and the cumulative exposure time (C × T).[15] Alkylating agents, such as 1,3-bis-(2-chloroethyl)-1-nitrosourea (BCNU) and procarbazine, are given in high doses to produce a peak concentration because of a steep dose-response curve.[16,17] Cell cycle-specific agents, such as methotrexate (MTX), are given by prolonged infusion to expose cells as they enter a specific cell cycle phase.[16]

Table 7–4. **Drug and Tumor Properties That Increase Drug Delivery to Tumor**

Drug properties
Lipid solubility
Weak protein binding
Low ionization
Tumor properties
Low plasma drug clearance and metabolism
Increased permeability and surface area of tumor capillaries
Increased tumor blood flow (lipid-soluble drugs)
Decreased tumor distance from capillaries

A single dose of drug will kill a fixed percentage of tumor cells over a dose range. Therefore, early treatment of small tumors is theoretically more likely to produce a cure.[15,16,18] In an in vivo rat brain tumor model, Gerosa and colleagues[19] demonstrated that treatment with sequential therapy of BCNU and 5-fluorouracil (5-FU) produced long-term survival and occasional cures, while BCNU delivered alone produced no long-term survival or cures. However, the median survival of the BCNU and BCNU + 5-FU treatment groups were not different. 5-FU did not increase the median survival of the tumor-bearing rats but did have antitumor activity in clonogenic cell survival studies.[19] The results suggest that 5-FU is additive to BCNU in a minority of treated rats to produce cures. In adult glial tumors there is no controlled trial that shows multiagent chemotherapy is better than single-agent chemotherapy.

TUMOR DRUG RESISTANCE

Malignant glial tumors have regional differences in morphology and genotype. Tumor heterogeneity may be a spontaneous mutation in a clone of cells that produces cells of different genotypes.[20] Human tumor cells cloned in vitro from different areas of the same tumor may have different chemotherapeutic sensitivities to different drugs.[2] Rapidly dividing human tumor cells in tissue culture were typically hyperploid in karyotype and more sensitive to chemotherapy than were slowly dividing cells from different regions of the same malignant tumors. The slowly growing regions of malignant tumors and low-grade astrocytomas were near diploid in karyotype and were more resistant to drug.[21]

In Chapter 2, a variety of in vitro assay techniques to predict tumor cell chemotherapeutic drug sensitivity were reviewed. If patients are shown to be sensitive to or resistant to specific drugs in vitro, the physician is able to individualize appropriate therapy. However, the assays predict a positive clinical response in only 50% to 70% of patients. The assays predict drug resistance in 100% of patients but have not been used widely clinically because of their failure to predict positive clinical responses[2,7,8,22] Failure to predict a positive clinical response using in vitro assay systems may be because the assay systems lack a BBB[8] or the cells maintained in tissue culture may change genotypically or phenotypically if long-term culture is used.[23]

A nude mouse model was developed by Shapiro and associates[24] to test chemotherapeutic sensitivity. Human tumors were implanted in nude mice, and different tumors were sensitive to different drugs, with different regions of the same tumor having different chemotherapeutic sensitivities.[25] However, the in vivo response in nude mice did not reflect the patients' clinical response because only certain clones of the patients' heterogeneous original tumor grew in the in vivo nude mouse system. The growing cell clones in nude mice might not be the growing tumor cells in humans.[26] A nude rat model has been developed for in vivo chemosensitivity testing but will probably have the same limitations with nonrepresentative tumor growth.[27] Schold and Bigner[28] have written a comprehensive review of animal brain tumor models and their use in therapeutic studies.

Drug resistance may be an intrinsic property of tumor cells or may be acquired after treatment. In Chapter 2, drug resistance was divided into factors extrinsic or intrinsic to the tumor cell (see Table 2–6). Extrinsic factors included plasma protein drug binding, the delivery of adequate concentrations of drug through the BBB, and drug clearance from plasma. Intrinsic factors included the BTB, the ability of tumor to transport and retain drug, the increase or decrease in drug concentrations in tumor by metabolic processes, and the ability of tumor to repair drug-induced DNA damage. In a given tumor, there may be more than one mechanism of drug resistance, and mechanisms of drug resistance may vary in tumors of different histology and among tumors of identical histology.[29]

Nitrosoureas and procarbazine are the most active drugs for the treatment of malignant astrocytomas. Nitrosourea and procarbazine cytotoxicity are mediated by DNA alkylation at the O^6 position of guanine, followed by the formation of crosslinks between DNA strands or DNA strands and protein. Brain tumor cells have the enzyme O^6-methylguanine-DNA methyl transferase (MGMT) in varying quantities, and MGMT repairs DNA alkylation at the O^6 position (Table 7–5). The amount of MGMT in a brain tumor cell determines its intrinsic sensitivity or resis-

Table 7–5. **Mechanisms of Intrinsic Drug Resistance**

Drug	Mechanisms of Resistance
Nitrosoureas	Increased O^6-methylguanine-DNA methyl transferase
	Increased glutathione, glutathione-S-transferase-π
Procarbazine	Increased O^6-methylguanine-DNA methyl transferase
Cyclophosphamide	Increased inactivation of aldehyde dehydrogenase
	Increased glutathione, glutathione-S-transferase-π
Cisplatin and analogs	Decreased cellular drug uptake
	Increased DNA repair
	Increased activation of metallothionen
Vincristine, etoposide, doxorubicin	Increased MDR1 activation, P-glycoprotein

tance to nitrosoureas or procarbazine.[29–33] Extrinsic brain tumor resistance to nitrosoureas or procarbazine can be acquired by repeated drug exposure in vitro and in vivo in patients. MGMT is also present in oligodendroglioma, ependymoma, and medulloblastoma.[34,35] Early phase I and II clinical trials with the MGMT depletor O^6-benzylguanine are in progress.[36,37]

Reduced glutathione (GSH) is also important in the protection of tumor cells from nitrosourea-induced cytotoxicity. Low-grade astrocytomas have higher levels of GSH than do anaplastic astrocytomas, with glioblastomas having the lowest levels of GSH. GSH is higher in meningioma and normal brain than in astrocytoma or glioblastoma multiforme.[38] Glutathione-S-transferase-π (GST-π) is an enzyme that catalyzes the conjugation of GSH to electrophilic species. It is increased with increasing grades of astrocytic anaplasia, thus protecting to a greater degree the more malignant tumor cell from nitrosoureas. Nontoxic substrates for GST-π are being evaluated for their ability to deplete GST-π and potentiate nitrosourea cytotoxicity. Buthionine sulfoxime inhibits an enzyme necessary for the synthesis of GSH and is also being evaluated to increase nitrosourea cytotoxicity.[29]

Platinum compounds develop drug resistance by decreased intracellular drug uptake and accumulation, increased activation of the protein metallothionen, and increased DNA repair.[29] Cyclophosphamide resistance develops from increased inactivation of the enzyme aldehyde dehydrogenase and through increased GSH and GST-π.[29] Resistance to vincristine, etoposide, and doxorubicin is mediated through the *MDR1* gene and its protein product, P-glycoprotein. P-glycoprotein produces drug efflux from the tumor cell and is dependent on adenosine triphosphate (ATP) for energy. The development of MDR drug resistance is dependent on the amount of P-glycoprotein. MDR drug resistance can be intrinsic to the tumor or develop after exposure. Therapeutic possibilities to increase tumor drug sensitivity include the transfection of genes containing antisense oligonucleotides to the *MDR1* gene, or for nitrosoureas, the transfection of gene for alkyl transferases.[29,39]

Clinical Trials

Clinical chemotherapy trials are performed to establish the safe and effective doses of new drugs and to document their toxicity. The three common types of clinical trials are phase I, II, and III.

Phase I studies are the initial clinical studies with a new drug. The aim of the phase I study is to determine the maximum tolerated dose and establish the drug toxicity profile. Patients are entered in groups, typically of three patients, with gradual group dose escalation until the maximum tolerated dose is reached. Additional patients are then entered at the presumed maximum tolerated dose to assure safety and document toxicity. In some phase I studies, dose escalation is done in individual patients on subsequent chemotherapy cycles. Phase I trials may involve patients with more than one tumor type or more than one organ system. Phase I chemotherapy studies are usually performed in patients who have failed previous surgery, RT, and chemotherapy.

Phase II studies test a specific tumor type against a fixed dose of a drug, determined from phase I studies. The aim is to establish response rates, stability of response, and toxicity. Phase II studies are usually performed on patients who have failed other therapies.

Phase III trials are the most sophisticated trials, randomizing patients to the best "standard" therapy versus a new therapy or adding a new therapy to the "standard" therapy in one of the two trial arms. The aim of a phase III trial is to establish whether the new therapy is more effective than standard therapy. The standard therapy may be a placebo if there is no effective therapy for the tumor. Randomized designs might also test the timing of a new therapy, the use of adjuvant PCV (procarbazine, [N-(2-chloroethyl)-N'-cyclohexyl-N-nitrosourea (CCNU)] and vincristine chemotherapy with RT or on recurrence after RT failure for the treatment of anaplastic oligodendroglioma. Important outcome measures for phase III trials are response rate, duration of response, survival, and toxicity.

The phase III trial begins with a null hypothesis (Table 7–6). The usual null hypothesis is that the two treatments are equal with respect to the outcome measures chosen, with the alternative hypothesis that they are different. The hypothesis should be stated in writing at the study outset. Hypotheses formulated after the data are examined require different statistical treatment.[40] A phase III trial can be performed with the patient, or both the patient and physician, blind to treatment assignment; these are called *single-* or *double-blind trials*, respectively. It is essential to design the randomization with a set algorithm so research team members who have contact with the patients cannot bias patient allocation.[41]

In planning a phase III trial, the investigator must characterize the study population for demographic and clinical factors, such as age, gender, diagnosis, grade of tumor, and prior treatment, to maximally ensure balance of potential prognostic variables between treatment arms. The assignment of patients with a stratification scheme minimizes the likelihood that the two treatment arms will be different in important prognostic variables. Using a stratification scheme increases the entry number of patients to reach the same level of statistical significance.[41]

Inclusion and exclusion criteria must be developed for the trial. In Chapter 3, the selection and standardization of response criteria and the imaging modalities for response determination were discussed. When the treatment arms to be compared

Table 7–6. **Planning a Phase III Randomized Chemotherapy Trial**

Steps

(1) Formulate a null hypothesis and alternative hypothesis.
(2) Develop treatment arms.
(3) Characterize the population variables to ensure balance between treatment arms.
(4) Choose determinable outcome measures—are they continuous or dichotomous?
(5) Develop inclusion and exclusion criteria.
(6) Anticipate side effects.
(7) Determine drug dose modifications for toxicity.
(8) Develop standardized response criteria.
(9) Anticipate confounding variables and dropout rate
(10) Design an unbiased randomization scheme
(11) If necessary, stratify randomization scheme, remembering that the purpose of randomization is to distribute variables equally.
(12) Choose a statistical test(s), appropriate for outcome measure(s)—get statistical consultation!
(13) Choose type I and type II error to determine sample size.
(14) Plan interim analyses?
(15) Write protocol.
(16) Develop database.
(17) Complete human use form with informed consent.
(18) Perform study.
(19) Collect data in database.
(20) Perform statistical analysis of data.
(21) Write paper.

are known, the stratification of variables planned, confounding variables anticipated, dropout rate estimated, and an outcome measure (or measures) chosen, a plan for statistical analysis can be developed.[41] The statistical analysis method is chosen based on whether the predictor and outcome variables are continuous or dichotomous. Outcome variables such as median survival, response rate, or duration of response are continuous variables. The number of patients living longer than 180 days is a dichotomous variable.[41]

The t test is usually used to determine whether the mean value of a continuous outcome variable in one treatment group differs from that of another treatment group. This test is often used in survival analysis of two treatments. The z statistic can be used to compare the proportion of two subjects who have a dichotomous outcome. For instance, the z statistic can be used to test the proportion of men who develop myelosuppression, less than 1500 neutrophils, on one chemotherapy drug versus another drug. After selection of the appropriate statistical test, the alpha (type I) and beta (type II) error need to be chosen for the study.[42] The type I error is the probability of rejecting the null hypothesis, if it is true. The hypothesis is one-tailed if it specifies the direction of the association between the predictor and outcome variables, and it is two-tailed if only an association is presumed to exist.[40] The type I error is usually set between 0.01 and 0.10, depending on the level of reasonable doubt the investigator is willing to accept. A type II error occurs if the investigator fails to reject a null hypothesis that is false. A type II error is usually set between 0.05 and 0.20. In general, the investigator should use a low type I error when it is important to avoid a type I (false-positive) error and a low type II error when it is important to avoid a type II (false-negative) error. A low type I or II error requires a larger sample size to reject the null hypothesis.[40]

When the data are analyzed, the P value is determined and the null hypothesis is rejected if the P value is less than the type I error. If the P value is accepted, it does not mean that there is no difference in the two treatments; rather, the difference observed in the sample is small compared with what may have occurred by chance.[40] If another study with similar treatments is planned, a larger sample size may be needed to detect the smaller-than-expected difference.

A meta-analysis is a statistical method of combining several small trials to answer a question that remains unanswered from each of the small trials.[43] To evaluate the addition of chemotherapy to RT, Fine and colleagues[43] performed a meta-analysis on 16 randomized trials involving 3000 patients with malignant glioma. The estimated increase in survival for patients treated with both RT and chemotherapy was 10.1% at 1 year (95% confidence interval [CI], 6.8%–13.3%), and 8.6% at 2 years (95% CI, 5.2%–12.0%). The absolute increases in survival (treated minus control) convert into relative increases in survival (treated minus control divided by control) of 23.4% at 1 year (95% CI, 15.8%–30.9%) and 52.4% at 2 years (95% CI, 31.7%–73.2%). The survival advantage was thought to be present for both anaplastic astrocytoma and glioblastoma multiforme, although the trial was unable to analyze data separately from each of the two tumor types. An indirect measure of statistical analysis was used to group studies by predominant tumor type, glioblastoma or anaplastic astrocytoma. Seven studies had more than 75% of patients with glioblastoma, and these trials were assumed to be representative of glioblastoma. In this group, there was a survival advantage for the RT-plus-chemotherapy group at all time points, ranging from 2.5% to 11.3%, with the advantage greatest at 24 months. Trials with a significant proportion of anaplastic astrocytoma were analyzed separately. The survival advantage was again present for chemotherapy at all time points, with the advantage being greatest at the early time points of 6 months and 1 year and decreasing thereafter. The survival advantage was also present for both BCNU and CCNU when analyzed separately.[43] The greater the similarity among small trials in terms of inclusion criteria, exclusion criteria, randomization, blinding, stratification, treatment, response criteria, response determination, and follow-up, the more meaningful the statistical meta-analysis can be in defining subgroups of patients with important prognostic variables who will benefit from chemotherapy.

The generalization of results from a randomized clinical trial to the population at large, with the identical disease, has to be done cautiously. Winger and colleagues[44] examined the median length of survival of 197 patients with supratentorial glioblastoma multiforme (n=135) or anaplastic glioma (n=62) in whom randomization to chemotherapy was performed after RT. At diagnosis, 197 patients were eligible for the study. At the start of RT, 134 (68%) were eligible for the study; at the completion of RT 6 weeks later, 93 (47%) were eligible; and at randomization 8 weeks later, 78 patients (40%) were eligible for the study. A total of 55 of the 78 patients agreed to participate in the study. Of the eligible patients, 23 refused to participate (18 of the 23 patients refused chemotherapy, and five did not want an investigational drug). A total of 84 patients (43%) became ineligible because of deterioration in neurologic status; 23 (12%) because radiotherapy did not conform to specifications; eight (4%) because significant medical problems precluded participation, and four (2%) because they refused radiotherapy. The median survival of the study patients was 60 weeks versus 25 weeks for the patients who did not participate in the study. The median survival was 50 weeks for the 23 patients who met the criteria for randomization but who chose not to be randomized. This group had a significantly lower Karnofsky performance status prior to randomization than patients who agreed to participate in the study.[44] Therefore, it is important to use survival data from clinical trials cautiously and offer clinical trials to patients when appropriate.

Individual phase III chemotherapy trials will be discussed in chapters on specific tumor types (Chapters 8 to 15).

PROGNOSTIC FACTORS

When planning clinical brain tumor trials, it is important to be aware of important prognostic variables so they can be distributed evenly through stratification among treatment arms if necessary. Eagan and Scott[45] evaluated the prognostic significance of six factors in patients who had failed RT and were about to undergo chemotherapy. Age, gender, tumor grade, onstudy performance score, time to progression from histological diagnosis, and prior chemotherapy exposure did not correlate with response to therapy. Not surprisingly, tumor regression after chemotherapy correlated with prolonged time to progression and survival. In this study, tumor grade did not correlate with response, time to progression, or survival.

In another study, by Grant and colleagues,[46] age was found to be strongly predictive of chemotherapy response. A partial response (PR) occurred in 39% of patients younger than 40 years of age, 17% of patients 40 to 69 years of age, and 5% of those 60 years old or older ($p<0.001$). The median survival of those younger than 60 years of age was 43 weeks, with a median survival of 24 weeks for patients 60 years old or older ($p<0.001$). Patients 60 years old or older have less chance of responding to chemotherapy. This confirms work of the Brain Tumor Cooperative Group (BTCG), in which patients younger than 40 years of age postsurgery were compared with patients older than 60 years of age postsurgery. In this randomized trial, patients were divided into those having no further therapy and those having RT, chemotherapy, or both. Patients younger than 40 years old had an 18-month survival rate of 64% versus an 8% survival rate in patients older than 60 years old.[47,48] Therefore, a trial with a greater proportion of elderly patients is less likely to show the null hypothesis to be false or, alternatively, larger numbers will be required to do so. If the study population is young, the results may not be applicable to the majority of patients who develop glioma in the fifth and sixth decades of life.

Brain Cancer Chemotherapy Drugs and Toxicity

ALKYLATING AGENTS

Nitrosoureas are lipid-soluble drugs that are cell-cycle nonspecific and readily cross the BBB (Table 7–7). They act by alkylating DNA at the O^6 position of guanine

Table 7–7. **Brain Tumor Chemotherapy**

Drug	Mechanism of Action	Route	Dose	Principal Toxicity
Alkylating Agents *Nitrosoureas*				
ACNU	Alkylate DNA and form DNA-DNA crosslinks	IV	100–150 mg/m^2	Myelosuppression, pulmonary toxicity
BCNU	Alkylate DNA and form DNA-DNA crosslinks	IV	200–250 mg/m^2	Myelosuppression, pulmonary toxicity
CCNU	Alkylate DNA and form DNA-DNA crosslinks	PO	100–130 mg/m^2	Myelosuppression, pulmonary toxicity
Methyl-CCNU	Alkylate DNA and form DNA-DNA crosslinks	PO	130–220 mg/m^2	Myelosuppression, pulmonary toxicity
PCNU	Alkylate DNA and form DNA-DNA crosslinks	IV	60–100 mg/m^2	Myelosuppression, pulmonary toxicity
Streptozotocin	Alkylate DNA and form DNA-DNA crosslinks	IV	500–1500 mg/m^2	Myelosuppression
Fotemustine	Alkylate DNA and form DNA-DNA crosslinks	IV	100 mg/m^2	Myelosuppression
Other				
Procarbazine	Alkylate DNA and form DNA-DNA crosslinks Inihibit RNA and protein systhesis	PO	100–150 mg/m^2 for 28 days	Myelosuppression, fatigue
Cyclophosphamide	Alkylate DNA and form DNA-DNA crosslinks	IV	500–900 mg/m^2	Myelosuppression, cystitis, hepatic
Ifosfamide	Alkylate DNA and form DNA-DNA crosslinks	IV	1200–3000 mg/m^2	Myelosuppression, encephalopathy
Cisplatin	Binds DNA forming inter and intrastrand crosslinks	IV	40–100 mg/m^2	Myelosuppression, ototoxicity, renal, peripheral neuropathy
Diaziquone	Alkylating agent	IV	10–20 mg/m^2	Myelosuppression
Temozolomide	Alkylating agent	PO	150–200 mg/m^2	Myelosuppression
Antimetabolites				
Methotrexate	Inhibits dihydrofolate reductase, blocks pyrimidine and purine synthesis	IV IT	200–1200 mg/m^2 8–12 mg	Myelosuppression, mucositis, renal, leukoencephalopathy
5-Fluorouracil	Blocks pyrimidine synthesis	IV	1000 mg/m^2	Myelosuppression, mucositis, cerebellar

Continued on following page

Table 7–7. *—continued*

Drug	Mechanism of Action	Route	Dose	Principal Toxicity
Cytosine arabinoside	Inhibits DNA polymerase	IV IT	100–300 mg/m^2 100 mg	Myelosuppression, nausea, cerebellar leukoencephalopathy
Thioguanine	Inhibits purine biosynthesis	PO	40–100 mg/m^2	Myelosuppression
Naturally Occurring Compounds				
Vincristine	Inhibits microtubule assembly	IV	1.4–2.0 mg/m^2	Peripheral neuropathy
Etoposide	Inhibits topoisomerase II and produces DNA strand breaks	IV PO	50–140 mg/m^2 50 mg/m^2	Myelosuppression
Taxol	Stabilize microtubules	IV	210–240 mg/m^2	Myelosuppression, peripheral neuropathy, nausea, arthralgias
Topotecan	Topoisomerase I inhibitor	IV	1.5 mg/m^2 daily × 5	Myelosuppression, lethargy, nausea, vomiting
Doxorubicin	Inhibits topoisomerase II DNA cleavage	IV	15–75 mg/m^2	Myelosuppression, cardiac toxicity
Other				
Dexamethasone	Anti-edema, cytolytic for lymphoma	PO, IV	0.5–100 mg	Cushing's syndrome, ulcers, myopathy, psychosis, tremor
Hydroxyurea	Anti-edema, cytolytic for lymphoma	PO	300–1000 mg/m^2	Skin discoloration
Tamoxifen	Protein kinase C inhibitor	PO	240 mg/m^2	Myelosuppression, lethargy, nausea, vomiting

and then forming DNA or DNA-protein crosslinks. The common nitrosoureas are [(4-amino-2 methyl-5' primidinyl) methyl-1-(chloroethyl)-1-nitrosourea hydrochloride] (ACNU), BCNU, CCNU, methyl-CCNU, [1-(2-chloroethyl)-2-(2,6-dioxo-3 piperidyl)-1-nitrosourea] (PCNU), chlorozotocin, streptozotocin, and fotemustine. BCNU is the most frequently used drug in the treatment of malignant glioma. CCNU and methyl-CCNU can be given orally, with CCNU the second most commonly prescribed nitrosourea. The major systemic side effect of nitrosoureas is myelosuppression, which is dose-related and occurs late, 4 to 6 weeks after chemotherapy. The most feared complication is pulmonary fibrosis, also dose-related, which occurs at lower cumulative drug doses in smokers than in nonsmokers. Patients should be followed with pulmonary function tests prior to and during nitrosourea chemotherapy. If pulmonary function changes occur secondary to use of nitrosoureas, they are frequently reversible after stopping the chemotherapy. Rare late complications include renal failure and the development of acute myelogenous leukemia. No neurotoxicity is present, unless the nitrosoureas are delivered intra-arterially or in high doses intravenously with autologous bone marrow rescue.

Procarbazine is a lipid-soluble, cell-cycle nonspecific, monoamine oxidase inhibitor that crosses the BBB and alkylates DNA at the O^6 position of guanine. It also affects RNA and protein synthesis. It is used to treat malignant astrocytoma, oligodendroglioma, and primary central nervous system lymphoma (PCNSL). The major systemic side effect of procarbazine is dose-related myelosuppression. Common side effects are fatigue and herpes zoster.[49] Rash, muscle cramps, and hepatic dysfunction are rarely seen. Encephalopathy and ataxia have been reported. Interestingly, procarbazine is effective after nitrosourea failure even though both alkylate DNA at the O^6 position.[50]

Diaziquone (AZQ) is a lipid-soluble alkylating agent that crosses the BBB. In a randomized malignant glioma trial, it was as effective as BCNU, with the AZQ group having a median survival of 325 days and the BCNU group, 379 days.[51] The principal side effect is dose-related myelosupression.

Cyclophosphamide is a prodrug, requiring hepatic activation to a hydroxy derivative for cytotoxicity. It is an alkylating agent and has activity against malignant glioma, primitive neuroectodermal tumor (PNET), medulloblastoma, and germinoma. It is used most often in combination with vincristine for malignant glioma after initial chemotherapy failure.[52] Its major systemic toxicites are myelosuppression and hemorrhagic cystitis; the latter can be eliminated by appropriate hydration. Neurotoxicity is rare. Second malignancies are rarely reported. Ifosfamide is related to cyclophosphamide. It produces less myelotoxicity but can produce an encephalopathy. It is used to treat medulloblastoma and PNET.

Cisplatin (CDDP) is a water-soluble compound that does not cross the BBB well. It binds directly to DNA, forming interstrand and intrastrand crosslinks. The drug's major role has been in medulloblastoma, PNET, and germinoma, in combination with other drugs. Its major systemic toxicities are myelosuppression, renal failure, and ototoxicity. The renal toxicity can be significantly lessened by appropriate hydration. Common neurotoxic side effects are severe emesis and an axonal sensory neuropathy. The peripheral neuropathy may progress even after the drug has been stopped. Reversibility is slow. Its role in malignant astrocytoma as a single agent is minimal. CDDP has also been given intra-arterially (see later section on intra-arterial chemotherapy).

Carboplatin is a CDDP analog with greater myelotoxicity and less renal and ototoxicity than its parent compound. It has the same spectrum of activity as CDDP. Carboplatin is given in combination with etoposide to patients with malignant astrocytoma after initial chemotherapy failure.[53] It is a marginally active regimen.

Temozolomide is a new alkylating agent and is a methylated second-generation imidazotetrazine. In early phase II trials it is active against recurrent malignant gliomas.[54] It is taken orally at monthly intervals with a major systemic toxicity of myelosuppression.

ANTIMETABOLITES

Methotrexate (MTX) is a water-soluble, cell cycle-specific drug that does not cross the BBB well. It is an analog of folic acid. MTX binds to dihydrofolate reductase, inhibiting the production of tetrahydrofolate. (Tetrahydrofolate is necessary for the synthesis of purines and pyrimidines.) Its clinical role is in the treatment of medulloblastoma, PNET, and PCNSL. In PCNSL, it has been used in both IA BBBD and intravenous (IV) high-dose single-agent, multimodality, and multiagent chemotherapy regimens. It is also used intrathecally to treat meningeal spread of systemic cancer. MTX systemic toxicities include myelosuppression, mucositis, immuno-suppression, and nephrotoxicity, especially in high doses. Intrathecal (IT) MTX toxicity includes a transient aseptic meningitis, a permanent myelopathy, and leukoencephalopathy. The myelopathy is idiosyncratic, and the leukoencephalopathy occurs most frequently when the IT MTX is given in combination with RT. The leukoencephalopathy also occurs with high-dose systemic MTX.

5-Fluorouracil (5-FU) is a fluoropyrimidine that competes with uracil for thymidylate synthetase, an enzyme that is necessary for the synthesis of the pyrimidine thymidine. Thymidine is necessary for both DNA and RNA synthesis. 5-FU crosses the BBB but has no significant activity either as a single agent or in combination with BCNU in the treatment of malignant glioma. Its major toxicities are myelosuppression and mucositis. Neurologic toxicity includes an acute pancerebellar syndrome.

Cytosine arabinoside (Ara-C) is a cell cycle-specific drug. Its metabolite competes with deoxycytidine and inhibits DNA polymerase. Ara-C crosses the BBB and is used for the treatment of PCNSL and intrathecally for neoplastic meningitis. Its principal systemic toxicities are myelosuppression and nausea. In high IV doses, it produces a pancerebellar syndrome, seizures, and encephalopathy. Intrathecally, it can cause transient aseptic meningitis. After multiple IT Ara-C doses, usually in conjunction with RT, a permanent leukoencephalopathy may occur.

Thioguanine (6-TG) is a purine analog that requires hepatic activation for activity. It inhibits purine biosynthesis, which is necessary for DNA synthesis. 6-TG makes DNA more sensitive to strand breakage. It is used in some combination chemotherapy regimens for malignant glioma and medulloblastoma. Systemic side effects are myelosuppression and immuosuppression.

NATURALLY OCCURRING COMPOUNDS

Vincristine is a water-soluble drug that does not cross the intact BBB. It inhibits microtubule assembly and function. It is used in combination with procarbazine and CCNU to treat malignant glioma, anaplastic oligodendroglioma, anaplastic mixed oligo-astrocytoma, and PCNSL. It is used in other multi-agent drug combinations to treat PNET, medulloblastoma, and germinoma. Its major toxicity is neural, with a dose-related axonal peripheral and autonomic neuropathy that includes constipation, impotence, and orthostatic hypotension. It can cause a paralytic ileus, often misdiagnosed as an acute abdomen.

Etoposide (VP-16) binds to tubulin and inhibits microtubular assembly. It inhibits topoisomerase II by binding it in a stable complex with DNA. It is used in combination with carboplatin for therapy of malignant gliomas and in some germinoma and PNET regimens. VP-16 produces myelosuppression but not neurotoxicity.

Doxorubicin is an antibiotic that inhibits topoisomerase II DNA cleavage, impairing DNA synthesis. It does not cross the BBB but has been used in the treatment of PCNSL. Its major systemic toxicities are myelosuppression and cardiomyopathy. It does not often produce neurotoxicity.

OTHER

Dexamethasone is a corticosteroid used for its anti-edema effect in most brain tumors. It is cytotoxic in PCNSL. Systemic toxicities include immunosuppression, diabetes, weight gain, hirsutism, acne, ulcers, osteoporosis, Cushing's syndrome, hypokalemia, and hypernatremia. Central nervous system (CNS) side effects include psychosis, depression, anxiety, and tremor. Peripheral nervous system toxicity is manifested as a mild to severe myopathy that resolves very slowly after steroid withdrawal. It may limit the access of chemotherapeutic agents to tumors by stabilizing the blood-tumor barrier.

Innovative Approaches for Chemotherapy

HIGH-DOSE INTRAVENOUS CHEMOTHERAPY WITH AUTOLOGOUS BONE MARROW TRANSPLANT

High-dose chemotherapy with autologous bone marrow is an innovative chemotherapy approach (Table 7–8). The rationale for high-dose IV chemotherapy is that brain tumors have a steep dose-response

Table 7–8. **Innovative Approaches for Chemotherapy**

High-dose IV chemotherapy with bone marrow rescue
IA chemotherapy
IA chemotherapy with BBBD
IV or IA chemotherapy with BTBD
Intratumoral chemotherapy
Drug encapsulated liposomes
Metabolic therapies
Differentiating agents

curve to alkylating agents, and with sufficient drug exposure relatively resistant cells become sensitive.[16,55,56] The major dose-limiting toxicity of high-dose therapy with alkylating agents is bone marrow suppression, and autologous bone marrow rescue provides the means to maximize single-dose administration.[55] Most drugs produce a cytotoxic effect by a log-linear relationship, killing a fixed percentage of cells over a range of doses, followed by a flattening of the curve in the upper dose ranges.[15,16,18,55] Therefore, within the log-linear portions of the curve, small increases in drug dose may produce large changes in tumor cell kill, whereas in the flat portion of the curve, tumor cell kill increases marginally, with a high likelihood of increased toxicity.[55]

High-dose BCNU and other alkylating agents have been used in both adjuvant[57–61] and recurrent settings[57,62–65] for the treatment of malignant glioma. In the three largest trials of adjuvant high-dose BCNU with autologous bone marrow rescue, the median survival was 17, 17.5, and 26 months, with a 22% to 56% 2-year survival.[58–60] In the trial by Johnson and colleagues,[59] with the longest median survival of 26 months, a further data update reveals a median survival of approximately 18 months (Messerschmidt GL, personal communication, 1987). The median age of patients entered on the three trials was only 27, 34, and 46. Toxic deaths occurred in 11 of 65 (16%) patients.

In the recurrent setting, the two largest trials had 28 and 27 patients, both with a median age of 38, and an average response rate of 45%.[57,64] There were occasional long duration responses in both studies, with seven patients being disease free from 15 to 84 months. An average of 25% of patients from the two trials had toxic deaths. Two recent reviews[66,67] concerning high-dose chemotherapy both see promise for the modality in the adjuvant setting. In summary, high-dose chemotherapy with autologous bone marrow transplantation is an expensive therapy with good scientific rationale. However, considering the young age of patients on bone marrow rescue trials and their age-associated increased median survival, autologous bone marrow rescue probably has no effect on median survival, with a toxic fatality rate between 15% and 25%.

In the pediatric age group, high-dose chemotherapy has been used to treat a variety of tumors including hemispheral malignant astrocytomas, brainstem astrocytomas, medulloblastomas, and ependymomas.[68,69] The largest number of patients treated has been with malignant astrocytoma, a total of 28 in the three trials. The overall response rate was 10 of 29 (34%) patients. In the largest trial, Heideman and associates[70] concluded that high-dose chemotherapy was no more effective than conventional treatment in pediatric malignant gliomas. The role of high-dose chemotherapy in other tumors in the pediatric age group will require larger trials in a research setting.

INTRA-ARTERIAL CHEMOTHERAPY

The rationale for intra-arterial (IA) infusion of chemotherapy or monoclonal antibodies is to increase the exposure of tumor cells to therapeutic agents and decrease systemic toxicity. The quantitative advantage of IA over IV delivery of a drug depends directly on the clearance of the drug from the plasma and is inversely proportional to the flow in the capillary bed. It is defined by the formula:

$$\text{Regional advantage (Ra)} = 1 + \text{Clearance (Cl)/Flow(F)}$$

where there is no metabolism of the drug in the tissue. The clearance of a drug is largely fixed; it is possible to decrease the arterial flow and increase drug exposure time in the capillaries and, therefore, passage across the BBB.[71,72] IA carotid infusion of [^{14}C] BCNU in monkeys produced 2.2 to 2.8 times greater tissue BCNU levels, than IV infusion of identical doses.[73] [^{13}N]cisplatinum was infused intra-arterially during PET, and Ra was 1.1 and 2.5 in two patients with glioblastoma.[74] Intra-arteral BCNU and CDDP have been delivered in clinical trials by infraophthalmic[75–79] and supraophthalmic catheter placement.[80,81] The supraophthalmic location was used to decrease arterial tumor flow and the risk of retinal toxicity.[80,81] The supraophthalmic catheter placement is more likely to cause drug streaming and unequal drug distribution in the tumor bed.[82]

The BTCG entered 315 patients with malignant astrocytoma in a randomized phase III trial of adjuvant infraophthalmic IA versus intravenous BCNU with or without 5-FU. The initial course of BCNU was delivered before RT was performed, with subsequent courses at 6-week intervals. Actuarial analysis demonstrated reduced survival for the IA BCNU group (p=0.03). On subset analysis of the anaplastic astrocytoma patients, whereas the survival of the IA BCNU group was worse than those receiving IV BCNU (p=0.002), the glioblastoma patients in the two groups did not differ in survival. Serious toxicity was seen in the IA BCNU group, with 10% of patients developing irreversible encephalopathy and 15% developing ipsilateral blindness. Neuropathologically, IA BCNU produced brain white matter leukoencephalopathy and hemorrhagic necrosis, and a hemorrhagic retinal vasculopathy.[77] In the controlled trial, IA BCNU and RT were delivered concurrently. The concurrent delivery was probably potentiated white matter toxicity. IA BCNU and RT were given sequentially in phase I and II studies; in these studies, white matter leukoencephalopathy was also seen frequently but was less often symptomatic.[75]

In a BTCG study of recurrent malignant gliomas, patients were randomized to IA CDDP versus IV PCNU. There was "modest advantage" in the IV PCNU treatment group.[78] The Southwest Oncology Group (SWOG) was unable to complete a randomized trial of two courses of IA CDDP, before or concomitant with RT, because of arterial catheterization and toxicity difficulties.[79] There appears to be a lower incidence of irreversible encephalopathy after IA CDDP than after IA BCNU, but there are more frequent seizures, including status epilepticus, cortical blindness, extraocular muscle palsies, and hearing loss.[83–87]

In phase I and II trials, infraophthalmic IA CDDP has been combined with IA etoposide adjuvantly for the treatment of high-grade glioma and metastatic tumor before and after RT.[88] The median survival for malignant glioma patients in the combined IA CDDP and etoposide trial was 14 months. Twelve of 28 patients with metastases responded to IA CDDP and etoposide, with a median survival in responders of 7 months.[88] IA CDDP has also been combined with IA BCNU for the treatment of recurrent gliomas[89] and with IA bleomycin in the treatment of progressive malignant brain tumors and metastases.[90] In the recurrent glioma trial, alternating IA CDDP with BCNU, only five of the original 43 patients received a second course of BCNU. A total of 22 patients progressed after their initial courses of IA BCNU or CDDP, and 14 patients were removed from the study, because of IA BCNU (n=2) or CDDP (n=9) toxicity, catheterization intolerance (n=2), or an unrelated medical condition (n=1).[89] IA bleomycin with IA CDDP produced short-duration responses in nine of 15 patients with either primary or metastatic brain tumors.[90] In a large phase II trial of 56 patients with recurrent malignant astrocytoma, infraophthalmic IA BCNU was combined with oral procarbazine and IV vincristine. The median survival in the anaplastic astrocytoma group (n = 35) was 20 months, and in the glioblastoma group (n = 23), median survival was 30 months.[91] In summary, IA chemotherapy has a strong scientific rationale in the treatment of malignant glial tumors if the clearance of the infused drug from the plasma is rapid and the arterial flow is low. The current drugs used for arterial chemotherapy do not achieve sufficient Ra to overcome the intrinsic resistance of most glial tumors and are too toxic to surrounding cerebral gray and white matter.

IA BBBD AND CHEMOTHERAPY

Chapter 2 discusses the scientific basis of osmotic BBBD. A shortcoming of IA mannitol BBBD is the greater degree of BBB opening in normal brain than in either tumor or brain adjacent to tumor.[92] In spite of the theoretical shortcomings of IA BBBD, Neuwelt and colleagues[93] treated

17 patients with PCNSL with IA mannitol BBBD and IA MTX every 28 days for 12 cycles. Oral procarbazine and dexamethasone were given for 14 days of every 28-day cycle. The median survival was 44.5 months, with RT given only on disease recurrence. No CNS toxicity was present. In assessing this trial, it is uncertain what percentage of the therapeutic effect is related to the IA BBBD and the additional exposure from IA MTX, or alternatively, to the combination of MTX, procarbazine, and dexamethasone. A multi-institution phase II trial of IA BBBD with MTX in PCNSL is ongoing. DeAngelis and colleagues[94] have achieved similar treatment results in PCNSL, using IT MTX, multiagent IV MTX and Ara-C chemotherapy, and RT (see Chapter 12).

Neuwelt and coworkers[95] also used IA BBBD with IA MTX, and concurrent systemic procarbazine and cyclophosphamide in 38 patients with glioblastoma, after surgery and RT. The predicted median survival was 17.5 months. Three patients had acute strokes related to the catheterization procedure, 22 had transient neurologic worsening, and 21 had seizures.

RMP-7, a bradykinin analog, and leukotriene C4 have been infused intra-arterially in rats with RG-2 tumors, with selective opening of the BTB and not the BBB.[96] Carboplatin was given intra-arterially to rats after IA RMP-7 or IA saline. RMP-7 increased the transport of [^{14}C] carboplatin to tumors 2.7-fold, and the survival rate of rats was 10% in untreated controls, 37% without RMP-7, and 74% with RMP-7. RMP-7 does not have the theoretical shortcomings of IA mannitol BBBD, and it is about to enter clinical trials in glioma.[96]

INTRATUMORAL CHEMOTHERAPY

Intratumoral infusion of chemotherapeutics, biologic response modifiers, radioisotopes, and immunotoxins are being explored to increase the exposure of the tumor to the therapeutic agent. Theoretically, intratumoral infusions will bypass the BBB to achieve prolonged intracerebral therapeutic levels while minimizing systemic exposure and toxicity.[97] The technology for intratumoral infusion is varied and includes (1) direct intratumoral injections through a catheter, (2) drug injection through an implanted reservoir, (3) an implanted reservoir connected to a subcutaneous implantable infusion pump, and (4) biodegradable polymer matrices loaded with drug and implanted in the walls of the resection cavity. A recent review[97] describes each of these methods in detail and reviews the clinical trials. Direct catheter intratumoral injections and injections through an implanted reservoir bypass the BBB but still may have to traverse the space from the injection site in tumor to the surrounding tumor and brain adjacent to tumor. This space may include cysts, edema, hemorrhage, and necrosis before reaching tumor. When an infusion pump is connected to a reservoir, it drives the drug through tissue by pressure, in addition to diffusion and bulk flow.

One of the earliest matrix intratumoral trials was with MTX delivered through a spongostan sponge in multimodality therapy with surgery, RT, and systemic chemotherapy. The treatment group that received all four types of treatment including intratumoral MTX had no better median survival than the group that received the other three therapies with no intratumoral MTX.[98]

Brem and colleagues[99–101] used a drug loaded polymer directly implanted in the tumor cavity after surgical resection. The polymer releases drug load over a time interval, depending on the characteristics of the polymer matrix. The implanted polymer matrix is not subject to blockage, repeated infection exposure from injection, or patient compliance difficulties. The disadvantages of the polymer matrix include these: fixed dose of drug is being used, drug release cannot be modified, and the system is not refillable.[99]

Early experiments in rats demonstrated good BCNU penetration: 10 mm from the loaded polymer disc at 3 and 7 days. No significant pathologic changes occurred in normal primate brain implanted with the BCNU loaded polymer.[99,100] In a phase III placebo-controlled, double-blind trial, patients with recurrent glioma were randomized to a polymer loaded with 3.85% BCNU or empty placebo polymer. The BCNU-polymer group had a median survival of 31 weeks compared with 23 weeks for the placebo group ($p=0.007$). In the glioblastoma group, 6-month survival was increased by more than 50% ($p=0.02$). In the polymer-implanted group, CNS toxicity did not increase.[101] The authors have demonstrated that BCNU polymers are more effective than placebo and are safe but not that they are more effective than IV BCNU therapy.

DRUG-ENCAPSULATED LIPOSOMES

Sterically stabilized liposomes are small particles (<100 nm) with a mixed lipid composition that are delivered intravenously. A drug is encapsulated in the internal aqueous space of the liposome. Systemically, the liposomes have selective tumor localization, and it is hoped that they will localize intracerebrally with reduced systemic exposure.[102] Fischer rats were implanted with a malignant sarcoma in the right parietal region and treated with either doxorubicin-encapsulated liposomes or free doxorubicin. The encapsulated liposomes achieved 14-fold higher tumor levels and a significant increase in survival.[102] No human brain tumor trials have been carried out.

METABOLIC THERAPIES

Lonidamine is a drug that interferes with aerobic glycolysis by inhibiting a mitochondrially bound hexokinase. It decreases energy production capabilities, hopefully limiting cell growth and the ability to repair potentially lethal damage, induced by either RT or other chemotherapeutic agents.[103,104] In tissue culture with BCNU, lonidamine has been shown to increase BCNU cytotoxicity.[104] In a phase II recurrent glioma trial of 10 patients, two patients with anaplastic glioma (one oligoastrocytoma) had a partial radiologic and clinical response to lonidamine lasting 94 and 88 weeks. Three patients had stable disease (SD) for 16 to 26 weeks, and five progressed.[105] When lonidamine was added to RT in the treatment of single brain metastasis, no advantage in the lonidamine and RT arm was observed.[106]

A second type of metabolic manipulation, and possibly the prototype for metabolic manipulation in the future, is the insertion of a gene for an enzyme using a viral vector.[107] D-amino acid oxidase (DAAO) is an enzyme that catalyzes the conversion of the substrate D-alanine to H_2O_2 and the subsequent generation of free radicals. The enzyme cloned from yeast has been packaged in a plasmid and inserted in vitro in cultured 9L cells. Exposure of cells to D-alanine resulted in a dose-dependent cell kill. Intracranial 9L tumors that constitutively expressed the DAAO gene were treated with D-alanine. D-alanine treatment resulted in a significant reduction in tumor growth rates. D-alanine will cross into brain, mostly where there is disruption of the BBB, and thus should not be taken up into normal brain. The H_2O_2 generated is membrane permeable and should produce a significant bystander effect. The prevention of free-radical cytotoxicity with free-radical scavengers has become important in neurologic diseases, such as Parkinson's disease, amyotrophic lateral sclerosis, and stroke. In tumor therapy, the generation of free radicals may have important metabolic effects.

DIFFERENTIATING AGENTS

Differentiating agents induce malignant cell differentiation.[108] They have played a minor role in cancer therapeutics, but interest in this type of drug is increasing. Retinoids are the most interesting of this class of compounds, directly inducing cell differentiation in vitro. They also inhibit cell growth, possibly by stimulating transforming growth factor (TGF-β).[108] Trans-retinoic acid and cis-retinoic acid have both been used in clinical trials of malignant glioma.[109–111] Trans-retinoic acid was used orally every day to treat 30 patients with recurrent malignant astrocytoma (14 glioblastoma multiforme, 14 anaplastic astrocytoma, two other glioma), after RT and chemotherapy failure with only 3 PR in 25 evaluable patients.[109] In a second trial, seven of nine evaluable patients with malignant glioma were responders, with 1 complete response (CR), 1 PR, and 5 SD, with the median survival more than 9 months.[110] Yung and colleagues[111] treated 23 patients with cis-retinoic acid orally with 2 PR and 8 SD, with median time to progression of 25.4 weeks in these 10 patients.

Phenylacetate is another differentiating agent, a naturally occurring plasma component produced in the beta oxidation of fatty acids. In vitro studies with phenylacetate in medulloblastoma and glioma cell lines resulted in a dose-dependent decline in DNA synthesis and cell proliferation. Cells accumulated at a G_0/G_1 interphase in the cell cycle. In addition, two of the glioma cell lines had morphologic changes, with increased glial fibrillary acidic protein (GFAP) expression.[112] The exact role of phenylacetate and retinoids in brain tumor chemotherapy still needs to be defined.

IMMUNOTHERAPY

Principles

Malignant glioma frequently has rapid tumor progression despite surgery, RT, and chemotherapy. Immunotherapy is another potential therapeutic modality for the treatment of gliomas, particularly on recurrence, when there may be infiltrating tumor cells. Immunotherapy is not presently a curative therapy but is administered in combination with other therapies. The intact BBB is impermeable to immunoglobulins and cytokines and places the brain behind an immunologic closed door. In addition, surgery, RT, chemotherapy, and steroids may significantly depress the immune system. Most gliomas do not produce a significant lymphocytic response when infiltrating brain. The presence of a lymphocytic response has been correlated with a better prognosis by some investigators.[113] Brain tumors effect both systemic and local immune function. In patients with brain tumors, there is an impaired peripheral blood lymphocyte blastogenic response to phytohemagglutinin and phorbol esters.[114] Patients with brain tumors also have suppressed humoral antibody-mediated cytotoxicity and cell-mediated cytotoxicity.[9]

Humoral B-cell antibodies are occasionally present in glioma tissue, but their ability to produce anti-glioma antibodies participating in complement- or antibody-dependent cell-mediated cytotoxicity is doubtful.[115] Brain tumor cells possess cytoplasmic, cell surface, and extracellular antigens.[9,115] Tenascin is a glial antigen expressed on the extracellular surface of gliomas.[115,116] Mel-14 is a neuroectodermal surface antigen on many tumors including melanoma, neuroblastoma, glioma, and fetal brain tissue.[115,117] Monoclonal antibodies have been developed to both of these antigens and labeled with Iodine-131 (^{131}I) for tumor localization and treatment.[116–118]

Host cellular immune responses against brain tumors fall into two categories, major histocompatibility (MHC)-restricted and non-MHC-restricted. For a glioma antigenic determinant to produce a host response, the glioma cell with antigenic determinant must be associated with an MHC class 2 molecule and bind to antigen-presenting cells. The cell complex must then be recognized by a T-cell receptor, with activation of the T cell. The activated T cell must stimulate cytotoxic lymphocytes and helper T cells. Both of these cells must access the tumor site and then cause tissue destruction for effective MHC-mediated cell cytotoxicity. The mechanisms of non-MHC lymphocyte mediated brain tumor lysis are not known.[115] Tumor-infiltrating lymphocytes surrounding glial tumors have decreased responsiveness.[119]

Glioma cells also secrete growth factors and cytokines that effect the immune system. In Chapter 2 it was discussed that TGF-β2 is secreted by glioma cells, and there is increased expression with increasing degree of anaplasia.[120,121] TGF-β2 suppresses T-lymphocyte activation within malignant gliomas.[120] In vitro, the suppression of T-lymphocyte activation can be reversed with a phosphorothioate-antisense oligodeoxynucleotide.[122] TGF-β2 also has other immunosuppressive actions, which may be partially reversed by

IL-2.[115] IL-10 is expressed in gliomas and is more common in invasive tumors.[123] It inhibits the synthesis of a variety other cytokines, including IL-1, interferon (INF- α), TNF, and IL-6 by activated macrophages.[115]

In summary, humoral and cell-mediated immunity are suppressed in patients with gliomas. All of the common brain tumor treatments—surgery, RT, chemotherapy, and steroids—frequently further suppress the immune system. In addition, gliomas secrete cytokines and growth factors that impair the immune system. Labeled monoclonal antibodies and antisense oligodeoxynucleotides offer some hope for successful immunotherapy. Most clinical immunotherapy trials have evaluated the treatment of recurrent malignant astrocytoma.

Types

Many small predominantly phase I and II trials for the treatment of recurrent malignant gliomas have been performed.[9,124] Most immunotherapy trials fall into 5 categories: restorative (active nonspecific), passive, adoptive, active specific, and genetic modification (Table 7–9).[9,124]

RESTORATIVE (ACTIVE NONSPECIFIC)

Restorative immunotherapy nonspecifically stimulates the patient's deficient immune system to mount an immune response against the tumor. Early clinical trials were with bacille Calmette-Guérin (BCG),[125] BCG cell walls,[126] *Corynebacterium parvum,*[127] OK432,[128] levamisole,[129] and α-1 thymosine.[130] There were no responses in any patients given these agents. Jaeckle and colleagues[131] administered *Serratia marcescens* extract subcutaneously to 19 patients with recurrent malignant astrocytoma. Two patients had CR lasting 63 and more than 77 weeks, and four patients had SD, ranging from 7 to more than 58 weeks. Side effects were mild and of two types: (1) local, consisting of injection site tenderness and induration, and less commonly, (2) systemic flu-like symptoms and hypotension. These results are more encouraging than those from previous restorative trials. In addition to bacterial extracts, mumps and rabies virus vaccines have been used without effect.[132,133]

Other proteins used to nonspecifically stimulate the immune system are the interferons, interleukins, and TNF-α. The three major types of INF—INF-α, INF-β, and INF-γ—all have been used in clinical trials in glioma patients. INF-α and -β have direct antiproliferative effects on human glioma cells in vitro and when implanted in nude mice.[9,115,124] INF-α has been used in leukocyte, lymphoblastoid, and recombinant forms and has been given intramuscularly, intravenously, intrathecally, and intratumorally. The best results were with lymphoblastoid INF-α administered intravenously or intramuscularly, over an 8-week period. Seven of 17 patients had tumor regression.[134] After therapy initiation, approximately 50% of patients had reversible confusion, memory loss, and lethargy, often lasting weeks. INF-α therapy was interrupted for CNS toxicity in six patients, secondary infections in five patients, leukopenia and/or thrombocytopenia in four patients, and elevated SGOT in two patients. In another trial, INF-α was given by intratumoral injection in conjunction with RT, CDDP, and vincristine chemotherapy. Eight patients were reoperated for presumed tumor recurrence. Seven had no residual tumor but were thought to have tumor necrosis secondary to the intratumoral INF-α injections.[135]

INF-β is the most active of the three interferons against brain tumors. The response rate in IV infusions of INF-β has varied between 0% in four trials, to 45% in one trial.[124] Recent trials with IV recombinant INF-β administered intravenously have all had a response rate of 15% to 25%.[124,136,137] Intratumoral INF-β produced no responses in 20 patients.[138]

INF-γ has limited antiproliferative activity compared with INF-α and -β. It is a potent regulator of gene expression and function. Mahaley[139] conducted a clinical

Table 7–9. **Types of Immunotherapy**

Immunotherapy	Reference Number
Restorative (Active Nonspecific)	
Bacterial components	
BCG	125,126
Corynebacterium parvum	127
Serratia marcescens	131
OK432 (streptococcus pyogenes)	128
Viruses	
Rabies	132
Mumps	133
Other	
Levamisole	129
α-1 thymosine	130
Cytokines	
IFN-α, IFN-β, IFN-γ	134–139
Interleukins	161
TNF-α	124
Passive	
Polyclonal antibodies	140
Monoclonal antibodies	142
Monoclonal antibodies coupled to:	
Radionuclide	116,118,141,145–147
Immunotoxin	148–151
Chemotherapeutic agents	152
Boron	153
Adoptive	
Cytotoxic lymphocytes	154–156
Lymphokine activated killer cells	157–160,162
Antigen stimulated lymphocytes	163,164
Active Specific	
Autologous tumor immunization	165–167
Anti-idiotypic antibody	168
Genetic Modification	
Antisense oligodeoxynucleotides	122,123
Lymphocyte transfection	169

trial in 15 patients, with only one response. Toxicity was severe and included fever, chills, nausea, vomiting, elevated liver enzymes, and hypotension. Trials of INF-γ have been abandoned. If given in lower doses or with other cytokines with different toxicities, it may still have a role in controlling gene expression.

Interleukin-1, interleukin-2, and TNF-α and -β all have potent immunomodulatory actions in vitro, but all have significant systemic toxicities preventing their clinical use.[124]

PASSIVE

Passive immunotherapy involves the transfer of sera containing antiglioma antibodies or monoclonal antibodies. In 1965, Day and associates[140] performed the first clinical immunotherapy trial of malignant glioma patients with a polyclonal rabbit antiglioma sera without efficacy. They were able to document glioma tissue localization. Problems with polyclonal rabbit antiglioma serum include low yield from the antiserum globulin, normal tissue cross reactivity, and heterogeneity of antibody-specific affinity.[115] Monoclonal antibodies were developed with the advent of hybridoma technology and can be produced in high quantity and homogeneity. These antibodies are specific for a single antigenic determinant on malignant brain tumors and have been developed to surface antigens, extracellular matrix proteins, growth factor receptors, and gene products.[141] They localize in tumor and produce high tumor to brain ratios. Monoclonal antibodies react with antigens that are not tumor-specific antigens but are "self" antigens that cross-react with normal tissue. Fragments of antibody, $F(ab)_2$, have been produced that more easily cross the BBB with rapid tissue distribution and clearance, yet retain the ability to localize in tumor.[117,141] Native or unlabeled monoclonal antibodies produce their antitumor effect by antibody-mediated cellular cytotoxicity or by binding complement.[124] In clinical trials, they have been ineffective.[142]

Monoclonal antibodies will be used in the future to localize tumor and deliver another more toxic substance to tumor. Monoclonal antibodies have been labeled with radioisotopes, plant and bacterial toxins, chemotherapeutic agents, chemotherapy-containing liposomes, interferons, photosensitizers, and boron.[143] The BBB presents obstacles for delivery of labeled monoclonal antibodies, and BBBD may be used to open tight junctions.[144] Drug and tumor properties in Table 7–4, must be considered for monoclonal antibody delivery. Monoclonal antibodies may cross-react with normal tissue, or an immune response may develop to the anti-mouse antibody, preventing multiple administrations. ^{131}I-labeled anti-tenascin monoclonal antibody, 81C6, localizes to tumor and is cytotoxic to D54 human glioma implanted subcutaneously,[145] and intracerebrally in nude rats.[116] IA delivery of 81C6 was no more effective than IV delivery in nude rats implanted with D54 human glioma.[146] Brady and colleagues[147] performed a small phase I to II trial of IA I^{125}-labeled anti-EGFR 425 monoclonal antibody in patients with recurrent malignant glioma. The results were difficult to interpret, with a few responses reported.

Highly potent peptide toxins have been linked to monoclonal antibodies and hormones to form immunotoxins.[148] These toxins are from plants or bacteria; three of the most common are ricin, from the castor oil plant; pseudomonas; and diphtheria exotoxin. Other plant toxins similar to ricin are pokeweed antiviral protein and saporin.[148] These toxins bind to the cell through the monoclonal antibody. They then enter the cell, catalytically inactivate the ribosomes, and produce cell death. Transferrin receptors are expressed on all replicating cells. Three different anti-transferrin monoclonal-toxin conjugates (saporin, pokeweed anti-viral protein, and momordin) were tested against three glioma cell lines. Protein synthesis was inhibited in all cell lines with all toxins. The saporin conjugate showed the highest efficiency and was tested in a clonogenic assay against the glioma cell lines, producing at least a 5-log cell kill.[149] Anti-transferrin receptor immunotoxins were directed against pediatric glioblastoma and medulloblastoma cell lines and produced cell killing at low concentrations.[150] Oldfield[151] has used an anti-transferrin monoclonal antibody covalently linked to a genetically engineered diphtheria toxin for the treatment of malignant brain tumors. The genetic engineering removed the portion of the diphtheria toxin that binds to normal cells. The immunotoxin was injected intratumorally in 16 patients (13 with malignant gliomas, one with oligodendroglioma, and two with metastatic tumors). To enhance immunotoxin delivery, a convection system was used. Twelve patients were evaluable, and five had greater than a 90% reduction in tumor. Larger clinical trials are planned.

Monoclonal antibodies have been linked to MTX and loaded into liposomes. They have been directed against glioma cells in tissue culture, with 100-fold increase in glioma cell cytoxicity compared with MTX alone.[152] Boron compounds have also been linked to monoclonal antibodies for delivery to the tumor cell. Neutrons will then need to be directed at the tumor to release a high-energy α particle for cytotoxicity.[153]

ADOPTIVE

Adoptive immunotherapy involves the transfer of autologous or allogeneic-sensitized immune cells to an immunodeficient host. Early trials[154–156] of intratumoral autologous white blood cells were without significant effect. Recent adoptive immunotherapy trials of malignant glioma have focused on the intratumoral delivery of lymphokine-activated killer (LAK) cells. LAK cells are produced by the incubation of peripheral blood lymphocytes with IL-2. The LAK cells produced have cytolytic activity against autologous tumors and other tumors but not normal brain tissue.[157]

Initial reports of clinical trials of intratumoral LAK cells, with IL-2 delivered through an Ommaya reservoir connected to a ventricular catheter, were positive. Jacobs and colleagues[158] reported eight of ten patients stable or improving. In the largest trial, Ingram and colleagues[159] reported 76 of 83 patients responding, with 18 patients having no evidence of tumor at follow-up. Subsequent reports were less optimistic. Merchant and colleagues[160] treated 29 patients, five at the time of initial craniotomy and 24 at recurrence. In the five adjuvantly treated patients, the median time of recurrence was 12 months. In the 24 patients treated on recurrence, the median time to progression was 4 months, and the median survival time was 8 months. All patients developed worsening of neurological deficits in the days after therapy. Significant cerebral edema was seen radiographically around the treatment site in both patients and animal models.

In another trial, three glioma patients treated with parenteral IL-2 had increased cerebral edema with neurological deterioration. Seven patients with extracranial cancer also received IL-2, and there was no neurological deterioration. Magnetic resonance imaging in six of seven patients with extracranial cancer showed increased water content in gray and white matter.[161] Lillehei and colleagues[162] treated 20 patients with recurrent malignant astrocytoma with LAK plus IL-2 intratumorally. Eleven patients were evaluable, with median survival of 18 weeks, after treatment. The use of steroids or previous chemotherapy did not influence survival. The initial optimism for LAK therapy has faded because early response rates could not be documented. In addition, all patients were treated with one or more surgical resections, further complicating interpretation of the results of LAK therapy. Immediate neurological complications were significant, and the therapy is expensive.

Antigen-stimulated lymphocytes have also been injected intratumorally and intrathecally.[163,164] A total of 31 patients with glioblastoma were treated with autologous lymphocytes and lymphoblastoid INF, with a median survival of 17 weeks and only one patient responding.[163] An IT autologous lymphocyte infusion study was also performed in patients with malignant glioma.[164]

ACTIVE SPECIFIC

Active specific immunotherapy involves immunization with autologous or allogeneic tumor cells or with tumor antigens to stimulate an immune response against the patient's glioma. In two early trials,[165,166] autologous tumor cells were injected subcutaneously. There were no responses in five and 62 patients in the two trials, respectively. Mahaley and colleagues[167] immunized 20 patients with live irradiated glioma cells. Patients where also treated with BCG and levamisole, restoratively. Many patients developed antibodies against the glioma cells. There was prolonged survival in nine patients, with only three patients developing cutaneous hypersensitivity reactions. The results with autologous tumor injection have been disappointing. The tumor-associated antigens that are reinjected may be part of the host and may not generate a significant immune response. Attempts at tumor membrane modification are being made.[124]

Anti-idiotypic antibodies are antibodies that are antigenically similar to known glioma antigens. They induce reactivity to the antigen and may be useful in future tumor vaccines in the future.[168]

GENETIC MODIFICATION

A phosphorothioate-antisense oligodeoxynucleotide to TGF-β2 has been used to reverse the cellular immune suppression produced by TGF-β2.[122,123] It is to be hoped that this antisense oligodeoxynucleotide can be transfected into glioma cells and increase immunity. In another molecular biology study, cDNA for mouse INF-γ was inserted into a cytotoxic T-lymphocyte genome, with increased INF release and increased cytotoxicity for a glioma cell line.[169]

CHAPTER SUMMARY

The chemotherapeutic and immunotherapeutic treatment of brain tumors has been, for the most part, a major disappointment during the past 30 years. During this time, an understanding of the fundamental scientific principles of drug and biologic response modifier delivery have been discovered. Tumor drug resistance is a function of drug delivery to tumor, the BBB and the BTB, and intrinsic and acquired drug resistance. Intrinsic and acquired resistance to nitrosoureas from MGMT is being treated in clinical trials with methyltransferase depletors, and antisense oligodeoxynucleotides to MGMT are being investigated.

The advances in phase III clinical trial design should allow us to plan more effective and economical phase III clinical trials, with the ability to accept or reject a null hypothesis. A phase III clinical trial is in process to answer the question of whether adjuvant chemotherapy is beneficial in the treatment of anaplastic oligodendroglioma. The application of statistical meta-analysis to 16 malignant glioma trials of 3000 patients has shown a survival advantage with the addition of chemotherapy to RT for both glioblastoma multiforme and anaplastic astrocytoma. The absolute increases in survival from the meta-analysis were small, with a 10% increase at 1 and 2 years. This explains why phase III chemotherapy trials with 400 to 600 patients have often been only intermittently able to reject the null hypothesis that chemotherapy is not additive to RT.

The survival of patients with PCNSL appears to have improved markedly with (1) IA BBBD and IA MTX, with oral procarbazine and dexamethasone and with (2) multiagent multimodality therapy, with IT and IV MTX, RT, and IV Ara-C.

Brain tumors have decreased humoral and cell-mediated immunity and secrete growth factors and cytokines that further suppress the immune system. TGF-β2 secreted by gliomas suppresses T-lymphocyte activation, which can be reversed with a phosphorothioate-antisense oligodeoxynucleotide developed with molecular biology techniques. The recent intratumoral immunotherapy trial with a genetically engineered anti-transferrin diphtheria immunotoxin offers hope in an otherwise disappointing series of clinical studies with monoclonal antibodies.

It is hoped that with the addition of molecular biologic techniques to our understanding of drug delivery, tumor resistance, and immunologic mechanisms, the outcome of patients with brain tumors will improve over the next 20 years.

REFERENCES

1. Groothuis, DR, and Blasberg, RG: Rational brain tumor chemotherapy. The interaction of drug and tumor. Neurol Clin 3(4):801–816, 1985.
2. Shapiro, WR, and Shapiro, JR: Principles of brain tumor chemotherapy. Semin Oncol 13(1): 56–69, 1986.
3. Blasberg, RG, and Groothuis, DR: Chemotherapy of brain tumors: physiological and pharmacokinetic considerations. Semin Oncol 13(1): 70–82, 1986.
4. Obbens, EAMT, and Shapiro, WR: Brain tumor chemotherapy. In Pinedo, HM, Longo, DL, and Chabner, BA (eds): Cancer Chemotherapy and Biological Response Modifiers Annual 15. Elsevier Science B.V., Amsterdam, The Netherlands, 1994, pp 628–645.
5. Freeman, AI, Fenstermacher, J, Shapiro, W, et al: Forbeck forum on improved drug delivery to brain tumors. Selective Cancer Therapeutics 6(3):109–118, 1990.
6. Shapiro, WR: Treatment of neuroectodermal brain tumors. Ann Neurol 12:231–237, 1982.

7. Greenberg, HS: Treatment of primary malignant brain tumors. In Klawans, HL, Goetz, CG, and Tanner, CM (eds): Textbook of Clinical Neuropharmacology and Therapeutics, ed. 2. Raven Press, New York, 1992, pp 335–348.
8. Fine, HA: Chemotherapy of astrocytomas in adults. In Black, PM, Schoene, WC, and Lampson, LA (eds): Astrocytomas: Diagnosis, Treatment, and Biology. Blackwell Scientific Publications, Boston, pp 86–109, 1993.
9. Jaeckle, KA: Immunotherapy of malignant gliomas. Semin Oncol 21(2):249–259, 1994.
10. Reese, TS, and Karnovsky, MJ: Fine structural localization of a blood-brain barrier to exogenous peroxidase. J Cell Biol 34:207–217, 1967.
11. Vick, N, Khandekar, JD, and Bigner, DD: Chemotherapy of brain tumors. The "blood-brain barrier" is not a factor. Arch Neurol 34: 523–526, 1977.
12. Ghersi-Egea, JF, Minn, A, and Siest, G: A new aspect of the protective function of the blood-brain barrier: activities of four drug-metabolizing enzymes in isolated rat brain microvessels. Life Sci 42:2515–2523, 1988.
13. Levin, VA, Landahl, HD, and Patlak, CS: Drug delivery to CNS tumors. Cancer Treat Rep 65 (Suppl 2):19–25, 1981.
14. Levin, VA, Patlak, CS, and Landahl, HD: Heuristic modeling of drug delivery to malignant brain tumors. J Pharmacokinet Biopharm 8:257–296, 1980.
15. Schold, SC Jr: Chemotherapy of primary central nervous system neoplasms. Semin Neurol 1:189–202, 1981.
16. Skipper, HE, and Schabel, FM Jr: Quantitative and cytokinetic studies in experimental tumor systems. In Holland, SF, and Frei, E III (eds): Cancer Medicine, ed. 2. Lea and Febiger, Philadelphia, 1982, pp 663–685.
17. Rosenblum, ML, Gerosa, MA, Dougherty, DV, and Wilson, CB: Improved treatment of a brain-tumor model. Part 1: Advantages of single over multiple-dose BCNU schedules. J Neurosurg 58:177–182, 1983.
18. Bogdahn, U: Chemosensitivity of malignant brain tumors. Preliminary results. J Neurooncol 1:149–166, 1983.
19. Gerosa, MA, Dougherty, DV, Wilson, CB, and Rosenblum, ML: Improved treatment of a brain-tumor model. Part 2: Sequential therapy with BCNU and 5-fluorouracil. J Neurosurg 58: 368–373, 1983.
20. Schnipper, LE: Clinical implications of tumor-cell heterogeneity. N Engl J Med 14:1423–1431, 1986.
21. Shapiro, JR, Pu, PY, and Shapiro, WR: Resistant cell types in human gliomas. In Salmon, SE, and Trent, JM (eds): Human Tumor Cloning. Grune and Stratton, Orlando, 1984, pp 133–142.
22. Kornblith, PL, Smith, BH, and Leonard, LA: Response of cultured human brain tumors to nitrosoureas: correlation with clinical data. Cancer 47:255–265, 1981.
23. Shapiro, JR, and Shapiro, WR: Clonal tumor cell heterogeneity. Prog Exp Tumor Res 27:49–66, 1984.
24. Shapiro, WR, Basler, GA, Chernik, NL, and Posner, JB: Human brain tumor transplantation into nude mice. J Natl Cancer Inst 62: 447–453, 1979.
25. Basler, GA, and Shapiro, WR: Brain tumor research with nude mice. In Fogh, J, and Giovanella, B (eds): The Nude Mouse in Experimental and Clinical Research. Academic Press, Inc., New York, 1982, pp 475–490.
26. Horten, BC, Basler, GA, and Shapiro, WR: Xenograft of human malignant glial tumors into brains of nude mice. A histopathological study. J Neuropath Exp Neurol 450:493–511, 1981.
27. Saris, SC, Bigner, SH, and Bigner, DD: Intracerebral transplantation of a human glioma line in immunosuppressed rats. J Neurosurg 60:582–588, 1984.
28. Schold, SC Jr, and Bigner, DD: A review of animal brain tumor models that have been used for therapeutic studies. In Walker, MD (ed): Oncology of the Nervous System. Martinus Nijhoff Publishers, Boston, 1983, pp 31–63.
29. Phillips, PC: Antineoplastic drug resistance in brain tumors. Neurol Clin 9(2):383–404, 1991.
30. Schold, SC Jr, Brent, TP, and von Hofe, E, et al: O^6-alkylguanine-DNA alkyltransferase and sensitivity to procarbazine in human brain-tumor xenografts. J Neurosurg 70:573–577, 1989.
31. Hotta, T, Saito, Y, Fujita, H, et al: O^6-alkylguanine-DNA alkyltransferase activity in human malignant glioma and its clinical implications. J Neurooncol 21:135–140, 1994.
32. Citron, M, Decker, R, Chen, S, et al: O^6-methylguanine-DNA methyltransferase in human normal and tumor tissue from brain, lung, and ovary. Cancer Res 51:4131–4134, 1991.
33. Mineura, K, Izumi, I, Watanabe, K, and Kowada, M: Influence of O^6-methylguanine-DNA methyltransferase activity on chloroethylnitrosourea chemotherapy in brain tumors. Int J Cancer 55:76–81, 1993.
34. Mineura, K, Izumi, I, Kuwahara, N, and Kowada, M: O^6-methylguanine-DNA methyltransferase activity in cerebral gliomas. A guidance for nitrosourea treatment? Acta Oncol 33(1):29–32, 1994.
35. Silber, JR, Mueller, BA, Ewers, TG, and Berger MS: Comparison of O^6-methylguanine-DNA methyltransferase activity in brain tumors and adjacent normal brain. Cancer Res 53:3416–3420, 1993.
36. Marathi, UK, Kroes, RA, Dolan, ME, and Erickson, LC: Prolonged depletion of O^6-methylguanine-DNA methyltransferase activity following exposure to O^6-benzylguanine with or without streptozotocin enhances 1,3-bis(2-chloroethyl)-1-nitrosourea sensitivity *in vitro*. Cancer Res 53:4281–4286, 1993.
37. Chen, J-M, Zhang, Y-P, Moschel, RC, and Ikenaga, M: Depletion of O^6-methylguanine-DNA methyltransferase and potentiation of 1,3-bis

(2-chloroethyl)-1-nitrosourea antitumor activity by O^6-benzylguanine *in vitro*. Carcinogenesis 14(5):1057–1060, 1993.
38. Kudo, H, Mio, T, Kokunai, T, et al: Quantitative analysis of glutathione in human brain tumors. J Neurosurg 72:610–615, 1990.
39. Rothenberg, M, and Ling, V: Multidrug resistance: molecular biology and clinical relevance. J Natl Cancer Inst 81(12):907–910, 1989.
40. Browner, WS, Newman, TB, Cummings, SR, and Hulley, SB: Getting ready to estimate sample size: Hypotheses and underlying principles. In Hulley, SB, and Cummings, SR (eds): Designing Clinical Research. Williams and Wilkins, Baltimore, 1988, pp 128–138.
41. Hulley, SB, Feigal, D, Martin, M, and Cummings, SR: Designing a new study: IV. Experiments. In Hulley, SB, and Cummings, SR (eds): Designing Clinical Research. Williams and Wilkins, Baltimore, 1988, pp 110–127.
42. Browner, WS, Black, D, Newman, TB, and Hulley, SB: Estimating sample size and power. In Hulley SB, Cummings SR (eds): Designing Clinical Research. Williams and Wilkins, Baltimore, 1988, pp 139–150.
43. Fine, HA, Dear, KBG, Loeffler, JS, et al: Meta-analysis of radiation therapy with and without adjuvant chemotherapy for malignant gliomas in adults. Cancer 71:2585–2597, 1993.
44. Winger, MJ, Macdonald, DR, Schold, SC Jr, and Cairncross, JG: Selection bias in clinical trials of anaplastic glioma. Ann Neurol 26:531–534, 1989.
45. Eagan, RT, and Scott, M: Evaluation of prognostic factors in chemotherapy of recurrent brain tumors. J Clin Oncol 1:38–44, 1983.
46. Grant, R, Liang, BC, Page, MAet al: Age influences chemotherapy response in astrocytomas. Neurology 45:929–933, 1995.
47. Walker, MD, Alexander, E Jr, Hunt, WE, et al: Evaluation of BCNU and/or radiotherapy in the treatment of anaplastic gliomas: a cooperative clinical trial. J Neurosurg 49:333–343, 1978.
48. Walker, MD, Green, SB, Byar ,DP, et al: Randomized comparisons of radiotherapy and nitrosoureas for the treatment of malignant glioma after surgery. N Engl J Med 303:1323–1329, 1980.
49. Liang, BC, Newton, HB, Junck, L, and Greenberg, HS: Herpes zoster and procarbazine therapy in patients with malignant glioma. Int J Oncology 5:97–100, 1994.
50. Newton, HB, Junck, L, Bromberg, J, et al: Procarbazine chemotherapy in the treatment of recurrent malignant astrocytomas after radiation and nitrosourea failure. Neurology 40:1743–1746, 1990.
51. Schold, SC Jr, Herndon, JE, Burger, PC, et al: Randomized comparison of diaziquone and carmustine in the treatment of adults with anaplastic glioma. J Clin Oncol 11:77–83, 1993.
52. Longee, DC, Friedman, HS, Albright, RE Jr, et al: Treatment of patients with recurrent gliomas with cyclophosphamide and vincristine. J Neurosurg 72:583–588, 1990.
53. Buckner, JC, Brown, LD, Cascino, TL, et al: Phase II evaluation of infusional etoposide and cisplatin in patients with recurrent astrocytoma. J Neurooncol 9:249–254, 1990.
54. O'Reilly, SM, Newlands, ES, Glaser, MG, et al: Temozolomide: a new oral cytotoxic chemotherapeutic agent with promising activity against primary brain tumours. Eur J Cancer 29A(7):940–942, 1993.
55. Cheson, BD, Lacerna, L, Leyland-Jones, B, et al: Autologous bone marrow transplantation. Ann Inter Med 110:51–65, 1989.
56. Rosenblum, ML, and Gerosa, MA: Stem cell sensitivity. Prog Exp Tumor Res 28:1–17, 1984.
57. Phillips, GL, Wolff, SN, Fay, JW, et al: Intensive 1,3-Bis (2-chloroethyl)-1-nitrosourea (BCNU) monochemotherapy and autologous marrow transplantation for malignant glioma. J Clin Oncol 4:639–645, 1986.
58. Wolff, SN, Phillips, GL, and Herzig, GP: High-dose carmustine with autologous bone marrow transplantation for the adjuvant treatment of high-grade gliomas of the central nervous system. Cancer Treat Rep 71:183–185, 1987.
59. Johnson, DB, Thompson, JM, Corwin, JA, et al: Prolongation of survival for high-grade malignant gliomas with adjuvant high-dose BCNU and autologous bone marrow transplantation. J Clin Oncol 5:783–789, 1987.
60. Mbidde, EK, Selby, PJ, Perren, TJ, et al: High dose BCNU chemotherapy with autologous bone marrow transplantation and full dose radiotherapy for grade IV astrocytoma. Br J Cancer 58:779–782, 1988.
61. Biron, P, Vial, C, Cauvin, F, et al: Strategy including surgery, high dose BCNU followed by ABMT and radiotherapy in supratentorial high grade astrocytomas: A report of 98 patients. In Dicke, KA, Armitage, JO, and Dicke-Evinger, MJ (eds): Autologous Bone Marrow Transplantation: Proceedings of the Fifth International Symposium. The University of Nebraska Medical Center, Omaha, 1991, pp 637–642.
62. Hochberg, FH, Parker, LM, Takvorian, T, et al: High-dose BCNU with autologous bone marrow rescue for recurrent glioblastoma multiforme. J Neurosurg 54:455–460, 1981.
63. Nomura, K, Watanabe, T, Nakamura, O, et al: Intensive chemotherapy with autologous bone marrow rescue for recurrent malignant gliomas. Neurosurg Rev 7:13–22, 1984.
64. Takvorian, T, Parker, LM, Hochberg, FH, Canellos, GP: Autologous bone-marrow transplantation: Host effects of high-dose BCNU. J Clin Oncol 1:610–620, 1983.
65. Giannone, L, and Wolff, SN: Phase II treatment of central nervous system gliomas with high-dose etoposide and autologous bone marrow transplantation. Cancer Treat Rep 71:759–-761, 1987.
66. Fine, HA, and Antman, KH: High-dose chemotherapy with autologous bone marrow transplantation in the treatment of high grade astrocytomas in adults: therapeutic rationale and clinical experience. Bone Marrow Transplantation 10:315–321, 1992.

67. Petersdorf, SH, and Livingston, RB: High dose chemotherapy for the treatment of malignant brain tumors. J Neurooncol 20:155–163, 1994.
68. Finlay, JL, August, C, Packer, R, et al: High-dose multi-agent chemotherapy followed by bone marrow 'rescue' for malignant astrocytomas of childhood and adolescence. J Neurooncol 9:239–248, 1990.
69. Kalifa, C, Hartmann, O, Demeocq, F, et al: High-dose busulfan and thiotepa with autologous bone marrow transplantation in childhood malignant brain tumors: a phase II study. Bone Marrow Transplant 9:227–233, 1992.
70. Heideman, RL, Douglass, EC, Krance, RA, et al: High-dose chemotherapy and autologous bone marrow rescue followed by interstitial and external-beam radiotherapy in newly diagnosed pediatric malignant gliomas. J Clin Oncol 11:1458–1465, 1993.
71. Fenstermacher, JD, and Cowles, AC. Theoretic limitations of intracarotid infusions in brain tumor chemotherapy. Cancer Treat Rep 61:519–526, 1977.
72. Collins, JM: Pharmacologic rationale for regional drug delivery. J Clin Oncol 2:498–504, 1984.
73. Levin, VA, Kabra, PM, and Freeman-Dove, MA: Pharmacokinetics of intracarotid artery 14C BCNU in the squirrel monkey. J Neurosurg 48: 587–593, 1987.
74. Ginos, JZ, Cooper, AJ, Dhawan, V, et al: (13N) cisplatin PET to assess pharmacokinetics of intra-arterial versus intravenous chemotherapy for malignant brain tumors. J Nucl Med 28: 1844–1852, 1987.
75. Greenberg, HS, Ensminger, WD, Chandler, WF, et al: Intra-arterial BCNU chemotherapy for treatment of malignant gliomas of the central nervous system. J Neurosurg 61:423–429, 1984.
76. Johnson, DW, Parkinson, D, Wolpert, SM, et al: Intracarotid chemotherapy with 1,3-bis-(2-chloroethyl)-1-nitrosourea (BCNU) in 5% dextrose in water in the treatment of malignant glioma. Neurosurgery 20:577–583, 1987.
77. Shapiro, WR, Green, SB, Burger, PC, et al: A randomized comparison of intra-arterial versus intravenous BCNU, with or witout intravenous 5-fluorouracil, for newly diagnosed patients with malignant glioma. J Neurosurg 76:772–781, 1992.
78. Hiesiger, EM, Green, SB, Shapiro, WR, et al: Results of a randomized trial comparing intra-arterial cisplatin and intravenous PCNU for the treatment of primary brain tumors in adults: Brain Tumor Cooperative Group trial 8420A. J Neurooncol 25:143–154, 1995.
79. Mortimer, JE, Crowley, J, Eyre, H, et al: A phase II randomized study comparing sequential and combined intraarterial cisplatin and radiation therapy in primary brain tumors. Cancer 69: 1220–1223, 1992.
80. Foo, S-H, Choi, I-S, Berenstein, A, et al: Supraophthalmic intracarotid infusion of BCNU for malignant glioma. Neurology 36:1437–1444, 1986.
81. Kapp, JP, and Vance, RB: Supraophthalmic carotid infusion for recurrent glioma: Rationale, technique, and preliminary results for cisplatin and BCNU. J Neuro-Oncol 3:5–11, 1985.
82. Saris, SC, Blasberg, RG, Carson, RE, et al: Intravascular streaming during carotid artery infusions. Demonstration in humans and reduction using diastole-phased pulsatile administration. J Neurosurg 74:763–772, 1991.
83. Newton, HB, Page, MA, Junck, L, and Greenberg, HS: Intra-arterial cisplatin for the treatment of malignant gliomas. J Neurooncol 7:39–45, 1989.
84. Mahaley, MS Jr, Hipp, SW, Dropcho, EJ, et al: Intracarotid cisplatin chemotherapy for recurrent gliomas. J Neurosurg 70:371–378, 1989.
85. Dropcho, EJ, Rosenfeld, SS, Morawetz, RB, et al: Preradiation intracarotid cisplatin treatment of newly diagnosed anaplastic gliomas. J Clin Oncol 10:452–458, 1992.
86. Maiese, K, Walker, RW, Gargan, R, and Victor, JD: Intra-arterial cisplatin-associated optic and otic toxicity. Arch Neurol 49:83–86, 1992.
87. van Gelder, T, Geurs, P, Kho, GS, et al: Cortical blindness and seizures following cisplatin treatment: both of epileptic origin? Eur J Cancer 29A:1497–1498, 1993.
88. Madajewicz, S, Chowhan, N, Iliya, A, et al: Intracarotid chemotherapy with etoposide and cisplatin for malignant brain tumors. Cancer 67:2844–2849, 1991.
89. Rogers, LR, Purvis, JB, and Lederman, RJ, et al: Alternating sequential intracarotid BCNU and cisplatin in recurrent malignant glioma. Cancer 68:15–21, 1991.
90. Feun, LG, Savaraj, N, Lee, Y-Y, et al: A pilot clinical and pharmacokinetic study of intracarotid cisplatin and bleomycin. Selective Cancer Therapeutics 7(1):29–36, 1991.
91. Watne, K, Hannisdal, E, Nome, O, et al: Combined intra-arterial and systemic chemotherapy for recurrent malignant brain tumors. Neurosurgery 30:223–227, 1992.
92. Hiesiger, EM, Voorhies, RM, Basler, GA, et al: Opening the blood-brain and blood-tumor barriers in experimental rat brain tumors: The effect of intracarotid hyperosmolar mannitol on capillary permeability and blood flow. Ann Neurol 19:50–59, 1986.
93. Neuwelt, EA, Goldman, DL, Dahlborg,SA, et al: Primary CNS lymphoma treated with osmotic blood-brain barrier disruption: prolonged survival and preservation of cognitive function. J Clin Oncol 9:1580–1590, 1991.
94. DeAngelis, LM, Yahalom, J, Thaler, HT, and Kher, U: Combined modality therapy for primary CNS lymphoma. J Clin Oncol 10:635–643, 1992.
95. Neuwelt, EA, Howieson, J, Frenkel, EP, et al: Therapeutic efficacy of multiagent chemotherapy with drug delivery enhancement by blood-brain barrier modification in glioblastomas. Neurosurgery 19:573–582, 1986.
96. Inamura, T, Nomura, T, Bartus, RT, and Black, KL: Intracarotid infusion of RMP-7, a bradykinin analog: a method for selective drug

delivery to brain tumors. J Neurosurg 81:752–758, 1994.
97. Walter, KA, Tamargo, RJ, Olivi, A, et al: Intratumoral chemotherapy. Neurosurgery 37:1128–1145, 1995.
98. Diemath, HE: Local use of cytostatic drugs following removal of glioblastomas. Wien Klin Wochenschr 99:674–676, 1987.
99. Grossman, SA, Reinhard, C, Colvin, OM, et al: The intracerebral distribution of BCNU delivered by surgically implanted biodegradable polymers. J Neurosurg 76:640–647, 1992.
100. Brem, H, Tamargo, RJ, Olivi, A, et al: Biodegradable polymers for controlled delivery of chemotherapy with and without radiation therapy in the monkey brain. J Neurosurg 80:283–290, 1994.
101. Brem, H, Piantadosi, S, Burger, PC, et al: Placebo-controlled trial of safety and efficacy of intraoperative controlled delivery by biodegradable polymers of chemotherapy for recurrent gliomas. The Polymer-brain Tumor Treatment Group. Lancet 345:1008–1012, 1995.
102. Siegal, T, Horowitz, A, and Gabizon, A: Doxorubicin encapsulated in sterically stabilized liposomes for the treatment of a brain tumor model: biodistribution and therapeutic efficacy. J Neurosurg 83:1029–1037, 1995.
103. Schiffer, D, Sales, S, Soffietti, R: Lonidamine in malignant brain tumors. Semin Oncol 18(2):38–41, 1991.
104. Kyritsis, AP: Chemotherapy for malignant gliomas. Oncology (Huntingt) 7:93–100, 1993.
105. Carapella, CM, Paggi, MG, Cattani, F, et al: The potential role of lonidamine (LND) in the treatment of malignant glioma. Phase II study. J Neurooncol 7:103–108, 1989.
106. DeAngelis, LM, Currie, VE, Kim, J-H, et al: The combined use of radiation therapy and lonidamine in the treatment of brain metastases. J Neurooncol 7:241–247, 1989.
107. Stegman, LD, Zheng, H, Neal, E, et al: A novel suicide gene therapy strategy with the H2O2-generating enzyme D-amino acid oxidase. Proceedings of the 88th Annual Meeting of the American Association for Cancer Research (AACR), San Diego, California, A2562, 1997.
108. Parkinson, DR, Smith, MA, Cheson, BD, et al: Trans-retinoic acid and related differentiation agents. Semin Oncol 19(6):734–741, 1992.
109. Yung, WKA, Scott, C, Fischbach, AJ, et al: All trans-retinoic acid: a phase II Radiation Therapy Oncology Group study (RTOG-9113) in patients with recurrent malignant astrocytoma. Proc Annu Meet Am Soc Clin Oncol 13:A495, 1994.
110. Atiba, J, Jamil, S, Meyskens, FL Jr, et al: Transretinoic acid (tRA) in the treatment of malignant gliomas (MG): a phase II study. Proc Annu Meet Am Soc Clin Oncol 13:A501, 1994.
111. Yung, WKA, Simaga, M, and Levin, VA: 13-cis retinoic acid: a new and potentially effective agent for recurrent malignant astrocytomas. Proc Ann Meet Am Soc Clin Oncol 12:A497, 1993.
112. Stockhammer, G, Manley, GT, Johnson, R, et al: Inhibition of proliferation and induction of differentiation in medulloblastoma- and astrocytoma-derived cell lines with phenylacetate. J Neurosurg 83:672–681, 1995.
113. Palma, L, Di Lorenzo, N, and Guidetti, B: Lymphocytic infiltrates in primary glioblastomas and recidivous gliomas. Incidence, fate, and relevance to prognosis in 228 operated cases. J Neurosurg 49:854–861, 1978.
114. Brooks, WH, Latta, RB, Mahaley, MS, et al: Immunobiology of primary intracranial tumors. Part 5: Correlation of a lymphocyte index and clinical status. J Neurosurg 54:331–337, 1981.
115. Sawamura, Y, de and Tribolet, N: Immunobiology of brain tumors and implications for immunotherapy. In Kay, AH, and Laws, ER Jr (eds): Brain Tumors. An Encyclopedic Approach. Churchill Livingstone, New York, 1995, pp 113–124.
116. Lee, Y, Bullard, DE, Humphrey, PA, et al: Treatment of intracranial human glioma xenografts with ^{131}I-labeled anti-tenascin monoclonal antibody 81C6. Cancer Res 48: 2904–2910, 1988.
117. Colapinto, EV, Humphrey, PA, Zalutsky, MR, et al: Comparative localization of murine monoclonal antibody mel-14 F(ab')2 fragment and whole IgG2a in human glioma xenografts. Cancer Res 48:5701–5707, 1988.
118. Zalutsky, MR, Moseley, RP, Coakham, HB, et al: Pharmacokinetics and tumor localization of ^{131}I-labeled anti-tenascin monoclonal antibody 81C6 in patients with gliomas and other intracranial malignancies. Cancer Res 49:2807–2813, 1989.
119. Yoshida, S, Tanaka, R, Ono, M, et al: Analysis of mixed lymphocyte-tumor culture in patients with malignant brain tumor. J Neurosurg 71:398–402, 1989.
120. Maxwell, M, Galanopoulos, T, Neville-Golden, J, and Antoniades, HN: Effect of the expression of transforming growth factor-β2 in primary human glioblastomas on immunosuppression and loss of immune surveillance. J Neurosurg 76:799–804, 1992.
121. Yamada, N, Kato, M, Yamashita, H, et al: Enhanced expression of transforming growth factor-β and its type-I and type-II receptors in human glioblastoma. Int J Cancer 62:386–392, 1995.
122. Jachimczak, P, Bogdahn, U, Schneider, J, et al: The effect of transforming growth factor-β2-specific phosphorothioate-anti-sense oligodeoxynucleotides in reversing cellular immunosuppression in malignant glioma. J Neurosurgery 78:944–951, 1993.
123. Nitta, T, Hishii, M, Sato, K, and Okumura, K: Selective expression of interleukin-10 gene within glioblastoma multiforme. Brain Res 649:122–128, 1994.
124. Wen, PY: Clinical experience with immunotherapy. In Black, PM, Schoene, WC, and Lampson, LA (eds): Astrocytomas: Diagnosis, Treatment, and Biology. Blackwell Scientific Publications, Boston, 1993, pp 123–147.

125. DeCearvalho, S, Kaufman, A, and Pineda, A: Adjuvant chemo-immunotherapy in central nervous system tumors. In Salmon, J (ed): Adjuvant Therapy of Cancer. Elsevier/North Holland, Amsterdam, The Netherlands, pp 495–502, 1977.
126. Bergquist, BJ, Mahaley, MS Jr, Steinbok, P, and Dudka, L: Treatment of a brain tumor with BCG cell wall preparation. Surg Neurol 13: 197–201, 1980.
127. Selker, RG, Wolmark, N, Fisher, B, and Moore, P: Preliminary observations on the use of *corynebacterium parvum* in patients with primary intracranial tumors: effect on intracranial pressure. J Surg Oncol 10:299–303, 1978.
128. Saito, T, Tanaka, R, Sekiguchi,K, et al: Local immunotherapy with OK-432 for malignant gliomas: Immunohistochemical analysis of chronological changes of tumor tissues. No To Shinkei 40:609–615, 1988.
129. Fischer, SP, Lindermuth, J, Hash, C, and Shenkin, HA: Levamisole in the treatment of glioblastoma multiforme. J Surg Oncol 28:214–216, 1985.
130. Baskies, AM, and Chretien, PB: Thymosine a-1 in malignant gliomas: Augmentation of immune reactivity in a phase I study. Surg Forum 33:522–524, 1982.
131. Jaeckle, KA, Mittelman, A, and Hill, FH: Phase II trial of serratia marcescens extract in recurrent malignant astrocytoma. J Clin Oncol 8: 1408–1418, 1990.
132. Yumitori, K, Handa, H, Yamashita, J, et al: Treatment of malignant glioma with mumps virus. No Shinkei Geka 10:143–147, 1982.
133. Filipo, FV: A trial of rabies vaccine treatment of patients with glioblastoma multiforme. Zh Vopr Neirokhir 3:38–40, 1988.
134. Mahaley, MS Jr, Urso, MB, Whaley, RA, et al: Immunobiology of primary intracranial tumors. Part X: Therapeutic efficacy of interferon in the treatment of recurrent gliomas. J Neurosurg 63:719–725, 1985.
135. Jereb, B, Petric-Grabnar, G, Klun, B, et al: Addition of IFN-α to treatment of malignant brain tumors. Acta Oncologica 33(6):651–654, 1994.
136. Yung, WKA, Prados ,M, Levin, VA, et al: Intravenous recombinant interferon beta in patients with recurrent malignant gliomas: A phase I/II study. J Clin Oncol 9:1945–1949, 1991.
137. Allen, J, Packer, R, Bleyer, A, et al: Recombinant interferon beta: A phase I-II trial in children with recurrent brain tumors. J Clin Oncol 9:783–788, 1991.
138. Fetell, MR, Housepian, EM, Oster, MW, et al: Intratumor administration of β-interferon in recurrent malignant gliomas. A phase I clinical and laboratory study. Cancer 65:78–83, 1990.
139. Mahaley, MS Jr, Bertsch, L, and Cush, S: Systemic gamma-interferon therapy for recurrent gliomas. J Neurosurg 69:826–829, 1988.
140. Day, ED, Lassiter, S, Woodhall, B, et al: The localization of radioantibodies in human brain tumors. I. Preliminary exploration. Cancer Res 25:773–778, 1965.
141. Bullard, DE, Wikstrand, CJ, Humphrey, PA, et al: Specific imaging of human brain tumor xenografts utilizing radiolabelled monoclonal antibodies (MAbs). Nucl Med 25:210–215, 1986.
142. Nanda, A, Liwnicz, B, Atkinson, BF, et al: Monoclonal antibodies with cytoxic reactivities against human gliomas. J Neurosurg 71:892–897, 1989.
143. Mahaley, MS Jr: Neuro-oncology index and review (adult primary brain tumors). Radiotherapy, chemotherapy, immunotherapy, photodynamic therapy. J Neurooncol 11:85–147, 1991.
144. Neuwelt, EA, Specht, HD, Barnett, PA, et al: Increased delivery of tumor-specific monoclonal antibodies to brain after osmotic blood-brain barrier modification in patients with melanoma metastatic to the central nervous system. Neurosurgery 20:885–895, 1987.
145. Lee, Y-S, Bullard, DE, Zalutsky, MR, et al: Therapeutic efficacy of antiglioma mesenchymal extracellular matrix ^{131}I-radiolabeled murine monoclonal antibody in a human glioma xenograft model. Cancer Res 48:559–566, 1988.
146. Lee, Y, Bullard, DE, Wikstrand, CJ, et al: Comparison of monoclonal antibody delivery to intracranial glioma xenografts by intravenous and intracarotid adminstration. Cancer Res 47: 1941–1946, 1987.
147. Brady, LW, Woo, DV, Karlsson, U, et al: Radioimmunotherapy of human gliomas using I-125 labeled monoclonal antibody to epidermal growth factor receptor. Proc ASCO 7:83, 1988.
148. Frankel, AE: Immunotoxin therapy of cancer. Oncology 7(5):69–78, 1993.
149. Vooijs, WC, Krouwer, HGJ, Marx, JJ, and de Gast, GC: Efficacy of different transferrin-toxin conjugates on human glioma cell lines. J Neurooncol 28:95, 1996.
150. Martell, LA, Agrawal, A, Ross, DA, and Muraszko, KM: Efficacy of transferrin receptor-targeted immunotoxins in brain tumor cell lines and pediatric bran tumors. Cancer Res 53: 1348–1353, 1993.
151. Oldfeld, EH: Recombinant immunotoxin perfusion of malignant brain tumors: The results of a clinical trial. J Neurooncol 28:49, 1996.
152. Kito, A, Yoshida, J, and Kageyama, N: Liposomes coupled with monoclonal antibodies against glioma-associated antigen for targeting chemotherapy of glioma. J Neurosurg 71:382–387, 1989.
153. Nowak, TP: Monoclonal antibodies: prospects for specific immunotherapy for gliomas. Am J Clin Oncol 10:278–280, 1987.
154. Trouillas, P, and Lapras, CL: Active immunotherapy of cerebral tumor. 20 cases. Neurochirurgie 16:143–170, 1970.
155. Takakura, K, Miki, Y, Kubo, Oet al: Adjuvant immunotherapy for malignant brain tumors. Jpn J Clin Oncol 2:109–120, 1972.
156. Young H, Kaplan A, Regelson W: Immunotherapy with autologous white cell infusions ("lymphocytes") in the treatment of recurrent

glioblastoma multiforme: a preliminary report. Cancer 40:1037–1044, 1977.

157. Yoshida, S, Takai, N, Ono, K, et al: Observations on the local administration of autologous lymphokine activated killer cells and recombinant interleukin-2 in patients with malignant gliomas. No To Shinkei 40:119–125, 1988.
158. Jacobs, SK, Wilson, DJ, Kornblith, PL, and Grimm, EA: Interleukin-2 and autologous lymphokine-activated killer cells in the treatment of malignant glioma. J Neurosurg 64:743–749, 1986.
159. Ingram, M, Buckwalter, JG, Jacques, DB, et al: Immunotherapy for recurrent malignant glioma: An interim report on survival. Neurol Res 12:265–273, 1990.
160. Merchant, RE, Ellison, MD, and Young, HF: Immunotherapy for malignant glioma using human recombinant interleukin-2 and activated autologous lymphocytes. A review of preclinical and clinical investigations. J Neurooncol 8:173–188, 1990.
161. Saris, SC, Patronas, NJ, Rosenberg, SA, et al: The effect of intravenous interleukin-2 on brain water content. J Neurosurg 71:169–174, 1989.
162. Lillehei, KO, Mitchell, DH, Johnson, SD, et al: Long-term follow-up of patients with recurrent malignant gliomas treated with adjuvant adoptive immunotherapy. Neurosurgery 28:16–23, 1991.
163. Vaquero, J, Martinez, R, Oya, S, et al: Intratumoral injection of autologous lymphocytes plus human lymphoblastoid interferon for the treatment of glioblastoma. Acta Neurochir (Wien) 98:35–41, 1989.
164. Neuwelt, EA, Clark, K, Kirkpatrick, JB, and Toben, H: Clinical studies of intrathecal autologous lymphocyte infusions in patients with malignant glioma. A toxicity study. Ann Neurol 4:307–312, 1978.
165. Bloom, WH, Carstairs, KC, Crompton, MR, and McKissock, W: Autologous glioma transplantation. Lancet 2:77–78, 1960.
166. Bloom, HJ, Peckham, MJ, Richardson, AE, et al: Glioblastoma multiforme: A controlled trial to assess the value of specific active immunotherapy in patients treated by radical surgery and radiotherapy. Br J Cancer 27:253–267, 1973.
167. Mahaley, MS Jr, and Fleming, H: Immunotherapy for malignant tumors. BNI Quarterly 2:32–42, 1986.
168. Cheung, NK, Canete, A, Cheung ,IY, et al: Disialoganglioside GD2 anti-idiotypic monoclonal antibodies. Int J Cancer 54:499–505, 1993.
169. Nishikara, K: A novel experimental approach to immunotherapy against malignant brain tumor with the mouse IFN-gamma gene transfer. Nippon Geka Hokan 58:18–42, 1989.

Chapter 8

MALIGNANT ASTROCYTOMA

Malignant astrocytomas are devastating tumors that strike adults during their productive years of life, shorten life acutely, and often disable people physically and emotionally during that shortened life span. During the past 25 years, treatment advances for malignant gliomas have not kept pace with those for other central nervous system (CNS) or systemic neoplasms. Their heterogeneity and invasiveness provide particular problems for physicians treating patients with malignant astrocytoma. The comprehensive management of these patients is best handled by a neuro-oncology team consisting of a neurosurgeon, neuro-oncologist, radiation oncologist, neuroradiologist, neuropathologist, and oncologist. Lastly and very importantly, a nurse practitioner is needed to coordinate care among specialties, deliver chemotherapy, and with a social worker, provide patient and family counseling.

HISTORY AND NOMENCLATURE

The first operative excision of an astrocytoma from brain with antiseptic technique and general anesthesia was performed in late 1884 by Richard Godlee.[1] The patient presented with "violent paroxysms of lancinating pain in the head," "attacks of uncontrollable vomiting," and "twitchings in the fingers and thumb of the left hand, which occurred many times a day." "An incision an inch long was made into the gray matter" of a distended ascending frontal convolution, and Godlee removed a "hard glioma about the size of a walnut."

The earliest histological classification of brain tumors was developed by Bailey and Cushing,[2] in 1926 (see Table 1–1). The most malignant astrocytic glial neoplasm was the spongioblastoma multiforme, now known as *glioblastoma multiforme*. Astrocytoma was the most differentiated neoplasm and was divided into astrocytoma fibrillare and astrocytoma protoplasmaticum. In this three-tiered classification system, the glial neoplasm of intermediate histology was called *astroblastoma*. Bailey and Cushing[2] correlated the histology of these neoplasms with biologic behavior. The Bailey and Cushing[2] classification was followed by the Kernohan and Sayre[3] system, a four-tiered schema developed in 1950. Astrocytomas were graded I through IV based on dedifferentiation of cellular elements and increasing degrees of anaplasia rather than on the embryologic cell of origin used as the basis for the Bailey and Cushing classification. In this system, grades III and IV were malignant astrocytomas and both had vascular proliferation and necrosis. The distinction between the two grades was subjective and imprecise.[3] In 1950, Ringertz[4] developed a three-tiered system for glioma in which tumors were called *astrocytoma, intermediate type,* and *glioblastoma multiforme.* A problem with the Bailey-Cushing,[2] Kernohan-Sayre,[3] and Ringertz[4] classification systems is that they are continuous-variable systems. A descriptor such as Kernohan grade III merges imperceptibly with the next category, grade IV. Labeling is, therefore, subjective with significant individual variability. A grade III astrocytoma of Kernohan was roughly equivalent to an intermediate-type astrocytoma of Ringertz, and a grade IV astrocytoma of Kernohan was equal to a glioblastoma or Ringertz (see Table 1–4).

In 1988, Daumas-Duport and colleagues[5] developed a discrete grading system depending on the presence or absence of four variables: nuclear atypia, mitosis, endothelial proliferation, and necrosis. If no criteria were present, the tumor was a grade I; if one criterion, grade II; if two criteria, grade III; and three or four criteria, grade IV. Pathologic grading with the Daumas-Duport[5] method is less likely to be subject to individual variability.

The pathologic classification system used for malignant astrocytomas in this chapter and in the text in general, is the 1993 World Health Organization (WHO) classification system.[6] It is a three-tiered continuous variable system, graded II through IV, with a grade I designation reserved for pilocytic astrocytoma, discussed in Chapter 9. Grades II to IV are used as follows: grade II, low grade astrocytoma (LGA); grade III, anaplastic astrocytoma; and grade IV, glioblastoma multiforme. Grade II is also discussed in Chapter 9. Grades III and IV are classified as malignant astrocytomas and are discussed in this chapter. Other grading systems currently in use are presented in Chapter 1 and Table 1–4.

EPIDEMIOLOGY

In the United States in 1991, primary brain tumors were diagnosed in approximately 16,000 people, with 35% to 45% of these tumors malignant astrocytoma.[7] The average annual incidence rate for glioma in adults was 5.0 to 5.4 per 100,000 per year. If malignant gliomas were 65% of all gliomas, then the incidence rate was 3.3 per 100,000 per year.[7,8] Age-specific rates of malignant astrocytoma increased from two per 100,000 per year at ages 35 to 44 years to reach a maximum of 17 per 100,000 per year in ages 75 to 84 years (see Chapter 1).[8] In the 35 to 44 age group, LGA was more common than malignant astrocytoma by a ratio of 1.5:1, but in the 75 to 84 age group, the ratio was closer to 1:1. In a second study, the ratio of astrocytoma to glioblastoma was 5:2 in children younger than 14 years and 0.37:1 in adults older than 45 years.[9]

Anaplastic astrocytoma and glioblastoma are more common in men than women. The male to female ratio of malignant astrocytoma varies between 1.06 and 2.0 in published series.[7,9–16] Whereas in African Americans, astrocytoma and malignant astrocytoma represent only 37% of the primary brain tumors, in whites, astrocytoma and malignant astrocytoma account for greater than 50% of primary brain tumors.[17]

The incidence of primary malignant brain tumors has been reported to have increased dramatically in the past 25 years, particularly in developed countries.[16,18,19] Between 1960 and 1985, the incidence of malignant brain tumors increased by 40% in the general population and 100% in the elderly (those older than 65 years of age).[16,18,19,20] The subject of debate has been whether the increased incidence is due to better diagnostic imaging or an increase in disease frequency. A recent population study of both malignant and nonmalignant brain neoplasms in Rochester, Minnesota, found a nonsignificant increase in incidence from 9.5 to 12.5 per 100,000 per year for the time periods of 1950 to 1969 and 1970 to 1989. This increase was attributed to an increase in pituitary adenomas, not benign or malignant astrocytomas.[7] It appears that most of the increase was due to better diagnostic imaging with computed tomography (CT) and magnetic resonance imaging (MRI).

Inherited diseases have been associated with an increased incidence of malignant astrocytoma. The epidermal nevus syndrome is an inherited syndrome with linear skin nevi and is associated with an increased incidence of malignant glioma. The Li-Fraumeni syndrome is a familial syndrome of young closely related family members who develop cancer. Families with this syndrome have p53 germline mutations on chromosome 17. Affected individuals are heterozygous for the allele, and the mutation results in a faulty protein. The common tumors associated with this syndrome are breast, lung, colon, and osteogenic sarcoma. Some families with Li-Fraumeni syndrome have an increased incidence of anaplastic astrocytoma.[21] In Neurofibromatosis Type I (NF1) and Neurofibromatosis Type II (NF2), gliomas do not appear to be increased in frequency.[22]

When families with multifocal glioma, unifocal glioma with a second primary malignancy, or a history of familial cancer were examined for p53 germline mutations, there was a 12% incidence of p53 germline mutations.[23] If all three factors—multifocal glioma, second primary malignancy, and family history of cancer—were present, there was a 67% rate of p53 germline mutations. The Johns Hopkins Brain Tumor Registry has identified 59 families with multiple malignant astrocytic tumors in one or two generations. There were no multiple generation families. There were 20 parent-child pairs, 27 sibling pairs, and nine husband-wife pairs.[24,25] These findings were thought to be most consistent with a common environmental or toxic exposure, particularly in the husband-wife pairs in which 33% were diagnosed within 1 year of each other.[24,25]

BIOLOGY

Chromosomal Changes

The development of malignant astrocytoma is associated with a series of allelic changes involving both the loss of tumor-suppressor genes and gain of proto-oncogenes.[26–28] The earliest change in the development of LGA is the loss of genetic material on chromosomes 6, 13, 17p, and 22. These changes are presumably associated with the biologic change from normal astrocytes to astrocytoma (see Fig. 2–4).

If a tumor dedifferentiates to an anaplastic astrocytoma or presents de novo, additional allelic changes are present with frequent loss of chromosomes 9p and 19q. These latter changes are seen infrequently in grade II astrocytoma and appear commonly in grade III astrocytoma. The 9p21 chromosome region controls for cyclin-dependent kinase (CDK4), which inhibits cell proliferation. $p16^{INK4}$ is a cell-cycle regulator that binds to and inactivates CDK4. It is absent in 50% of high-grade tumors. The loss of 9p and $p16^{INK4}$ removes inhibitory controls to growth.[29] The replacement of a p16/*CDKN2* gene in a U-373 glioma cell line in which there is a homozygous deletion of the gene suppresses growth, suggesting p16/*CDKN2* is a tumor-suppressor gene.[30] Allelic loss of 19q is seen in 46% of grade III tumors and only 11% of grade II tumors.[28]

The most frequent chromosomal abnormality, present only in glioblastoma multiforme, is a loss of chromosome 10.[26,27] The region of chromosome 10 that functions as a tumor suppressor gene has been identified (see Chapter 2). A second chromosomal change is the amplification or rearrangement of the epidermal growth factor receptor (EGFR) gene. The amplification can occur from extra copies of chromosome 7 or duplication of the *EGFR* region on chromosome 7.[31–34] EGF overexpression was common in glioblastoma with a clinical history of less than three months and no previous history of LGA. In the patients reported (see Chapter 2) there was a low incidence of p53 mutations. In glioblastomas presenting initially as LGA or anaplastic astrocytoma there was a high incidence of p53 mutations and frequent overexpression of EGF receptors. Other genes amplified in glioblastoma include *MDM2,* N-*myc,* and the *gli* gene.[31,33,35] Reduced expression of the deleted colorectal carcinoma gene on 18q is seen frequently in glioblastoma.[36]

The chromosomal changes are targets for future gene therapy, with transfection of absent genes in areas of allelic loss and antisense oligodeoxynucleotides for regions of amplification.

Growth Factors

Malignant astrocytoma growth and invasion are influenced by growth factors, which are normally under the control of proto-oncogenes and tumor-suppressor genes. Malignant brain tumor cells generally lose their dependence on exogenous growth factors while developing the machinery to synthesize and respond to endogenously produced growth factors.[37] These growth factors act through autocrine, paracrine, and intracrine mechanisms to stimulate themselves and neighboring malignant glioma cells (see Table 2–1, Fig. 2–2). Epidermal growth factor is growth stimulatory to human glioma cells, but the level of expression of its receptor does not mediate its response.[38] A monoclonal antibody to EGFR has been labeled with iodine-131 and delivered intra-arterially through the internal carotid artery to treat malignant astrocytomas. There were occasional nondurable tumor regressions.[39,40] Basic fibroblast growth factor increases in astrocytoma cells with increase in malignancy and stimulates glioma cells through an autocrine mechanism.[41]

IGF-1 mRNA stimulates glioma cell growth in culture. This can be inhibited through transfection of an antisense IGF-1 expression construct with a viral vector.[42] Platelet-derived growth factor (PDGF) is composed of two polypeptide chains that can be combined to form three isoforms, PDGF-AA, -AB, and -BB.[43] The A chain is expressed in almost all astrocytic tumors, and the B chain is expressed in only 50% of anaplastic astrocytomas.[44–47] PDGF-α and PDGF-β receptors are present on glioma cells, and PDGF-β receptor is present on endothelial cells, suggesting an autocrine mechanism of stimulation for PDGF-α on malignant glioma cells and a paracrine stimulation of PDGF-β on endothelial cells.[44,47] The PDGF-B chain is identical to the simian virus *sis* oncogene. When the human homologue c-*sis* of the simian sarcoma virus oncogene was used as the template for an antisense oligodeoxynucleotide and was transfected into A172 glioma cells, there was dose-dependent inhibition of cell proliferation. However, c-*sis* was expressed on only a minority of gliomas, so the therapeutic potential is limited.[48]

Transforming growth factors (TGFs) produce phenotypic transformation of normal cells, producing a gain in anchorage-independent cell growth.[49] The transforming growth factors TGF-α and TGF-β and their receptors have increased expression with increasing malignancy.[50–53] Whereas TGF-β_1 inhibits normal brain cell and glial cell growth, it stimulates astrocytoma cells to migrate and invade.[53,54] TGF-β_2 functions as a cytokine to mediate suppression of T-lymphocyte activation. TGF-β_2 function can be suppressed by an antisense oligodeoxynucleotide.[55]

Cell Surface Receptors and Malignant Astrocytoma Growth and Invasion

Protein kinase C (PKC) is a serine kinase receptor expressed on LGA to a greater extent than on anaplastic glioma or glioblastoma multiforme.[56] PKC has an extracellular ligand-binding domain. It activates a phospholipase enzyme to phosphorylate substrate, and with calcium, activates the second messenger, pyruvate kinase. PKC controls cell activity through the transcriptional control elements, c-*fos* and c-*jun*, and when PKC binds tumor promoting phorbol esters, glioma cell growth is stimulated.[56,57] PKC is stimulated by EGF and FGF and inhibited by tamoxifen, which inhibits DNA glioma cell synthesis and cell proliferation.[58]

Malignant glioma cell invasion into the surrounding white matter of the brain is mediated by cell surface adhesion molecules and their transmembrane receptors, which interact with components of the extracellular matrix (ECM) and the vascular basement membrane.[59,60] Adhesion molecules and their receptors expressed on the surface of glioma cells belong to four structural classifications, based on chemistry: (1) the integrins, (2) the immunoglobulin superfamily, (3) selectins, and (4) CD44 (see Table 2–4).[59] Adhesion molecules are upregulated by interaction with components of the ECM and by growth factors and cytokines, such as TNF-α, INF-γ and IL1-β.[61] CD44H is an adhesion molecule with its receptor expressed on normal brain and glial tumors of all grades. The receptor binds with hyaluronic acid, a major component of the ECM, and may contribute to the invasive character of astrocytomas (see Table 2–3).[62]

Adhesion molecules and their transmembrane receptors also play an important role in the production and secretion of proteases, which catabolize the ECM and facilitate glioma cell migration. Proteases and their precursors are released by glioma cells and bind to their cell surface receptors. When activated, they degrade the Natural inhibitors of serine and cysteine proteases have been recognized (see Table 2–5).[60] High levels of the matrix metalloproteinase (MMP), a type IV collagenase, have been found in malignant gliomas. Inhibitors of glioma cell migration, TIMP-1 and TIMP-2, are also present in malignant gliomas.[63] Northern blot analysis of TIMP-1 and TIMP-2 transcripts showed lower levels of these transcripts in anaplastic astrocytoma and glioblastoma multiforme than in meningioma or normal brain.[63] The discovery of a protease unique to gliomas and cloning of an inhibitor or regulatory factor would greatly facilitate treatment of gliomas.

Growth Kinetics

The growth kinetics of malignant astrocytoma have been studied with S-phase bromodeoxyuridine (BUdR) labeling, with an index ranging from 9.1% to 46.5%.[64] The labeling was found to vary from very low in necrotic areas to 46.5% in the most actively growing regions of tumor. Malignant astrocytoma S-phase duration and tumor doubling times have been determined with double-labeling techniques. BUdR and iododeoxyuridine (IudR) were infused at 3-hour intervals preoperatively, and tissue was stained postoperatively with two monoclonal antibodies, one that stains BUdR-labeled cells alone, and the second that stains both BUdR and IUdR. S-phase duration or DNA synthesis time ranged from 6 to 10 hours, and doubling times varied from 2 days to more than 1 month.[65,66] Hoshino and colleagues[66] correlated labeling index with biologic behavior, but other studies of both de novo and recurrent gliomas reported no correlation of labeling index with biologic behavior.[67,68]

PATHOLOGY

Malignant astrocytomas are divided into anaplastic astrocytoma (grade III) and glioblastoma multiforme (grade IV) on the basis of their histopathologic features. They are located most frequently in the deep white matter of the cerebral hemispheres, with 30% to 40% of tumors involving the frontal, temporal, and parietal lobes alone or in combination. The occipital lobe is involved in approximately 15% of cases, and the basal ganglia, thalamus, pineal, brainstem, and cerebellum are involved less frequently (Table 8–1).[69] Both anaplastic astrocytoma and glioblastoma multiforme have significant regional variability or heterogeneity. The tumor is graded pathologically by its most anaplastic region. Anaplastic regions may be dedifferentiated regions of astrocytoma or may arise de novo.[6,70–73]

An anaplastic astrocytoma has mitotic activity, increased cellularity, and cellular pleomorphism. Vascular proliferation and necrosis are absent in anaplastic astrocytoma. Glioblastoma multiforme is the most malignant tumor in the astrocytic series, and it is identified histologically by the presence of vascular proliferation and necrosis. Anaplastic astrocytoma often dedifferentiates to glioblastoma multiforme on recurrence.

Table 8–1. **Glioblastoma: Location of Tumor by Percentage in 495 Patients**

Location	%	Location	%	Location	%
Frontal	19.6%	Frontotemporal	2.8%	Frontotemporoparietal	1.6%
Temporal	16.8%	Temporoparietal	5.8%	Temporoparieto-occipital	10.9%
Parietal	14.6%	Parieto-occipital	4.8%	Frontoparieto-occipital	0.6%
Occipital	2.8%	Frontoparietal	6.2%		
Bifrontal	3.6%				
		Bilateral multiple lobes	2.6%		
		Thalamus/basal ganglia/upper brainstem	3.2%		
		Pons	1.6%		
		Cerebellum	0.4%		
		Spinal cord	1.2%		

Adapted from Roth and Elvidge,[69] p 738, with permission.

Anaplastic astrocytoma and glioblastoma multiforme are composed of poorly differentiated pleomorphic small, round, or fusiform cells and occasional giant cells.[6] These tumors express glial fibrillary acidic protein (GFAP) less consistently than the more differentiated astrocytoma. At surgery, glioblastoma multiforme often appears circumscribed with varied coloration due to necrosis and hemorrhage. The tumor may invade the leptomeninges and disseminate through the ventricular system. Two rarer histologic variants of the glioblastoma multiforme exist: a giant-cell glioblastoma composed of bizarre giant cells with an eosinophilic cytoplasm, and the gliosarcoma, which has a malignant sarcomatous component in addition to the malignant glial component (Fig. 8–1a,b).[6]

A structural classification for astrocytoma was developed describing the relation of tumor to surrounding brain.[73] Type I tumors are solid tumors with no infiltration of surrounding brain. Type II tumors have a solid portion and independent tumor cells infiltrating normal brain. The majority of anaplastic astrocytoma and glioblastoma have a type II structure. Type III tumors are composed of individual tumor cells that infiltrate normal brain. Gliomatosis cerebri in its classic form is the diffuse infiltration of the brain by neoplastic glial cells corresponding to a type III structure.[6] It requires imaging or pathologic evidence of infiltration of mul-

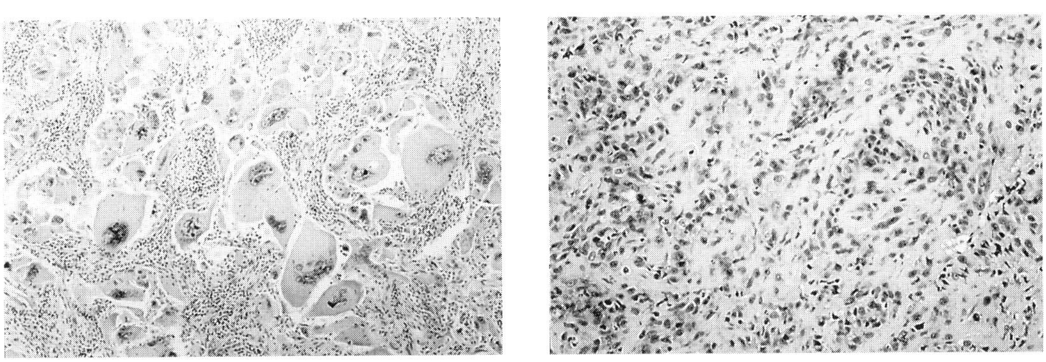

A B

Figure 8–1. *(A)* Giant cell glioblastoma multiforme. Bizarre multinucleated cells are hallmark of the neoplasm. They are interspersed with clusters of smaller-sized neoplastic astrocytes. Mitotic figures, vascular endothelial proliferation and necrosis are also features of this high-grade glioma. H&E stain. Mag. ×200. (Courtesy of Mila Blaivas, MD, PhD, Department of Pathology, University of Michigan Medical School, Ann Arbor, MI). *(B)* Gliosarcoma. Highly malignant neoplasm with numerous mitotic figures is biphasic and is formed by glioblastoma (clusters of larger cells) and a fibrosarcoma (collagenous connective tissue of the background with malignant fibroblasts). H&E stain. Mag. ×200. (Courtesy of Mila Blaivas, MD, PhD, Department of Pathology, University of Michigan Medical School, Ann Arbor, MI).

tiple lobes of the brain. Gliomatosis cerebri has the biologic behavior of a grade III or IV astrocytoma.

CLINICAL SYMPTOMS

Malignant astrocytoma produces symptoms and signs of mass effect, local brain infiltration, tissue destruction, and increased intracranial pressure. The symptoms of patients with anaplastic astrocytoma or glioblastoma multiforme are dependent on the anatomic location of the tumor. Malignant cerebral astrocytoma does not often grow into the ventricular pathways. When it produces increased intracranial pressure, it is usually due to mass effect. Basal ganglia, thalamic, brainstem, and cerebellar malignant astrocytoma are more likely to produce ventricular obstruction with hydrocephalus and increased intracranial pressure.

The most frequent initial symptom in two adult glioblastoma multiforme series was headache in 37% and 39% of cases (Table 8–2).[10,69] Headache was also the most frequent symptom at diagnosis in 73% to 86% of patients (Table 8–3).[10,69] The second most frequent initial symptom was seizures in 16% to 18% of patients, which was present in 26% to 32% of patients at diagnosis.[10,69] Whereas headaches were present for an average of 4.4 months

Table 8–2. **Glioblastoma: Initial Symptom in 704 Patients***

Initial Symptom	Percentage of Patients
Headache	38.2
Seizure	17.5
Motor weakness	7.9
Mental status change	7.4
Dysphasia	5.4
Visual symptoms	4.3
Altered consciousness	2.2
Sensory loss	2.2
Gait disturbance	1.5
Other	13.4

*Combined from two series.[10,69]

Table 8–3. **Glioblastoma: Symptom at Presentation in 708 Patients***

Symptom at Presentation	Percentage of Patients
Headache	77.7
Seizure	29.2
Motor weakness	42.7
Mental status change	41.5
Dysphasia	29.2
Visual symptoms	38.9
Altered consciousness	35.7
Sensory loss	14.2
Gait disturbance	18.5
Nausea and vomiting	32.8

*Combined from two series[10,69]

before diagnosis, seizures were present for an average of 1 year.[69] Symptom duration was less than 6 months in 70% of patients with glioblastoma multiforme.[10]

In patients with LGA, the two most common symptoms at diagnosis were seizures in approximately 60% of patients, followed by headache in 40%. The symptom duration was often years.[75–78] The difference in presenting symptoms reflected differences in growth pattern and kinetics. LGA grows and infiltrates brain slowly, with irritation of surrounding brain, and malignant astrocytoma divides rapidly, with tissue destruction. Approximately 6% of patients with anaplastic astrocytoma and glioblastoma multiforme presented with the acute onset of symptoms secondary to intracranial hemorrhage.[79] These patients present a difficult management problem and have a poor prognosis.

The most common presenting neurologic signs in patients with glioblastoma multiforme at presentation were hemiparesis in 61%[1] to 83%, papilledema in 32% to 66%, confusion in 18% to 40%, and aphasia in 25% to 32% of patients.[69,74] Confusion and mental status difficulties are more common with bilateral tumors. Only 1% of patients with glioblastoma were neurologically normal at presentation. This is significantly lower than in LGA.[69]

DIFFERENTIAL DIAGNOSIS

The differential diagnosis of an adult presenting with less than a 6-month history of headache, seizures, and other focal symptoms and signs is small. LGA, anaplastic oligodendroglioma, anaplastic mixed oligoastrocytoma, supratentorial primitive neuroectodermal tumor (PNET), anaplastic ependymoma, primary central nervous system lymphoma (PCNSL), and metastatic tumor are included in the differential diagnosis. Brain abscess, thromboembolic and hemorrhagic vascular process, parasitic cyst, and multiple sclerosis (MS) must also be considered.

In anaplastic astrocytoma and glioblastoma multiforme, MRI often reveals decreased signal on T_1-weighted images before contrast infusion (Fig. 8–2a). CT scans most often show a large, irregular, low-density area. Contrast enhancement on MRI or CT is heterogeneous with a serpiginous pattern, a solid mass enhancing heterogeneously, or rarely, a variable thick ringlike enhancing rim with a necrotic center. The area of T_2-weighted abnormality or edema is slightly larger than the enhancing abnormality (Fig. 8–2b). However, 30% of patients with anaplastic astrocytoma, and 4% of patients with glioblastoma do not have contrast enhancement on CT.[80]

LGA typically presents with seizures, has a longer duration of symptoms, and infrequently has contrast enhancement.[77,81,82] Anaplastic oligodendroglioma, mixed oligoastrocytoma, supratentorial PNET, and anaplastic supratentorial ependymoma cannot be reliably differentiated from malignant astrocytoma preoperatively based on symptoms, signs, or imaging characteristics.

PCNSL has a more rapid onset of symptoms, with an average duration of symptoms of 2 weeks to 2.5 months. Cognitive changes are the most frequent presenting symptom in 36% of patients.[83,84] MRI and CT scans show dense homogeneous contrast enhancement. Whereas a multiplicity of lesions is unusual in malignant astrocytoma (3% to 7.5%), it is frequent in PCNSL (30%).[84–86] Brain metastasis must also be differentiated from malignant astrocytoma. Brain metastases present with a history of less than 2 months' duration. They occur at the gray-white junction or in watershed zones and are spherical in shape. If small in size, they enhance homogeneously; when large in size, they have a smooth, ringlike enhancing rim with a necrotic center. Vasogenic edema is usu-

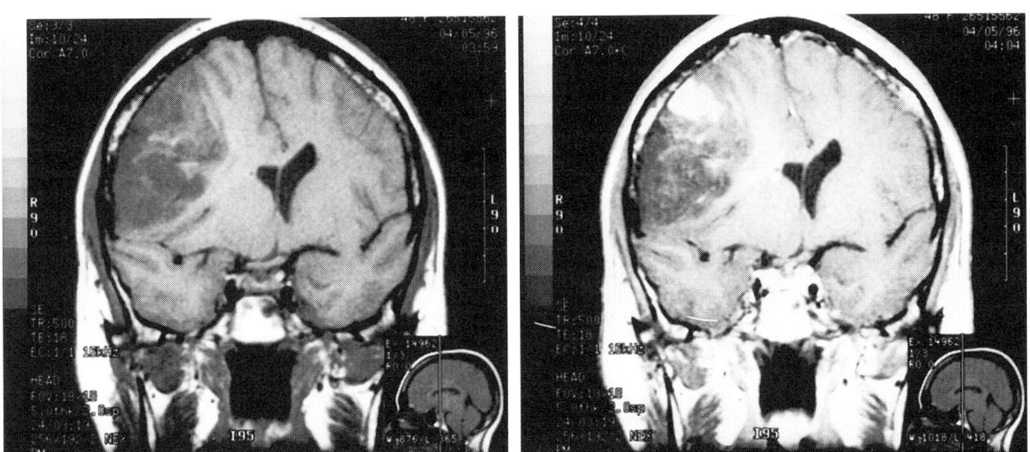

Figure 8–2. Glioblastoma multiforme: *(A)* T_1-weighted MRI shows large right frontal heterogeneous mass with predominantly hypointense signal; there is a small central hyperintense hemorrhagic area. *(B)* After gadolinium heterogeneous contrast enhancement; note subfalcian herniation compression of ventricular system, and hemispheric edema, right to left shift.

ally more extensive than in malignant astrocytoma, and multifocality is present in 50% of cases.[87,88]

Brain abscess presents most often with a more acute history accompanied by fever, with evidence of a systemic infectious process, often in the lung. On imaging studies, brain abscess typically has a thin rim with uniform contrast enhancement, in contrast to malignant astrocytoma, which has a variable-thickness rim with "fingers" projecting into the center of the necrotic area.

Cerebral infarct and hemorrhage present with the acute onset of symptoms. Cerebral infarct typically enhances in the days after stroke, with the enhancement heterogeneous and serpiginous similar to a malignant astrocytoma. The enhancing abnormality resolves in 6 to 8 weeks with occlusive vascular disease and progress with malignant astrocytoma. If there is a significant diagnostic question, corticosteroids should not be used because they may also change the imaging picture of a malignant astrocytoma and cloud the decision-making process. Hemorrhagic vascular disease may be confused with the apoplectic presentation of hemorrhagic tumor. On CT and MRI scans, the hemorrhage may obscure contrast enhancement leading to the incorrect diagnosis. Tumoral hemorrhage most often has marked signal heterogeneity, pronounced edema, and nonhemorrhagic enhancing tumor tissue.[89]

Cysticercosis, the most common parasitic cyst, frequently presents with seizures and typically occurs in the southwestern United States and Mexico. Calcified cystic lesions are seen frequently in cysticercosis. The lesions are often multiple, and most often do not have extensive edema.

MS may be confused with malignant astrocytoma. Patients with MS may have had previous subtle neurologic symptoms in the past, with multifocal signs on examination. MS very rarely presents with headache or seizures. MS lesions are typically periependymal in location and enhance heterogeneously and serpiginously, similar to malignant astrocytoma. The contrast enhancement pattern in MS changes over time, with new contrast lesions appearing and old enhancing lesions resolving. Evoked-response studies and cerebrospinal fluid (CSF) analysis may provide further evidence for the diagnosis of MS.

DIAGNOSTIC WORKUP

MRI, with and without contrast enhancement, is the initial diagnostic imaging procedure of choice in patients suspected of having a malignant astrocytoma.[90–92] MRI with thin 3-mm slices provides maximum anatomic detail. Multiplanar image sequences should include T_1-weighted sagittal and axial planes before contrast infusion and sagittal, axial, and coronal planes after contrast infusion. T_2-weighted axial and coronal images are needed. MRI is a more sensitive diagnostic procedure for tumor identification than CT and provides more anatomic detail. The margin of the T_2-weighted abnormality on MRI scans is a more accurate, although imperfect, measure of the boundary of the malignant astrocytoma.[93–95] Frequently, isolated malignant astrocytoma cells extend beyond the edge of the T_2-weighted high-signal abnormality into brain that is imaged as normal. MRI is not specific for histologic grade of astrocytoma.[93]

Malignant astrocytoma is usually hypointense on T_1-weighted images and most typically enhances heterogeneously and serpiginously after contrast infusion. There may be areas of solid contrast enhancement within a more serpiginous pattern, or the lesion may enhance solidly, with the degree of enhancement varying within the solid portion of enhancement (see Fig. 3–1A to C). Less commonly, malignant astrocytoma enhances in a ringlike pattern. The ring is usually variable in thickness, with small fingerlike extensions into the necrotic center or out from the rim. On T_1-weighted sequences with contrast, the enhancing tumor can be distinguished from the hypointense signal of edema. On T_2-weighted sequences, the edema is hyperintense and cannot be distinguished from tumor.[96]

Malignant astrocytoma cysts typically are hypointense on T_1-weighted sequences and hyperintense on T_2-weighted sequences (see Fig. 3–2). Acute intratumoral hemorrhage is seen acutely as increased signal on T_1-weighted images, and over time evolves into an area of decreased signal, although more slowly than nontumoral hemorrhage (see Fig. 3–3).[89]

Astrocytic neoplasms graded histologically using a modified 1979 WHO classification (see Table 1–4) were scored retrospectively for a number of MRI imaging criteria. Three criteria were significantly higher in glioblastoma multiforme than anaplastic astrocytoma: (1) heterogeneity of contrast enhancement, (2) central necrosis in tumor, and (3) the extent of flow voids. The anatomic extent of tumor, signal heterogeneity before contrast, the presence or absence of hemorrhage, edema or mass effect, border definition, and bilaterality of disease were not significantly different in anaplastic astrocytoma and glioblastoma multiforme.[97]

CT is an acceptable alternative to MRI in the diagnostic workup of a suspected malignant astrocytoma. On precontrast imaging studies, the tumor most often is hypodense or isodense when compared with normal brain. After contrast infusion, enhancement patterns are similar to those seen in MRI, with contrast infusion allowing distinction between tumor and edema. Cysts appear as decreased density, and hemorrhage appears as increased density before contrast. Hemorrhage does not change significantly with contrast, although surrounding tumor may enhance and hemorrhage may obscure tumor enhancement.

Contrast enhancement on MRI and CT is not specific for tumor and can be seen in any process that disrupts the blood-brain barrier (BBB). After treatment with radiation therapy (RT), radiation necrosis can produce an image identical to that of tumor on either CT or MRI.[98] (^{18}F)-2-fluoro-2-deoxyglucose positron emission tomography (FDG-PET) may be helpful in differentiating recurrent tumor from radiation necrosis.

FDG-PET has been evaluated in the preoperative workup of patients with suspected malignant glioma. Glucose utilization did not correlate with tumor grade or size,[99] and subsequent histology was more predictive of survival than glucose utilization.[100] FDG-PET has also been used preoperatively to localize the area of maximum glucose utilization to aid the neurosurgeon in performing a biopsy of a tumor with the most aggressive biologic behavior.[101–103] FDG-PET has not been compared with MRI or MRI plus PET for its additive role in tissue diagnosis. After surgical resection, patients with hypermetabolic areas on postoperative FDG-PET scans have early recurrence of tumor.[104] FDG-PET measurement of glucose utilization was not influenced by corticosteroid treatment.[104] FDG-PET is the best noninvasive method to differentiate between radiation necrosis and recurrent tumor (see Fig. 3–6).[105] In patients heavily pretreated with high-dose interstitial or accelerated fraction RT, FDG-PET may be misleading, and surgical resection is needed for definitive diagnosis.[106] In summary, the role of PET in the preoperative management of patients with suspected malignant astrocytomas has not been established. It is the best noninvasive technique for the evaluation of radiation necrosis versus tumor recurrence.

Single photon emission computed tomography (SPECT) has also been evaluated preoperatively for grading of astrocytoma malignancy and localizing the area of maximum ^{201}Tl uptake for biopsy.[107–110] After treatment, SPECT has also been used to diagnose tumor recurrence and differentiate tumor recurrence from radiation necrosis.[111,112] Several studies have found a correlation between tumor uptake of ^{201}Tl and the subsequent grade of the surgically resected tumor.[107–110,201] Tl uptake was unaffected by steroids.[108] SPECT ^{201}Tl has not been as useful as FDG-PET in distinguishing radiation necrosis from recurrent tumor.[112]

Angiography is no longer a routine preoperative examination for patients with suspected malignant astrocytoma. Angiography has the capability of visualizing large and small blood vessels supplying an astrocytoma. The preoperative use of angiography is restricted to ruling out the presence of an arteriovenous malformation after an acute intracerebral hemorrhage. Magnetic resonance angiography is a noninvasive procedure able to visualize large arterial vessels supplying a meningioma or, rarely, a malignant astrocytoma, but it is not helpful in evaluating small blood vessel supply to a tumor. Its role is expanding, and it is frequently used in place of angiography.

Echo-planar MRI is a new technique that can provide blood flow maps of tumor and will hopefully provide information about diffusion of contrast into tumor and allow better resolution of tumor and edema.[113]

TREATMENT

Symptomatic

ANTICONVULSANTS

Valproic acid, diphenylhydantoin and carbamazepine should be used for the symptomatic treatment of seizures. Diphenylhydantoin and carbamazepine have produced the Stevens-Johnson syndrome in the setting of radiation therapy and corticosteroid intake. There is no evidence that prophylactic anticonvulsants are helpful in preventing seizures.

CORTICOSTEROIDS

Malignant astrocytoma grows rapidly and often presents with increased intracranial pressure. Dexamethasone is the most frequently used corticosteroid, and is used in a dosage of 1 to 4 mg 4 times a day. If the initial dose used is ineffective, the dose should be doubled.[114] After the first week of steroid treatment, patients do not require dexamethasone on an every 6-hour schedule; in fact, they can take the dose three times a day. Dexamethasone should be tapered, beginning in the postoperative period as the clinical situation permits, usually continuing a small dose of 0.5 to 1.0 mg two times a day through the completion of RT.

UNSTABLE PATIENTS

In unstable patients with markedly increased intracranial pressure or herniation, intubation and hyperventilation to lower the $Paco_2$ level to 20 to 25 mm Hg are indicated.[115] IV hyperosmolar mannitol is given in a dosage of 1.5 to 2.0 g/kg for 10 to 20 minutes. After bolus administration, it is continued in a dosage of 10 to 20 g/h until the increased intracranial pressure resolves. Furosemide increases the mannitol effect and is usually given in a dose of 80 mg.[114]

The development of hydrocephalus is unusual except in malignant basal ganglia, thalamic, and posterior fossa astrocytomas. If patients develop hydrocephalus from deep midline growth, temporary ventricular drainage or a ventriculoperitoneal shunt may be necessary.

Surgery

The initial treatment of choice in the management of malignant supratentorial astrocytoma is surgical resection of the maximal tumor possible, with as little damage to the surrounding normal brain as possible.[10,13,69,115–120] The selection and planning of the surgical procedure, including intraoperative localization of tumor, microsurgical techniques, and intra-operative electrophysiologic mapping, are discussed in Chapter 4. The benefits of extensive surgical resection include more accurate histologic diagnosis;[121] tumor cytoreduction; improvement in symptoms and signs; decreased tumor burden for RT, chemotherapy, or immunotherapy; and tissue for special proliferative and experimental studies.[117,118]

In a retrospective study, patients with complete resection had fewer neurologic complications and no greater risk of being neurologically impaired than patients with biopsy or less extensive resection.[116] The mortality rate was 3.3% for patients in this series. In another small retrospective study, whereas gross total surgical resection produced a significant improvement in neurologic[122] and Karnofsky performance status,[123] subtotal resection did not. In a prospective randomized chemotherapeutic trial of intravenous (IV) 1-(2-chloroethyl)-2-(2,6-dioxo-3 piperidyl)-1-nitrosourea (PCNU) versus IV 1,3-bis-(2-chloroethyl)-1-nitrosourea (BCNU) in 334 patients with malignant glioma and in an overlap retrospective trial of 263 patients from the same institution, multivariate analysis found a significant survival advantage for patients treated with gross total resection compared with other surgical treatment.[119,124] In a retrospective study of 285 patients with malignant astrocytoma using multivariate analysis, the extent of resection correlated with survival. Patients with gross total resection lived longer than subtotal resection, and those with any resection lived longer than patients who underwent only a biopsy procedure.[125] In a prospective Brain Tumor Cooperative Group (BTCG) study, patients with gross total resection had increased survival, and the smaller the residual tumor after surgery, the longer patients lived.[120,126] In these studies, a wide range of prognostic variables was examined, and age, tumor grade, and Karnofsky performance status were more strongly correlated with survival than the extent of resection.[13,119,124,125]

The principle of maximal surgical resection for malignant astrocytoma has been debated strongly for the past decade. There are multiple prospective randomized[127] and retrospective studies[128–133] in which the extent of surgical resection has not been found to be a significant prognostic factor. In 1988, Coffey and colleagues[128] reported on 91 malignant astrocytoma patients diagnosed by stereotactic biopsy and treated with varying doses of RT. A total of 45 patients with glioblastoma completed adequate RT and had a median survival of 29.5 weeks. A smaller group of 22 patients with lobar tumors treated surgically with only biopsy received adequate RT and had a median survival of 46.9 weeks. Patients with anaplastic astrocytoma treated with adequate RT had a median survival of 74 weeks. The authors found no difference between these patients and their historical controls with subtotal resection and RT. However, the survival in their biopsy- and adequately treated RT patients was worse than in the BTCG trials that prospectively analyzed a randomized population to RT, with or without chemotherapy.[11,13]

In a prospective randomized study of malignant astrocytoma patients treated with RT, with or without procarbazine (PCV) chemotherapy, no difference was found between the group treated with gross total resection and that with subtotal resection, with biopsy patients excluded from analysis.[127] In a series of prospective studies, patients with any resection had a better survival than the biopsy group in univariate analysis but not in multivariate analysis. However, a greater proportion of young patients had extensive surgery.[130] In 222 tumor biopsies of patients with both low- and high-grade astrocytomas, there were five deaths (2.7%) in patients with glioblastoma multiforme.[134]

The definitive answer to the question of surgical biopsy versus extensive resection is not available. A randomized trial to answer the question is unlikely to occur because of physician and patient biases and the extensive stratification by tumor location that would be necessary. It is not surprising that the extent of surgery is insignificant in many trials because the three most important prognostic variables in this disease are the pretreatment variables: age, histology, and preoperative Karnofsky performance status. In studies that question the use of radical resection, there is a trend favoring radical resection over biopsy[131,133] or statistical benefit from resection in univariate analysis but not multivariate analysis.[130] In conclusion, prudent maximal surgical resection is a sound neuro-oncologic principle with no increase in morbidity and an improvement in functional performance status. It allows more accurate histologic diagnosis, improves neurologic symptoms and signs, reduces tumor bulk, and allows time for other therapy. It also provides tissue for proliferative indices and other experimental studies.

REOPERATION

The indications for reoperation of malignant astrocytoma after initial treatment with surgery, RT, and chemotherapy are not firmly established. The most significant predictive variable of survival after reoperation was a preoperative Karnofsky performance status of 60, 70, or more (Table 8–4).[135–138] Other identifiable prognostic variables include young age,[137,138] prolonged interval between operations,[135,139] and extent of the second surgical resection.[136] The median survival for glioblastoma multiforme after reoperation varied from 14 to 36 weeks, with a shorter median duration of survival when patients were

Table 8–4. **Malignant Astrocytoma: Prognostic Factors for Reoperation**

Preoperative Karnofsky performance status
Time interval between operations
Young age
Extent of resection on second operation

treated with only surgical reoperation[135] and no subsequent therapy.[135–139] The median survival for anaplastic astrocytoma after reoperation in three series varied from 56 to 88 weeks.[136–138]

In summary, reoperation is best performed when the Karnofsky status is more than 60, the patient is young, and the surgical resection will provide time for further therapy.

Radiation Therapy

WHOLE BRAIN RADIATION THERAPY (WBRT)

External-beam RT is the single most effective treatment for malignant astrocytoma. For randomized prospective clinical studies document the effectiveness of adjuvant WBRT for the treatment of malignant astrocytoma (Table 8–5).[11,127,140,141] In a randomized study of the Brain Tumor Study Group (BTSG), WBRT increased survival from 14 weeks with surgery alone to 36 weeks with surgery and WBRT.[140] In a second BTSG study, surgery with adjuvant WBRT was associated with a longer median survival of 36 weeks than surgery and adjuvant N-(2-chloroethyl)-N'-cyclohexyl-N-nitrosourea (CCNU) chemotherapy with a median survival of 24 weeks.[11]

The BTSG analyzed RT dose and found a relationship between increasing the dose of WBRT from 5000 to 6000 cGy and increasing survival, with a median survival of 28 weeks at a dose of 5000 cGy, 36 weeks at 5500 cGy, and 42 weeks at 6000 cGy (Fig. 8–3).[142] A further increase in WBRT dose to 7000 cGy did not appear to produce a further survival increase.[143] An earlier study[144] found patients treated with WBRT and a focal boost to 8000 cGy had a 55-week median survival.

In the 18-week period after completion of a trial of 5000-cGy WBRT, with a 1000-cGy focal boost for malignant astrocytoma, approximately 50% of patients deteriorated,

Table 8–5. **Malignant Astrocytoma: Randomized Whole Brain Radiation Therapy Trials***

Trial	Total Patients	Treatment	Median Survival (Weeks)	1-Year Survival (%)
BTSG 69–01[140]	222	Supportive care	14	3
		WBRT	36	12
		BCNU	19	24
		WBRT+BCNU	35	32
BTSG 72–01[11]	358	Methyl-CCNU	24	15
		WBRT	36	35
		WBRT + methyl-CCNU	42	37
		WBRT + BCNU	51	50
Andersen[141]	108	Supportive care	15*	0*
		WBRT	20*	17*
Sandberg-Wohlheim et al[127]	171	WBRT + PCV	62	58*
		PCV	42	43*

*Estimated from survival curve.

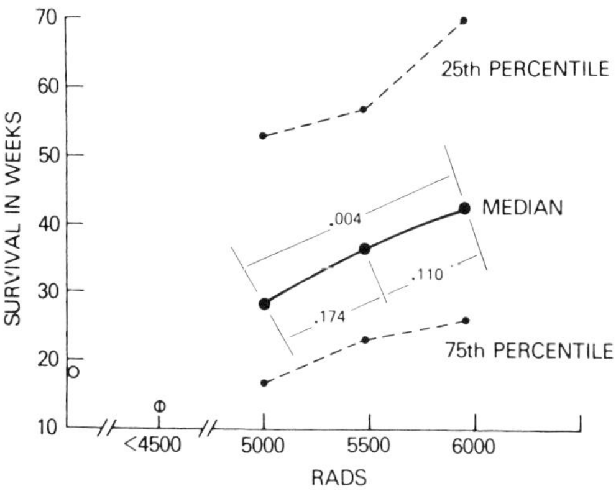

Figure 8–3. The median survival of patients receiving no radiotherapy (○), less than 4500 rads (⦶), and 5000, 5500, or 6000 rads (●) as well as survival at the 25th and 75th percentile and the Gehan-Wilcoxon test p value for significance. (From Walker et al,[142] p 1729, with permission.)

and 50% of the remaining patients did not improve. They had a median time to disease progression of 31 weeks. The other 50% of these patients improved without a change in therapy and had a median time to tumor progression of 73 weeks.[145] Late delayed sequelae after WBRT included asymptomatic narrowing of large vessels, radiation necrosis, and secondary neoplasia.[146,147] Radiation necrosis was the major risk, and the process was progressive and irreversible. The pathologic process was centered in the white matter and was secondary to both small blood vessel injury and occlusion and demyelination in white matter.[147]

Two studies[148,149] looked at tumor recurrence after WBRT and found that tumor recurred within 2 cm of the original site in 90% and 78% of cases, supporting the use of focal RT. Multifocal recurrence occurred in 6% of patients in one study and 5% in a second trial.[148,150] In the second study, multifocal recurrence occurred in 5% of patients with glioblastoma multiforme and 8.6% of anaplastic astrocytoma.[150]

FOCAL EXTERNAL-BEAM RADIATION THERAPY

After reports that recurrence after WBRT failure was almost entirely at the original site,[148,149] and with the increasing recognition of the incidence of CNS toxicity from WBRT,[147] focal external-beam radiation therapy (FEBRT) became the standard empirical approach. The FEBRT dose is delivered to the preoperative contrast-enhancing abnormality plus a margin, or the T_2-weighted MRI abnormality and a margin. The usual margin for the contrast-enhancing abnormality is 2.5 to 3.0 cm, and for the T_2-weighted abnormality, 1.5 to 2.0 cm. The development of computerized three-dimensional reconstruction of CT, MRI, PET, and SPECT images in cranial space allows one or more imaging modalities to be converted to three dimensions and a margin added around the data set to treat infiltrating cells. A computer then selects conformal radiation fields to optimally treat the tumor volume and minimize dose to normal brain.[151–154] The use of conformal techniques to treat malignant astrocytoma has decreased the amount of normal brain tissue radiated by up to 50%.[153,154]

Tumor recurrence after conformal FEBRT to 59.4 Gy has been almost entirely focal, with 100% of patients recurring within 2 cm of the original tumor site. Two patients had a second lesion both inside and outside the 2-cm margin, and two patients had a distant second lesion.[155] The change from WBRT to FEBRT did not change the pattern of treatment failure or alter the percentage of multifocal failure. Therefore, conformal FEBRT trials with dose escalation to 8000 and 8600 cGy are in progress.

NEW RADIATION THERAPY FRACTIONATION SCHEMES

Hyperfractionated RT decreases the dose of each fraction and increases the number of RT fractions. The aim is to deliver a higher dose of radiation in the same or shorter period of time. The size of each fraction is one of the primary factors in determining the frequency of late RT toxicity. Normal brain has a greater capacity to repair small fractionation sublethal RT damage than tumor, and thus dose escalation is possible. The smaller size of each fraction does not decrease tumor cell kill significantly, and the increased number of fractions allows time for redistribution of tumor cells into sensitive cell-cycle phases. The decreased dose per fraction will make tumor cell killing less oxygen dependent.[156]

Hyperfractionated RT trials with twice-daily fractions to doses of 61, 71, and 80 Gy found median survivals of 46, 38, and 45 weeks.[157] A second trial with twice-daily fractions to hyperfractionated doses of 65, 72, 77, and 82 Gy found the optimum dose to be 72 Gy.[158]

Superfractionated RT is a form of hyperfractionated RT in which the radiation dose is delivered three times a day. Two superfractionation RT trials for malignant astrocytoma were performed, with 76 and 88.8 cGy fractions three times a day, to 4500 cGy and 4760 cGy, followed by a conventionally fractionated 1000-cGy boost.[159,160] No significant difference was found when compared with single daily-fraction RT.

Accelerated-fraction RT delivers larger doses with fewer fractions over a shorter period of time. The accelerated course may be delivered with a conventional or hyperfractionated protocol. Accelerated or hypofractionated RT has been used to treat patients with malignant astrocytoma, with significant improvements in Karnofsky performance status, but no overall increase in survival when compared with 6-week single-daily fraction RT.[161–164] Treatment time shortens considerably, with an attendant cost saving.

Low-dose hyperfractionation (64 and 72 Gy), high-dose hyperfractionation (76 and 81 Gy) and accelerated hyperfractionation focal RT have been used in malignant gliomas.[165] All patients were treated with IV BCNU concurrent with and after RT. No significant survival difference was found in any of the treatment arms. Median survival was 12.6 months for low hyperfractionation, 12.4 months for high-dose hyperfractionation, and 11.6 months for accelerated hyperfractionation. This does not appear significantly different than single daily-dose RT trials. When analysis was performed according to tumor type, anaplastic astrocytoma or glioblastoma, and treatments grouped according to low-dose, high-dose or accelerated hyperfractionation, anaplastic astrocytoma had a nonsignificant trend to longer survival at 64 and 72 Gy, and glioblastoma multiforme at 72 and 76 Gy. In conclusion, no convincing evidence exists that hyperfractionation, with or without dose escalation or accelerated-fraction RT, leads to increased survival or fulfillment of its theoretical advantages.

HEAVY PARTICLE RADIATION THERAPY

Heavy particle beams consisting of neutrons, heavy charged particles such as helium and neon ions, and pi-mesons have been used alone or as boost therapy with conventional photon radiation. The rationale for heavy particle RT is its lower oxygen enhancement ratio, which may work better in hypoxic malignant astrocytoma cells, and a more significant direct-damaging effect on DNA that is less repairable than with photon RT.[166–168] Early clinical trials with whole brain neutron-beam RT in the treatment of patients with malignant astrocytoma produced no increase in survival compared with conventional fractionation. Postmortem examination showed tumor sterilization in many cases, with widespread radiation necrosis of normal brain.[166,167]

After the toxicity seen with whole brain neutron-beam RT, the Radiation Therapy Oncology Group (RTOG) developed a randomized clinical trial comparing 50-Gy WBRT with a 15-Gy conventional photon boost with 50-Gy WBRT with a neutron-boost dose equivalent to a 15-Gy photon boost. This trial included patients with glioblastoma multiforme and anaplastic astrocytoma. In the patients with glioblastoma multiforme, no difference in survival in the two treatment arms was found. Whereas all autopsied photon patients had persistent tumor, nine of 12 neutron patients had no viable tumor.[168,169] In the anaplastic astrocytoma group, whereas the photon-boost arm had a median survival of 26.3 months, the neutron boost arm had median survival ofonly 15.8 months. An unproven concern of the investigators was the neutron boost produced late RT necrosis in patients with glioblastoma and shortened survival in the anaplastic astrocytoma patients.[169] Neutrons have also been combined with misonidazole, a hypoxic cell sensitizer, in the treatment of malignant astrocytoma without significant effect.[170]

Heavy charged particles from which electrons are stripped can be accelerated to energy levels that allow them to be stopped precisely in targeted tissue. They have the same theoretical advantages as neutron-beam RT. The median survival in a trial of 17 patients with glioblastoma treated with photon WBRT and helium or neon heavy particle boost was 13.9 months. Eleven patients with anaplastic astrocytoma had a median survival of 7.6 months.[171] These preliminary studies were obviously not a clinical advance.

Boron neutron capture therapy (BNCT) is a form of heavy particle RT that has stimulated interest in the treatment of malignant astrocytoma. In BNCT, the nonradioactive boron-10 (^{10}B) atom captures slow neutrons with 4000 times more affinity than other atoms present in tissues. After capture, the boron compound is unstable and splits into two heavy charged particles, with the release of high and low energy (Fig. 8–4). The high energy is deposited in tissue over short distances. The critical issues for clinical application are effective distribution of ^{10}B to the tumor and a sufficient number of slow thermal neutrons.[172] Boron sulfhydryl and the compound, $Na_2B_{12}H_{11}SH$ have been shown to concentrate in high-grade gliomas but do not pass an intact BBB.[173–175] In clinical trials in Japan, 116 patients with brain tumors were infused with $Na_2B_{12}H_{11}SH$ intra-arterially, with thermal neutrons delivered superficially, less than 6 cm from the brain surface with a nuclear reactor.[176–178] One patient with glioblastoma survived more than 18 years, and six patients with anaplastic astrocytoma lived more than 9 years. These results are exciting, but a controlled clinical trial is needed.[179]

$$^{10}\mathrm{B} + \text{thermal neutron} \rightarrow [^{11}\mathrm{B}] \rightarrow {}^{4}\mathrm{He} + {}^{7}\mathrm{Li} + \gamma$$

Figure 8–4. Boron neutron capture therapy involves the exposure of a boron-containing tumor to a low-energy or thermal neutron. This capture results in the generation of alpha particles and lithium ions, both high–linear energy transfer with a path length of 10–14 μM. The path length is approximately one cell diameter, and theoretically the radiation effect is limited to tumor cells that have taken up boron.

Malignant astrocytoma has also been treated with postoperative interstitial implantation of californium-252, a neutron emitter, followed by 6000 to 7000 cGy in photon RT, to a total tumor dose of between 8100 and 9100 cGy. The median survival of 10 months, and 18-month survival of 28%, were not better than conventional photon RT.[180]

PHOTODYNAMIC THERAPY

Photodynamic therapy is an experimental treatment modality that depends on the interaction of a photosensitizing agent localized in malignant tissue, typically the hematoporphyrin derivative (HPD) or dihematoporphyrin (DHE), oxygen, and a light source.[181] In humans, infusion studies have shown selective uptake in all grades of glioma, greatest in most malignant tumors, with lesser amounts of HPD or DHE in brain adjacent tumor.[182,183] In phase I and II clinical trials, recurrent malignant astrocytomas were infused with HPD or DHE intravenously, with intratumoral placement of an argon pump dye laser coupled to an optical fiber.[183–185] In the most recent study with DHE, no surgical resection was performed before the photodynamic therapy. All six malignant astrocytomas had an almost complete disappearance of contrast enhancement on post-therapy scans, and all patients developed cerebral edema at the treatment site. The edema was often symptomatic, with the symptoms resolving spontaneously within 1 week. MRI spectroscopy in three patients showed marked energy depletion in tumor 1 day after therapy when compared with pretreatment values. Four patients recurred at 2, 6, 8, and 27 weeks, and two have continued response at 35 and 45 weeks.[184] It is possible that the decreased contrast enhancement that was transitory in at least three patients was not due to tumor necrosis but instead to increased interstitial edema pressure. The role of photodynamic therapy in the treatment of brain tumors is still evolving.

INTERSTITIAL BRACHYTHERAPY

Interstitial brachytherapy is the stereotactic placement into tumors of radio-isotope seeds, most commonly iodine-125 (^{125}I) or iridium-192 (^{192}Ir). These seeds release low-dose rate radiation for the duration of implantation. Low-dose rate irradiation is different than photon radiation, which is intermittent and of a high-dose rate.[187,188] In tissue culture, low-dose rate irradiation has effectively killed glioma cells.[189,190] Interstitial brachytherapy delivers a large dose of radiation to the tumor volume with rapid fall-off of radiation in surrounding tissue. Its radiobiologic advantages are a low oxygen enhancement ratio, time for accumulation of malignant cells in a sensitive phase of the cell cycle, and decreased repair of sublethal damage because of continuous delivery.[187,190]

Interstitial brachytherapy has been used as adjuvant therapy and as treatment for tumor recurrence in malignant astrocytoma. Interstitial brachytherapy has significant size and geography limitations, which limit its widespread utilization. The tumor must be unilateral and less than 5 cm in diameter. Malignant astrocytomas in the insula region are difficult technically, and dangerous neurologically, to implant. Thalamic and other deep tumors cannot be implanted because of the difficulty in resecting radiation necrosis. This eliminates approximately 75% of patients with malignant astrocytoma from consideration for this type of therapy.[191]

In an adjuvant randomized phase III trial of the BTCG, patients with malignant astrocytoma were randomized postoperatively to FEBRT and interstitial brachytherapy or FEBRT alone.[192] Patients treated with interstitial brachytherapy had better median survival of 15.8 months compared with that of the conventional FEBRT group, which was of 13.6 months ($p= 0.08$). The difference was 2.2 months (personal communication, Sylvan Green, MD, 1996). After interstitial brachytherapy, up to 40% of patients require another surgery for removal of radiation necrosis.[187] In summary, 25% of patients will be eligible for an adjuvant therapy that prolongs life by 2.2 months and requires up to two additional operations and hospitalizations.

As mentioned earlier, interstitial brachytherapy has been used to treat recurrent malignant astrocytoma.[186,187,190] In one series, 66 patients had recurrent glioblastoma, and 45 had recurrent high-grade nonglioblastoma. The median survival from the date of implantation was 49 weeks in the recurrent glioblastoma group, with a 3-year survival of 15%. In the recurrent high-grade nonglioblastoma cohort, the median survival was 52 weeks, with a 3-year survival of 24%.[187]

Interstitial brachytherapy has also been combined with interstitial hyperthermia in two phase I/II trials for the treatment of glioblastoma, with median survival of 88 and 41 weeks in the two trials.[193,194] Despite the positive randomized trial of the BTCG with a significant benefit for adjuvant interstitial brachytherapy, enthusiasm for this technique seems to be waning. The benefit for patients with glioblastoma, although significant, seems marginal when considering the likelihood of two operations and hospitalizations and the cost.

The Northern California Oncology Group (NCOG) has achieved better survival results for patients with anaplastic astrocytoma treated with conventional FEBRT and 5 hydroxyurea followed by PCV chemotherapy than with those treated with interstitial brachytherapy. The median survival was 157 weeks compared with 142 weeks with an adjuvant interstitial boost.[195]

Tumor recurrence after interstitial radiation was within 2 cm of the primary site in 77% and 88% of patients in two studies.[196,197] In two other studies, the rate of distant recurrence was higher at 25% and 46%.[198,199] It is still uncertain whether interstitial brachytherapy has a higher proportion of distant recurrences than FEBRT. If better local control were to be achieved, a higher rate of distant spread would be expected, and possibly at a longer time interval.

STEREOTACTIC RADIOSURGERY

Stereotactic radiosurgery (SR) uses narrowly collimated stereotactic beams of ionizing radiation in high-dose single fractions to treat small (i.e., less than 3 cm) targets.[200] The initial radiosurgery system developed by Leksell[201] was the gamma knife, which used approximately 200 cobalt-60 sources. Recently, the linear accelerator, commonly used in radiation oncology, has been modified to deliver small photon beams to a target. The ionizing radiation source used in gamma knife and linear accelerator radiosurgery differ, but both techniques are capable of delivering a single high dose of ionizing radiation to a small target, with a very sharp dose falloff that spares normal surrounding tissue.[200]

SR has been used as an adjuvant boost after conventional FEBRT to 5940 cGy for the treatment of newly diagnosed glioblastoma multiforme. SR maximum doses ranged from 1250 to 2500 cGy. A total of 69 patients were treated with a median survival of 19.7 months, and a 2- and 3-year survival of 31% and 20%, respectively.[202,203] Recurrence was found in 33 patients, 85% of which was outside the boost volume and 15% of which was local. A total of 27 patients (43.5%) underwent reoperation because of increasing mass effect, a percentage similar to that seen other interstitial brachytherapy trials. A total of 14 patients with anaplastic astrocytoma were treated, with 11 patients remaining alive at more than 1 year. Two deaths occurred at 7 months, one attributed to amyotrophic lateral sclerosis, and a second from a seizure in a patient with no evidence of tumor at postmortem examination.[202,203] A second trial treated 31 glioblastoma patients with FEBRT of 50 to 66 Gy and a SR boost with a central dose of 15 to 35 Gy. A median survival of 9.5 months and a 1-year survival of 37% were reported.[204,205]

SR has also been used for recurrent gliomas. Fourteen of 19 evaluable treated patients died, with a median survival of 7 months. Five patients, four who failed SR, were alive, with a median time to progression of 9 months.[206] SR dose has also been fractionated into 6 to 10 fractions of 5 Gy each to more effectively sterilize tumor.[207,208] A total of 22 patients who failed previous FEBRT with a median dose of 55 Gy were treated with fractionated 30- to 50-Gy SR on recurrence, with a median survival of 9.8 months.[208]

Patients who are eligible for SR are in a prognostically favorable group because of the selection criteria for SR.[191,209] When SR eligible patients were selected from RTOG non-SR trials, the patients eligible for SR had a median survival of 14.4 months versus 11.7 months ($p=0.047$) for the patients not eligible for SR. Only 9% of the 775 patients entered on the RTOG non-SR trials were eligible for SR. These trials were performed before the widespread availability of SR. A controlled trial randomizing eligible patients to FEBRT, with or without SR, is needed to define the role of adjuvant SR.

RADIOSENSITIZERS

Radiosensitizers are compounds that increase the therapeutic effect of RT. The four main classes of radiosensitizers are (1) nitroimidazoles, which increase tissue oxygenation and decrease the hypoxic fraction of the tumor increasing radiosensitivity; (2) perfluorochemicals, which carry oxygen to tissue; (3) halogenated pyrimidines, which are incorporated into tumor DNA instead of thymidine and increase tumor radiosensitivity; and (4) chemotherapeutic agents.[210] These compounds can be used with all forms of RT discussed in this chapter.

Misonidazole and metronidazole are two nitroimadazoles that have been used clinically in multiple clinical trials without improvement in survival.[210–216] Fluosol-DA is perfluorochemical emulsion that carries administered oxygen to tissue and decreases tissue hypoxia. It has been administered to patients with malignant astrocytoma. A preliminary report suggests that this might possibly increase survival, with a median survival of 64 weeks in 18 patients, 15 with glioblastoma multiforme and three with anaplastic astrocytoma.[217]

Halogenated pyrimidines are incorporated into dividing tumor cells instead of thymidine and increase the radiation sensitivity of tumor. Neurons and glia do not have a significant mitotic rate, do not incorporate BUdR or IUdR, and are not sensitized to RT. The halogenated pyrimidine BUdR has been infused intravenously for 96 hours, or 12 of 24 hours, for 4 consecutive days each week, and by continuous intra-arterial (IA) infusion through an implanted pump for the treatment of malignant astrocytoma during RT.[218,219] IV BUdR provided no increase in survival for patients with glioblastoma, but showed promise in anaplastic astrocytoma, with almost a 4-year median survival. IA BUdR was evaluated in a total of 62 patients with malignant astrocytoma who were treated in two phase I/II trials of IA BUdR infusion beginning 2 weeks before RT and continuing throughout RT. BUdR was given intra-arterially because of its regional advantage of 11 to 16. In the second trial, 5-fluorouracil (5-FU) was also infused intra-arterially to decrease the endogenous synthesis of thymidine by tumor cells. The median survival of all patients was 18 months, with 58 of 62 patients with glioblastoma multiforme by the 1993 WHO classification.[220]

The chemotherapeutic agents hydroxyurea, 5-FU, and cisplatin (CDDP) have also been used as radiosensitizers.[210] Tissue culture experiments with these compounds have shown increased radiation cytotoxicity in nonchemotherapeutic doses.

RADIOPROTECTORS

Radioprotectors are drugs that provide protection for CNS parenchymal and vascular elements but not neoplasms. Pentobarbital anesthesia in irradiated tumor-bearing rats has been shown to provide radioprotection to the normal brain, with animals under pentobarbital anesthesia living longer than those treated with RT alone.[221–223] Phosphorothioate compounds are water-soluble radioprotective compounds that must be administered directly into the CSF.[224]

Chemotherapy

ADJUVANT

The aim of adjuvant chemotherapy combined with surgery and RT is to increase cell kill, and achieve a cure. Chemotherapy administered in the adjuvant setting has the least remaining tumor cells to treat. Acquired tumor cell resistance will not have developed. The scenario for adjuvant chemotherapy cytoreduction is shown in Table 7–2. Starting in the 1970s, adjuvant chemotherapy was evaluated in randomized phase III multi-institution clinical trials by the BTSG and others.[140,225] Survival was used as the primary endpoint in these trials because of difficulties in measuring disease progression and differentiating residual tumor from postoperative changes and radiation necrosis.

The first BTSG trial (69–01) randomized patients to one of four arms after surgery: (1) supportive care, (2) BCNU, (3) WBRT, (4) WBRT and BCNU (Table 8–6).[140] The median survival of the WBRT and combined WBRT and BCNU groups was prolonged compared with the supportive care group. The 18-month survival with combined WBRT and BCNU was significantly greater than that for RT alone (19% versus 4 %). The surgery and BCNU arms were inferior to both WBRT arms. The second BTSG trial (72-01) was also a four-arm trial comparing (1) CCNU, (2) WBRT, (3) WBRT and CCNU, and (4) WBRT and BCNU. The median survival of the three groups with WBRT was superior to that of CCNU alone, confirming the benefit of WBRT in trial 69-01. In this trial (72-01), the 18-month survival pattern for the two combined WBRT and chemotherapy arms showed a trend similar to the 69-01 trial, but no statistically significant improvement over WBRT alone was found.[11] The next BTSG trial (75-01) evaluated the adjuvant therapy arms (1) BCNU, (2) methylprednisolone, (3) procarbazine, and (4) BCNU and methylprednisolone. Procarbazine was equal in chemotherapeutic effectiveness to BCNU, and methylprednisolone was inferior to either BCNU or procarbazine.[13] Subsequent trials of the BTCG, the successor to the BTSG, found streptozotocin equal to BCNU (trial 77-02), and combination chemotherapy with BCNU and procarbazine or BCNU and hydroxyurea, alternating with procarbazine and VM-26, no more effective than BCNU alone (80-01).[120,226]

Other cooperative groups have also contributed importantly in the evaluation of adjuvant chemotherapy. The Southwest Oncology Group (SWOG) performed two trials with randomization between CCNU and combined CCNU and procarbazine in one trial. In the second three-arm trial, randomization was between BCNU and combined procarbazine and dacarbazine. No significant difference was noted in survival in the treatment arms of these trials.[227,228] The NCOG randomized patients with either glioblastoma multiforme or anaplastic astrocytoma to chemotherapy with BCNU or the combination chemotherapy regimen of PCV after RT and hydroxyurea. In anaplastic astrocytoma patients, PCV produced a significantly longer time to progression of 126 weeks and median survival of 157 weeks; use of BCNU had an 82-week median time to progression and a 62-week median survival.[195] No difference was found in the two treatments in patients with glioblastoma. The Duke Cancer Consortium randomized patients to IV BCNU or IV 2,5-diaziridinyl 3,6-bis (carboethoxyamino) 1,4-benzoquinone (AZQ) and found no significant difference between the two treatments, although the AZQ survival curve was consistently below the BCNU survival curve.[229]

Individual adjuvant chemotherapy trials fail to show an increase in median survival in the chemotherapy arms. A marginal increase in 18-month survival is seen in occasional trials with chemotherapy. To assess the effect of adding chemotherapy to RT, Fine and colleagues[230] performed a meta-analysis of 16 randomized chemotherapy trials involving 3000 patients. The estimated increase in survival was small, with a 10.1% (95% CI: 6.8% to 13.3%) increase at 1 year, and 8.6% (95% CI: 5.2% to 12.0%) at 2 years. The survival advantage was present for both glioblastoma multiforme and anaplastic astrocytoma and for both chemotherapeutic agents analyzed, BCNU and CCNU.[230]

In summary, adjuvant nitrosourea or procarbazine chemotherapy appears to be of modest benefit, and the combination chemotherapy regimen of PCV may be superior for anaplastic astrocytoma. The generalization of clinical trial results to the population of patients with malignant astrocytoma must be done cautiously because such patients may not be representative of the cohort as a whole (see section on clinical chemotherapy trials in Chapter 7).[231]

SINGLE AGENT

The chemotherapy treatment of patients with malignant astrocytoma, particularly glioblastoma, has been disappointing, with little gain since the initial trials of the BTSG. No single chemotherapeutic agent in a randomized trial has been shown to increase the median survival of patients with recurrent malignant astrocytoma. An interpretation of the lack of change in median survival is that the response rate (CR + PR) for any single drug is at or below 50%. The most commonly used single agents are the nitrosoureas, procarbazine, etoposide, and AZQ. Other agents include platinum compounds, lovastatin, methotrexate (MTX), edatrexate, VM-26, temozolomide, tamoxifen, taxol, and topotecan.[232–250] The results of these trials are listed in Table 8–7. A good response rate for a malignant astrocytoma clinical trial is 40% (CR + PR + SD), with a median duration of response of 26 to 30 weeks. A good response rate for a glioblastoma multiforme trial is lower, with a 25% to 35% response rate for a median duration of 20 to 24 weeks. The response rate for the anaplastic astrocytoma trials is higher, with a good response rate of 50% to 60% and a median duration of response of 30 to 40 weeks.[251]

MULTIAGENT

The advantages of multiagent chemotherapy in the treatment of malignant astrocy-

Table 8–6. **Malignant Astrocytoma: Randomized Multimodality Chemotherapy**

Trial	Total Patients	Treatment	Patients per Treatment	Median Survival (Weeks)	18-Month Survival (%)
Reagan et al[225] (1975)	63	WBRT	22	50	37*
		CCNU	22	28	13*
		WBRT + CCNU	19	52	22*
BTSG 69–01[140] (1978)	222	Supportive care	31	14	0
		BCNU	51	19	4
		WBRT	68	36	4
		WBRT+BCNU	72	35	19
BTSG 72–01[11] (1980)	547	Methyl-CCNU	111	31	20
		WBRT	118	37	19
		WBRT + methyl-CCNU	120	49	29
		WBRT + BCNU	118	43	30
BTSG 75–01[13] (1983)	609	WBRT + methyl-prednisone	156	41	16
		WBRT + BCNU	147	50	26.5
		WBRT + procarbazine	153	43	29
		WBRT + BCNU + methyl-prednisone	153	41	23
Chang et al[143] (1983)	626	WBRT	167	43	19
		WBRT + 1000 cGy FB	114	37	22
		WBRT + BCNU	185	43	29
		WBRT + methyl-CCNU + DTIC	160	42	24
SWOG[227] (1983)	115	WBRT + CCNU	56	55	36*
		WBRT + CCNU+ procarbazine	59	50	24*
SWOG[228] (1986)	243	WBRT + BCNU	82	45	26*
		WBRT + procarbazine	83	31	17*
		WBRT + DTIC	78	49	28*

Continued on following page

toma are uncertain. Multiagent adjuvant chemotherapy with PCV produced a longer median duration of response and survival than BCNU in a randomized trial for the treatment of anaplastic astrocytoma but not of glioblastoma multiforme.[227] The longer duration response and survival may be due to the use of procarbazine. In other single-agent and randomized trials, procarbazine has produced a more durable response than BCNU.[13,236] A randomized trial for anaplastic astrocytomas comparing BCNU with procarbazine has not been carried out.

Table 8–6.—*continued*

Trial	Total Patients	Treatment	Patients Per Treatment	Median Survival (Weeks)	18–Month Survival (%)
BTCG 77–02[226] (1989)	557 (valid study group)	WBRT + BCNU	140	42	16
		WBRT + streptozotocin	136	42	24
		Hyperfractionated WBRT + BCNU	142	44	25
		WBRT (misonidazole) + BCNU	139	40	17
NCOG[195] (1990)	133	*GBM*			
		WBRT(HU) + BCNU	29	57	33*
		WBRT(HU) + PCV	38	50	33*
		AA			
		WBRT(HU) + BCNU	37	82	50*
		WBRT(HU) + PCV	36	157	68*
BTCG[120] (1989)	571	WBRT + BCNU	185	56	29
		WBRT + BCNU/ procarbazine	196	49	32
		WBRT + BCNU + HU/procarbazine VM-26	190	59	37
Duke[229] (1993)	251	WBRT + FB + AZQ	121	46	NA
		WBRT + FB + BCNU	128	54	NA
Mayo[119] (1993)	346	FEBRT + PCNU	168	47	25*
		FEBRT + BCNU	166	47	30*

* = estimated from curves.
/ = alternating.
AZQ = 2,5-diaziridinyl 3.6-bis (carboetaoxyamino) 1,4-benzoquinone.
DTIC = dacarbazine.
EORTC = European Organization for Research on Treatment of Cancer.
FB = focal boost.
FEBRT = focal external beam radiation therapy.
HU = hydroxyurea.
NA = not available.
SWOG = Southwest Oncology Group.
WBRT = whole brain radiation therapy.

The results for multiagent chemotherapy trials are listed in Table 8–8.[252–263] The most promising regimens are PCV; cyclophosphamide and vincristine; CDDP and VP-16; and meclorethamine, vincristine and procarbazine.[235,254,257,259,260] Similar results have been obtained in patients taking single-agent nitrosourea or procarbazine.[233,235,236]

INNOVATIVE APPROACHES

The experimental treatment of malignant astrocytomas with high-dose IV chemother-

Table 8-7. **Malignant Astrocytoma: Single-Agent Chemotherapy Trials (Adults)**

Drug	Total Patients	Dose	Responders CR + PR + SD (%)	Median Time to Responders Progression (Weeks)
BCNU[233]	57	80–90 mg/m² IV × 3d q 6 wk	47	39
BCNU[236]	31	150–300 mg/m² IV or IA × 1d q 6 wk	81	21 (all patients)
CCNU[233]	36	120–130 mg/m² q 6 wk	44	26
CCNU[234]	16	130 mg/m² q 6 wk	37.5	NA
Fotemustine[243]	21 (GBM)	100 mg/m² IV q 3 wk	67	NA
	9(AA)	100 mg/m² IV q 3 wk	89	NA
Procarbazine[233]	27	150 mg/m² × 28d q 56d	52	26
Procarbazine[235]	37 (GBM)	130–150 mg/m² × 28d q 56d	28	30
	46 (AA)	130–150 mg/m² × 28d q 56d	28	49
Procarbazine[236]	31	150 mg/m² × 28d q 56d	71	26 (all patients)
AZQ[237]	33	8mg/m²/d × 5d q 4 wk	45	NA
AZQ[238]	28	27.5–30 mg/m² IV q 3 wk	39	NA
AZQ[239]	20	8mg/m²/d × 5d q 4 wk	55	21
Carboplatin[240]	19	175 mg/m² weekly × 4, then 3 wk rest	47	8+
Etoposide[241]	18	50 mg/m² IV × 5d q 3 wk	50	16

Continued on following page

apy with autologous bone marrow transplant, IA chemotherapy, intratumoral chemotherapy, IA BBBD and chemotherapy, drug-encapsulated liposomes, metabolic therapies, and differentiating agents are discussed in Chapter 7.

Immunotherapy

Immunotherapeutic principles and treatment for malignant astrocytoma are discussed in Chapter 7. Immunotherapy has produced no significant advances in the treatment of malignant astrocytoma.

Gene Therapy

The insertion of genes into malignant astrocytomas is a scientific approach in its infancy, and holds tremendous promise. Some of the approaches being investigated for the treatment of malignant astrocytoma are gene transfer to replace chromosomal loss, to block transcription, to make a tumor more sensitive to administered drugs, to provide an enzyme that catalyzes the production of a cytotoxic product by itself or when substrate is infused, or to transfect a tumoricidal virus.

Table 8–7.—*continued*

Drug	Total Patients	Dose	Responders CR + PR + SD (%)	Median Time to Responders Progression (Weeks)
Etoposide[242]	15	600–1000 mg/m^2 IV q 3 wk	6	78
Etoposide[232]	46	50 mg/d continually	42	16
Methotrexate[244]	8	5–2200 mg/kg IA + leucovorin IA	75	88
Edatrexate[245]	16	80 mg/m2 IV weekly	87.5 (SD)	26
Temozolomide[246]	10	150 mg/m2/d × 5d q 4wk	80	26
Tamoxifen[247]	32	20 mg PO BID	22	26+
Tamoxifen[247]	32	20 mg PO BID	22	26+
Tamoxifen[248]	11	20–100 mg PO BID daily	36	52+
Taxol[249]	40	210–240 mg/m^2 IV	35	33
Topotecan[250]	12	15 mg/m2/d × 5 q 3 wk	16	NA

AA = anaplastic astrocytoma.
BID = twice daily.
d = day.
GBM = glioblastoma multiforme.
IA = intra-arterial.
IV = intravenous.
NA = not available.
PO = oral.
q = every.
SD = stable disease.

Clinical trials in patients with malignant astrocytoma have involved the transfection of a herpes virus thymidine kinase gene in a retroviral vector. The retroviral vector is incorporated only into proliferating cells. When ganciclovir is administered, it is phosphorylated by the transfected thymidine kinase gene intracellularly, with the production of toxic triphosphates and the resultant preferential death of the transfected malignant glioma cells.[264] In rats transfected with this gene and treated with ganciclovir, gliosarcomas regressed completely in 23 of 30 treated rats.[264] In another study using the herpes simplex virus vector, hrR3, which possesses an intact viral thymidine kinase gene, ganciclovir treatment produced long-term survival in 48% of rats implanted with 9L gliosarcoma.[265] A small human trial has been conducted at the National Institutes of Health with disappointing results.[266]

In another animal model, rats implanted with tumorigenic C6 glioma cells that express IGF-1 lose their tumorigenicity when transfected with antisense IGF cDNA.[267] Another approach has been to develop viruses that are replication competent and when transfected are cytotoxic to tumors but not to normal neurons or

Table 8–8. **Malignant Astrocytoma: Multiagent Chemotherapy Trials (Adults)**

Drug	Total Patients	Reponders CR + PR + SD (%)	Median Time to Reponders Progression (weeks)
BCNU/Procarbazine[252]	28	46	≈ 27
BCNU/DFMO[253]	10 (GBM)	30	24
	21 (AA)	57	NR
Procarbazine/CCNU/VCR[254]	30	27	39
Procarbazine/CCNU/VCR[255]	46	61	27
Procarbazine/Thiotepa/VCR[256]	20	20	32
Procarbazine/Mechlorethamine/VCR[257]	27	52	42
Procarbazine/VP-16/VCR[258]	11	73	48+
Cyclophosphamide/VCR[259]	10	70	34
Cisplatin/Etoposide[260]	33	31	≈ 26
AZQ/BCNU[261]	32 (GBM)	28	48a
	10 (AA)	80	68a
AZQ/Procarbazine[261]	42 (GBM)	31	28a
	10 (AA)	51.5	70a
TDPC-FuHu[262]	39 (GBM)	59.4	31
	38 (AA)	74	NA
TDPC-FuHu[263]	31 (GBM)	42	13
	20 (AA)	80	32

a = median survival.
AA = anaplastic astrocytoma.
CR = complete response.
DFMO = difluoromethylornithine.
GBM = glioblastoma multiforme.
NA = not applicable.
NR = not reached.
PR = partial response.
SD = stable disease.
TPDC-FuHu = thioguanine, procarbazine, dibromodulcitol, CCNU, 5-fluorouracil, hydroxyurea.
VCR = vincristine.

astrocytes.[268] It is hoped that these and other avenues of scientific investigation will lead to clinical trials yielding positive results.

PROGNOSIS AND COMPLICATIONS

Prognosis

The most important prognostic variables for survival for patients with malignant astrocytoma entered on randomized trials are age, tumor histology, and preoperative Karnofsky performance status (Tables 8–5 to 8–7).[10,13,119,120,124,125,226,227,229,269] In some trials, the duration of symptoms,[10,13] the extent of the surgical resection,[119,124,125] and the residual tumor postoperatively[120,126] have been found to be prognostically important (Table 8–9).

The prognosis for elderly patients older than age 70 years was poor, with a median survival of 2.9 months. Patients older than age 80 years did not appear to benefit from RT.[269] In patients with glioblastoma and anaplastic astrocytoma treated with nitrosourea-based chemotherapy on recurrence, age was found to be predictive of response, time to progression, survival, and risk of myelosuppressive complications (Figs. 8–8 and 8–9).[270]

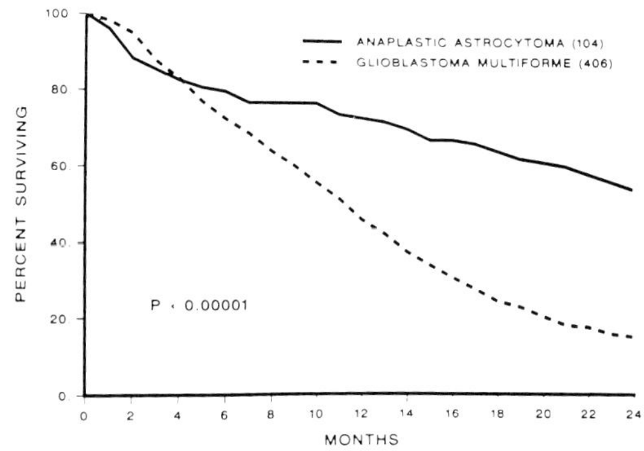

Figure 8–6. Graph showing the effect of tumor histology on survival. An anaplastic astrocytoma has a markedly prolonged survival percentage when compared to a glioblastoma multiforme. Numbers in parentheses denote numbers of patients in each age group. (From Shapiro et al,[120] p 7, with permission.)

Complications

Deep venous thrombosis (DVT) is a frequent complication in the management of patients with malignant astrocytoma. In the first month after surgery, the incidence of DVT or pulmonary embolism in patients with malignant astrocytoma was 1%.[271] During the total time course of the illness, the incidence of DVT in two retrospective series was 19% and 28%.[272,273] A retrospective analysis of 381 malignant glioma patients found a 36.7% incidence of clinical phlebitis in those who did not

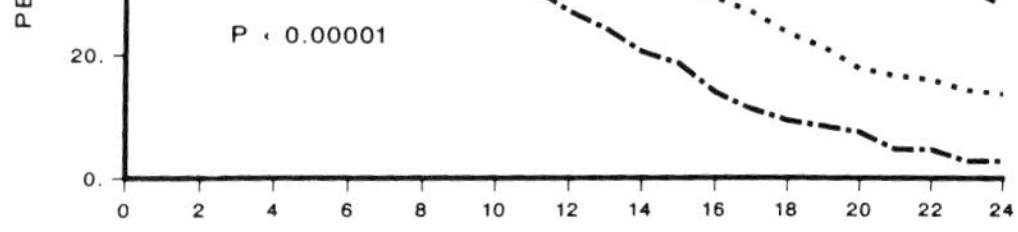

Figure 8–5. Graph showing the effect of age on survival from the time of randomization in a random multimodality trial. Note decreasing survival with increasing age. Numbers in parentheses denote numbers of patients in each age group. (From Shapiro et al,[120] p 7, with permission.)

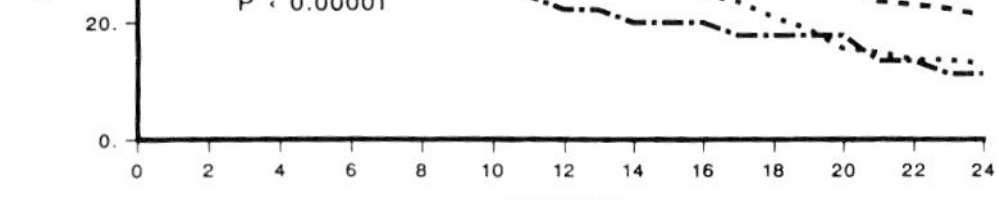

Figure 8–7. Graph showing the effect of preoperative Karnofsky performance status on survival from time of randomization in a multimodality trial. Note increasing survival with better Karnofsky score. Numbers in parentheses denote numbers of patients in each age group. (From Shapiro et al,[120] p 7, with permission.)

Table 8–9. **Malignant Astrocytoma: Prognostic Variables for Survival**

Most Important
Age
Tumor histology
Preoperative Karnofsky performance status
Others
Extent of surgical resection
Residual tumor postoperatively

receive anticoagulant prophylaxis and a 10% incidence in those treated with anticoagulants.[274] Whereas untreated patients had a 25% incidence of DVT in the first 6 weeks, treated patients had a 3% incidence. The incidence of DVT of 25% and 3% in untreated and treated patients,respectively, is much higher than the 1% reported for DVT and pulmonary embolism in the month after surgery. Anticoagulant prophylaxis must be considered before surgery and again in the postoperative period.

Meningeal spread of malignant astrocytoma has been found in up to 21% of cases examined at autopsy. Two thirds of these patients were diagnosed antemortem with positive CSF cytology.[275] Back pain with or without radicular symptoms, mental status changes, cranial nerve palsies, myelopathy or cauda equina syndrome, and headache with symptomatic hydrocephalus are common presenting symptoms.[275–278] Contrast-enhanced MRI may aid in the detection of meningeal tumor spread. Malignant astrocytoma can also present with

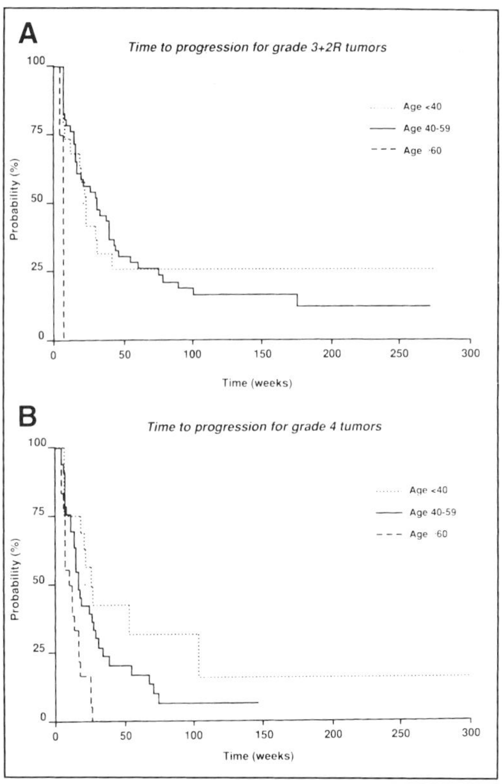

Figure 8–8. The effect of age on time to progression after nitrosourea-based chemotherapy. Time to progression is decreased in *(A)* recurrent grade 2 (2R), grade 3, and *(B)* grade 4 tumors in patients greater than 60 years of age. (From Grant et al,[270] p 931, with permission.)

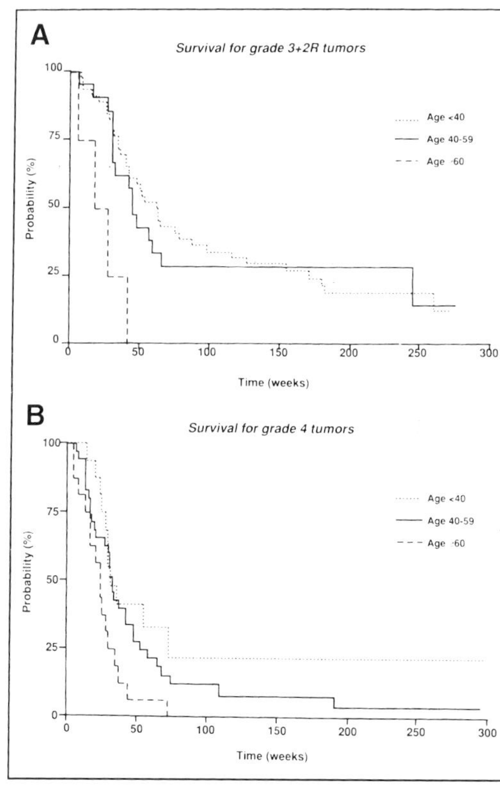

Figure 8–9. The effect of age on survival after nitrosourea-based chemotherapy. Survival is decreased *(A)* recurrent grade 2 (2R), grade 3, and *(B)* grade 4 tumors with patients greater than 60 years of age. (From Grant et al,[270] p 932, with permission.)

meningeal dissemination.[275] In a series of 12 patients with meningeal gliomatosis, eight had spinal subarachnoid seeding, nine had lateral ventricular invasion, three spinal cord compression, and 10 had hydrocephalus.[276] Patients with meningeal dissemination of glioblastoma did not respond to therapy and died in a median of 8 weeks. Three of five patients with anaplastic astrocytoma responded to treatment, with RT to areas of bulky disease, and IT chemotherapy in two of the responders.[276]

Malignant astrocytoma rarely metastasizes systemically to the viscera, lymph nodes, skeleton, and bone marrow.[279] Multifocal malignant gliomas developed in three of 37 adolescents treated for acute lymphoblastic leukemia with prophylactic cranial RT and IT MTX.[280] Malignant gliomas are known to develop after cranial RT for other diseases.[281]

Quality of Life

The assessment of quality of life for patients with malignant astrocytoma has become increasingly important, with aggressive multimodality therapies, the prospect of increased survival, and societal change.[282] Karnofsky performance status has been the measure of quality of life used in most malignant astrocytoma trials, but it does not address important psychosocial concerns such as emotional function, self-image, interactions with family, work, and daily activity. These factors are the reasons to survive and must be assessed to measure the needs of patients and adequately understand the risk-benefit ratio of therapies.

Two quality-of-life instruments, the Ferrans and Powers Quality of Life Index and the Psychosocial Adjustment to Illness Scale-Self Report have been used with patients with malignant brain tumor.[283] The Ferrans and Powers index measures health and functioning, socioeconomic aspects, psychological and spiritual aspects, and family. The Psychological Adjustment to Illness Scale has 46 questions that quantify healthcare orientation, vocational environment, domestic environment, sexual relationships, extended family relationships, social environment, and psychological distress. Quality-of-life measurements in patients with malignant astrocytoma were affected adversely by divorce, female gender, bilateral tumor, poor Karnofsky performance status, and chemotherapy with these two quality-of-life instruments.[283]

Another measurement tool for quality-of-life assessment is the Functional Assessment of Cancer Therapy (FACT) scale, for which a brain subscale has been developed.[284] The brain subscale is a 20-item questionnaire that can be completed in 10 to 15 minutes. It makes a series of statements that are categorically grouped: physical well-being, social and family well-being, relationship with doctor, emotional well-being, functional well-being, and additional concerns. Patients are asked how true each statement is on a scale of 0 to 4.

These tests can be given to patients during therapy to better assess patient response to therapy and complications of therapy and to quantify a therapy's impact on quality of life.

CHAPTER SUMMARY

Malignant astrocytoma is the most common adult brain tumor, accounting for 35% to 45% of the 16,000 brain tumors diagnosed in the United States each year. They are more common in men than women, and the incidence rate increases beginning in the fourth decade of life. The development of malignant astrocytoma is associated with a series of allelic changes, with both the loss of presumed tumor-suppressor genes and gain of proto-oncogenes.

Growth and invasion of malignant astrocytoma is influenced by growth factors, which are normally under genetic control. Malignant astrocytoma tumor cells produce their own growth factors that stimulate themselves through autocrine and intracrine processes and stimulate their neighbors through paracrine mechanisms. Growth factors and cytokines influence the expression and secretion of adhesion molecules by glioma cells. Adhesion molecules bind to their cell-surface receptors and interact with ECM proteins and their inhibitors to control the process of tumor invasion.

Pathologically, malignant astrocytoma is a heterogeneous tumor with significant regional variability. Regional variability makes treatment difficult, with certain regions of a tumor sensitive to a specific treatment and other regions of the same tumor resistant.

The most common presenting symptoms of malignant astrocytoma are headache and seizures. The differential diagnosis includes LGA, anaplastic oligodendroglioma and mixed glioma, supratentorial PNET, anaplastic ependymoma, PCNSL, metastatic tumor, brain abscess, thromboembolic stroke, hemorrhagic vascular process, parasitic cyst, and MS. Multiplanar MRI, with and without contrast enhancement, is the imaging procedure of choice to differentiate between these disease processes.

The initial treatment of choice in the management of malignant astrocytoma is surgical resection of the maximal tumor possible, with as little trauma to surrounding brain as possible. Extensive surgical resection provides accurate histological diagnosis, tumor cytoreduction, improved symptoms and signs, decreased tumor burden for further therapy, and tissue for experimental studies. In some clinical trials, the extent of surgical resection and lack of tumor on postoperative scan have correlated with a good outcome.

WBRT has been the single most effective treatment for malignant astrocytoma. Recurrence was almost entirely focal. Therefore, FEBRT is currently the treatment of choice, and this change has not produced a change in the recurrence pattern of tumor. Altered fractionation and dose per fraction, heavy particle RT, and photodynamic therapy have all been attempted with little success. Adjuvant interstitial brachytherapy has been shown to significantly increase median survival in a randomized trial. However, the significance of a 2.5-month increase in survival, requiring an average of 1.5 additional hospitalizations and operations per patient, with the additional economic and psychosocial cost, have decreased interest in this procedure. In addition, only 25% to 30% of patients are eligible because of size and location limitations. SR has been evaluated as an adjuvant treatment with mixed results in two trials.

Adjuvant chemotherapy in a meta-analysis of 3000 patients in 16 randomized trials has shown an increase in survival by approximately 10% at 1 and 2 years when chemotherapy is added to RT. No adjuvant single drug, single drug, or multiple drug chemotherapy regimen has shown a convincing increase in median survival. PCV multiagent chemotherapy has been reported to be more effective than BCNU in the treatment of anaplastic astrocytoma but not glioblastoma multiforme. Many innovative chemotherapy approaches have been attempted and the most promising has been intratumoral therapy.

Gene therapy is an extremely promising therapeutic avenue for further development in the next decade.

The most important prognostic variables for survival in patients entered on randomized clinical trials for the treatment of malignant astrocytoma are age, Karnofsky performance status, and histology. The extent of surgical resection correlated with survival in some trials but not in others. DVT is a very common complication of malignant astrocytoma, and anticoagulant prophylaxis should be considered in all patients.

Quality-of-life assessment has become increasingly important to help measure outcome in patients treated with multimodality aggressive therapies, with the possibility of increased survival. The Karnofsky performance status measure is inadequate by itself to measure psychosocial concerns.

Progress in treatment for malignant astrocytomas has been inexorably slow over the past 25 years despite the devotion and efforts of many physicians and scientists, the expenditure of millions of dollars, and loss of hundreds of thousands of patient lives.

REFERENCES

1. Bennett, H, and Godlee, RJ: Excision of a tumour from the brain. Lancet 2:1090–1091, 1884.

2. Bailey, P, and Cushing, H: A Classification of the Tumors of the Glioma Group on a Histogenetic Basis with a Correlated Study of Prognosis. JB Lippincott Company, Philadelphia, 1926.
3. Kernohan, JW, and Sayre, GP: Atlas of Tumor Pathology: Tumors of the Central Nervous System. Armed Forces Institute of Pathology, Washington, 1952.
4. Ringertz, N: Grading of gliomas. Acta Pathol Microbiol Scand 27:51–64, 1950.
5. Daumas-Duport, C, Scheithauer, BW, O'Fallon, J, and Kelly, P: Grading of astrocytomas. A simple and reproducible method. Cancer 62:2152–2165, 1988.
6. Kleihues, P, Burger, PC, and Scheithauer, BW: Histological Typing of Tumours of the Central Nervous Sytem, Ed 2. World Health Organization, Springer-Verlag, Berlin, 1993.
7. Radhakrishnan, K, Mokri, B, Parisi, JE, et al: The trends in incidence of primary brain tumors in the population of Rochester, Minnesota. Ann Neurol 37:67–73, 1995.
8. Schoenberg, BS, Schoenberg, DG, Christine, BW, and Gomez, MR: The epidemiology of primary intracranial neoplasms of childhood. A population study. Mayo Clin Proc 51:51—56, 1976.
9. Cohen, A, and Modan, B: Some epidemiologic aspects of neoplastic diseases in Israeli immigrant population. 3. Brain tumors. Cancer 22: 1323–1328, 1968.
10. Frankel, SA, and German, WJ: Glioblastoma multiforme. Review of 219 cases with regard to natural history, pathology, diagnostic methods, and treatment. J Neurosurg 15:489–503, 1958.
11. Walker, MD, Green, SB, Byar, DP, et al: Randomized comparisons of radiotherapy and nitrosoureas for the treatment of malignant glioma after surgery. N Engl J Med 303:1323–1329, 1980.
12. Annegers, JF, Schoenberg, BS, Okazaki ,H, and Kurland, LT: Epidemiologic study of primary intracranial neoplasms. Arch Neurol 38:217–219, 1981.
13. Green, SB, Byar, DP, Walker, MD, et al: Comparisons of carmustine, procarbazine, and high-dose methylprednisolone as additions to surgery and radiotherapy for the treatment of malignant glioma. Cancer Treat Rep 67:121–132, 1983.
14. Mahaley, MS Jr, Mettlin, C, Natarajan, N, et al: National survey of patterns of care for brain-tumor patients. J Neurosurg 71:826–836, 1989.
15. Trojanowski, T, Peszynski, J, Turowski, K, et al: Quality of survival of patients with brian gliomas treated with postoperative CCNU and radiation therapy. J Neurosurg 70:18–23, 1989.
16. Mao, Y, Desmeules, M, Semenciw, RM, et al: Increasing brain cancer rates in Canada. Can Med Assoc J 145:1583–1591, 1991.
17. Ohaegbulam, SC, Saddeqi, N, and Ikerionwu, S: Intracranial tumors in Enugu, Nigeria. Cancer 46:2322–2324, 1980.
18. Greig, NH, Ries, LG, Yancik, R, and Rapoport, SI: Increasing annual incidence of primary malignant brain tumors in the elderly. J Natl Cancer Inst 82:1621–1624, 1990.
19. Davis, DL, Lilienfeld, AD, Gittelsohn, A, and Scheckenbach, ME: Increasing trends in some cancers in older Americans: Fact or artifact? Toxicol Ind Health 2:127–144, 1986.
20. Davis, DL, Hoel, D, Fox, J, and Lopez, A: International trends in cancer mortality in France, West Germany, Italy, Japan, England and Wales, and the USA. Lancet 336:474–481, 1990.
21. Lynch, HT, Krush, AJ, Harlan, WL, and Sharp, EA: Association of soft tissue sarcoma, leukemia, and brain tumors in families affected with breast cancer. Am Surg 39:199–206, 1973.
22. Huson, SM, and Upadhyaya, M: Neurofibromatosis 1. Clinical management and genetic counselling. In: Huson, SM, and Hughes, RAC (eds): The Neurofibromatoses. A Pathogenetic and Clinical Overview. Chapman & Hall Medical, London, 1994, pp 355–381.
23. Kyritsis, AP, Bondy, ML, Xiao, M, et al: Germline p53 gene mutations in subsets of glioma patients. J Natl Cancer Inst 86:344–349, 1994.
24. Lossignol, D, Grossman, SA, Sheidler, VR, et al: Familial clustering of malignant astrocytomas. J Neurooncol 9:139–145, 1990.
25. Grossman, SA, Osman, M, Hruban, RH, and Piantadosi, S: Familial gliomas: The potential role of environmental exposures. Proc ASCO 14:A291, 1995.
26. Collins, VP, and James, CD: Molecular genetics of primary intracranial tumors. Curr Opin Oncol 2:666–672, 1990.
27. James, CD, Mikkelsen, T, Cavenee, WK, and Collins, VP: Molecular genetic aspects of glial tumour evolution. Cancer Surveys 9(4):631–644, 1990.
28. von Deimling, A, Bender, B, Jahnke, R, et al: Loci associated with malignant progression in astrocytomas: A candidate on chromosome 19q. Cancer Res 54:1397–1401, 1994.
29. Nishikawa, R, Furnari, FB, Lin, H, et al: Loss of P16 ^{INK4} expression is frequent in high grade gliomas. Cancer Res 55:1941–1945, 1995.
30. Arap, W, Nishikawa, R, Furnari, FB, Cavenee WK, and Huang H-J: Replacement of the p16/CDKN2 gene suppresses human glioma cell growth. Cancer Res 55:1351–1354, 1995.
31. Bigner, SH, Burger, PC, Wong, AJ, et al: Gene amplification in malignant human gliomas: Clinical and histopathologic aspects. J Neuropathol Exp Neurol 47:191–205, 1988.
32. Hurtt, MR, Moossy, J, Donovan-Peluso, M, and Locker, J: Amplification of epidermal growth factor receptor gene in gliomas: Histopathology and prognosis. J Neuropathol Exp Neurol 51:84–90, 1992.
33. Fuller, GN, and Bigner, SH: Amplified cellular oncogenes in neoplasms of the human central nervous system. Mutation Research 276:299–306, 1992.
34. Olson, JJ, James, CD, Krisht, A, et al: Analysis of epidermal growth factor receptor gene amplification and alteration in stereotactic biopsies of brain tumors. Neurosurgery 36:740–748, 1995.
35. Reifenberger, G, Liu, L, Ichimura, K, et al: Amplification and overexpression of the *MDM2*

gene in a subset of human malignant gliomas without *p53* mutations. Cancer Res 53:2736–2739, 1993.
36. Scheck, AC, and Coons, SW: Expression of the tumor suppressor gene *DCC* in human gliomas. Cancer Res 53:5605–5609, 1993.
37. Salomon, DS, Brandt, R, Ciardiello, F, and Normanno, N: Epidermal growth factor-related peptides and their receptors in human malignancies. Crit Rev Oncol Hematol 19:183–232, 1995.
38. Hoi Sang, U, Espiritu, OD, Kelley PY, et al: The role of the epidermal growth factor receptor in human gliomas: I. The control of cell growth. J Neurosurg 82:841–846, 1995.
39. Epenetos, AA, Courtenay-Luck, N, Pickering, D, et al: Antibody guided irradiation of brain glioma by arterial infusion of radioactive monoclonal antibody against epidermal growth factor receptor and blood group A antigen. Br Med J 290:1463–1466, 1985.
40. Kalofonos, HP, Pawlikowska, TR, Hemingway, A, et al: Antibody guided diagnosis and therapy of brain gliomas using radiolabeled monoclonal antibodies against epidermal growth factor receptor and placental alkaline phosphatase. J Nucl Med 30:1636–1645, 1989.
41. Morrison, RS, Yamaguchi, F, Bruner, JM, et al: Fibroblast growth factor receptor gene expression and immunoreactivity are elevated in human glioblastoma multiforme. Cancer Res 54: 2794–2799, 1994.
42. Trojan, J, Blossey, BK, Johnson, TR, et al: Loss of tumorigenicity of rat glioblastoma directed by episome-based antisense cDNA transcription of insulin-like growth factor I. Proc Natl Acad Sci USA 89:4874–4878, 1992.
43. Beitz, JG, Kim, IS, Calabresi, P, and Frackelton, AR Jr: Human microvascular endothelial cells express receptors for platelet-derived growth factor. Proc Natl Acad Sci USA 88:2021–2025, 1991.
44. Hermanson, M, Funa, K, Hartman, M, et al: Platelet-derived growth factor and its receptors in human glioma tissue: Expression of messenger RNA and protein suggests the presence of autocrine and paracrine loops. Cancer Res 52:3213–3219, 1992.
45. Mapstone, T, McMichael, M, and Goldthwait, D: Expression of platelet-derived growth factors, transforming growth factors, and the ros gene in a variety of primary human brain tumors. Neurosurgery 28:216–222, 1991.
46. Mapstone, TB: Expression of platelet-derived growth factor and transforming growth factor and their correlation with cellular morphology in glial tumors. J Neurosurg 75:447–451, 1991.
47. Mauro, A, Bulfone, A, Turco, E, and Schiffer, D: Coexpression of platelet-derived growth factor (PDGF) B chain and PDGF B-type receptor in human gliomas. Childs Nerv Syst 7:432–436, 1991.
48. Nitta, T, and Sato, K: Specific inhibition of c-sis protein synthesis and cell proliferation with antisense oligodeoxynucleotides in human glioma cells. Neurosurgery 34:309–314, 1994.
49. Rutka, JT, Rosenblum, ML, Stern, R, et al: Isolation and partial purfication of growth factors with TGF-like activity from human malignant gliomas. J Neurosurg 71:875–883, 1989.
50. Linggood, RM, Hsu, DW, Efird, JT, and Pardo, FS: TGF α expression in meningioma - tumor progression and therapeutic response. J Neurooncol 26:45–51, 1995.
51. Schlegel, U, Moots, PL, Rosenblum, MK, et al: Expression of transforming growth factor alpha in human gliomas. Oncogene 5:1839–1842, 1990.
52. Maxwell, M, Galanopoulos, T, Neville-Golden, J, and Antoniades, HN: Effect of the expression of transforming growth factor-β2 in primary human glioblastomas on immunosuppression and loss of immune surveillance. J Neurosurg 76:799–804, 1992.
53. Yamada, N, Kato, M, Yamashita, H, et al: Enhanced expression of transforming growth factor-b and its type-I and type-II receptors in human glioblastoma. Int J Cancer 62:386–392, 1995.
54. Merzak, A, McCrea, S, Koocheckpour, S, and Pilkington, GJ: Control of human glioma cell growth, migration and invasion *in vitro* by transforming growth factor β1. Br J Cancer 70:199–203, 1994.
55. Jachimczak, P, Bogdahn, U, Schneider, J, et al: The effect of transorming growth factor-β2-specific phosphorothioate-anti-sense oligodeoxynucleotides in reversing cellular immunosuppression in malignant glioma. J Neurosurg 78:944–951, 1993.
56. Benzil, DL, Finkelstein, SD, Epstein, MH, and Finch, PW: Expression pattern of α-protein kinase C in human astrocytomas indicates a role in malignant progression. Cancer Res 52:2951–2956, 1992.
57. Couldwell, WT, Antel, JP, Apuzzo, MLJ, and Yong, VW: Inhibition of growth of established human glioma cell lines by modulators of the protein kinase-C system. J Neurosurg 73:594–600, 1990.
58. Pollack, IF, Randall, MS, Kristofik, MP, et al: Effect of tamoxifen on DNA synthesis and proliferation of human malignant glioma lines *in vitro*. Cancer Res 50:7134–7138, 1990.
59. Couldwell, WT, de Tribolet, N, Antel, JP, et al: Adhesion molecules and malignant gliomas: Implications for tumorigenesis. J Neurosurg 76:782–791, 1992.
60. De Clerck, YA, Shimada, H, Gonzalez-Gomez, I, and Raffel, C: Tumoral invasion in the central nervous system. J Neurooncol 18:111–121, 1994.
61. Rosenman, SJ, Shrikant, P, Dubb, L, et al: Cytokine-induced expression of vascular cell adhesion molecule-1 (VCAM-1) by astrocytes and astrocytoma cell lines. J Immunol 154:1888–1899, 1995.
62. Nagasaka, S, Tanabe, KK, Bruner, JM, et al: Alternative RNA splicing of the hyaluronic acid receptor CD44 in the normal human brain and in brain tumors. J Neurosurg 82:858–863, 1995.

63. Mohanam, S, Wang, SW, Rayford, A, et al: Expression of tissue inhibitors of metalloproteinases: negative regulators of human glioblastoma invasion *in vivo*. Clin Exp Metastasis 13:57–62, 1995.
64. Yoshii, Y, Maki, Y, Tsuboi, K, et al: Estimation of growth fraction with bromodeoxyuridine in human central nervous system tumors. J Neurosurg 65:659–663, 1986.
65. Asai, A, Shibui, S, Barker, M, et al: Cell kinetics of rat 9L brain tumors determined by double labeling with iodo- and bromodeoxyuridine. J Neurosurg 73:254–258, 1990.
66. Hoshino, T, Ito, S, Asai, A, et al: Cell kinetic analysis of human brain tumors by in situ double labeling with bromodeoxyuridine and iododeoxyuridine. Int J Cancer 50:1–5, 1992.
67. Bookwalter, JW III, Selker, RG, Schiffer, L, et al: Brain-tumor cell kinetics correlated with survival. J Neurosurg 65:795–798, 1986.
68. Ritter, AM, Sawaya, R, Hess, KR, et al: Prognostic significance of bromodeoxyuridine labeling in primary and recurrent glioblastoma multiforme. Neurosurgery 35:192–198, 1994.
69. Roth, JG, and Elvidge, AR: Glioblastoma multiforme: A clinical survey. J Neurosurgery 17: 736–750, 1960.
70. Giangaspero, F, and Burger, PC: Correlations between cytologic composition and biologic behavior in the glioblastoma multiforme. A postmortem study of 50 cases. Cancer 52:2320–2333, 1983.
71. Burger, PC: Malignant astrocytic neoplasms: Classification, pathologic anatomy, and response to treatment. Semin Oncol 13(1):16–26, 1986.
72. Bruner, JM: Neuropathology of malignant gliomas. Semin Oncol 21(2):126–138, 1994.
73. Daumas-Duport, C: Histoprognosis of gliomas. Adv Tech Stand Neurosurg 21:43–76, 1994.
74. Jelsma, R, and Bucy, PC: The treatment of glioblastoma multiforme of the brain. J Neurosurg 27:388–400, 1967.
75. Whitton, AC, and Bloom, HJ: Low grade glioma of the cerebral hemispheres in adults: A retrospective analysis of 88 cases. Int J Radiat Oncol Biol Phys 18:783–786, 1990.
76. Lunsford, LD, Somaza, S, Kondziolka, D, and Flickinger, JC: Survival after stereotactic biopsy and irradiation of cerebral nonanaplastic, nonpilocytic astrocytoma. J Neurosurg 82:523–529, 1995.
77. Pollack, IF, Claassen, D, Al-Shboul, Q, et al: Low-grade gliomas of the cerebral hemispheres in children: An alnalysis of 71 cases. J Neurosurg 82:536–547, 1995.
78. Janny, P, Cure, H, Mohr, M, et al: Low grade supratentorial astrocytomas. Management and prognostic factors. Cancer 73:1937–1945, 1994.
79. Kondziolka, D, Bernstein, M, Resch, L, et al: Significance of hemorrhage into brain tumors: Clinicopathological study. J Neurosurg 67:852–857, 1987.
80. Chamberlain, MC, Murovic, JA, and Levin, VA: Absence of contrast enhancement on CT brain scans of patients with supratentorial malignant gliomas. Neurology 38:1371–1374, 1988.
81. Piepmeier, JM: Observations on the current treatment of low-grade astrocytic tumors of the cerebral hemispheres. J Neurosurg 67:177–181, 1987.
82. Silverman, C, and Marks, JE: Prognostic significance of contrast enhancement in low-grade astrocytomas of the adult cerebrum. Radiology 139:211–213, 1981.
83. DeAngelis, LM: Primary central nervous system lymphoma. In Gilman, S, Goldstein, G, and Waxman, S (eds): Neurobase. Arbor Publishing Company, San Diego, 1996.
84. Hochberg, FH, and Miller, DC: Primary central nervous system lymphoma. J Neurosurg 68: 835–853, 1988.
85. Barnard, RO, and Geddes, JF: The incidence of multiforcal cerebral gliomas. A histologic study of large hemisphere sections. Cancer 60:1519–1531, 1987.
86. Murray, K, Kun, L, and Cox, J: Primary malignant lymphoma of the central nervous system. Results of treament of 11 cases and review of the literature. J Neurosurg 65:600–607, 1986.
87. Sze, G, Milano, E, Johnson, C, and Heier, L: Detection of brain metastases: Comparison of contrast-enhanced MR with unenhanced MR and enhanced CT. Am J Neuroradiol 11:785–791, 1990.
88. Davis, PC, Hudgins, PA, Peterman, SB, and Hoffman, JC Jr: Diagnosis of cerebral metastases: double-dose delayed CT vs contrast-enhanced MR imaging. Am J Neuroradiol 12: 293–300, 1991.
89. Atlas, SW, Grossman, RI, Gomori, JM, et al: Hemorrhagic intracranial malignant neoplasms: Spin-echo MR imaging. Radiology 164:71–77, 1987.
90. Bragg, DG, and Osborn, AG: CNS imaging of neoplasms. Int J Radiat Oncol Biol Phys 21: 841–845, 1991.
91. Jaeckle, KA: Neuroimaging for central nervous system tumors. Semin Oncol 18(2):150–157, 1991.
92. Byrne, TN: Imaging of gliomas. Semin Oncol 21(2):162–171, 1994.
93. Zimmerman, RA: Imaging of adult central nervous system primary malignant gliomas. Staging and follow-up. Cancer 67:1278–1283, 1991.
94. Price, AC, Runge, VM, Allen, JH, et al: Primary glioma: diagnosis with magnetic resonance imaging. J Comput Tomogr 10:325–334, 1986.
95. Kelly, PJ, Daumas-Duport, C, Scheithauer, BW, et al: Stereotactic histologic correlations of computed tomography- and magnetic resonance imaging-defined abnormalities in patients with glial neoplasms. Mayo Clin Proc 62:450–459, 1987.
96. Jolesz, FA, Schwartz, RB, and Guttmann, CRG: Diagnostic imaging of intracranial gliomas. In Black, PM, Schoene, WC, and Lampson, LA (eds): Astrocytomas: Diagnosis, Treatment, and Biology. Blackwell Scientific Publications, Boston, 1993, pp 37–49.
97. Asari, S, Makabe, T, Katayama, S, et al: Assessment of the pathological grade of astrocytic gliomas using an MRI score. Neuroradiology 36:308–310, 1994.

98. Forsyth, PA, Kelly, PJ, Cascino, TL, et al: Radiation necrosis or glioma recurrence: is computer-assisted stereotactic biopsy useful? J Neurosurg 82:436–444, 1995.
99. Tyler, JL, Diksic, M, Villemure, JG, et al: Metabolic and hemodynamic evaluation of gliomas using positron emission tomography. J Nucl Med 28:1123–1133, 1987.
100. Junck, L, Strawderman, M, Ross, DA, et al: Prognostic value of PET-FDG scans in untreated gliomas. Neurology 45(4):A387, 1995.
101. Hanson, MW, Glantz, MJ, Hoffman, JM, et al: FDG-PET in the selection of brain lesions for biopsy. J Comput Assist Tomogr 15(5):796–801, 1991.
102. Herholz, K, Pietrzyk, U, Voges, J, et al: Correlation of glucose consumption and tumor cell density in astrocytomas. A stereotactic PET study. J Neurosurg 79:853–858, 1993.
103. Levivier, M, Goldman, S, Pirotte, B, et al: Diagnostic yield of stereotactic brain biopsy guided by positron emission tomography with [^{18}F]fluorodeoxyglucose. J Neurosurg 82:445–452, 1995.
104. Glantz, MJ, Hoffman, JM, Coleman, RE, et al: Identification of early recurrence of primary central nervous system tumors by [^{18}F]fluorodeoxyglucose positron emission tomography. Ann Neurol 29:347–355, 1991.
105. Doyle, WK, Budinger, TF, Valk, PE, et al: Differentiation of cerebral radiation necrosis from tumor recurrence by [^{18}F]FDG and ^{82}Rb positron emission tomography. J Comput Assist Tomogr 11(4):563–570, 1987.
106. Janus, TJ, Kim, EE, Tilbury, R, et al: Use of [^{18}F]fluorodeoxyglucose positron emission tomography in patients with primary malignant brain tumors. Ann Neurol 33:540–548, 1993.
107. Slizofski, WJ, Krishna, L, Katsetos, CD, et al: Thallium imaging for brain tumors with results measured by a semiquantitative index and correlated with histopathology. Cancer 74:3190–3197, 1994.
108. Black, KL, Hawkins, RA, Kim, KT, et al: Use of thallium-201 SPECT to quantitate malignancy grade of gliomas. J Neurosurg 71:342–346, 1989.
109. Vertosick, FT Jr, Selker, RG, Grossman, SJ, and Joyce, JM: Correlation of thallium-201 single photon emission computed tomography and survival after treatment failure in patients with glioblastoma multiforme. Neurosurgery 34:396–401, 1994.
110. Kaplan, WD, Takvorian, T, Morris, JH, et al: Thallium-201 brain tumor imaging: a comparative study with pathologic correlation. J Nucl Med 28:47–52, 1987.
111. Alexander, E III, Loeffler, JS, Schwartz, RB, et al: Thallium-201 technetium-99m HMPAO single-photon emission computed tomography (SPECT) imaging for guiding stereotactic craniotomies in heavily irradiated malignant glioma patients. Acta Neurochir (Wien) 122:215–217, 1993.
112. Carvalho, PA, Schwartz, RB, Alexander, E III, et al: Detection of recurrent gliomas with quantitative thallium-201/technetium-99m HMPAO single-photon emission computerized tomography. J Neurosurg 77:565–570, 1992.
113. Pardo, FS, Aronen, HJ, Kennedy, D, et al: Functional cerebral imaging in the evaluation and radiotherapeutic treatment planning of patients with malignant glioma. Int J Radiat Oncol Biol Phys 30(3):663–669, 1994.
114. Posner, JB: Management of brain metastases. Rev Neurol (Paris) 148(6–7):477–487, 1992.
115. Black, PM: Brain tumors (first of two parts). N Engl J Med 324(21):1471–1476, 1991.
116. Fadul, C, Wood, J, Thaler, H, et al: Morbidity and mortality of craniotomy for excision of supratentorial gliomas. Neurology 38:1374–1379, 1988.
117. Salcman, M: Surgical resection of malignant brain tumors: Who benefits? Oncology 2:47–63, 1988.
118. Berger, MS: Malignant astrocytomas: Surgical aspects. Seminars in Oncology 21:172–185, 1994.
119. Dinapoli, RP, Brown, LD, Arusell, RM, et al: Phase III comparative evaluation of PCNU and carmustine combined with radiation therapy for high-grade glioma. J Clin Oncol 11:1316–1321, 1993.
120. Shapiro, WR, Green, SB, Burger, PC, et al: Randomized trial of three chemotherapy regimens and two radiotherapy regimens in postoperative treatment of malignant glioma. Brain Tumor Cooperative Group Trial 8001. J Neurosurg 71:1–9, 1989.
121. Glantz, MJ, Burger, PC, and Herndon, JE II: Influence of the type of surgery on the histologic diagnosis in patients with anaplastic gliomas. Neurology 41:1741–1744, 1991.
122. Ciric, I, Ammirati, M, Vick, N, and Mikhael, M: Supratentorial gliomas: Surgical considerations and immediate postoperative results. Gross total resection versus partial resection. Neurosurgery 21:21–26, 1987.
123. Ammirati, M, Vick, N, Liao, Y, et al: Effect of the extent of surgical resection on survival and quality of life in patients with supratentorial glioblastomas and anaplastic astrocytomas. Neurosurgery 21:201–206, 1987.
124. Devaux, BC, O'Fallon, JR, and Kelly, PJ: Resection, biopsy, and survival in malignant glial neoplasms. A retrospective study of clinical parameters, therapy, and outcome. J Neurosurg 78:767–775, 1993.
125. Winger, MJ, Macdonald, DR, and Cairncross, JG: Supratentorial anaplastic gliomas in adults. The prognostic importance of extent of resection and prior low-grade glioma. J Neurosurg 71:487–493, 1989.
126. Wood, JR, Green, SB, and Shapiro, WR: The prognostic importance of tumor size in malignant gliomas: A computed tomographic scan study by the Brain Tumor Cooperative Group. J Clin Oncol 6:338–343, 1988.
127. Sandberg-Wollheim, M, Malmström, P, Strömblad, L-G, et al: A randomized study of chemotherapy with procarbazine, vincristine, and loumstine with and without radiation ther-

apy for astrocytoma grades 3 and/or 4. Cancer 68:22–29, 1991.
128. Coffey, RJ, Lunsford, LD, and Taylor, FH: Survival after stereotactic biopsy of malignant gliomas. Neurosurgery 22:465–473, 1988.
129. Nazzaro, JM, and Neuwelt, EA: The role of surgery in the management of supratentorial intermediate and high-grade astrocytomas in adults. J Neurosurg 73:331–344, 1990.
130. Curran, WA Jr, Scott, CB, Horton, J, et al: Does extent of surgery influence outcome for astrocytoma with atypical or anaplastic foci (AAF)? A report from three Radiation Therapy Oncology Group (RTOG) trials. J Neurooncol 12:219–227, 1992.
131. Quigley, MR, and Maroon, JC: The relationship between survival and the extent of the resection in patients with supratentorial malignant gliomas. Neurosurgery 29:385–389, 1991.
132. Duncan, GG, Goodman, GB, Ludgate, CM, and Rheaume, DE: The treatment of adult supratentorial high grade astrocytomas. J Neurooncol 13:63–72, 1992.
133. Kreth, FW, Warnke, PC, Scheremet, R, and Ostertag, CB: Surgical resection and radiation therapy versus biopsy and radiation therapy in the treatment of glioblastoma multiforme. J Neurosurg 78:762–766, 1993.
134. Bernstein, M, and Parrent, AG: Complications of CT-guided stereotactic biopsy of intra-axial brain lesions. J Neurosurg 81:165–168, 1994.
135. Young, B, Oldfield, EH, Markesbery, WR, et al: Reoperation for glioblastoma. J Neurosurg 55: 917–921, 1981.
136. Ammirati, M, Galicich, JH, Arbit, E, and Liao, Y: Reoperation in the treatment of recurrent intracranial malignant gliomas. Neurosurgery 21:607–614, 1987.
137. Harsh, GR IV, Levin, VA, Gutin, PH, et al: Reoperation for recurrent glioblastoma and anaplastic astrocytoma. Neurosurgery 21:615–621, 1987.
138. Landy, HJ, Feun, L, Schwade, JG, et al: Retreatment of intracranial gliomas. Southern Med J 87:211–214, 1994.
139. Dirks, P, Bernstein, M, Muller, PJ, and Tucker, WS: The value of reoperation for recurrent glioblastoma. Can J Surg 36:271–275, 1993.
140. Walker, MD, Alexander, E Jr, Hunt ,WE, et al: Evaluation of BCNU and/or radiotherapy in the treatment of anaplastic gliomas. A cooperative clinical trial. J Neurosurg 49:333–343, 1978.
141. Andersen, AP: Postoperative irradiation of glioblastomas. Results in a randomized series. Acta Radiologica Oncology 17:475–484, 1978.
142. Walker, MD, Strike, TA, and Sheline, GE: An analysis of dose-effect relationship in the radiotherapy of malignant gliomas. Int J Radiat Oncol Biol Phys 5:1725–1731, 1979.
143. Chang, CH, Horton, J, Schoenfeld, D, et al: Comparison of postoperative radiotherapy and combined postoperative radiotherapy and chemotherapy in the multidisciplinary management of malignant giomas. A joint Radiation Therapy Oncology Group and Eastern Cooperative Oncology Group study. Cancer 52:997–1007, 1983.
144. Salazar, OM, Rubin, P, McDonald, JV, and Feldstein, ML: High dose radiation therapy in the treatment of glioblastoma multiforme: A preliminary report. Int J Radiat Oncol Biol Phys 1:717–727, 1976.
145. Hoffman, WF, Levin, VA, and Wilson, CB: Evaluation of malignant glioma patients during the postirradiation period. J Neurosurg 50:624–628, 1979.
146. Leibel, SA, and Sheline, GE: Radiotherapy in the treatment of cerebral astrocytomas. In Thomas, DG (ed): Neuro-Oncology: Primary Malignant Brain Tumors. Johns Hopkins Series in Contemporary Medicine and Public Health. Johns Hopkins University Press, Baltimore, 1990, pp 193–221.
147. Shapiro, WR: Therapy of adult malignant brain tumors: What have the clinical trials taught us? Semin Oncol 13:38–45, 1986.
148. Hochberg, FH, and Pruitt, A: Assumptions in the radiotherapy of glioblastoma. Neurology 30:907–911, 1980.
149. Wallner, KE, Galicich, JH, Krol, G, et al: Patterns of failure following treatment for glioblastoma multiforme and anaplastic astrocytoma. Int J Radiat Oncol Biol Phys 16:1405–1409, 1989.
150. Choucair, AK, Levin, VA, Gutin, PH, et al: Development of multiple lesions during radiation therapy and chemotherapy in patients with gliomas. J Neurosurg 65:654–658, 1986.
151. Glatstein, E, Lichter, AS, Fraass, BA, et al: The imaging revolution and radiation oncology: use of CT, ultrasound, and NMR for localization, treatment planning and treatment delivery. Int J Radiat Oncol Biol Phys 11:299–314, 1985.
152. Fraass, BA, and McShan, DL: 3-D treatment planning: I Overview of a clinical planning system. In Bruinvis, IAD (ed): The Use of Computers in Radiation Therapy. Elsevier Science Publishers BV, Amsterdam, 1987, pp 521–524.
153. Thornton, AF Jr, Hegarty, TJ, Ten Haken, RK, et al: Three-dimensional treatment planning of astrocytomas: a dosimetric study of cerebral irradiation. Int J Radiat Oncol Biol Phys 20: 1309–1315, 1991.
154. Ten Haken, RK, Thornton, AF Jr, Sandler, HM, et al: Quantitative assessment of the addition of MRI to CT-based, 3-D treatment planning of brain tumors. Radiother Oncol 25:121–133, 1992.
155. Liang, BC, Thornton, AF Jr, Sandler, HM, and Greenberg, HS: Malignant astrocytomas: focal tumor recurence after focal external beam radiation therapy. J Neurosurg 75:559–563, 1991.
156. Jeremic, B, Grujicic, D, Antunovic, V, et al: Hyperfractionated radiation therapy (HFX RT) followed by multiagent chemotherapy (CHT) in patients with malignant glioma: A phase II study. Int J Radiat Oncol Biol Phys 30:1179–1185, 1994.
157. Fulton, DS, Urtasun, RC, Scott-Brown, I, et al: Increasing radiation dose intensity using hyperfractionation in patients with malignant

glioma. Final report of a prospective phase I-II dose response study. J Neurooncol 14:63–72, 1992.
158. Curran, W, Scott, C, Nelson, D, and Sause, W: Results from RTOG phase I/II twice-daily RT dose escalation trials for malignant glioma (83-02) and brain metastases (85-28). J Neurooncol 12:239, 1992.
159. Ludgate, CM, Douglas, BG, Dixon, PF, et al: Superfractionated radiotherapy in grade III, IV intracranial gliomas. Int J Radiat Oncol Biol Phys 15:1091–1095, 1988.
160. Shin, KH, Muller, PJ, and Geggie, PHS: Superfractionation radiation therapy in the treatment of malignant astrocytoma. Cancer 52:2040–2043, 1983.
161. Hercbergs, AA, Tadmor, R, Findler, G, et al: Hypofractionated radiation therapy and concurrent cisplatin in malignant cerebral gliomas. Rapid palliation in low performance status patients. Cancer 64:816–820, 1989.
162. González González, D, Menten, J, Bosch, DA, et al: Accelerated radiotherapy in glioblastoma multiforme: A dose searching prospective study. Radiother Oncol 32:98–105, 1994.
163. Shenouda, G, Souhami L, Freeman, CR, et al: Accelerated fractionation for high-grade cerebral astrocytomas. Preliminary treatment results. Cancer 67:2247–2252, 1991.
164. Marcial-Vega, VA, Wharam, MD, Leibel, S, et al: Treatment of supratentorial high grade gliomas with split course high fractional dose postoperative radiotherapy. Int J Radiat Oncol Biol Phys 16:1419–1424, 1989.
165. Werner-Wasik, M, Scott, CB, Nelson, DF, et al: Final report of a phase I/II trial of hyperfractionated and accelerated hyperfractionated radiation therapy with carmustine for adults with supratentorial malignant gliomas. Radiation Therapy Oncology Group Study 83–02. Cancer 77:1535–1543, 1996
166. Cohen, L, and Awschalom, M: Fast neutron radiation therapy. Ann Rev Biophys Bioeng 11:359–390, 1982.
167. Cohen, L, Hendrickson, FR, Kurup, PD, et al: Clinical evaluation of neutron beam therapy. Current results and prospects, 1983. Cancer 55:10–17, 1985.
168. Griffin, TW, Davis, R, Laramore, G, et al: Fast neutron radiation therapy for glioblastoma multiforme. Am J Clin Oncol 6:661–667, 1983.
169. Laramore, GE: Neutron radiotherapy for high grade gliomas: The search for the elusive therapeutic window. Int J Radiat Oncol Riol Phys 19:493–495, 1990.
170. Kurup, PD, Pajak, TF, Hendrickson, FR, et al: Fast neutrons and misonidazole for malignant astrocytomas. Int J Radiat Oncol Biol Phys 11:679–686, 1985.
171. Castro, JR, Saunders, WM, Austin-Seymour, MM, et al: A phase I-II trial of heavy charged particle irradiation of malignant glioma of the brain: A Northern California Oncology Group study. Int J Radiat Oncol Biol Phys 11:1795–1800, 1985.
172. Barth, RF, Soloway, AH, and Fairchild, RG: Boron neutron capture therapy of cancer. Cancer Res 50:1061–1070, 1990.
173. Finkel, GC, Poletti, CE, Fairchild, RG, et al: Distribution of ^{10}B after infusion of $Na_2{}^{10}B_{12}H_{11}SH$ into a patient with malignant astrocytoma: Implications for boron neutron capture therapy. Neurosurgery 24:6–11, 1989.
174. Haselsberger, K, Radner, H, Gössler, W, et al: Subcellular boron-10 localization in glioblastoma for boron neutron capture therapy with $Na_2B_{12}H_{11}SH$. J Neurosurg 81:741–744, 1994.
175. Stragliotto, G, and Fankhauser, H: Biodistribution of boron sulfhydryl for boron neutron capture therapy in patients with intracranial tumors. Neurosurgery 36:285–293, 1995.
176. Hatanaka, H, Kamano, S, Amano, K, et al: Clinical experience of boron-neutron capture therapy for gliomas - A comparison with conventional chemo-immuno-radiotherapy. In Hatanaka, H (ed): Boron-Neutron Capture Therapy for Tumors. Nishimura Co., Ltd., Niigata, Japan, 1986, pp 349–379.
177. Hatanaka, H, and Urano, Y: Eighteen autopsy cases of malignant brain tumors treated by boron-neutron capture therapy between 1968 and 1985. In Hatanaka, H (ed): Boron-Neutron Capture Therapy for Tumors. Nishimura Co., Ltd., Niigata, Japan, 1986, pp 381–416.
178. Hatanaka, H, Amano, K, Kanemitsu, H, et al: Boron uptake by human brain tumors and quality control of boron compounds. In Hatanaka, H (ed): Boron-Neutron Capture Therapy for Tumors. Nishimura Co., Ltd., Niigata, Japan, 1986, pp 77–106.
179. Dorn, RV III: Boron neutron capture therapy (BNCT): A radiation oncology perspective. Int J Radiat Oncol Biol Phys 28:1189–1201, 1994.
180. Patchell, RA, Maruyama, Y, Tibbs, PA, et al: Neutron interstitial brachytherapy for malignant gliomas: A pilot study. J Neurosurg 68:67–72, 1988.
181. Manyak, MJ, Russo, A, Smith, PD, and Glatstein, E: Photodynamic therapy. J Clin Oncol 6:380–391, 1988.
182. Hill, JS, Kaye, AH, Sawyer, WH, et al: Selective uptake of hematoporphyrin derivative into human cerebral glioma. Neurosurgery 26:248–254, 1990.
183. Powers, SK, Cush, SS, Walstad, DL, and Kwock, L: Stereotactic intratumoral photodynamic therapy for recurrent malignant brain tumors. Neurosurgery 29:688–696, 1991.
184. Laws, ER Jr, Cortese, DA, Kinsey, JH, et al: Photoradiation therapy in the treatment of malignant brian tumors: A phase I (feasibility) study. Neurosurgery 9:672–678, 1981.
185. Perria, C, Carai, M, Falzoi, A, et al: Photodynamic therapy of malignant brain tumors: Clinical results of, difficulties with, questions about, and future prospects for the neurosurgical applications. Neurosurgery 23:557–563, 1988.
186. Bernstein, M, Laperriere, N, Leung, P, and McKenzie, S: Interstitial brachytherapy for malignant brain tumors: Preliminary results. Neurosurgery 26:371–380, 1990.

187. Scharfen, CO, Sneed, PK, Wara, WM, et al: High activity iodine-125 interstitial implant for gliomas. Int J Radiat Oncol Biol Phys 24:583–591, 1992.
188. Marin, LA, Smith, CE, Langston, MY, et al: Response of glioblastoma cell lines to low dose rate irradiation. Int J Radiat Oncol Biol Phys 21: 397–402, 1991.
189. McLaughlin, PW, Mancini, WR, Stetson, PL, et al: Halogenated pyrimidine sensitization of low dose rate irradiation in human malignant glioma. Int J Radiat Oncol Biol Phys 26:637–642, 1993.
190. Nehls, DG, Shetter, AG, and Rossman, KJ: Interstitial irradiation of malignant tumors. BNI Quarterly 1(1):34–39, 1985.
191. Wilson, CB, Larson, DA, and Gutin, PH: Radiosurgery: A new application? J Clin Oncol 10:1373–1374, 1992.
192. Green, SB, Shapiro, WR, Burger, PC, et al: A randomized trial of interstitial radiotherapy (RT) boost for newly diagnosed malignant glioma: Brain Tumor Cooperative Group (BTCG) Trial 8701. Proc Annu Meet Am Soc Clin Oncol 13:A486, 1994.
193. Sneed, PK, Stauffer, PR, Gutin, PH, et al: Interstitial irradiation and hyperthermia for the treatment of recurrent malignant brain tumors. Neurosurgery 28:206–215, 1991.
194. Stea, B, Rossman, K, Kittelson, J, et al: Interstitial irradiation versus interstitial thermoradiotherapy for supratentorial malignant gliomas: A comparative survival analysis. Int J Radiat Oncol Biol Phys 30:591–600, 1994.
195. Levin, VA, Silver, P, Hannigan, J, et al: Superiority of post-radiotherapy adjuvant chemotherapy with CCNU, procarbazine, and vincristine (PCV) over BCNU for anaplastic gliomas: NCOG 6G61 final report. Int J Radiat Oncol Biol Phys 18:321–324, 1990.
196. Sneed, PK, Gutin, PH, Larson, DA, et al: Patterns of recurrence of glioblastoma multiforme after external irradiation followed by implant boost. Int J Radiat Oncol Biol Phys 29(4):719–727, 1994.
197. Agbi, CB, Bernstein, M, Laperriere, N, et al: Patterns of recurrence of malignant astrocytoma following stereotactic interstitial brachytherapy with iodine-125 implants. Int J Radiat Oncol Biol Phys 23:321–326, 1992.
198. Heros, DO, Renkens, K, Kasdon, DL, and Adelman, LS: Patterns of recurrence in glioma patients after interstitial irradiation and chemotherapy: Report of three cases. Neurosurgery 22: 474–478, 1988.
199. Loeffler, JS, Alexander, E III, Wen, PJ, et al: Results of stereotactic brachytherapy used in the initial management of patients with glioblastoma. J Natl Cancer Inst 82:1918–1921, 1990.
200. Loeffler, JS, Alexander, E III, Kooy HM, et al: Radiosurgery for brain metastases. In: Devita, VT, Hellman, S, and Rosenberg, SA (eds) PPO Updates: Cancer. Principles & Practice of Oncology, Volume 5(2). Philadelphia, JB Lippincott, pp 1–12, 1991.
201. Leksell, L: The stereotaxic method and radiosurgery of the brain. Acta Chir Scand 102:316–319, 1951.
202. Loeffler, JS, Alexander, E III, Shea, WM, et al: Radiosurgery as part of the initial management of patients with malignant gliomas. J Clin Oncol 10:1379–1385, 1992.
203. Addesa, A, Shrieve, D, Alexander, E, et al: Stereotactic radiosurgery as primary adjuvant treatment for glioblastoma multiforme: The JCRT update. Proc ASCO 14:A274, 1995.
204. Mehta, MP, Masciopinto, J, Rozental, J, et al: Stereotactic radiosurgery for glioblastoma multiforme: Report of a prospective study evaluating prognostic factors and analyzing long-term survival advantage. Int J Radiat Oncol Biol Phys 30:541–549, 1994.
205. Masciopinto, JE, Levin, AB, Mehta, MP, and Rhode, BS: Stereotactic radiosurgery for glioblastoma: A final report of 31 patients. J Neurosurg 82:530–535, 1995.
206. Chamberlain, MC, Barba, D, Kormanik, P, and Shea, WMC: Stereotactic radiosurgery for recurrent gliomas. Cancer 74:1342–1347, 1994.
207. Brenner, DJ, Martel, MK, and Hall, EJ: Fractionated regimens for stereotactic radiotherapy of recurrent tumors in the brain. Int J Radiat Oncol Biol Phys 21:819–824, 1991.
208. Laing, RW, Warrington, AP, Graham, J, et a;: Efficacy and toxicity of fractionated stereotactic radiotherapy in the treatment of recurrent gliomas (phase I/II study). Radiotherapy Oncol 27:22–29, 1993.
209. Curran, WJ Jr, Scott, CB, Weinstein, AS, et al: Survival comparison of radiosurgery-eligible and -ineligible malignant glioma patients treated with hyperfractionated radiation therapy and carmustine: A report of Radiation Therapy Oncology Group 83–02. J Clin Oncol 11:857–862, 1993.
210. Loeffler, JS: Radiotherapy in managing malignant gliomas: Current role and future directions. Advances in Oncology 8:14–21, 1992.
211. Urtasun, R, Band, P, Chapman, JD, et al: Radiation and high-dose metronidazole in supratentorial glioblastomas. N Engl J Med 294:1364–1367, 1976.
212. Phillips, TL, Wasserman, TH, Johnson, RJ, et al: Final report on the United States phase I clinical trial of hypoxic cell radiosensitizer, misonidazole (Ro-07–0582; NSC #261037). Cancer 48:1697–1704, 1981.
213. Urtasun, R, Feldstein, ML, Partington, J, et al: Radiation and nitroimidazoles in supratentorial high grade gliomas: A second clinical trial. Br J Cancer 46:101–108, 1982.
214. Nelson, DF, Schoenfeld, D, Weinstein, AS, et al: A randomized comparison of misonidazole sensitized radiotherapy plus BCNU and radiotherapy plus BCNU for treatment of malignant glioma after surgery; preliminary results of an RTOG study. Int J Radiat Oncol Biol Phys 9:1143–1151, 1983.
215. EORTC Brain Tumour Group: Misonidazole in radiotherapy of supratentorial malignant brain gliomas in adult patients: A randomized dou-

ble-blind study. Eur J Cancer Clin Oncol 19:39–42, 1983.
216. Stadler, B, Kärcher, KH, Kogelnik, HD, and Szepesi, T: Misonidazole and irradiation in the treatment of high-grade astrocytomas: Further report of the Vienna study group. Int J Radiat Oncol Biol Phys 10:1713–1717, 1984.
217. Evans, RG, Kimler, BF, Morantz, RA, et al: A phase I/II study of the use of fluosol as an adjuvant to radiation therapy in the treatment of primary high-grade brain tumors. Int J Radiat Oncol Biol Phys 19:415–420, 1990.
218. Kinsella, TJ, Mitchell, JB, Russo, A, et al: Continuous intravenous infusions of bromodeoxyuridine as a clinical radiosensitizer. J Clin Oncol 2:1144–1150, 1984.
219. Phillips, TL, Levin, VA, Ahn, DK, et al: Evaluation of bromodeoxyuridine in glioblastoma multiforme: A Northern California Cancer Center phase II study. Int J Radiat Ocol Biol Phys 21:709–714, 1991.
220. Greenberg, HS, Chandler, WF, Ensminger, WD, et al: Radiosensitization with carotid intra-arterial bromodeoxyuridine ± 5-fluorouracil biomodulation for malignant gliomas. Neurology 44:1715–1720, 1994.
221. Oldfield, EH, Friedman, R, Kinsella, T, et al: Reduction in radiation-induced brain injury by use of pentobarbital or lidocaine protection. J Neurosurg 72:737–744, 1990.
222. Olson, JJ, Friedman, R, Orr, K, et al: Enhancement of the efficacy of x-irradiation by pentobarbital in rodent brain-tumor model. J Neurosurg 72:745–748, 1990.
223. Olson, JJ, Friedman, R, Orr, K, et al: Cerebral radioprotection by pentobarbital: Dose-response characteristics and association with GABA agonist activity. J Neurosurg 72:749–758, 1990.
224. Spence, AM, Edmondson, SW, Krohn, KA, et al: Toxicity and biodistribution of the radioprotectors, WR2721, WR77913, and WR3689, in the CNS following intraventricular or intracisternal administration. Int J Radiat Oncol Biol Phys 12:1653–1660, 1986.
225. Reagan, TJ, Bisel, HF, Childs, DS Jr, et al: Controlled study of CCNU and radiation therapy in malignant astrocytoma. J Neurosurg 44:186–190, 1976.
226. Deutsch, M, Green, SB, Strike, TA, et al: Results of a randomized trial comparing BCNU plus radiotherapy, streptozotocin plus radiotherapy, BCNU plus hyperfractionated radiotherapy, and BCNU following misonidazole plus radiotherapy in the postoperative treatment of malignant glioma. Int J Radiat Oncol Biol Phys 16:1389–1396, 1989.
227. Eyre, HJ, Quagliana, JM, Eltringham, JR, et al: Randomized comparisons of radiotherapy and CCNU versus radiotherapy, CCNU plus procarbazine for the treatment of malignant gliomas following surgery. A Southwest Oncology Group report. J Neurooncol 1:171–177, 1983.
228. Eyre, HJ, Eltringham, JR, Gehan, EA, et al: Randomized comparisons of radiotherapy and carmustine versus procarbazine versus dacarbazine for the treatment of malignant gliomas following surgery: A Southwest Oncology Group study. Cancer Treat Rep 70:1085–1090, 1986.
229. Schold, SC Jr, Herndon, JE, Burger, PC, et al: Randomized comparison of diaziquone and carmustine in the treatment of adults with anaplastic glioma. J Clin Oncol 11:77–83, 1993.
230. Fine, HA, Dear, KB, Loeffler, JS, et al: Meta-analysis of radiation therapy with and without adjuvant chemotherapy for malignant gliomas in adults. Cancer 71:2585–2597, 1993.
231. Winger, MJ, Macdonald, DR, Schold, SC Jr, and Cairncross JG: Selection bias in clinical trials of anaplastic glioma. Ann Neurol 26:531–534, 1989.
232. Fulton, D, Urtasun, R, and Forsyth, P: Phase II study of prolonged oral therapy with etoposide (VP16) for patients with recurrent malignant glioma. J Neurooncol 27:149–155, 1996.
233. Wilson, CB, Gutin, P, Boldrey, EB, et al: Single-agent chemotherapy of brain tumors. A five-year review. Arch Neurol 33:739–744, 1976.
234. European Organization for Research on Treatment of Cancer (EORTC) Brain Tumor Group: Evaluation of CCNU, VM-26 plus CCNU, and procarbazine in supratentorial brain gliomas. J Neurosurg 55:27–31, 1981.
235. Rodriguez, LA, Prados, M, Silver, P, and Levin, VA: Reevaluation of procarbazine for the treatment of recurrent malignant central nervous system tumors. Cancer 64:2420–2423, 1989.
236. Newton, HB, Bromberg, J, Junck, L, et al: Comparison between BCNU and procarbazine chemotherapy for treatment of gliomas. J Neurooncol 15:257–263, 1993.
237. EORTC Brain Tumour Cooperative Group: Effect of AZQ (1,4-cyclohexadiene-1,4-diacarbamic acid-2,5-bis(1-aziridinyl)-3,6-dioxodiethylester) in recurring supratentorial malignant brain giomas - a phase II study. Eur J Cancer Clin Oncol 21:143–146, 1985.
238. Haid, M, Khandekar, JD, Christ, M, et al: Aziridinylbenzoquinone in recurrent, progressive glioma of the central nervous system. A phase II study by the Illinois Cancer Council. Cancer 56:1311–1315, 1985.
239. Feun, LG, Yung, W-KA, Leavens, ME, et al: A phase II trial of 2,5,-diaziridinyl3,6-bis(carboethoxy amino)1,4-benzoquinone(AZQ, NSC 182986) in recurrent primary brain tumors. J Neurooncol 2:13–17, 1984.
240. Walker, RW, Dantis, E, and Shapiro, WR: Treatment of recurrent glioma with carboplatin (CBDCA). Proc Am Soc Clin Oncol 6:72, 1989.
241. Tirelli, U, D'Incalci, M, Canetta, R, et al: Etoposide (VP-16–213) in malignant brain tumors: A phase II study. J Clin Oncol 2:432–437, 1984.
242. Finn, GP, Bozek, T, Souhami, RL, et al: High-dose etoposide in the treatment of relapsed primary brain tumors. Cancer Treat Rep 69:603–605, 1985.
243. Frenay, M, Giroux, B, Khoury, S, et al: Phase II study of fotemustine in recurrent supratentor-

ial malignant giomas. Eur J Cancer 27:852–856, 1991.
244. Djerassi, I, Kim, JS, and Reggev, A: Response of astrocytoma to high-dose methotrexate with citrovorum factor rescue. Cancer 55:2741–2747, 1985.
245. Drinkard, L, Olopade, F, Krauss, S, et al: A phase II trial of edatrexate (ETX) in progressive malignant glioma (PMG). Proc Annu Meet Am Soc Clin Oncol 13:A517, 1994.
246. O'Reilly, SM, Newlands, ES, Glaser, MG, et al: Temozolomide: A new oral cytotoxic chemotherapeutic agent with promising activity against primary brain tumours. Eur J Cancer 29A:940–942, 1993.
247. Vertosick, FT Jr, Selker, RG, Pollack, IF, Arena, V: The treatment of intracranial malignant gliomas using orally administered tamoxifen therapy: Preliminary results in a series of "failed" patients. Neurosurgery 30:897–903, 1992.
248. Couldwell, WT, Weiss, MH, DeGiorgio, CM, et al: Clinical and radiographic response in a minority of patients with recurrent malignant gliomas treated with high-dose tamoxifen. Neurosurgery 32:485–490, 1993.
249. Prados, M, Schold, C, Spence, A, et al: Phase II study of taxol in patients (PTS) with recurrent malignant glioma: North American Brain Tumor Consortium. Proc Am Soc Clin Oncol 14:146, 1995.
250. Eisenhauer, EA, Wainman, N, Boos, G, et al: Phase II trials of topotecan in patients (PTS) with malignant glioma and soft tissue sarcoma. Proc Am Soc Clin Oncol 13:175, 1994.
251. Berger, MS, Leibel, SA, Bruner, JM, et al: Primary central nervous system tumors of the supratentorial compartment. In Levin, VA (ed): Cancer in the Nervous System. Churchill Livingstone, New York, 1996, pp 57–126.
252. Levin, VA, Crafts, DC, Wilson, CB, et al: BCNU (NSC-409962) and procarbazine (NSC-77213) treatment for malignant brain tumors. Cancer Treat Rep 60:243–249, 1976.
253. Prados, M, Rodriguez, L, Chamberlain, M, et al: Treatment of recurrent gliomas with 1,3-bis(2-chloroethyl)-1-nitrosourea and α-difluoromethylornithine. Neurosurgery 24:806–809, 1989.
254. Gutin, PH, Wilson, CB, Kumar, ARV, et al: Phase II study of procarbazine, CCNU, and vincristine combination chemotherapy in the treatment of malignant brain tumors. Cancer 35:1398–1404, 1975.
255. Levin, VA, Edwards, MS, Wright, DC, et al: Modified procarbazine, CCNU, and vincristine (PCV 3) combination chemotherapy in the treatment of malignant brain tumors. Cancer Treat Rep 64:237–241, 1980.
256. Ameri, A, Poisson, M, Chen, QM, and Delattre, JY: Treatment of recurrent malignant supratentorial gliomas with the association of procarbazine, thiotepa and vincristine: A phase II study. J Neurooncol 17:43–46, 1993.
257. Coyle, T, Baptista, J, Winfield, J. et al: Mechlorethamine, vincristine, and procarbazine chemotherapy for recurrent high-grade glioma in adults: A phase II study. J Clin Oncol 8:2014–2018, 1990.
258. Hellman, RM, Calogero, JA, and Kaplan, BM: VP-16, vincristine and procarbazine with radiation therapy or treatment of malignant brain tumors. J Neurooncol 8:163–166, 1990.
259. Longee, DC, Friedman, HS, Albright, RE Jr, et al: Treatment of patients with recurrent gliomas with cyclophosphamide and vincristine. J Neurosurg 72:583–588, 1990.
260. Buckner, JC, Brown, LD, Cascino, TL, et al: Phase II evaluation of infusional etoposide and cisplatin in patients with recurrent astrocytoma. J Neurooncol 9:249–254, 1990.
261. Schold, SC Jr, Mahaley, MS Jr, Vick, NA, et al: Phase II diaziquone-based chemotherapy trials in patients with anaplastic supratentorial astrocytic neoplasms. J Clin Oncol 5:464–471, 1987.
262. Levin, VA, and Prados, MD: Treatment of recurrent gliomas and metastatic brain tumors with a polydrug protocol designed to combat nitrosourea resistance. J Clin Oncol 10:766–771, 1992.
263. Rostomily, RC, Spence, AM, Duong, D, et al: Multimodality management of recurrent adult malignant gliomas: Results of a phase II multiagent chemotherapy study and analysis of cytoreductive surgery. Neurosurgery 35:378–388, 1994.
264. Ram, Z, Culver, KW, Walbridge, S, et al: *In situ* retroviral-mediated gene transfer for the treatment of brain tumors in rats. Cancer Res 53:83–88, 1993.
265. Boviatsis, EJ, Park, JS, Sen-Esteves, M, et al: Long-term survival of rats harboring brain neoplasms treated with ganciclovir and a herpes simplex virus vector that retains an intact thymidine kinase gene. Cancer Res 54:5745–5751, 1994.
266. Oldfield, EH: Advantages and limitations of experimental therapy of patients with malignant brain tumors with a retroviral vector containing the gene for thymidine kinase and intravenous ganciclovir. J Neurooncol 28:61, 1996.
267. Trojan, J, Johnson, TR, Rudin, SD, et al: Treatment and prevention of rat glioblastoma by immunogenic C6 cells expressing antisense insulin-like growth factor I RNA. Science 259:94–96, 1993.
268. Martuza, R, Mineta, T, Yazaki, T, et al: Replication-competent viruses for tumor therapy. J Neurooncol 28:61, 1996.
269. Meckling, S, Dold, O, Forsyth, PAJ, et al: Malignant supratentorial glioma in the elderly: Is radiotherapy useful? Neurology 47:901–905, 1996.
270. Grant, R, Liang, BC, Page, MA, et al: Age influences chemotherapy response in astrocytomas. Neurology 45:929–933, 1995.
271. Levi, ADO, Wallace, MC, Bernstein, M, and Walters, BC: Venous thromboembolism after brain tumor surgery: A retrospective review. Neurosurgery 28:859–863, 1991.
272. Cheruku, R, Tapazoglou, E, Ensley, J, et al: The incidence and significance of thromboembolic

complications in patients with high-grade gliomas. Cancer 68:2621–2624, 1991.
273. Quevedo, JF, Buckner, JC, Schmidt, JL, et al: Thromboembolism in patients with high-grade glioma. Mayo Clin Proc 69:329–332, 1994.
274. Ruff, RL, and Posner, JB: Incidence and treatment of peripheral venous thrombosis in patients with glioma. Ann Neurol 13:334–336, 1983.
275. Yung, WA, Horten, BC, and Shapiro, WR: Meningeal gliomatosis: A review of 12 cases. Ann Neurol 8:605–608, 1980.
276. Grant, R, Naylor, B, Junck, L, and Greenberg, HS: Clinical outcome in aggressively treated meningeal gliomatosis. Neurology 42:252–254, 1992.
277. Vertosick, FT Jr, and Selker, RG: Brain stem and spinal metastases of supratentorial glioblastoma multiforme: A clinical series. Neurosurgery 27:516–522, 1990.
278. Awad, I, Bay, JW, and Rogers, L: Leptomeningeal metastasis from supratentorial malignant gliomas. Neurosurgery 19:247–251, 1986.
279. Lampl, Y, Eshel, Y, Gilad, R, and Sarova-Pinchas, I: Glioblastoma multiforme with bone metastase and cauda equina syndrome. J Neurooncol 8:167–172, 1990.
280. Fontana, M, Stanton, C, Pompili, A, et al: Late multifocal gliomas in adolescents previously treated for acute lymphoblastic leukemia. Cancer 60:1510–1518, 1987.
281. Shapiro, S, Mealey, J Jr, and Sartorius, C: Radiation-induced intracranial malignant gliomas. J Neurosurg 71:77–82, 1989.
282. Aiken, RD: Quality-of-life issues in patients with malignant gliomas. Seminars in Oncology 21: 273–275, 1994.
283. Weitzner, MA, Meyers, CA, and Byrne, K: Psychosocial functioning and quality of life in patients with primary brain tumors. J Neurosurg 84:29–34, 1996.
284. Weitzner, MA, Meyers, CA, Gelke, CK, et al: The Functional Assessment of Cancer Therapy (FACT) scale. Development of a brain subscale and revalidation of the general version (FACT-G) in patients with primary brain tumors. Cancer 75:1151–1161, 1995.

Chapter 9

PILOCYTIC ASTROCYTOMA, LOW-GRADE ASTROCYTOMA, AND OTHER "BENIGN" NEUROEPITHELIAL NEOPLASMS

This chapter discusses most "benign" neuroepithelial tumors with a grade I or II biologic behavior. These tumors were classified pathologically in Table 1–2. Pilocytic astrocytoma is discussed initially and has a grade I biologic behavior, although its histological appearance may appear more aggressive. Astrocytoma or low-grade astrocytoma (LGA) is covered next and has a grade II biologic behavior. The names used to describe this tumor vary with the grading system. In the Kernohan or Mayo St. Anne grading system, this tumor is called a *grade II astrocytoma*; in the Ringertz or 1979 World Health Organization (WHO) grading system, an *astrocytoma*; and in the University of California, San Francisco system, a *mildly anaplastic astrocytoma* (Table 1–4). The chapter concludes with descriptions of the rarer "benign" neuroepithelial neoplasms: subependymal giant cell astrocytoma, pleomorphic xanthoastrocytoma, gangliocytoma and ganglioglioma, desmoplastic infantile ganglioglioma, dysembryoplastic neuroepithelial tumor (DNET), and central neurocytoma. Oligodendroglioma and oligoastrocytoma are covered in Chapter 10, and ependymoma and choroid plexus papilloma in Chapter 11. Oligodendroglioma, oligo-astrocytoma, ependymoma, and choroid plexus papilloma are other benign neuroepithelial neoplasms and are discussed in Chapters 10 and 11.

PILOCYTIC ASTROCYTOMA

History and Nomenclature

Pilocytic astrocytoma was initially described in 1918 by Ribbert.[1] Bailey and Cushing[2] included it in their initial brain tumor classification in 1926, under the name *spongioblastoma* (see Fig. 1–1). In 1931, Penfield[3] called these tumors *piloid astrocytomas* to describe the elongated bipolar or multipolar cells. He and others thought the term *spongioblastoma* was inappropriate because it implied malignant behavior, yet the tumor behaved benignly.[3] Kagan[4] and Rubinstein[5] named this same tumor *astrocytoma of the juvenile type* because of the age group in which it occurred and to differentiate it from more malignant glial neoplasms. The 1993 WHO[6] classification system groups all "piloid" tumors with a biphasic pattern of tightly packed bipolar cells intermixed with looser microcystic areas of protoplasmic astrocytes as *pilocytic astrocytomas*. These tumors typically occur in children and are located in midline structures, the optic nerve, hypothalamus, thalamus, brainstem, and cerebellum. In adults they are located more often in the cerebral hemispheres in the temporoparietal region.[6]

Epidemiology

A total of 75% to 80% of pilocytic astrocytomas occur in the first two decades of life, with a peak incidence at age 10.[6,7] Most of the remainder occur in young adults in the third, or less commonly, the fourth decade of life.[7,8] Cerebellar pilocytic astrocytoma represents 4.7% of all intracranial gliomas.[9] Cerebral pilocytic astrocytoma accounted for 3% of adult gliomas and slightly less than 1% of all brain tumors operated on at the Institute of Neurosurgery in Rome.[10]

Biology

The biologic behavior of pilocytic astrocytoma is benign, or grade I. In allelic deletion studies of pilocytic astrocytoma, four of 20 patients had allelic loss on chromosome 17q.[11] The neurofibromatosis-1 (*NF1*) gene is located on chromosome 17q. Other loci known to contain abnormalities in LGA (17p), anaplastic astrocytoma (19q), and glioblastoma multiforme (10) have been normal in patients with pilocytic astrocytoma.[12–14]

Bromodeoxyuridine (BUdR)-labeling index measurements of S-phase in 50 tumors have been consistently low (mean labeling index, 1.05%).[15] The Ki-67 labeling index in 20 juvenile pilocytic astrocytomas (three optic nerve, 17 cerebellar) had a mean labeling index of 0.93%.[16] DNA flow cytometry studies were diploid in 19 of 20 patients in one study[16] and 18 of 34 in a second study,[17] with 11 aneuploid, four aneuploid-polyploid, and one tetraploid. No correlation was found between ploidy and pathologic grading, pathologic features, or survival.[17]

Glucose metabolism was significantly higher in (^{18}F)-2-fluoro-2-deoxyglucose positron emission tomography (FDG-PET) studies in five patients with juvenile pilocytic astrocytoma than in other more aggressive LGAs and was similar to that in anaplastic astrocytoma.[18] The authors suggested that the increased glucose utilization might be related to increased expression of a glucose transporter.

Pathology

Pilocytic astrocytoma is often located in the midline structures: the optic nerve, hypothalamus, thalamus, brainstem, and cerebellum. In adults, the tumor is usually located in the cerebral hemispheres in the medial temporoparietal region.[6] On gross examination, pilocytic astrocytomas are yellowish to grayish-pink translucent masses, which often contain a single large or multiple small cysts.[9,19] A single mural tumor nodule is frequently located in the wall of large cysts in tumors of the cerebellar and cerebral hemispheres. The mural nodule is reddish-brown, friable, and may have areas of hemorrhage and calcification. The margins of the pilocytic astrocytoma are thought to be distinct both macroscopically and microscopically,[20] although one study found white matter infiltration in 64% of cases.[8]

Microscopically, two distinct pathological varieties exist: the "juvenile" form described by Russell and Rubenstein,[21] and the "adult" variant described by Clark.[19] The juvenile pilocytic astrocytoma has a biphasic pattern in which cellular regions of unipolar and bipolar "piloid" cells are mixed with hypocellular microcystic regions (see Fig. 1–5). The piloid cells often sheath blood vessels while forming whorls, streams, and other patterns. The cellular pleomorphism is mild to moderate, with occasional mitoses. Rosenthal fibers (rod- or club-shaped eosinophilic structures) are contained within the pilocytic cell processes. Glomeruloid capillary and endothelial proliferation is not uncommon and may be responsible for magnetic resonance imaging (MRI) and computed tomography (CT) contrast enhancement.[6] The fibrillar cytoplasmic processes and Rosenthal fibers within the cells immunostain with glial fibrillary acidic protein (GFAP). Pilocytic astrocytoma can grow into the subarachnoid space and produce a desmoplastic meningeal reaction.[6]

The "adult" variant has monotonous areas of densely packed broad, bipolar, fibrillar cells without microcystic regions.[19,21] Pilocytic astrocytoma has a grade I biologic behavior despite histological features of nuclear pleomorphism and glomeruloid capillary and endothelial proliferation. Anaplastic degeneration, characterized by frequent mitoses, is very uncommon but occurs more frequently in the adult variant.[21] Anaplastic pilocytic astrocytoma has a grade III biologic behavior.[6]

Clinical Symptoms

The clinical manifestations of pilocytic astrocytoma are similar to those of other focal brain tumors, and they depend on the location of tumor in brain. Juvenile pilocytic astrocytoma of the lateral cerebellum presents with the symptoms of appendicular ataxia followed by truncal unsteadiness and then increased intracranial pressure. When the tumor develops in the cerebellar vermis, truncal unsteadiness develops earlier, followed more quickly by increased intracranial pressure. The clinical signs include papilledema; gait ataxia; appendicular dysmetria; nystagmus; and cranial nerve palsies, most frequently of the sixth cranial nerve. Brainstem gliomas are pilocytic in pathology in 20% of cases and most frequently arise in the pons. These tumors typically present with cranial nerve, cerebellar and pyramidal tract signs, and symptoms and signs associated with increased intracranial pressure.

Whereas optic nerve pilocytic astrocytoma commonly presents with proptosis, chiasmal tumor presents with decreased vision.[22–24] The neurological findings are visual loss with central scotomas, papilledema, and optic atrophy. Peripheral field defects are common, but a bitemporal hemianopsia occurs in less than half of patients.[25] If the chiasmal lesion extends into the hypothalamus, an endocrinopathy may occur, typically with diabetes insipidus or precocious puberty. The diencephalic syndrome occurs with symptoms of failure to thrive, wasting, and seeming overalertness.[25] Obstructive hydrocephalus can be present from third ventricular obstruction. The tumor frequently spreads along white matter tracts into the midbrain.

The most common symptoms at presentation of pilocytic astrocytoma of the cerebral hemispheres are seizures or headache, each in approximately 50% of patients.[10,17,19,20] Visual disturbances and symptomatic weakness are each present in 20% of cases. Symptoms developed insidiously, and were present for a mean of 14 months and 3.7 years before surgical diagnosis, in two series of cerebral pilocytic astrocytomas.[10,19] Neurologic signs, in order of frequency, are papilledema, hemianopsia, and pyramidal tract.[10,19,20] The progression of symptoms and signs is usually slow unless hydrocephalus or a mural nodule hemorrhage develops.

Differential Diagnosis

The differential diagnosis of pilocytic astrocytoma depends on the location of the mass. Pilocytic astrocytoma of the cerebellum must be differentiated from medulloblastoma, ependymoma, and other more aggressive astrocytomas.[26] Pilocytic astrocytoma is the most common astrocytic neoplasm of the cerebellum in children. On CT and MRI scans, all pilocytic astrocytomas are sharply demarcated and smoothly marginated, except when located in the optic nerve or chiasm. They also lack edema. If a tumor is cystic with an enhancing mural nodule, a pilocytic astrocytoma is more likely (Fig. 9–1).[26] Brainstem pilocytic astrocytoma may be difficult to differentiate clinically from more aggressive brainstem astrocytomas unless they are cystic or enhance. Brainstem pilocytic astrocytoma enhances less often, than pilocytic tumors elsewhere. Aggressive brainstem astrocytoma tends to be hypodense on CT scans and has decreased signal on T_1-weighted MRI. It extends along the axis of the brainstem and involves the middle cerebellar peduncle and spinal cord. Locally, the tumor may produce pontine hypertrophy. Stereotactic biopsy, with or without resection, provides the definitive answer.

Optic chiasm (i.e., suprasellar) and hypothalamic pilocytic tumors must be differentiated from craniopharyngioma, germinoma, invasive pituitary adenoma, lymphoma, histiocytosis X, and primitive neuroectodermal tumor (PNET). Rare, nontumorous conditions in the differential diagnosis are fungal granuloma, tuberculoma, and retro-orbital opto-chiasmatic arachnoiditis.[26] Craniopharyngioma is more common than optic chiasm glioma and presents with symptoms and signs associated with increased intracranial pressure due to third ventricular or foramen of Monro obstruction. Visual field deficits are common and are seen in 50% to 90% of patients, with neuroendocrine defects in 90%.[26] Craniopharyngioma can often be distinguished radiographically as a cyst containing a homogeneous enhancing mass. Suprasellar germinoma often presents insidiously with endocrine dysfunction, such as diabetes insipidus and growth hormone insufficiency. Although certain radiographic features are helpful, such as the cyst in a craniopharyngioma, a

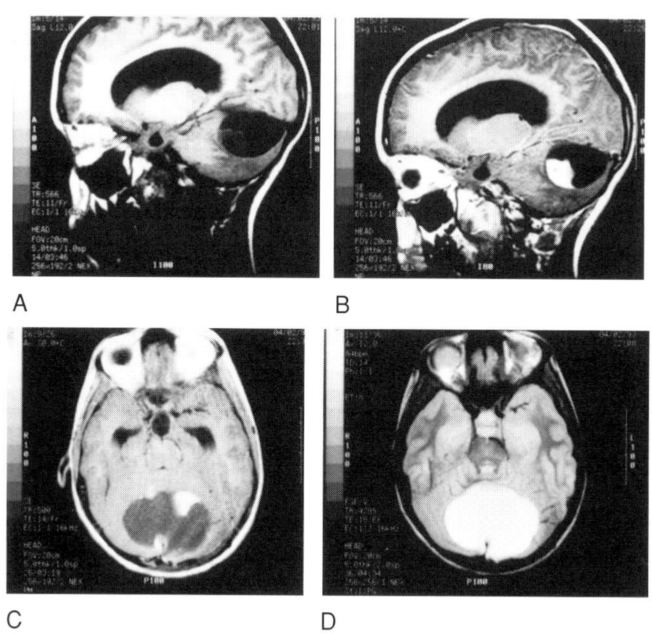

Figure 9–1. Pilocytic astrocytoma *(A)* Precontrast sagittal T_1-weighted MRI showing superior cerebellar cyst sharply demarcated from normal brain. *(B)* postcontrast T_1-weighted sagittal MRI, and *(C)* axial MRI. Both show an enhancing nodule. *(D)* T_2-weighted MRI with hyperintense signal of tumor and cyst.

biopsy is advocated at all times before therapy.[27]

The differential diagnosis for cerebral pilocytic astrocytoma includes LGA, ganglioglioma, oligodendroglioma, pleomorphic xanthoastrocytoma, DNET, and rarely, brain abscess and metastasis. Pilocytic astrocytoma should be easily distinguished on imaging studies from LGA and oligodendroglioma by their sharp margins and displacement rather than infiltration of brain.[17,26] They should be distinguishable from brain abscess and metastasis because of their lack of edema.[17] Ganglioglioma is difficult to distinguish radiologically from pilocytic astrocytoma because it can occur in the midline; however, it more typically presents in the cerebral hemispheres. They are often cystic, occasionally calcified, and enhance in approximately 50% of the cases.[28] Pleomorphic xanthoastrocytoma is a tumor of juveniles, similar to pilocytic astrocytoma, often presenting with seizures, but it is typically superficial in location adjacent to the leptomeninges. It often has an underlying cyst.[6] DNET is diagnosed almost exclusively in children undergoing epilepsy surgery for intractable seizures.

Diagnostic Workup

The procedure of choice for patients with a history and examination compatible with a pilocytic astrocytoma is MRI, with and without contrast administration. A noncontrast- and contrast-enhanced CT is an acceptable alternative. MRI is particularly helpful if the tumor is in the optic pathways or posterior fossa. On MRI or CT scans, pilocytic astrocytoma is seen as a discrete, circumscribed mass that does not infiltrate surrounding brain and is not associated with significant edema.[17,18,26,29] In juveniles, it is typically located in the midline around the ventricular system. On T_1-weighted MRI scans, it is seen as isointense or hyperintense; on T_2-weighted MRI scans, it is always hyperintense (see Fig. 9–1). Contrast enhancement is common only in the mural nodule and is most often homogeneous.[17,18,26,29] The pilocytic tumor is hypodense or isodense on CT scan before contrast infusion, and it enhances similarly to MRI.[26] Cysts are common in the tumors and vary from one large cyst to many small cysts. Calcification is present in 11% to 40% of tumors on imaging studies and is better visualized with CT.[26,30]

In a series of 56 patients with pilocytic astrocytoma and a median age of 17 years, the most common location was cerebral in 32%, followed by thalamus or basal ganglia in 21%, and cerebellar in 20% (Table 9–1).[8]

Treatment

SYMPTOMATIC

If seizures are the presenting symptom, they must be treated with anticonvulsants, preferably diphenylhydantoin or carbamazepine monotherapy. Most patients will not have significant local mass effect, but obstructive hydrocephalus is common in hypothalamic, brainstem, and cerebellar pilocytic astrocytomas. Dexamethasone is often used to temporize before surgery, but temporary ventricular drainage or a ventriculoperitoneal shunt is often appropriate.

SURGERY

Surgery is the cornerstone of therapy for pilocytic astrocytoma. The goal of the surgical resection is to evacuate the cyst contents and remove all contrast-enhanced tissue on MRI or CT.[10,30] This includes not

Table 9–1. **Pilocytic Astrocytoma: Tumor Location**

Location	Percentage
Cerebral	32
Basal ganglia thalamus	21
Cerebellar	20
Brainstem	12
Third ventricle or hypothalamus	9
Optic nerve or chiasm	4
Spinal cord	2

only the enhancing mural nodule but also any enhancing cyst wall.[30,31] Cerebellar hemisphere, optic nerve, and cerebral pilocytic astrocytomas can typically be resected completely, with a cure rate approaching 100%.[7,17,19,20,32,33] In a series of 51 pilocytic astrocytomas, 18 had a gross total or radical subtotal resection with a 10-year survival rate of 100%. Whereas patients with a subtotal resection had a 10-year survival rate greater than 80%, patients with biopsy alone had a 10-year survival of 44%.[17] Shaw and colleagues[32] reported similar percentages of 10-year survivors for the three types of surgical procedures in a series of 41 patients. If there is a gross total resection of tumor, no further therapy is needed.[7,17,20,31–33] Patients should have an imaging study done postoperatively to document complete resection, with neurological examinations and serial imaging studies over the next 10 years. Although long-term survival of patients with pilocytic astrocytoma is decreased incomplete resection, it is still better than with other LGA. The use of radiotherapy (RT) postoperatively after subtotal resection is a contentious matter among physicians treating patients with pilocytic astrocytoma.

RADIATION THERAPY

Most series fail to find benefit from RT after subtotal excision of pilocytic astrocytoma.[17,20,32–35] Wallner and colleagues[7] advocate postoperative RT for patients age 4 years or older. The recommended dose is 45 to 60 Gy. Their rationale is the tumor will never be smaller than it is postoperatively, and RT kills a fixed percentage of cells. Shaw and coworkers[32] suggest RT may be appropriate for patients with pilocytic astrocytoma after subtotal resection based on a study comparing four patients who did not receive RT, with 27 patients who were irradiated. The 5-year survival in the RT-treated group was 85% compared with 50% in the four patients who did not receive RT. In the total treated population of 41 patients, there was no difference between the surgery and RT group and the surgery alone group.[32]

In summary, the evidence is meager that RT benefits subtotally resected pilocytic astrocytomas in the postoperative setting. The best course may be to observe the patient with frequent neurological examinations and serial scans. If there is tumor progression, RT should be considered. If the cyst fluid reaccumulates, a catheter can be placed in the cyst and attached to an Ommaya-type device. The role of SR has not yet been defined.

CHEMOTHERAPY

Chemotherapy has been used for patients with recurrent tumor after surgery and RT and in those who have multifocal spread of their neoplasm. Brown and associates[36] treated 11 patients with progressive disease (PD) after surgery (n=4) and after surgery and RT (n=7) with various chemotherapeutic regimens. Five patients had radiographic response and three had SD, with a median time to progression of only 7.5 months. Mamelak and colleagues[37] treated 10 patients with recurrent multifocal spread of hypothalamic pilocytic glioma with 10 different chemotherapy regimens. Multicentric disease stabilized or regressed in seven patients, with a median follow-up of 31 months.

Packer and coworkers[25,38] treated 13 children younger than 5 years of age with chemotherapy after surgery using a combination of actinomycin D and vincristine. These children had chiasmatic and hypothalamic pilocytic astrocytomas. A concern was that RT would cause growth failure and endocrinopathy. The treatment stabilized or produced disease regression in 80% of newly diagnosed children, delaying the need for RT for an average of 3 years. More recently, Packer and colleagues[25,39] used the combination of carboplatinum and vincristine, with 60% of children having a radiographic response. Petronio and associates[40] treated six children with hypothalamic and chiasmal glioma, with a five-drug combination including procarbazine, lomustine, and vincristine. Five of six patients had PR or SD, and there was more than 2.5 years median time to progression.

Prognosis and Complications

Pilocytic astrocytomas that are completely surgically resected have a cure rate approaching 100%.[7,17,19,20,32,33] After subtotal resection, the 10-year survival rate is greater than 80%; with only a stereotactic biopsy, 10-year survival is reduced to 44%.[17,32] Pilocyctic astrocytoma occasionally pursues a more aggressive course with local progression or multifocal spread, which can include the neuraxis.[36,37] In a series of 90 patients with pilocytic astrocytoma, 11 patients developed multifocal spread of the tumor. Ten of 33 (30%) patients with hypothalamic tumors had multifocal spread. Only one of the other 57 patients with pilocytic tumors had multifocal spread.[37] Fifty percent of patients with multifocal spread develop neuraxis dissemination. When recurrence occurs, the tumor usually has identical histology to the original tumor.[37] Degeneration to a malignant pilocytic astrocytoma is rare but does occur.[6,9,17,19,21,35]

The complications of pilocytic astrocytoma are related to the location of the tumor. Chiasmal and hypothalamic tumors produce a high incidence of endocrinopathy. Hydrocephalus occurs with deep midline tumors of the chiasm, hypothalamus, thalamus, brainstem, and cerebellum. Patients with cerebral pilocytic tumors may present with or develop intractable seizures. If tumor removal and antiepileptic therapy fail to control the seizures, resection of the epileptic focus should be considered.[31]

LOW-GRADE ASTROCYTOMA

History and Nomenclature

Astrocytoma was one of the original tumors in the Bailey and Cushing[2] classification scheme created in 1926. Astrocytoma was classified as fibrillary or protoplasmic by Bailey and Cushing[2] (see Fig. 1–1). The median survival of protoplasmic and fibrillary astrocytomas in the Bailey and Cushing[2] series was 67 and 86 months, respectively (see Table 1–1). It is thought that protoplasmic and fibrillary astrocytomas have an identical prognosis.[6] Kernohan and Sayre[41] introduced a grading system for astrocytomas: grades I and II are the low-grade astrocytomas, and grades III and IV are the high-grade astrocytomas. Grades I and II included both pilocytic tumors and nonpilocytic LGA. Increasing malignancy was associated with increasing cellularity, nuclear and cellular pleomorphism, and the appearance of mitoses, endothelial proliferation, and necrosis in higher grades of malignancy. Ringertz[42] introduced a three-tiered classification system of astrocytoma, anaplastic astrocytoma, and glioblastoma. An astrocytoma in the Ringertz system was roughly equivalent to grades I and II in the Kernohan and Sayre system. Two newer grading systems, Daumas-Duport[43] and the 1993 WHO classification,[6] classify pilocytic astrocytomas separately from other astrocytomas because of their benign biologic behavior. In the 1993 WHO classification of 1993,[6] LGA is classified as grade II, as in the Daumas-Duport classification system (see Table 1–3). Whereas the WHO classification is a continuous grading system, the Daumas-Duport classification is a discrete system that depends on the presence or absence of four variables: nuclear atypia, mitoses, endothelial proliferation, and necrosis. In the Daumas-Duport system, if none of the variables are present, the tumor is grade 1; if one of the pathological features is present, the tumor is grade II; if two histological criteria are present, it is grade III; and if more than two variables are present, it is grade IV.

Epidemiology

LGA accounts for 10% to 20%[44–49] of brain tumors in adults and 8% to 25% in children.[49,50] It tends to occur in younger patients than high-grade astrocytomas do, and approximately two thirds of patients with LGA are younger than than 40 years of age.[49,51] The average annual adult incidence rate of gliomas is 5.4 per 100,000 population per year, and if LGA is proportionally 15% of these, then the incidence rate of LGA is 0.8 per 100,000 per year.[52] The gender distribution (males:females) in series varied from 1:1[45,46,50,54,55] to 3:2.[48,53] A characteristic tumor in NF1 is low-grade optic nerve glioma.

Biology

Astrocytoma acquires a series of sequential allelic changes with the deletion and amplification of genetic material, both in its development and in its evolution to a more malignant state.[55,56] The earliest chromosomal changes present in LGA are the loss of genetic material on chromosomes 6, 13, 17p and 22, presumably associated with the change from normal glia to LGA. If the LGA dedifferentiates to a more malignant phenotype, additional chromosomal changes often occur (see Fig. 2–4).

LGA proliferative potential has been measured in two series, with the intravenous (IV) infusion of BUdR before surgery. The labeling index varied between 2.0% and 6.7% in one series[57] and between less than 1% and 9.3% in the other series.[58] Ito and colleagues[58] found the labeling index was less than 1% in 50 of 69 primary LGA and 14 of 18 recurrent LGAs. A Cox proportional hazard analysis of influence found that labeling index and extent of surgery predicted progression-free survival and survival.[59] Ki-67 antibody labeling index of 9 LGA varied from 0% to 2.7%, with a mean of 0.81%.[16]

LGA is a slow-growing tumor but is not considered benign because of infiltration through white matter. It is also surrounded by a rigid, bony structure, the skull, which cannot expand.

Pathology

LGA is composed of neoplastic astrocytes, which diffusely infiltrate brain. Macroscopically, the tumor is yellow-white or gray and has indistinct margins with normal brain.[6] The tumor can be firm and rubbery or soft and gelatinous, depending on the fibrillarity of the neoplasm. Cysts may be seen. Microscopically, diffuse infiltration of brain, but not destruction, leads to blurring of the normal gray-white junction and the trapping of the pre-existing cells in the infiltrating process.[6] LGA is often histologically uniform with a slight increase in cellularity and nuclear pleomorphism when compared with normal brain. There are no mitoses, endothelial proliferation, or necrosis. Despite its relative histological uniformity, flow cytometric and cytogenetic analysis demonstrate both cellular and regional heterogeneity, which may play a role in tumor progression.[60]

The three predominant histological variants are fibrillary, protoplasmic, and gemistocytic. The fibrillary astrocytoma is the most common variant. Biopsy specimens vary from isolated tumor cells sprinkled through intact parenchyma with hyperchromatic nuclei and scant cytoplasm to more cellular lesions with glial fibrillary processes in the cytoplasm. LGA stains positively for GFAP. The protoplasmic cell type has a small cell body and few glial processes and less GFAP staining. The gemistocytic astrocytoma is composed of cells with large eosinophilic cell bodies with angular short cell processes. The nuclei are usually eccentrically placed. The gemistocytic astrocytoma is associated with a poorer prognosis than either the fibrillary or protoplasmic astrocytoma. It has a greater tendency to dedifferentiate to an anaplastic tumor.[6]

Clinical Symptoms

LGA produces symptoms by local infiltration and mass effect and by an increase in intracranial pressure. The most common presenting symptom in three adult and one pediatric series with LGA was seizures, occurring in approximately 60% of patients.[45,48,50,53] The second most common symptom in the four series was headache, varying in frequency from 38% to 46%. Weakness or visual abnormalities occurred in 20% or fewer of cases, and other neurological deficits depended on tumor location.

Fried and coworkers[59] described a series of patients with intractable seizures and perilimbic neocortical astrocytomas. LGA accounted for 61% of the tumors, with mixed glial tumors (oligodendroglioma and ganglioglioma) accounting for 22% and anaplastic astrocytoma accounting for 17%. These perilimbic tumors had a benign tumor evolution, mean seizure history was 15 years, and mean follow-up from diagnosis was 17 years. Tumor resection without electrocorticography abolished seizures in 82% of cases.

LGA also occurs in the optic chiasm, hypothalamus, thalamus, brainstem, and cerebellum and has local symptoms referable to those areas. These deep midline tumors are less likely to present with seizures and more likely to present with symptoms and signs associated with increased intracranial pressure from obstructive hydrocephalus. In a series of infiltrative thalamic astrocytomas of all grades, 60% of patients presented with symptoms of headache, nausea, or vomiting, and 39% had papilledema. Only 12% had a clinical presentation with seizures.[61]

Differential Diagnosis

The differential diagnosis is limited in middle-aged adults who present with seizures and mild focal neurological signs on neurological examination, decreased signal on T_1-weighted MRI, and increased signal on T_2-weighted MRI. Other low-grade glial tumors included in the differential diagnosis are oligodendroglioma and mixed oligo-astrocytoma. In a series from the Royal Marsden Hospital in London, Whitton and Bloom[45] found that LGA was 2.5 times more common than oligodendroglioma, and mixed oligo-astrocytomas accounted for less than 5% of tumors. In recent years oligoastrocytoma has become a more frequent pathologic diagnosis. All three tumors present with the same symptoms and signs in approximately similar frequency. Oligodendroglioma is more likely to be calcified than LGA, but LGA is 2.5 times more common. Pilocytic astrocytoma has to be considered, but in its typical juvenile form it has an enhancing mural nodule. Pleomorphic xanthoastrocytoma is another tumor that is common in young adults and most frequently presents with seizures. It is typically superficial in location, adjacent to the leptomeninges, and may be associated with an underlying cyst.[6,62] Gangliocytoma and ganglioglioma are mixed neuroepithelial tumors. When they are located in the cerebral hemispheres, they are often in the frontal and temporal lobes. Patients present with a 6- to 10-year clinical history of seizures.[63] On MRI or CT scans, a solid and cystic component is often present, with spotty enhancement in the solid component.[64] DNET is a benign cortical neuroepithelial tumor. It is diagnosed almost exclusively in children or young adults who undergo epilepsy surgery for intractable seizures.[65,66]

LGA must also be distinguished from astrocytomas with more aggressive biologic behavior, anaplastic astrocytoma and glioblastoma multiforme. Chamberlain and colleagues[67] found an absence of CT contrast enhancement in more than 30% of patients with anaplastic astrocytoma and 4% of those with of glioblastoma multiforme. These numbers would probably be less with MRI. In addition, a percentage of LGA show preoperative contrast enhancement.[44,53,68] Initially, it was reported that these patients had a similar prognosis to those with nonenhancing LGA.[68] Two more recent series addressing the significance of enhancement as a prognostic variable have reached opposite conclusions.[44,53]

Diagnostic Workup

The diagnostic imaging procedure of choice is MRI, but CT is an acceptable alternative. Physicians involved in the care of patients with brain tumors have encountered a significant number of young patients who present with seizures, and CT with and without contrast is normal. When MRI is ordered, it reveals an area of increased signal on T_2-weighted images and an area of decreased signal on T_1-weighted sequences. A biopsy specimen is then taken and found to have an LGA.

LGA typically presents with decreased signal on T_1-weighted MRI that merges imperceptibly with brain with no distinct margin or boundary (Fig. 9–2).[48,50] On T_2-weighted images, there is an area of increased signal that is equal in size or slightly larger than T_1-weighted abnormality. On noncontrast CT, there is a hypodense area (Fig. 9–3). Typically, these tumors do not enhance with contrast agents on either CT or MRI; however, in three series of LGA, CT contrast enhancement occurred in 26%, 36%, and 41% of patients.[44,53,69] The series with 41% of LGAs enhancing included 17 more aggressive grade III tumors (using Daumas-Duport grading).[53]

LGA is a homogeneous lesion without contrast enhancement in 65% to 75% of cases. Neurosurgeons are without a guide to the optimal biopsy location. In addition, they want to avoid eloquent cortex with the biopsy and resection. FDG-PET has been used to select brain lesions for biopsy by looking for areas of increased glucose utilization. Increased glucose utilization has been correlated with tumor cell density.[69–71] FDG-PET and echo-planar MRI may be used in the future to measure cerebral blood flow before and after activation tasks to locate eloquent cortex and aid the neurosurgeon in resection.

Treatment

SYMPTOMATIC

If seizures are the presenting symptom, diphenylhydantoin or carbamezepine should be used, with every attempt at monotherapy. There is no evidence that prophylactic anticonvulsants are beneficial in preventing seizures. Whereas some investigators recommend initial tumor resection for patients with intractable seizures who are suspected of having a LGA,[72] others recommend removing the epileptic focus along with the tumor, with preoperative electrocardiographic mapping or electrocorticography during the tumor resection.[73,74] Packer and colleagues[72] reported that 75% of children with seizures who underwent LGA tumor

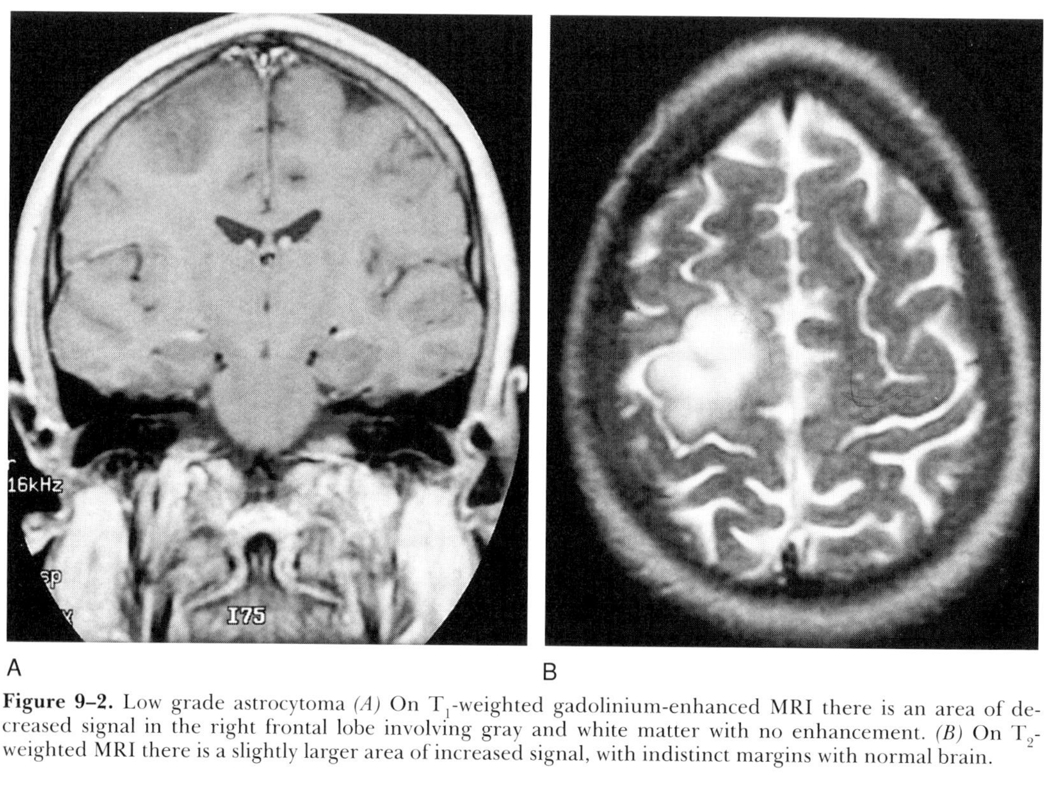

A B

Figure 9–2. Low grade astrocytoma *(A)* On T_1-weighted gadolinium-enhanced MRI there is an area of decreased signal in the right frontal lobe involving gray and white matter with no enhancement. *(B)* On T_2-weighted MRI there is a slightly larger area of increased signal, with indistinct margins with normal brain.

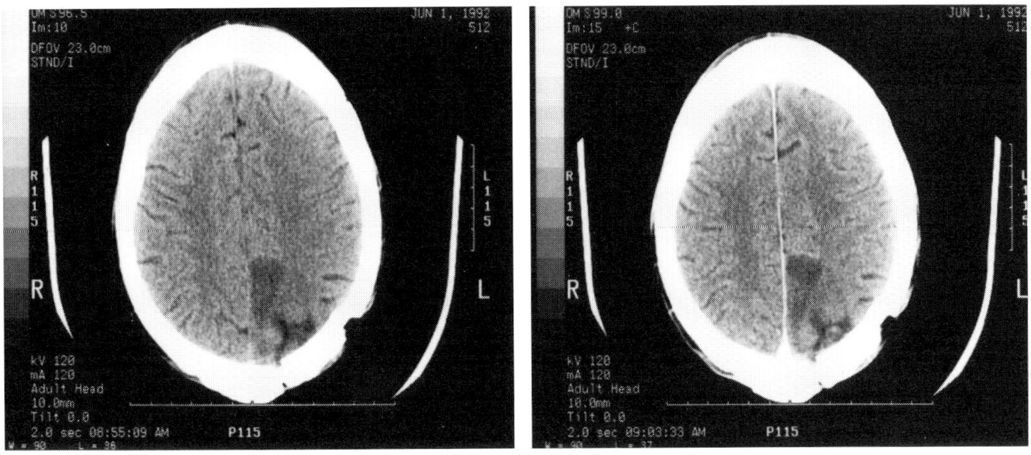

A B

Figure 9–3. Low grade astrocytoma. CT showing hypodense area in right frontal lobe white matter *(A)* before and *(B)* after contrast.

resection were seizure-free at 2 years. Patients who did best had less than a 1-year history of seizures and had a gross total resection. Berger and associates[74] agree with this approach but believe patients with intractable seizures should be monitored with intraoperative electrocorticography to identify and remove seizure foci near the neoplasm. A total of 88% of these patients were free of seizures, and 50% did not require epileptic drugs.

These tumors often infiltrate widely in the brain, producing increased intracranial pressure at diagnosis. This should be treated with corticosteroids, which produce some symptomatic relief in almost all patients. Dexamethasone is recommended in a dose of 2 to 4 mg 4 times day. Patients do not need to take it on a 6-hour schedule after the first few days, and in fact, can take dexamethasone two to three times day because of its relatively long half-life of 6 hours. If patients develop obstructive hydrocephalus from deep midline supratentorial or infratentorial LGA, temporary ventricular drainage or a ventriculoperitoneal shunt may be necessary.

SURGERY

A major area of controversy in the management of LGA is the unresolved question of when to perform surgery. Recht and colleagues[75] published a retrospective study of 26 patients who presented with a transient neurological event. The transient event was seizures in 23 of 26 patients. All patients had an MRI or CT study suggestive of an LGA. These patients were treated only with anticonvulsants until there was evidence of tumor growth, malignant tumor transformation, or intractable seizures (WAIT group). They were compared with 20 patients who presented similarly with a suspected LGA and had immediate surgical intervention (NO WAIT group). Other therapy was not specified. The median survival for both groups was 84 months, with no difference between the WAIT and NO WAIT groups. In the WAIT group, 15 patients eventually had surgery 4 to 129 months (median, 29 months) after diagnosis. In the WAIT group, seven of 15 patients older than 45 years of age had anaplastic tumors at surgery.

Recht and colleague's[75] analysis makes a strong case for watchful waiting in the patient who presents with a transient event and is suspected of having a LGA on imaging study. This conclusion is counterintuitive to the usual oncologic maxim of "making a diagnosis early and treating early." Clearly, with LGA, early diagnosis does not lead to cure. If the tumor is a more anaplastic neoplasm, it will progress in the next few months, and close follow-up enables the clinician to monitor growth and institute therapy. Are there treatable lesions that are being missed by waiting? All 15 lesions that required intervention in the WAIT group were gliomas. It is unlikely that any of these patients will have a brain abscess, and if they did, it would present quickly. What is to be gained by waiting? The patient postpones the risk of surgery and possible RT. The level of uncertainty that patients and physicians can live with varies widely; physicians have to individualize their approach to the patient. It is anticipated that all patients in the WAIT group will eventually have surgical intervention.

When surgery is performed, it is generally believed that there is a strong correlation between the extent of resection, postoperative tumor volume, and survival. However, no prospective randomized study has been performed to confirm this conclusion. Laws and associates[76] reported a series of 461 cases of LGA spanning 60 years in which patients who had biopsy or subtotal resection had a 5-year survival of 32% and a 15-year survival of 12%; patients who had gross total resection had a 5-year survival of 61% and a 15-year survival of 37%. Age was a stronger prognostic factor than extent of resection.[76]

In a retrospective study, Berger and coworkers[54] examined the preoperative tumor volume, the extent of resection, and recurrence in patients with LGA. For tumors greater than 10 cm^3, the greater the percent resection and the smaller the residual volume of tumor, the longer the time to recurrence. All patients who underwent 100% resection were disease-free at a mean follow-up of 54 months. Patients with a residual volume greater than 10 cm^3 had a recurrence rate of 46.2% and a time to progression of 30 months. The recurrence rate was less and the time to progression longer in operated patients, with a residual tumor volume of less than 10 cm^3. They had a 14.8% recurrence rate and time to progression of 50 months.

Kelly and colleagues[77] have shown that LGA tumor cells extended outside the noncontrast CT and T_2-weighted MRI abnormality (see Fig. 3–5). The T_2-weighted MRI abnormality matched the histological distribution of tumor cells more accurately than CT. The extension of tumor cells, outside imaged and resected areas, explains why these lesions eventually recur even after gross total resection.

Intraoperative ultrasound adds to preoperative imaging information, and a well-defined hyperechoic margin was seen with normal brain in 25 of 33 cases.[78] Eight patients had poorly defined ultrasound tumor margins with normal brain, and five of these patients had recurrent tumors and previous surgery.[78]

Stereotactic craniotomy has increased a neurosurgeon's ability to resect these diffusely infiltrating lesions. MRI or CT obtained with stereotactic frame in place localizes the abnormality in three- dimensional space with reference to the frame. A neurosurgeon can then pass operating instruments into the center of the tumor and resect the tumor from the center to the periphery according to coordinates on the imaging study. Kelly and colleagues[79–81], with sophisticated computer integration of preoperative imaging information and the stereotactic coordinates of the tumor, have developed a system that provides neurosurgeons with an image of the tumor in the operating microscope. In real time, neurosurgeons can visualize location of the operating instrument in the tumor being resected. This technique is particularly useful for resection of low-grade thalamic astrocytomas.

RADIATION THERAPY

A second significant area of controversy in LGA management is whether patients should receive adjuvant postoperative RT or whether RT should be deferred until recurrence. An important reason to defer RT is if its effect is marginal and its toxicity is significant. The Brain Tumor Cooperative Group (BTCG) attempted a randomized study of LGA patients after surgery to immediate RT or RT on recurrence or progression. They were unable to enter sufficient patients on trial because of patient and physician preferences, and the study was closed. Two clinical trials for LGA, designed by the European Organization for Research on Treatment of Cancer (EORTC) are currently in progress.

The most significant trial compares early postoperative RT with delayed RT on recurrence. The second trial randomizes patients with LGA to two different doses of RT, 45 and 59.4 Gy after surgery. The results from the second trial have been reported in abstract, and no difference is found in the 5-year survival of 47% in the 45 Gy group, the 5-year survival of 50% in the 59.4 Gy cohort.[82]

Until the EORTC reports its randomized trial of immediate versus delayed RT for LGA, clinicians must rely on retrospective studies comparing surgery with surgery plus RT and others of RT alone to provide treatment guidance (Table 9–2).[32,34,45,50,51,76,83–88] The largest study of 326 patients separated patients into two analysis groups: (1) surgery and RT greater than 4000 cGy (RT group), or (2) surgery and RT less than 4000 cGy (no RT group).[76] The RT group had a significantly better 5-year survival of 49% and a 15-year survival of 20% than the no RT group, which had a 34% 5-year survival and a 18% 15-year survival.[47,76]

In a later report from the same group[32], 121 patients with LGA or oligo-astrocytoma were divided into three treatment groups for analysis: (1) surgery alone (n=19), (2) surgery and low-dose RT (<53 Gy) (n=67), and (3) surgery and high-dose RT (>:53 Gy) (n=35). The 5-year survival rates were 32% for surgery, 47% for surgery and low-dose RT, and 68% for surgery and high-dose RT.[32] The 10-year survival rates were 11% for surgery, 21% for surgery and low-dose RT, and 39% for surgery and high-dose RT.

Leibel and associates[83] selected a group of LGA patients who had partial resection and RT, and compared this cohort with a group treated with only partial resection. The partial resection and RT survival rates were 46% and 35%, respectively, at 5 and 10 years compared with 19% and 11% survival rates in patients treated with partial resection alone. McCormack and coworkers[84] treated 48 patients with surgery and varying doses of RT (2400 to 6840 (median 5613) cGy), with a 5-year survival of 64%, and a 10-year survival of 48%.

In summary, most comparison studies suggest a survival advantage for surgery and RT. However, these studies are not controlled or randomized, and patient selection bias could be great.[47]

LGA anatomic recurrence patterns were examined after focal conformal RT in 46 patients. Eleven of 46 patients recurred, all within the area of abnormality on initial preoperative T_2-weighted MRI or CT.[89] Therefore, LGA is predominantly a focal disease despite tumor cells extending beyond the area of T^2-weighted signal abnormality on preoperative MRI scans.[77]

Tumor recurrence can be examined according to changes in histological grade of malignancy on recurrence. Tumors were graded according to the Ringertz system (see Table 1–4), and there were 72 astrocytomas at initial operation. At recurrence, 55% were anaplastic astrocytoma and 30% were glioblastoma, with a median time to recurrence of 30 months.[90] In another study, 14 of 25 (56%) LGAs dedifferentiated on recurrence. A total of 32% became glioblastoma and 24% became anaplastic astrocytoma during a median follow-up of 4.5 years.[88] In a pediatric study, 56 children were treated for LGA with focal RT. A median of 6.4 years after initial diagnosis, six patients had recurrence locally with more aggressive anaplastic astrocytoma.[91] Malignant dedifferentiation of an LGA previously was thought to be a rare event in children, and the more frequent occurrence reported in this study was believed to occur secondary to RT.

RT carries the potential risk of significant neurological or cognitive impairment. A total of 20 patients with LGA treated with early postoperative focal RT were compared with 21 patients with LGA who had surgery alone and l9 control patients with low-grade hematologic malignancies without CNS involvement. None of the patients in the three groups had significant neurological impairment, with a Karnofsky of 70 or greater in all patients. Patients in the two LGA groups had more cognitive impairment than the patients in the hematologic malignancy control group but they did not differ from each other in the degree of impairment.[92] A prospective study of patients with LGA receiving two different doses of focal RT,

Table 9–2. **Low-Grade Astrocytomas: Surgery ± Radiation Treatment**

Trial	Number of patients	Treatment	Survival Rate (Percentage) 5 Yr	10 Yr
Leibel et al[83] (1975)	35	Sa + RT (35–50 Gy)	19	15
	49		46*	35*
Laws et al[76] (1985)	461	S or S + RT (0–79 Gy)	36[b]	20[b]
	387	S or S + RT (40 Gy)	35[b]	10[b]
	74	S + RT (>40 Gy)	49[b]*	15[b]*
Garcia et al[34] (1985)	23	S	21	10[b]
	57	S + RT (35–61 Gy)	50	10[b]
Medbery et al[51] (1988)	50	Total Group	45	32
	25	S + RT (30–59 Gy)	22	13
	24	S + RT (>55 Gy)	55	45
Soffietti et al[85] (1989)	53	S	30	7
	21	S + RT (<Gy)	25	0
	11	S + RT (≥ 40 Gy)	9	9
Shaw et al[32] (1989)	19	S	32	11
	67	S + RT (<53 Gy)	47	21
	35	S + RT (>53 Gy)	68*	39*
Whitton and Bloom[45] (1990)	60	S + RT (50–55 Gy)	35	26
North et al[86c] (1990)	77	S or S + RT (50–55 Gy)	55	43
	66	S + RT (45–59 Gy)	66	NA
Vertosick et al[88] (1991)	25	S or S + RT (54–60 Gy)	65[b]	33[b]
McCormack et al[84] (1992)	53	S + RT (24–68 Gy)	64	48[b]
Shibamoto et al[87] (1993)	18	S	37	11
	101	S + RT (41–66 Gy)	60*	41*
Pollack et al[50d] (1995)	16a	S	95[b]	87[b]
	33a	S + RT (>50 Gy)	93[b]	93[b]

* = significant differences in groups.
a = Patients with subtotal resection only.
b = Estimate from graph.
c = 25 children included.
d = all children.
NA = not available.
RT = Radiation therapy.
S = Surgery.

5040 and 6480 cGy, found no cognitive change in either focal RT group.[93]

In summary, surgery with immediate postoperative RT appears to have a slight survival advantage in nonrandomized studies. Neuropsychological assessment after focal RT does not reveal significant cognitive impairment in adjuvant RT groups. However, if observation of patients who present with seizures and LGA does not adversely affect survival, an acceptable alternative is delaying RT in this population after biopsy until tumor growth occurs.

INTERSTITIAL RADIOTHERAPY

A total of 250 patients with grade II astrocytomas of 4 cm or less were treated with permanent and temporary Iodine-125 (^{125}I) implants and had 5- and 10-year survival rates of 61% and 51%, respectively.[94] The survival rates for interstitial brachytherapy do not seem better than the 68% 5-year, and 38% 10-year survival rates with high-dose (> 53 Gy) focal external-beam study.[32] In addition, the inclusion criteria for interstitial radiotherapy limits tumor size to 4 cm, and this tends to produce a more favorable outcome in the implant group.

CHEMOTHERAPY

A total of 60 patients with subtotally resected LGA were randomly assigned to receive focal RT or focal RT and CCNU every 6 weeks. The median survival for all patients was 4.45 years, with the RT group at 4.5 years and the RT and CCNU group at 7.4 years. The difference was not statistically significant.[46] At the present time, chemotherapy is not used in the adjuvant therapy of LGA. Chemotherapy should be considered at recurrence after RT, either as an LGA or as a more anaplastic tumor.

Prognosis and Complications

The prognosis for LGA treated with surgery and RT is a 5-year survival of slightly greater than 65% and a 10-year survival of approximately 40%. LGA occurs early in life, with a peak incidence in the third through fifth decades. Patients with LGA have, on the average, a greater shortening of predicted life span than patients with high-grade astrocytoma.

Favorable prognostic factors for survival in LGA include younger age, gross total resection, and extent of resection.[95] RT was a positive prognostic variable in a few series, and imaging contrast enhancement, a negative prognostic variable in others.

Eight cases of LGA were recently reported, with neuraxis dissemination at diagnosis.[96] Primary tumor sites were the hypothalamus in four patients, the brainstem or spinal cord in three, and the temporal lobe in one. All tumors spread along CSF pathways. The tumors responded to a variable combination of surgery, RT, and chemotherapy, and seven of eight patients survived a median of 15 months postdiagnosis.

Radiation-induced astrocytomas have been reported after cranial RT for nonmalignant conditions (i.e., tinea capitis), non-neural malignancies (i.e., acute lymphoblastic leukemia), and malignant neuroepithelial tumors (i.e., ependymoma and medulloblastoma).[97]

OTHER "BENIGN" NEUROEPITHELIAL NEOPLASMS

Subependymal Giant Cell Astrocytoma

Subependymal giant cell astrocytoma is a calcified intraventricular tumor arising from the walls of the lateral ventricles, occurring almost entirely in tuberous sclerosis.[6,98] These tumors grow very slowly and typically occur in the region of the head of the caudate. Macroscopically, they are gray to pinkish-red in color. Microscopically, they are composed of large plump cells with eosinophilic cytoplasm, which resemble astrocytes (see Fig. 1–7).[6] These tumors are pleomorphic and may have mitoses, endothelial proliferation, hemorrhage, and necrosis. Their biologic behavior is grade I, at variance with their histology. This is similar to pilocytic actrocytoma.[99] On electron microscopy, the cells have abundant cytoplasm and numerous astrocytic filaments. Some have neurofilaments.[21] On immunohistochemistry, almost all stain with the neuronal marker S-100, and 50% of the tumors stained with GFAP. These tumors are thought to arise from immature germinal matrix cells that have yet to differentiate into astrocytes or neurons.[100]

Subependymal giant cell astrocytoma becomes symptomatic by obstructing the foramen of Monro and producing obstructive hydrocephalus, with development of increased intracranial pressure. In neonatal patients who are thought to have tuberous sclerosis, cranial ultrasound can be used to diagnose the tumor on the ventricular wall.[101] This can be followed with CT to define the anatomy more clearly. Subependymal giant cell astrocytoma is frequently calcified, and on cranial radiographs the calcifications produce a pattern that has been referred to as "candle gutterings."[99]

When symptomatic, the treatment of choice for these tumors, is complete surgical resection, which will effect a cure. Subtotal resection may also produce a similar clinical outcome. In children with tuberous sclerosis, these tumors should be followed periodically after diagnosis with CT or MRI and subtotal resection. Use of CT and MRI permits diagnosis and treatment of presymptomatic hydrocephalus just before the development of symptoms. If hydrocephalus does not resolve with tumor removal, shunting may be necessary.

Pleomorphic Xanthoastrocytoma

Pleomorphic xanthoastrocytoma is a rare superficial cerebral hemisphere tumor that is typically located in the temporal lobe with extensive leptomenigeal involvement.[6,99] It may be associated with an underlying proteinaceous cyst.[6,21,62] Pleomorphic xanthoastrocytoma is a tumor of children and young adults. The tumor cells are pleomorphic GFAP-staining astrocytes that vary from typical fibrillary astrocytes to vacuolated lipid-laden multinucleated giant cells.[6,99] These cells are surrounded by reticulin because of the presence of a basement membrane (Fig. 1–6A). The tumor is well demarcated and has a grade II biologic behavior.[6] The usual clinical presentation is chronic seizures or headache.[21,62] CT often shows a cystic tumor with contrast enhancement of the solid portion.[102] The differential diagnosis for a cystic peripheral contrast-enhancing lesion includes pilocytic astrocytoma, LGA, glioblastoma multiforme, oligodendroglioma, oligo-astrocytoma, ganglioglioma, metastasis, and because of the peripheral location, meningioma. Gross total surgical removal is the treatment of choice. When surgical removal is complete, a cure may be effected. If this is not possible, local regrowth may occur and focal RT should be considered. The most important prognostic factor in survival is the completeness of resection.[62] A rare, more malignant variant exists, with a grade III biologic behavior and pathology revealing mitotic figures, endothelial proliferation, and necrosis (Fig. 1–6B).

Gangliocytoma and Ganglioglioma

Gangliocytoma is composed of two cell types, neoplastic ganglion cells and a minor component of normal supportive astrocytes (see Fig. 1–13A). The ganglioglioma differs from the gangliocytoma in that it is composed of both neoplastic ganglion cells and neoplastic astrocytes. They both occur in children and young adults in any CNS location but typically intracerebrally in the temporal lobe.[6] They also occur frequently in the spinal cord.[63] Gangliocytoma grows slowly and does not undergo anaplastic change. It has a grade I biologic behavior.[6] If symptomatic, the treatment of choice is complete resection.

Ganglioglioma is a firm grayish tumor that is more often cystic than gangliocytoma.[6] Microscopically, pathological identification is difficult because small biopsies may not contain neurons among astrocytes, or alternatively, the astrocytes may resemble neurons.[103] Larger samples contain an astrocytic component that should immunostain with GFAP and a neuronal component that stains with synaptophysin.[99,103] It has a grade II biologic behavior.[6] Ganglioglioma is graded by its astrocytic component; rarely, the astrocytic component has anaplastic features with a grade III biologic behavior.[6]

Seizures were the most common presenting symptom in 15 of 19 cases in one series of tumors in the cerebral hemisphere.[63] Headache was the presenting symptom in three patients with deep tumors. Twelve of 19 patients were neurologically normal, and the other seven had mild to moderate focal neurological deficits.[63] Nine tumors occurred in the brainstem, and unilateral cranial nerve abnormalities were common. Spinal cord ganglioglioma presented with back pain in 87% and 23 of 26 patients had associated weakness. Three patients presented with weakness alone.[63] CT scans usually demonstrated a hypodense or isodense, often cystic, abnormality with spotty contrast enhancement.[64]

The differential diagnosis includes gangliocytoma, pilocytic astrocytoma, pleomorphic xanthoastrocytoma, LGA, anaplastic astrocytoma, glioblastoma multiforme, oligodendroglioma, oligo-astrocytoma, and DNET. Gross total resection is the treatment of choice, regardless of tumor location. This can be accomplished much more frequently in the cerebral hemispheres and spinal cord than in the brainstem. Focal RT is generally administered to patients with subtotal resection, adjuvantly or at recurrence.[63] Chemotherapy is occasionally used to treat patients with anaplastic grade III ganglioglioma.[63]

Desmoplastic Infantile Ganglioglioma

Desmoplastic infantile ganglioglioma is a rare mixed neuronal and glial neoplasm of infancy.[6] Most cases occur before the age of 18 months to 2 years.[6,99] They invariably involve the meninges and may attain considerable size before diagnosis.[99] They contain a mixture of neuroepithelial cells that have astrocytic and neuronal differentiation.[6] They have a grade I biologic behavior. Patients present with seizures and occasionally symptoms of increased intracranial pressure. CT and MRI scans show a superficial cystic tumor with enhancement of the solid component.[104] The differential diagnosis includes medulloblastoma, ependymoma, pleomorphic xanthoastrocytoma, and superficial astrocytoma. The treatment of choice is gross total resection, and cure is anticipated.[105] RT and chemotherapy have been used after subtotal resection, but their role is not defined.

Dysembryoplastic Neuroepithelial Tumor

DNET is a benign, mixed neuronal glial neoplasm composed predominantly of neoplastic oligodendrocytes and neurons but also neoplastic astrocytes (see Fig. 1–14).[6] Pathologically, DNET may be confused with an oligodendroglioma if the neuronal component is inconspicuous.[6,99] The cortex surrounding the tumor is often dysplastic. Cystic change and calcification may be present.[6,66] The biologic behavior is grade I. This type of tumor occurs in children, with a median age at diagnosis of 6.6 years.[66] The presenting symptom is intractable complex partial seizures without neurological deterioration.[64,66] In one series, 12 of 14 tumors were equally divided between frontal and temporal locations.[66] CT scans showed hypodense lesions that were cystic in two thirds of the patients and had slight focal contrast enhancement in one third of the patients.[66] Nonenhanced MRI scans showed decreased signal on T_1-weighted images and increased signal on T_2-weighted images,[65,66] with variable contrast enhancement with gadolinium.[66] The clinical differential diagnosis includes oligodendroglioma, oligo-astrocytoma, ganglioglioma, hamartoma, pilocytic astrocytoma, pleomorphic xanthoastrocytoma, astrocytoma, and anaplastic astrocytoma.

Gross total resection is the treatment of choice. The long-term outcome of these patients is thought to be excellent with a cure likely.[64] DNET was described in 1988; therefore, long-term follow-up is not available. It is important to recognize DNET as distinct from oligodendroglioma or astrocytoma so RT and chemotherapy can then be avoided.

Central Neurocytoma

Central neurocytoma is the most common intraventricular tumor. It involves the septum pellucidum and the foramen of Monro in young adults.[6,99] The tumor has also been described in the cervical spinal cord.[106] It is composed of uniform round cells with clear cytoplasm and cell membranes, which mirror an oligodendroglioma. The neuronal differentiation is shown on electron microscopy, with axons, synapses, microtubules, and neurosecretory granules. It stains positively with the immunohistochemical marker synaptophysin, and may co-express GFAP.[6,99,107] The biologic behavior is Grade I.

Kim and colleagues[107] reported on a series of seven patients, with a median age of 24.6 years and a range of 15 to 38 years. The main symptoms and signs were associated with increased intracranial pressure consisting of headache (100%), papilledema (86%), and vomiting (71%).[107] CT imaged a cystic abnormality that varied from isodense to hyperdense with homogeneous contrast enhancement in all cases. Four patients had calcification in their tumors. MRI scans showed an isointense to hyperintense signal on both T_1- and T_2-weighted images, with gadolinium enhancement in the three cases in which it was administered.[107] The differential diagnosis includes intraventricular oligodendroglioma and ependymoma.

The treatment of choice is gross total resection, which should result in cure.[107] Central neurocytoma is gelatinous in consistency and well demarcated from normal adjacent brain.[108] Recently, a malignant variant of central neurocytoma has been described.[109] RT and chemotherapy should be considered for treatment of the malignant variant.

CHAPTER SUMMARY

The low-grade neuroepithelial tumors discussed in this chapter all tend to occur most frequently in the first four decades of life. Pilocytic astrocytoma is sharply demarcated from normal brain, and although the histology of the tumor is at times anaplastic, it has a grade I biologic behavior. It is cured by complete surgical resection.

LGA is a locally invasive tumor that cannot be excised surgically because of its infiltrative growth pattern. This type of tumor grows more slowly than anaplastic astrocytoma but produces neurological disability and death by infiltration of normal brain and by growth in a rigid skull. They have a grade II biologic behavior. When a patient presents with seizures, normal neurologic examination results, and a mass suspected to be a LGA, the appropriate timing of surgery is uncertain. RT is used postoperatively in the majority of patients, but it is appropriate to defer RT after gross total excision. The exact role of postoperative RT has not been answered in a randomized study. The EORTC has a study in progress comparing immediate RT with delayed postoperative RT on recurrence.

Subependymal giant cell astrocytoma is a grade I tumor that grows in the ventricular wall in patients with tuberous sclerosis. It is often asymptomatic and should not be treated unless symptomatic. Gangliocytoma, desmoplastic infantile ganglioglioma, DNET, and central neurocytoma are all benign grade I neoplasms, with a neuronal and astrocytic component. The tumors present with seizures or increased intracranial pressure and can be cured surgically.

Pleomorphic xanthoastrocytoma and ganglioglioma are both neoplasms with grade II biologic behavior. They occur in children and young adults and have a predilection for the temporal lobe. They present most frequently with seizures.

Pleomorphic xanthoastrocytoma and ganglioglioma are frequently enhancing cystic tumors. Gross total resection is the treatment of choice. If they regrow, RT should be considered.

REFERENCES

1. Ribbert, H: Über das spongioblastom und das gliom. Virchows Arch 225:195–213, 1918.
2. Bailey, P, and Cushing, H: A Classification of the Tumors of the Glioma Group on a Histogenetic Basis with a Correlated Study of Prognosis. JB Lippincott Company, Philadelphia, 1926, pp 146–153.
3. Penfield, W: The classification of gliomas and neuroglia cell types. Arch Neurol Psychiat 26: 745–753, 1931.
4. Kagan, H: Anorexia and severe inanition associated with a tumour involving the hypothalamus. Arch Dis Child 33:257–260, 1958.
5. Rubinstein, LJ: Tumors of the Central Nervous System. Armed Forces Institute of Pathology, Washington (Atlas of Tumor Pathology, second series, fascicle 6), 1972.
6. Kleihues, P, Burger, PC, and Scheithauer, BW: Histological Typing of Tumours of the Central Nervous System, Ed 2. World Health Organization, Springer-Verlag, 1993.
7. Wallner, KE, Gonzales, MF, Edwards, MSB, et al: Treatment results of juvenile pilocytic astrocytoma. J Neurosurg 69:171–176, 1988.
8. Coakley, KJ, Huston, J III, Scheithauer, BW, et al: Pilocytic astrocytomas: Well-demarcated magnetic resonance appearance despite frequent infiltration histologically. Mayo Clin Proc 70:747–751, 1995.
9. Zülch, KJ: Pilocytic Astrocytomas. Brain Tumors. Their Biology and Pathology, Ed. 3. Springer-Verlag, Berlin, 1986, pp 221–232.
10. Palma, L, and Guidetti, B: Cystic pilocytic astrocytomas of the cerebral hemispheres. Surgical experience with 51 cases and long-term results. J Neurosurg 62:811–815, 1985.
11. von Deimling, A, Louis, DN, Menon, AG, et al: Deletions on the long arm of chromosome 17 in pilocytic astrocytoma. Acta Neuropathol (Berl) 86:81–85, 1993.
12. James, CD, He, J, Carlbom, E, et al: Loss of genetic information in central nervous system tumors common to children and young adults. Genes Chrom Cancer 2:94–102, 1990.
13. Lang, FF, Miller, DC, Koslow, M, and Newcomb, EW: Pathways leading to glioblastoma multiforme: a molecular analysis of genetic alterations in 65 astrocytic tumors. J Neurosurg 81:427–436, 1994.
14. von Deimling, A, Louis, DN, von Ammon, K, et al: Evidence for a tumor suppressor gene on chromosome 19q associated with human astrocytomas, oligodendrogliomas, and mixed gliomas. Cancer Res 52:4277–4279, 1992.
15. Ito, S, Hoshino, T, Shibuya, M, et al: Proliferative characteristics of juvenile pilocytic astrocytomas determined by bromodeoxyuridine labeling. Neurosurgery 31:413–419, 1992.
16. Jay, V, Parkinson, D, Becker, L, and Chan, F-W: Cell kinetic analysis in pediatric brain and spinal tumors: A study of 117 cases with Ki-67 quantitation and flow cytometry. Pediatric Pathology 14:253–276, 1994.
17. Forsyth, PA, Shaw, EG, Scheithauer, BW, et al: Supratentorial pilocytic astrocytomas. A clinicopathologic, prognostic, and flow cytometric study of 51 patients. Cancer 72:1335–1342, 1993.
18. Fulham, MJ, Melisi, JW, Nishimiya, J, et al: Neuroimaging of juvenile pilocytic astrocytomas: An enigma. Radiology 189:221–225, 1993.
19. Clark, GB, Henry, JM, and McKeever, PE: Cerebral pilocytic astrocytoma. Cancer 56: 1128–1133, 1985.
20. Garcia, DM, and Fulling, KH: Juvenile pilocytic astrocytoma of the cerebrum in adults. A distinctive neoplasm with favorable prognosis. J Neurosurg 63:382–386, 1985.
21. Russell, DS, and Rubinstein, LJ: Pathology of Tumours of the Nervous System, Ed. 4. The Williams and Wilkins Company, Baltimore, 1997, pp 159–163.
22. Lloyd, LA: Gliomas of the optic nerve and chiasm in childhood. Trans Am Ophthalmol Soc 71:488–535, 1973.
23. Borit, A, and Richardson, EP Jr: The biological and clinical behaviour of pilocytic astrocytomas of the optic pathways. Brain 105:161–187, 1982.
24. Tenny, RT, Laws, ER Jr, Younge, BR, and Rush, JA: The neurosurgical management of optic glioma. Results in 104 patients. J Neurosurg 57: 452–458, 1982.
25. Packer, RJ: Chiasmatic Gliomas. In Gilman, S, Goldstein, G, and Waxman, S (eds): Neurobase. Arbor Publishing Corporation, San Diego, 1995.
26. Lee, Y-Y, Van Tassel, P, Bruner, JM, et al: Juvenile pilocytic astrocytomas: CT and MR characteristics. AJNR 10:363–370, 1989.
27. Flickinger, JC, Torres, C, and Deutsch, M: Management of low-grade gliomas of the optic nerve and chiasm. Cancer 61:635–642, 1988.
28. Haddad, SF, Moore, SA, Menezes, AH, and VanGilder, JC: Ganglioglioma: 13 years of experience. Neurosurgery 31:171–178, 1992.
29. Strong, JA, Hatten, HP Jr, Brown, MT, et al: Pilocytic astrocytoma: correlation between the initial imaging features and clinical aggressiveness. AJR Am J Roetgenol 161:369–372, 1993.
30. Campbell, JW, and Pollack, IF: Cerebellar astrocytomas in children. J Neurooncol 28:223–231, 1996.
31. Berger, MS, Leibel, SA, Bruner ,JM, et al: Primary central nervous system tumors of the supratentorial compartment. In Levin, VA (ed): Cancer in the Nervous System. Churchill Livingstone, New York, 1996, pp 57–126.

32. Shaw, EG, Daumas-Duport, C, Scheithauer, BW, et al: Radiation therapy in the management of low-grade supratentorial astrocytomas. J Neurosurg 70:853–861, 1989.
33. Shaw, EG, Scheithauer, BW, and O'Fallon, JR: Management of supratentorial low-grade gliomas. Oncology 7:97–107, 1993.
34. Garcia, DM, Fulling, KH, and Marks, JE: The value of radiation therapy in addition to surgery for astrocytomas of the adult cerebrum. Cancer 55:919–927, 1985.
35. Afra, D, Müller, W, Slowik, F, and Firsching, R: Supratentorial lobar pilocytic astrocytomas: Report of 45 operated cases, including 9 recurrences. Acta Neurochir (Wien) 81:90–93, 1986.
36. Brown, MT, Friedman, HS, Oakes, WJ, et al: Chemotherapy for pilocytic astrocytomas. Cancer 71:3165–3172, 1993.
37. Mamelak, AN, Prados, MD, Obana, WG, et al: Treatment options and prognosis for multicentric juvenile pilocytic astrocytoma. J Neurosurg 81:24–30, 1994.
38. Packer, RJ, Sutton, LN, Bilaniuk, LT, et al: Treatment of chiasmatic/hypothalamic gliomas of childhood with chemotherapy: An update. Ann Neurol 23:79–85, 1988.
39. Packer, RJ, Lange, B, Ater, J, et al: Carboplatin and vincristine for recurrent and newly diagnosed low grade gliomas of childhood. J Clin Oncol 11:850–856, 1992.
40. Petronio, J, Edwards, MSB, Prados, M, et al: Management of chiasmal and hypothalamic gliomas of infancy and childhood with chemotherapy. J Neurosurg 74:701–708, 1991.
41. Kernohan, JW, and Sayre, GP: Atlas of Tumor Pathology: Tumors of the Central Nervous System. Armed Forces Institute of Pathology, Washington, 1952.
42. Ringertz, N: Grading of gliomas. Acta Pathol Microbiol Scand 27:51–64, 1950.
43. Daumas-Duport, C, Scheithauer, BW, O'Fallon, J, and Kelly, P: Grading of astrocytomas. A simple and reproducible method. Cancer 62:2152–2165, 1988.
44. Piepmeier, JM: Observations on the current treatment of low-grade astrocytic tumors of the cerebral hemispheres. J Neurosurg 67:177–181, 1987.
45. Whitton, AC, and Bloom, HJG: Low grade glioma of the cerebral hemispheres in adults: A retrospective analysis of 88 cases. Int J Radiat Oncol Biol Phys 18:783–786, 1990.
46. Eyre, HJ, Crowley, JJ, Townsend, JJ, et al: A randomized trial of radiotherapy versus radiotherapy plus CCNU for incompletely resected low-grade gliomas: A Southwest Oncology Group study. J Neurosurg 78:909–914, 1993.
47. Macdonald, DR: Low-grade gliomas, mixed gliomas, and oligodendrogliomas. Seminars Oncology 21:236–248, 1994.
48. Lunsford, LD, Somaza, S, Kondziolka, D, and Flickinger, JC: Survival after stereotactic biopsy and irradiation of cerebral nonanaplastic, nonpilocytic astrocytoma. J Neurosurg 82:523–529, 1995.
49. Guthrie, BL, and Laws, ER Jr: Supratentorial low-grade gliomas. Neurosurg Clin N Am 1:37–48, 1990.
50. Pollack, IF, Claassen, D, Al-Shboul, Q, et al: Low-grade gliomas of the cerebral hemispheres in children: an analysis of 71 cases. J Neurosurg 82:536–547, 1995.
51. Medbery, CA III, Straus, KL, Steinberg, SM, et al: Low-grade astrocytomas: Treatment results and prognostic variables. Int J Radiat Oncol Biol Phys 15:837–841, 1988.
52. Radhakrishnan, K, Bohnen, NI, and Kurland, LT: Epidemiology of brain tumors. In Morantz, RA, and Walsh, J (eds): Brain Tumors: A Comprehensive Text. Marcel Dekker, New York, 1994, pp 1–18.
53. Janny, P, Cure, H, Mohr, M, et al: Low grade supratentorial astrocytomas. Management and prognostic factors. Cancer 73:1937–1945, 1994.
54. Berger, MS, Deliganis, AV, Dobbins, J, and Keles, GE: The effect of extent of resection on recurrence in patients with low grade cerebral hemisphere gliomas. Cancer 74:1784–1791, 1994.
55. Collins, VP, and James, CD: Molecular genetics of primary intracranial tumors. Curr Opin Oncol 2:666–672, 1990.
56. James, CD, and Collins, VP: Molecular genetic characterization of CNS tumor oncogenesis. Adv Cancer Res 58:121–142, 1992.
57. Yoshii, Y, Maki, Y, Tsuboi, K, et al: Estimation of growth fraction with bromodeoxyuridine in human central nervous system tumors. J Neurosurg 65:659–663, 1986.
58. Ito, S, Chandler, KL, Prados, MD, et al: Proliferative potential and prognostic evaluation of low-grade astrocytomas. J Neurooncol 19:1–9, 1994.
59. Fried, I, Kim, JH, and Spencer, DD: Limbic and Neocortical gliomas associated with intractable seizures: A distinct clinicopathological group. Neurosurgery 34:815–824, 1994.
60. Coons, SW, Johnson, PC, and Shapiro, JR: Cytogenetic and flow cytometry DNA analysis of regional heterogeneity in a low grade human glioma. Cancer Res 55:1569–1577, 1995.
61. Krouwer, HGJ, and Prados, MD: Infiltrative astrocytomas of the thalamus. J Neurosurg 82:548–557, 1995.
62. Kepes, JJ, Rubinstein, LJ, and Eng, LF: Pleomorphic xanthoastrocytoma: A distinctive meningocerebral glioma of young subjects with relatively favorable prognosis. A study of 12 cases. Cancer 44:1839–1852, 1979.
63. Lang, FF, Epstein, FJ, Ransohoff, J, et al: Central nervous system gangliogliomas. Part 2: Clinical outcome. J Neurosurg 79:867–873, 1993.
64. Castillo, M, Davis, PC, Takei, Y, and Hoffman, JC Jr: Intracranial glioma: MR, CT and clinical findings in 18 patients. AJR Am J Roentgenol 154:607–612, 1990.
65. Daumas-Duport, C, Schiethauer, BW, Chodkeiwicz, J-P, et al: Dysembryoplastic neuroepithelial tumor: A surgically curable tumor of young

patients with intractable partial seizures. Report of 39 cases. Neurosurgery 23:545–556, 1988.

66. Taratuto, AL, Pomata, H, Sevlever, G, et al: Dysembryoplastic neuroepithelial tumor: Morphological, immunocytochemical, and deoxyribonucleic acid analyses in a pediatric series. Neurosurgery 36:474–481, 1995.
67. Chamberlain, MC, Murovic, JA, and Levin, VA: Absence of contrast enhancement on CT brain scans of patients with supratentorial malignant gliomas. Neurology 38:1371–1374, 1988.
68. Silverman, C, and Marks, JE: Prognostic significance of contrast enhancement in low-grade astrocytomas of the adult cerebrum. Radiology 139:211–213, 1981.
69. Hanson, MW, Glantz, MJ, Hoffman, JM, et al: FDG-PET in the selection of brain lesions for biopsy. J Comput Assist Tomogr 15(5):796–801, 1991.
70. Herholz, K, Pietrzyk, U, Voges, J, et al: Correlation of glucose consumption and tumor cell density in astrocytomas. J Neurosurg 79:853–858, 1993.
71. Levivier, M, Goldman, S, Pirotte, B, et al: Diagnostic yield of stereotactic brain biopsy guided by positron emission tomography with [^{18}F]fluorodeoxyglucose. J Neurosurg 82:445–452, 1995.
72. Packer, RJ, Sutton, LN, Patel, KM, et al: Seizure control following tumor surgery for childhood cortical low-grade gliomas. J Neurosurg 80:998–1003, 1994.
73. Rasmussen, T: Surgery of epilepsy associated with brain tumors. Adv Neurol 8:227–239, 1975.
74. Berger, MS, Ghatan, S, Haglund, MM, et al: Low-grade gliomas associated with intractable epilepsy: seizure outcome utilizing electrocorticography during tumor resection. J Neurosurgey 79:62–69, 1993.
75. Recht, LD, Lew, R, and Smith, TW: Suspected low-grade glioma: Is deferring treatment safe? Ann Neurol 31:431–436, 1992.
76. Laws, ER Jr, Taylor, WF, Clifton, MB, and Okazaki, H: Neurosurgical management of low-grade astrocytoma of the cerebral hemispheres. J Neurosurg 61:665–673, 1984.
77. Kelly, PJ, Daumas-Duport, C, Scheithauer, BW, et al: Stereotactic histological correlations of computed tomography- and magnetic resonance imaging-defined abnormalities in patients with glial neoplasms. Mayo Clin Proc 62:450–459, 1987.
78. Le Roux, PD, Berger, MS, Wang, K, et al: Low grade gliomas: comparison of intraoperative ultrasound characteristics with preoperative imaging studies. J Neurooncol 13:189–198, 1992.
79. Kelly, PJ, Kall, BA, Goerss, S, and Earnest, F IV: Computer-assisted stereotaxic laser resection on intra-arterial brain neoplasms. J Neurosurg 64:427–439, 1986.
80. Kelly, PJ: Volumetric stereotactic surgical resection of intra-axial brain mass lesions. Mayo Clin Proc 63:1186–1198, 1988.
81. Kelly, PJ: Stereotactic biopsy and resection of thalamic astrocytomas. Neurosurgery 25:185–194, 1989.
82. Van Glabbeke, M, Karim, ABMF, Hamers, H, et al: No improvement in survival by an increased radiation dose given postoperatively to patients (pts) with low grade brain tumors: an EORTC randomized phase III study. Proc Am Soc Clin Oncol 14:145, 1995.
83. Leibel, SA, Sheline, GE, Wara, WM, et al: The role of radiation therapy in the treatment of astrocytomas. Cancer 35:1551–1557, 1975.
84. McCormack, BM, Miller, DC, Budzilovich, GN, et al: Treatment and survival of low-grade astrocytoma in adults, 1977–1988. Neurosurgery 31:636–642, 1992.
85. Soffietti, R, Chiò, A, Giordana MT, et al: Prognostic factors in well-differentiated cerebral astrocytomas in the adult. Neurosurgery 24:686–692, 1989.
86. North, CA, North, RB, Epstein, JA, et al: Low-grade cerebral astrocytomas. Survival and quality of life after radiation therapy. Cancer 66:6–14, 1990.
87. Shibamoto, Y, Kitakabu, Y, Takahashi, M, et al: Supratentorial low-grade astrocytoma. Correlation of computed tomography findings with effect of radiation therapy and prognostic variables. Cancer 72:190–195, 1993.
88. Vertosick, FT Jr, Selker, RG, and Arena, VC: Survival of patients with well-differentiated astrocytomas diagnosed in the era of computed tomography. Neurosurgery 28:496–501, 1991.
89. Pu, AT, Sandler, HM, Radany, EH, et al: Low grade gliomas: preliminary analysis of failure patterns among patients treated using 3D conformal external beam irradiation. Int J Radiat Oncol Biol Phys 31:461–466, 1995.
90. Müller, W, Afra, D, and Schröder, R: Supratentorial recurrences of gliomas. Morphological studies in relation to time intervals with astroctyomas. Acta Neurochir (Wien) 37:75–91, 1977.
91. Dirks, PB, Jay, V, Becker, LE, et al: Development of anaplastic changes in low-grade astrocytomas of childhood. Neurosurgery 34:68–78, 1994.
92. Taphoorn, MJB, Schiphorst, AK, Snoek, FJ, et al: Cognitive functions and quality of life in patients with low-grade gliomas: the impact of radiotherapy. Ann Neurol 36:48–54, 1994.
93. Hammack, J, Shaw, E, Ivnik, R, et al: Neurocognitive function in patients receiving radiation therapy (RT) for supratentorial low grade glioma (LGG): a North Central Cancer Treatment Group (NCCTG) prospective study. Proc Am Soc Clin Oncol 14:151, 1995.
94. Kreth, FW, Faist, M, Warnke, PC, et al: Interstitial radiosurgery of low-grade gliomas. J Neurosurg 82:418–429, 1995.
95. Scerrati, M, Roselli, R, Iacoangeli, M, et al: Prognostic factors in low grade (WHO grade II) gliomas of the cerebral hemispheres: the role of surgery. J Neurol Neurosurg Psychiatry 61:291–296, 1996.

96. Gajjar, A, Bhargava, R, Jenkins, JJ, et al: Low-grade astrocytoma with neuraxis dissemination at diagnosis. J Neurosurg 83:67–71, 1995.
97. Shapiro, S, Mealey, J Jr, and Sartorius, C: Radiation-induced intracranial malignant gliomas. J Neurosurg 71:77–82, 1989.
98. Boesel, CP, Paulson, GW, Kosmik, EJ, and Earle, KM: Brain hamartomas and tumors associated with tuberous sclerosis. Neurosurgery 4:410–417, 1979.
99. McKeever, PE, and Blaivas, M: The brain, spinal cord, and meninges. In Sternberg SS (ed): Diagnostic Surgical Pathology, Ed. 2. Raven Press, Ltd., New York, 1994, pp 409–492.
100. Nakamura, Y, and Becker, LE: Subependymal giant-cell tumor: astrocytic or neuronal? Acta Neuropathol (Berl) 60:271–277, 1983.
101. Hahn, JS, Bejar, R, and Gladson, CL: Neonatal subependymal giant cell astrocytoma associated with tuberous sclerosis: MRI, CT and ultrasound correlation. Neurology 41:124–128, 1991.
102. Kros, JM, Vecht, CJ, and Stefanko, SZ: The pleomorphic xanthoastrocytoma and its differential diagnosis: a study of five cases. Hum Pathol 22:1128–1135, 1991.
103. Miller, DC, Lang, FF, and Epstein, FJ: Central nervous system gangliogliomas. Part 1: pathology. J Neurosurg 79:859–866, 1993.
104. Taratuto, AL, Monges, J, Lylyk, P, and Leiguarda, R: Superficial cerebral astrocytoma attached to dura. Report of six cases in infants Cancer 54:2505–2512, 1984.
105. VandenBerg, SR, May, EE, Rubinstein, LJ, et al: Desmoplastic supratentorial neuroepithelial tumors of infancy with divergent differentiation potential ("desmoplastic infantile gangliogliomas"). Report on 11 cases of a distinctive embryonal tumor with favorable prognosis. J Neurosurg 66:58–71, 1987.
106. Tatter, SB, Borges, LF, and Louis, DN: Central neurocytomas of the cervical spinal cord. Report of two cases. J Neurosurg 81:288–293, 1994.
107. Kim, DG, Chi, JG, Park, SH, et al: Intraventricular neurocytoma: clinicopathological analysis of seven cases. J Neurosurg 76:759–765, 1992.
108. Nishio, S, Takeshita, I, Kaneko, Y, and Fukui, M: Cerebral neurocytoma. A new subset of benign neuronal tumors of the cerebrum. Cancer 70:529–537, 1992.
109. Yasargil, MG, von Ammon, K, von Deimling, A, et al: Central neurocytoma: histopathological variants and therapeutic approaches. J Neurosurg 76:32–37, 1992.

Chapter 10

OLIGODENDROGLIOMA AND OLIGO-ASTROCYTOMA

HISTORY AND NOMENCLATURE

Oligodendroglioma was initially classified in 1926 by Bailey and Cushing[1] and was considered to be a differentiated form of medulloblastoma. Three years later, Bailey and Bucy,[2] applying a new histological technique developed by Rio-Hortega, proved the presence of oligodendroglia in oligodendrogliomas, and reclassified the tumor to glial lineage. Oligodendroglioma is composed of oligodendroglia (>80%); if greater than 20% of the cells are astrocytic, the tumor is an oligo-astrocytoma.[3] Oligo-astrocytoma was first described pathologically in 1935 by Cooper.[4] Oligodendroglioma differentiates from an immature O1A progenitor cell. The O1A progenitor cell is a bipotential cell that also differentiates into a type 2A astrocyte.[5] The O1A bipotentiality may explain the oligo-astrocytoma.[6] Anaplastic variants of both oligodendroglioma and oligo-astrocytoma were described in the 1993 World Health Organization (WHO) classification with the additional pathological features of frequent mitoses, nuclear polymorphism, and vascular endothelial proliferation.[7]

EPIDEMIOLOGY

The incidence rate of oligodendroglioma in Rochester, Minnesota, is six cases per 100,000 per year (C.I.: 0.2 to 0.9) for the years 1950 to 1989.[8] Oligodendroglioma represented 3.2% of brain tumors and 11% of gliomas in this series.[8] The frequency of oligodendrogliomas among gliomas has varied from 4% to 15%.[8–11] The peak incidence of oligodendroglioma is in the fourth through sixth decades of life, with the youngest case diagnosed at 1 year of age and the oldest at 76 years.[11–14] In some series, there is a male preponderance,[9,12,14–16] with approximately 60% males. The tumor is confined to the frontal lobe in 17%, temporal lobe in 22%, parietal lobe in 11%, with 50% having involvement of multiple lobes. Fifty percent of tumors involve the frontal lobe, 42% the temporal lobe, and 32% the parietal lobe.[17]

The etiology of oligodendroglioma is unknown. A rare subtype, polymorphous oligodendroglioma, occurs in siblings with p53 gene mutations but without other familial tumors.[18] Oligodendroglioma is not typically a part of the phakomatoses.

BIOLOGY

Oligodendroglioma undergoes a series of chromosomal changes in development of malignancy from an oligodendroglial cell to an anaplastic oligodendroglioma. These changes have been discovered using molecular biologic techniques. Early changes in the malignant process include allelic loss of the short arm of chromosome 1p (p36 to p32) and in 50% of oligodendrogliomas, loss of a portion of the long arm of chromosome 19q (q13.2 to q13.4) (see Fig. 2–5).[19–21] Anaplastic oligodendroglioma shows additional chromosomal changes with loss of CDKN2 and MTS loci on 9p or amplification of CDK4 on 12q.[21] Chemotherapeutic response and survival in anaplastic oligodendroglioma has been correlated with 1p chromosomal deletions with or without 19q deletions.[21a] Allelic loss on 1p, 19q, and 9p with amplification on 12q makes it likely that tumor-suppressor genes are located on chromosomes with allelic loss and proto-oncogenes on chromosomes with amplification of genetic material. Oligodendroglioma and oligo-astrocytoma are generally slow-growing tumors, with their anaplastic variants having a considerably more aggressive biologic behavior. The MIB-1 monoclonal antibody to an antigenic site in the Ki-67 region labels from 1% to 10% of cells.[22] The determination of ploidy by flow cytometry has not been helpful prognostically in oligodendroglioma and oligo-astrocytoma,[23,24] although the S-phase fraction is reported to be predictive of survival.[24] The value of labeling indices in newly diagnosed astrocytoma has been questioned (see Chapter 2), so the utility of the S-phase fraction in predicting survival in oligodendroglioma needs further confirmation.

PATHOLOGY

Oligodendroglioma has hyperchromatic nuclei surrounded by clear artifactually swollen cytoplasm or perinuclear haloes with a "fried-egg appearance." The diagnosis depends on a homogeneous cell size, a delicate network of parenchymal vessels, and a tendency to infiltrate cortex.[11] The pathological classification of 1993 divides both oligodendroglioma and oligo-astrocytomas into two types, benign and anaplastic. Mitoses, nuclear polymorphism, and vascular endothelial proliferation are not rare in the benign oligodendroglioma and oligo-astrocytoma and are the hallmark of anaplastic oligodendroglioma and oligo-astrocytoma.[3,7] Celli and colleagues[3] reported a median survival of 84 months and a 5-year survival of 63% for patients with benign oligodendroglioma compared with a median survival of 35 months and a 5-year survival of 19% for patients with anaplastic oligodendroglioma. Oligo-astrocytoma generally has greater than 20% astrocytes,[3] although some series use 10%[24] and others describe the proportion of malignant astrocytic and oligodendroglial cells.[25,26]

Oligodendroglioma has also been classified by the Smith,[12,27] Kernohan,[17,25] and Mayo St. Anne[17,25,26] grading systems. Smith and colleagues[27] classified tumors into four different grades, A through D, based on the presence, absence, and degree (high and low) of five criteria: endothelial proliferation, necrosis, nuclear/cytoplasmic ratio, cell density, and pleomorphism. Whereas tumors graded A had all five features absent or low, tumors judged to be grade D had five features present or high. Grade B tumors showed pleomorphism, high cell density and increased nuclear/cytoplasmic ratio, and if in addition, endothelial proliferation was present, the tumor was graded C.[12,27] The authors found a significant age distribution of the tumors with 68% of grade A tumors occurring in patients younger age 40 years and 83% of grade D tumors in patients over age 40. The median survival for grades A through D was 94, 51, 45, and 17 months, respectively.[12,27]

The Kernohan[17,25] and Mayo St. Anne[17,25,26] oligodendroglioma grading systems are identical to their astrocytic counterpart, and are strongly associated with survival (see Table 1–4).[17,26] Patients with grade I or II oligodendroglial tumors (judged by either Kernohan or Mayo St. Anne grading system) had a median survival of 9.8 years and 5- and 10-year survival rates of 75% and 46%, respectively.

Table 10–1. **Influence of Oligodendroglial Pathological Grading on Median and 5- and 10-Year Survival Rates**

Study (year)	Tumor Type	Grade	Median Survival (months)	Survival Rate % 5-y	Survival Rate % 10-y
Ludwig et al[12] (1986)	O, OA	A	94	71	33*
		B	51	45	26*
		C	45	43	23*
		D	17	0	0*
Shaw et al[17] (1992)	ALL	I + II K	116	75	46
		III + IV K	47	41	20
Shimizu et al[34] (1993)	O, AO	O	147	68*	57*
		AO	50	36*	16*
Nijjar et al30 (1993)	O, AO	O	86*	73	32*
		AO	48	32	7
Kros et al[41] (1994)	O, AO	Low grade	55*	46*	14*
		Intermediate	23*	24*	0
		High grade	10*	16*	0
Shaw et al[25] (1994)	OA	I + II K	76	58	32
	AOA	III + IV K	34	36	9
Celli et al[3] (1994)	O, AO	O	84	63	NA
		AO	35	19	NA

* = estimated from graphs.
ALL = O, OA, AO, AOA.
AO = anaplastic oligodendroglioma.
AOA = anaplastic oligo-astrocytoma*.
K = Kernohan.
NA = not available.
O = oligodendroglioma.
OA = oligo-astrocytoma.

Patients with grade III and IV tumors had a median survival of 3.9 years and 5- and 10-year survival rates of 41% and 20%, respectively (Table 10–1).[17] Survival differences among Smith's intermediate grades B and C, or Kernohan's grade II and III, were not significantly different using a four-tiered grading system.[27]

Patients with oligo-astrocytomas graded I and II with the Kernohan system had a median survival of 6.3 years and 5- and 10-year survival rates of 58% and 32%, respectively. Patients with grade II and IV tumors had a median survival of 2.8 years and 5- and 10-year survival rates of 36% and 9%, respectively.[25] When median survival and 5- and 10-year survival rates are compared with those in the series by Shaw and coworkers[17,25] for oligodendroglioma and oligo-astrocytoma, prognosis appears to be slightly worse for patients with oligo-astrocytoma than for those having a similarly graded oligodendroglioma.

CLINICAL SYMPTOMS

Seizures were the most frequent initial clinical symptom in 50% to 75% of patients,[3,9,12,29,30] followed by headache in to 9% to 48%,[3,16,30] with up to 78% of patients having headache on diagnosis.[12] Clinical manifestations at diagnosis depended on the anatomic site of brain involvement, with seizures present in 61%, headaches in 29%, focal neurological deficit in 16%, impaired mentation in 16%, and multiple symptoms and signs in 78%.[30] The duration of symptoms prior to diagnosis varied from an acute intracerebral bleed to more than a decade of epilepsy. Oligodendroglial tumors are usually slowly progressive over years.[31] Whittle and Beaumont[29] classified patients' seizures into types: tonic clonic (32%), complex partial (16%), partial with secondary generalization (12%), partial motor (8%), and mixed seizure (32%). In this series[29] but not in others,[3,30] patients who presented with seizures were significantly younger than those who presented with other symptoms.

In a large series of retrospectively analyzed patients with oligodendroglioma, Celli and colleagues[3] classified patients into two groups: seizures as the presenting symptom with no neurological deficit (A) and other (B). Patients were treated with either surgery alone or surgery plus radiation. In group A, the 10 patients who did not receive radiation lived as long as the 30 patients treated with radiation; in group B, those who received radiation lived longer. The survival of the whole patient cohort, with and without radiation, is shown in Table 10–2. The results support a clinical approach of watchful waiting in patients with a presumed or newly diagnosed localized oligodendroglioma presenting with seizures alone and no focal signs.[3] In the study of low-grade glioma (LGA) by Recht and colleagues,[32] no advantage was found for early operative and postoperative intervention in patients presenting with seizures alone.

DIFFERENTIAL DIAGNOSIS

A total of 43% to 77% of oligodendrogliomas are calcified.[3,17,33,34] The percentage of oligo-astrocytoma with calcification is 14%.[25] Typically, computed tomography (CT) or magnetic resonance imaging (MRI) scans show an intrinsic frontal or temporal calcified nonenhancing mass with mild to moderate edema, with or without mass effect. The differential diagnosis includes low-grade astrocytoma, ganglioglioma, dysembryoplastic neuroepithelial tumor (DNET), or craniopharyngioma.[35] If the imaging abnormality lacks calcification and is nonenhancing with mild edema, the differential includes LGA, ganglioglioma, DNET, central neurocytoma, and the nonmalignant processes of multiple sclerosis (MS), encephalitis, or rarely, an infarct. Oligodendroglioma typically has either a type I or III structure of Daumas-Duport.[36] The time course of the clinical history, the associated neurological signs, and diagnostic workup (i.e., evoked potentials, CSF analysis, and Doppler ultrasound or angiography) are helpful in reaching a diagnosis.[31]

If the mass is calcified or noncalcified and moderately enhancing with moderate edema and mass effect, the differential diagnosis includes anaplastic astrocytoma, ganglioglioma, craniopharyngioma, and meningioma (if durally based). Rarely, an arteriovenous malformation may be confused with an oligodendroglioma, but MRI or arterial angiography scans should provide the correct answer.

Histologically, oligodendroglioma is easily confused with two tumors, central neurocytoma and DNET.[6,37] Both central neurocytoma and DNET are mixed neuronal and glial tumors, and the glial component contains oligodendroglia or oligodendroglial-like cells. Unlike oligodendroglioma, a neuronal component is present that immunostains with synaptophysin and neurofilament protein. Central neurocytoma is usually deep within the hemisphere, near the ventricular system.[7] DNET is most often in the temporal lobe, and microscopically includes admixed neurons and astrocytes adjacent to the dysplastic cortex.[37]

DIAGNOSTIC WORKUP

Plain radiographs of the skull may show calcification in the tumor, a midline shift of the calcified pineal gland, or calvarial erosion providing evidence of raised intracranial pressure.[31] CT is the definitive imaging technique for demonstration of calcification as increased signal.[35] The tumors are hypodense or isodense on CT scans and have poorly defined contrast enhancement in 50% of cases. The CT scan abnormalities most often have sharp margins with little edema. MRI scans most typically reveal hypointense lesions on T_1-weighted images and hyperintense lesions on T_2-weighted images (Fig. 10–1).

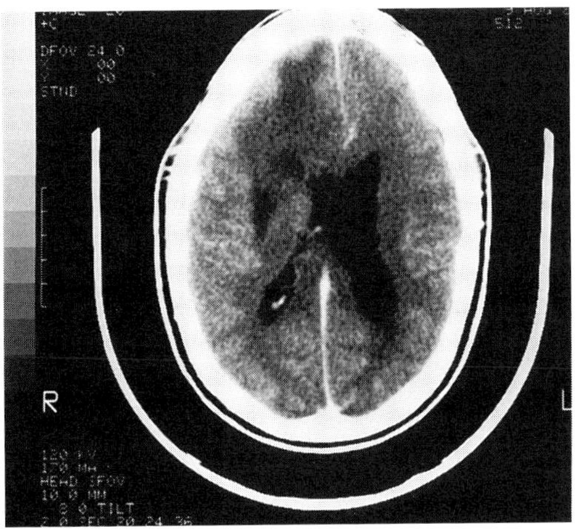

A

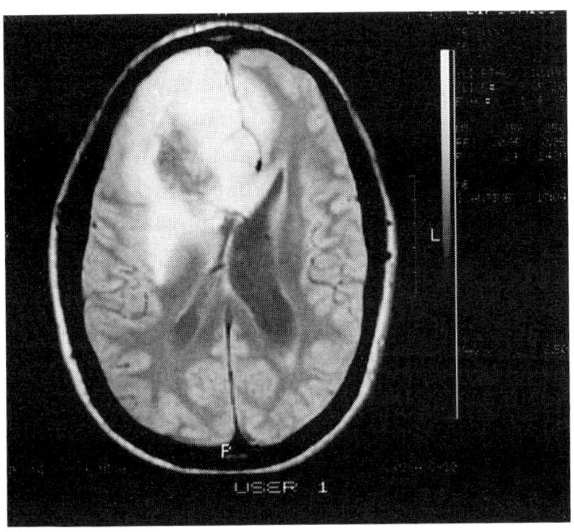

B

Figure 10–1. Oligodendroglioma. *(A)* Contrast-enhanced CT with decreased density predominantly in right frontal white matter without enhancement. Ventricular compression is present. *(B)* T_2-weighted MRI showing more extensive hyperintense signal in both right frontal gray and white matter spreading through the corpus callosum. Hyperintense signal showing diffuse edema.

Anaplastic oligodendroglioma and oligo-astrocytoma enhance more frequently (Fig. 10–2).[35] Anaplastic oligodendroglioma and oligo-astrocytoma are more likely to have hemorrhage or necrosis. On stereotactic biopsy, isolated tumor cells have been found to extend as far as the T2 prolongation on T_2-weighted MRI scans.[36] Rarely, oligodendroglioma presents as a contrast-enhancing leptomeningeal mass (primary leptomeningeal oligodendroglioma) without evidence of brain or spinal oligodendroglioma.[38]

In children, the typical CT findings are a noncalcified low-attenuation area with discrete margins with or without mass effect.[39] Enhancement is present in less than 25% of cases and calcification in less than 40%.

TREATMENT

Surgery

In patients who present with seizures, no neurological deficit, and a calcified, localized, nonenhancing abnormality typical of an oligodendroglioma, watchful waiting with frequent follow-up scans and anticonvulsant therapy is appropriate.[3,32] If the abnormality expands or seizures are refractory to drug therapy, biopsy with or without resection should be considered. Tissue typing, resection, and grading of the tumor will strongly influence subsequent management.

If the patient presents with focal neurological signs, an expanding mass, or evidence of increased intracranial pressure, biopsy and surgical resection, whenever possible, are indicated.

Radiation Therapy

The role of postoperative radiotherapy (RT) in the management of oligodendroglioma and oligo-astrocytoma is controversial. Since 1980, there have been 14 nonrandomized studies of RT in the treatment of oligodendroglioma and oligo-astrocytoma in which treatment assignment to surgery alone or surgery and RT

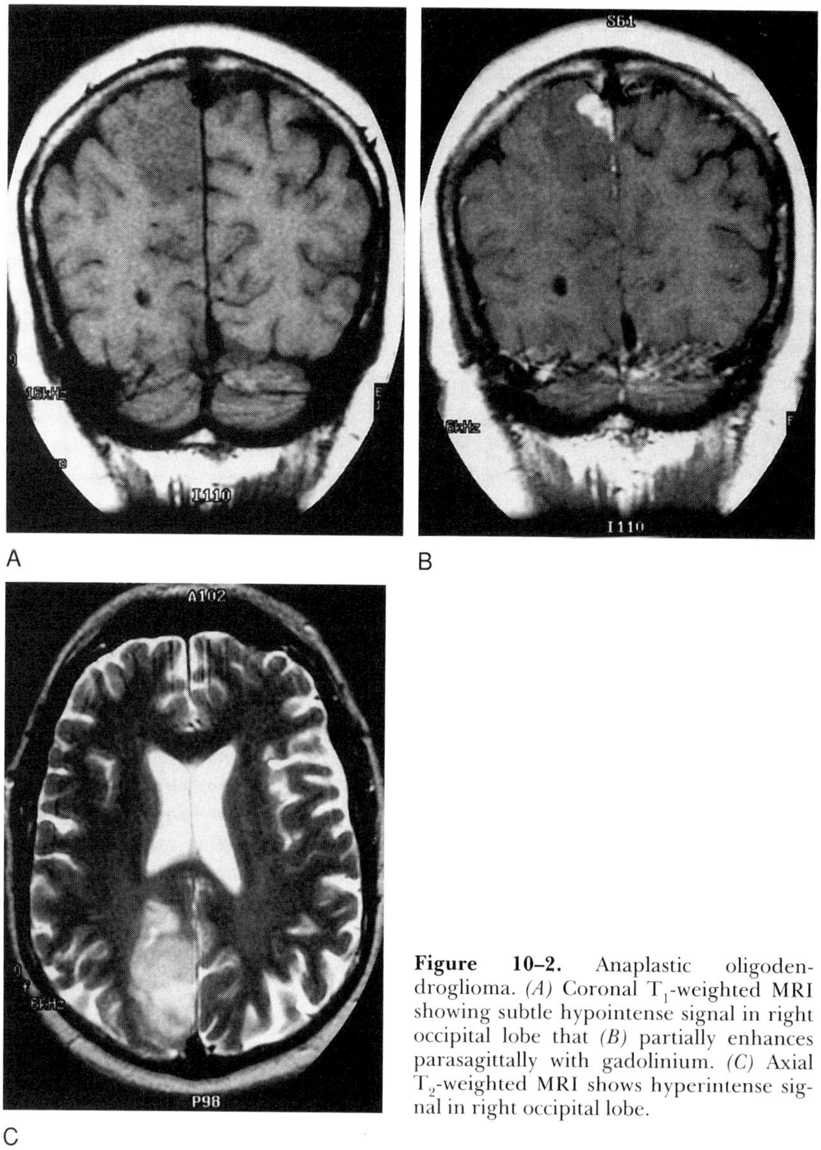

Figure 10–2. Anaplastic oligodendroglioma. *(A)* Coronal T_1-weighted MRI showing subtle hypointense signal in right occipital lobe that *(B)* partially enhances parasagittally with gadolinium. *(C)* Axial T_2-weighted MRI shows hyperintense signal in right occipital lobe.

has been at the discretion of the treating physician (Table 10–2). Nine studies[3,13,14,17,25,34,40,43,45] recommended immediate postoperative RT for incompletely resected tumors. Four studies found no benefit to postoperative RT,[10,30,41,44] and one[42] suggested that RT be deferred until evidence of tumor progression. A meta-analysis of seven studies and 425 patients[6,10,15,34,42–44] found a 14% improvement in postoperative 5-year survival in radiation-treated patients ($p<0.01$).[34] The number of patients needed for a prospective treatment trial would be 488 in order to demonstrate a 15% difference between two treatments with a power of 90% and type I error of 0.05.[34] The largest of the 13 individual studies was 170 patients, a sample size too small to demonstrate a 15% treatment difference between treatment arms.[13]

In many of these trials, treatment assignment was not balanced across variables. For example, in a study of 68 patients by Nijjar and colleagues,[30] 10 patients were treated with surgery alone; 50% of these had gross total resection, and 50% had subtotal resection. In the surgery and RT group of 58, 17% had gross total resection, 74% had subtotal resection, and 9% had biopsy. The surgery alone group, with a far greater proportion of gross total resection, had survival equal to the surgery plus RT group (see Table 10–2). It is expected that with small patient numbers and an unequal variable distribution in the two treatment arms, treatment differences might be obscured.[30] Bullard and colleagues[11] found no treatment differences between surgery and surgery plus RT in 71 patients. The study was balanced with respect to age, preoperative symptoms, Karnofsky score, and surgical procedure. The median survival of 4.5 years in the surgery alone group was not significantly different from the median survival of 5.2 years in the surgery plus RT group.

In summary, patients presenting with epilepsy alone and a circumscribed scanning abnormality presumed to be benign oligodendroglioma or oligo-astrocytoma can be followed closely with follow-up scans and anticonvulsant therapy. After gross total resection of a benign oligodendroglioma or oligo-astrocytoma, patients can also be observed. Patients with biopsy or minor subtotal resection should receive focal RT in doses greater than 5000 cGy.[3,13,14,17,25,34,40,43,45] Patients with anaplastic oligodendroglioma or oligo-astrocytoma, should receive focal RT to greater than 5000 cGy and should be considered strongly for multiagent chemotherapy (see below).

Chemotherapy

Anaplastic oligodendroglioma and oligo-astrocytoma are aggressive tumors that respond to procarbazine, CCNU, and vincristine (PCV) chemotherapy (Table 10–3).[26,46–49] In the most recent report from Cairncross and coworkers,[48] 18 of 19 consecutively treated patients with anaplastic oligodendroglioma responded (Tables 10–4 and 10–5). Ten patients with recurrent anaplastic oligodendroglioma were treated after one or more resections and RT. Eight patients received PCV, one received 1,3-bis-(2-chloroethyl)-1-nitrosourea (BCNU), and one received diaziquone. Two had a complete response (CR) and eight had a partial response (PR). Five patients were treated adjuvantly after surgery before RT, and there were three CRs and one PR. These responses have been durable with a range of 18 to 44 months.[48]

Kyritsis and colleagues[49] treated 17 patients who had anaplastic oligodendroglioma and 13 patients who had anaplastic oligo-astrocytoma with PCV chemotherapy. In the oligodendroglioma group, eight patients were treated adjuvantly with RT followed by PCV. All eight had a response (1 CR, 3 PR, 4 SD); seven progressed by 10 months (see Table 10–4). Of the eight patients with anaplastic oligodendroglioma who received chemotherapy for recurrence, seven responded (1 CR, 2 PR, 4 SD), with a median duration of response of 88 weeks. In the anaplastic oligo-astrocytoma group, all 12 patients treated adjuvantly had responses (2 CR, 3 PR, 7 SD), with a median response duration of 47+ weeks. The six patients with anaplastic oligo-astrocytomas treated on recurrence received a variety of chemotherapy regimens: one had PR and 5 SD, with a median time to progression of 6 months.[49] Responses were seen with (1) procarbazine; (2) nitrogen mustard, vincristine, procarbazine; (3) 6-thioguanine and BCNU; and (4) 5-fluorouracil, carboplatin, and procarbazine.[49] The durability of response for anaplastic oligodendroglioma was not equal to that found in the study by Cairncross and associates.[48] In the study by Kyritsis and colleagues,[49] patients additionally received RT. A randomized multi-institution trial in patients with newly diagnosed anaplastic oligodendroglioma is in progress. The two treatment arms are (1) RT and (2) PCV chemotherapy plus RT. Glass and colleagues,[26] like Kyritsis and coworkers,[49] found equal responses to PCV in anaplastic oligodendroglioma and oligo-astrocytoma.

PCV chemotherapy has been used to treat a small series of patients with benign oligodendroglioma at diagnosis. Eight pa-

Table 10–2. **Oligodendroglioma and Oligo-Astrocytoma: Median and 5- and 10-Year Survival Rates**

Study (year)	Tumor Type	Number of Cases	Treatment	Median Survival (months)	Survival Rate(%) 5-y	10-y
Chin et al[14] (1980)	O	11	S	NR	82	NR
		24	S + RT	NR	100	NR
Reedy et al[42] (1983)	O	21	S	NR	72*	NR
		27	S + RT	NR	70*	NR
Lindegaard et al[13] (1987)	ALL	62	S	26.5	27	12*
		108	S + RT	38.0	36	38*
Bullard et al[11] (1987)	O	34	S	54	47*	15*
	OA	37	S + RT	62	58*	13*
Wallner et al[43] (1988)	O	11	S	60*	55*	18
		14	S + RT (>4500 cGy)	132*	78*	56
Sun et al[44] (1988)	O	16	S	45	31	16
		30	S + RT	68*	57	43
Griffin et al[45] (1992)	O	14	S	NA	45	13
		27	S + RT	NA	78	43
Shaw et al[17] (1992)	ALL	19	S	127	63	55
		30	S + LDRT	55	46	23
		31	S + HDRT	96	61	36
		8	STR	24	25	25
		26	STR + RT	54	39	20

Continued on following page

tients were treated with 4 PR and 4 SD and a median duration of response of 35 months.[50] The role of chemotherapy in the treatment of both oligodendroglioma and anaplastic oligodendroglioma is to be defined.

PROGNOSIS AND COMPLICATIONS

Prognosis

The strongest prognostic factor for survival of patients with oligodendroglioma is tumor grade: there is a median survival of 9.8 years and 5- and 10-year survival rates of 75% and 46% for grade I and II tumors, respectively, compared with a median survival of 3.9 years and 5- and 10- year survival rates of 41% and 20% for grade III and IV tumors, respectively (using Kernohan or Mayo St. Anne classification systems).[17] Six other studies found a similar survival stratification using other pathological grading systems (see Table 10–1).[3,12,25,30,34,41] Other positive prognostic variables include age younger than 40 years[10,17,25,30,34,41] and calcification.[10,34] Negative prognostic factors include hemiparesis and intellectual changes.[10]

Table 10–2.—*continued*

Study (year)	Tumor Type	Number of Cases	Treatment	Median Survival (months)	Survival Rate(%) 5-y	10-y
Nijjar et al[30] (1993)	ALL	10	S	66	60	0
		58	S + RT	66	50	46
Shimizu et al[34] (1993)	ALL	8	S	41	25	NA
		23	S + RT	84	74	NA
Gannett et al[40] (1994)	O	14	S	47	51	36
	OA	27	S + RT	84	83	46
Kros et al[41] (1994)	O	10	S	23	22	NA
	OA	23	S + RT	45	46	NA
Shaw et al[25] (1994)	OA	33	S	38	36	21
	AOA	38	S + LDRT	72	71	34
			S + HDRT			
Celli et al[3] (1994)	ALL	28	S	37	36	NA
		77	S + RT	76	57	NA

* = estimated from graphs.
• = 8-y survival.
ALL = O, OA, AO, AOA.
AO = anaplastic oligodendroglioma.
AOA = anaplastic oligo-astrocytoma.
HDRT = high-dose radiation therapy.
LDRT = low-dose radiation therapy.
NA = not available.
NR = not reached.
O = Oligodendroglioma.
OA = oligo-astrocytoma.
RT = radiation therapy.
S = surgery.
STR = subtotal resection.

Complications

Oligodendroglioma occasionally disseminates through the CSF, seeding the cranial or spinal subarachnoid space, occasionally years after the primary tumor is treated. Systemic bony metastases have been described in patients with anaplastic oligodendroglioma heavily treated with surgery, radiation, and chemotherapy.[48,51] Patients with multiple craniotomies have had cervical lymph node metastases.[48]

Table 10–3. **PCV Chemotherapy**

Drug	Schedule and Dosage	Frequency of Delivery
Lomustine (CCNU)	Day 1: 100 mg/m^2 orally	Every 8 weeks [46–48]
Procarbazine (Matulane)	Days 8–21: 60 mg/m^2/d orally	
Vincristine	Days 8, and 29: 1.4 mg/m^2, intravenously	Every 6 weeks [26, 49]

PCV = procarbazine, lomustine, vincristine.

Table 10–4. **PCV Chemotherapy: Initial Treatment of Aggressive Oligodendroglioma and Oligo-Astrocytoma**

Study (year)	Cases	Tumor Types	Treatment (%)	SD × PR × CR %	Median Response Duration (weeks)
AO					
Cairncross et al[48] (1992)	5	AO (3) O (2)	PCV q 8 wk	80	42+
Glass et al[26] (1992)	3	AO	PCV q 6 wk + RT	100	50+
Kyritsis et al[49] (1993)	8	AO	RT + PCV q 6 wk	100	34
AOA					
Glass et al[26] (1992)	9	AOA	PCV q 6 wk ± RT	88	30+
Kyritsis et al[49] (1993)	12	AOA	RT + PCV q 8 wk	100	47+

AO = anaplastic oligodendroglioma.
AOA = anaplastic oligo-astrocytoma.
CR = complete response.
O = oligodendroglioma.
OA = oligo-astrocytoma.
PCV = procarbazine, lomustine, vincristine chemotherapy.
PR = partial disease.
RT = radiation therapy.
SD = stable disease.

Table 10–5. **PCV Chemotherapy at Recurrence**

Study (year)	Cases	Tumor Types	Treatment (%)	SD + PR + CR %	Median Response Duration (weeks)
Cairncross et al[48] (1992)	10	AO	PCV q 8 wk	100 (2 CR, 8 PR)	65+
Kyritsis et al[49] (1993)	12	AO	PCV q 6 wk	75 (1 CR, 2 PR, 650 SD)	88+

AO = anaplastic oligodendroglioma.
AOA = anaplastic oligo-astrocytoma.
CR = complete response.
O = oligodendroglioma.
OA = oligo-astrocytoma.
PCV = procarbazine, lomustine, vincristine chemotherapy.
PR = partial disease.
RT = radiation therapy.
SD = stable disease.

The complications of RT are described in Chapter 5. PCV chemotherapy is complicated by myelosuppression, with neutropenia and thrombocytopenia in up to 50% of cycles. Other frequent side effects include nausea and vomiting (70% to 80%), fatigue (50% to 75%), and mild to moderate vincristine neuropathy (70%).[31]

CHAPTER SUMMARY

Oligodendroglioma and oligo-astrocytoma are glial tumors that most likely arise from the bipotential immature O1A progenitor cell. A series of distinct chromosomal changes occurs during oligodendroglial cell dedifferentiation to benign oligodendroglioma (−1p, −19q), with further chromosomal changes on development of the anaplastic phenotype (−9p, +12q). The loss of 1p with or without 19q has been correlated with chemotherapy response and survival in anaplastic oligodendrogliomas. Clinically, the most common initial symptom in this slow-growing, often calcified tumor, is seizures (50% to 75%). The role of RT in the postoperative management of oligodendroglioma and oligo-astrocytoma is controversial. A recent meta-analysis of 425 patients reported a 14% improvement in 5-year survival in radiation-treated patients.[34] Anaplastic oligodendroglioma and oligo-astrocytoma are sensitive to PCV chemotherapy, both at the time of diagnosis and on tumor recurrence after RT. Median response durations vary between 10 months and 2 years. The best treatment is most likely a combination of radiation and PCV chemotherapy; a randomized trial of radiation with and without PCV chemotherapy is in progress.

REFERENCES

1. Bailey, P, and Cushing, H: A classification of the tumors of the glioma group on a histogenetic basis with a correlated study of prognosis. JB Lippincott Company, Philadelphia, 1926.
2. Bailey, P, and Bucy, PC: Oligodendrogliomas of the brain. J Pathol Bacteriol 32:735–751, 1929.
3. Celli, P, Nofrone, I, Palma, L, et al: Cerebral oligodendroglioma: prognostic factors and life history. Neurosurgery 35:1018–1035, 1994.
4. Cooper, ERA: The relation of oligocytes and astrocytes in cerebral tumours. J Pathol 41:259–266, 1935.
5. Linsky, ME, and Gilbert, MR: Glial differentiation. A review with implications for new directions in neuro-oncology. Neurosurgery 36:1–21, 1995.
6. Sarkar, C, Roy, S, and Tandon, PN: Oligodendroglial tumors. An immunohistochemical and electron microscopic study. Cancer 61:1862–1866, 1988.
7. Kleihues, P, Burger, PC, and Scheithauer, BW: Histological Typing of Tumours of the Central Nervous System, Second Edition. World Health Organization, Springer-Verlag, Berlin, 1993.
8. Radhakrishnan, K, Mokri, B, Parisi, JE, et al: The trends in incidence of primary brain tumors in the population of Rochester, Minnesota. Ann Neurol 37:67–73, 1995.
9. Horrax, G, and Wu, WQ: Post-operative survival of patients with intracranial oligodendroglioma with special reference to radical tumor removal: A study of 26 patients. J Neurosurg 8:473–479, 1951.
10. M¢rk, SJ, Lindegaard K-F, Halvorsen TB, et al: Oligodendroglioma: incidence and biological behavior in a defined population. J Neurosurg 63: 881–889, 1985.
11. Bullard, DE, Rawlings, E III, Phillips, B, et al: Oligodendroglioma. An analysis of the value of radiation therapy. Cancer 60:2179–2188, 1987.
12. Ludwig, CL, Smith, MT, Godfrey, AD, and Armbrustmacher, VW: A clinicopathological study of 323 patients with oligodendrogliomas. Ann Neurol 19:15–21, 1986.
13. Lindegaard, K-F, M¢rk, SJ, Eide, GE, et al: Statistical analysis of clinicopathological features, radiotherapy, and survival in 170 cases of oligodendroglioma. J Neurosurg 67:224–230, 1987.
14. Chin, HW, Hazel, JJ, Kim, TH, and Webster, JH: Oligodendrogliomas: I. A clinical study of cerebral oligodendrogliomas. Cancer 45:1458–1466, 1980.
15. Earnest, F III, Kernohan, JW, and Craig, WM: Oligodendrogliomas: a review of two hundred cases. Arch Neurol Psych 63:964–976, 1950.
16. Roberts, M, and German, WJ: A long term study of patients with oligodendrogliomas. Follow-up of 50 cases, including Dr. Harvey Cushing's series. J Neurosurg 24:697–700, 1966.
17. Shaw, EG, Scheithauer, BW, O'Fallon, JR, et al: Oligodendrogliomas: the Mayo Clinic experience. J Neurosurg 76:428–434, 1992.
18. Kros, JM, Lie, ST, and Stefanko, SZ: Familial occurrence of polymorphous oligodendroglioma. Neurosurgery 34(4):732–736, 1994.
19. Bello, MJ, Vaquero, J, de Campos, JM, et al: Molecular analysis of chromosome 1 abnormalities in human gliomas reveals frequent loss of 1p in oligodendroglial tumors. Int J Cancer 57(2): 172–175, 1994.
20. von Deimling, A, Nagel, J, Bender, B, et al: Deletion mapping of chromosome 19 in human gliomas. Int J Cancer 57(5):676–680, 1994.

21. Collins, VP: Molecular basis of glial oncogenesis. J Neurooncol 28:53, 1996.
21a. Cairncross, JG, Ueki, K, Zlatescu, MC, et al: Specific genetic predictors of chemotherapeutic response and survival in patients with anaplastic oligodendrogliomas. J Natl Cancer Inst 90: 1473–1479, 1998.
22. Karamitopoulou, E, Perentes, E, Diamantis, I, and Maraziotis, T: Ki-67 immunoreactivity in human central nervous system tumors: a study with MIB1 monoclonal antibody on archival material. Acta Neuropathol (Berl) 87(1):47–54, 1994.
23. Kros, JM, van Eden, CG, Vissers, CJ, et al: Prognostic relevance of DNA flow cytometry in oligodendroglioma. Cancer 69:1791–1798, 1992.
24. Coons, SW, Johnson, PC, Pearl, DK, and Olafsen, AG: Prognostic significance of flow cytometry deoxyribonucleic acid analysis of human oligodendrogliomas. Neurosurgery 34:680–687, 1994.
25. Shaw, EG, Scheithauer, BW, O'Fallon, JR, and Davis, DH: Mixed oligoastrocytomas: a survival and prognostic factor analysis. Neurosurgery 34: 577–582, 1994.
26. Glass, J, Hochberg, FH, Gruber, ML, et al: The treatment of oligodendrogliomas and mixed oligodendroglioma-astrocytomas with PCV chemotherapy. J Neurosurg 76:741–745, 1992.
27. Smith, MT, Ludwig, CL, Godfrey, AD, and Armbrustmacher, VW: Grading of oligodendrogliomas. Cancer 52:2107–2114, 1983.
28. Kros, JM, Troost, D, van Eden, CG, et al: Oligodendroglioma. A comparison of two grading systems. Cancer 61:2251–2259, 1988.
29. Whittle, IR, and Beaumont, A: Seizures in patients with supratentorial oligodendroglial tumours. Clinicopathological features and management considerations. Acta Neurochir (Wien) 135:19–24, 1995.
30. Nijjar, TS, Simpson, WJ, Gadalla, T, and McCartney, M: Oligodendroglioma. The Princess Margaret Hospital experience (1958–1984). Cancer 71:4002–4006, 1993.
31. Grant, R: Oligodendroglioma and oligo-astrocytoma. In Gilman, S, Goldstein, G, and Waxman, S (eds): Neurobase. Arbor Publishing Corporation, San Diego, 1996.
32. Recht, LD, Lew, R, and Smith, TW: Suspected low-grade glioma: Is deferring treatment safe? Ann Neurol 31:431–436, 1992.
33. Marcu, H, Vonofakos, D, and Hacker, H: Characteristic CT signs in oligodendrogliomas. In Wackenheim, A, and DuBoulay, GH (eds): Choices and Characteristics in Computerized Tomography. Kugler, Amsterdam, 1980, pp 93– 102.
34. Shimizu, KT, Tran, LM, Mark, RJ, and Selch, MT: Management of oligodendrogliomas. Radiology 186:569–572, 1993.
35. Lee, Y-Y, and Van Tassel, P: Intracranial oligodendrogliomas: imaging findings in 35 untreated cases. AJNR 10:119–127, 1989.
36. Kelly, PJ, Daumas-Duport, C, Scheithauer, Bwet al: Stereotactic histologic correlations of computed tomography- and magnetic resonance imaging-defined abnormalities in patients with glial neoplasms. Mayo Clin Proc 62:450–459, 1987.
37. Leung, SY, Gwi, E, Ng, HK, et al: Dysembryoplastic neuroepithelial tumor. A tumor with small neuronal cells resembling oligodendroglioma. Am J Surg Pathol 18(6):604–614, 1994.
38. Rogers, LR, Estes, ML, Rosenbloom, SA, and Harrold, L: Primary leptomeningeal oligodendroglioma: case report. Neurosurgery 36:166–169, 1995.
39. Tice, H, Barnes, PD, Goumnerova, L, et al: Pediatric and adolescent oligodenddrogliomas. AJNR 14:1293–1300, 1993.
40. Gannett, DE, Wisbeck, WM, Silbergeld, DL, and Berger, MS: The role of postoperative irradiation in the treatment of oligodendroglioma. Int J Radiat Oncol Biol Phys 30(3):567–573, 1994.
41. Kros, JM, Pieterman, H, van Eden, CG, and Avezaat CJJ: Oligodendroglioma: The Rotterdam-Dijkzigt experience. Neurosurgery 34:959–966, 1994.
42. Reedy, DP, Bay, JW, and Hahn, JF: Role of radiation therapy in the treatment of cerebral oligodendroglioma: an analysis of 57 cases and a literature review. Neurosurgery 13:499–503, 1983.
43. Wallner, KE, Gonzales, M, and Sheline, GE: Treatment of oligodendrogliomas with or without postoperative irradiation. J Neurosurg 68: 684–688, 1988.
44. Sun, ZM, Genka, S, Shitara, N, et al: Factors possibly influencing the prognosis of oligodendroglioma. Neurosurgery 22:886–891, 1988.
45. Griffin, BR, Silbergeld, DL, Berger, MS, et al: Oligodendrogliomas: postoperative radiotherapy increases survival. Int J Radiat Oncol Biol Phys 24(Suppl 1):142, 1992.
46. Cairncross, JG, and Macdonald, DR: Successful chemotherapy for recurrent malignant oligodendroglioma. Ann Neurol 23:360–364, 1988.
47. Macdonald, DR, Gaspar, LE, and Cairncross, JG: Successful chemotherapy for newly diagnosed aggressive oligodendroglioma. Ann Neurol 27: 573–574, 1990.
48. Cairncross, JG, Macdonald, DR, and Ramsay, DA: Aggressive oligodendroglioma: a chemosensitive tumor. Neurosurgery 31:78–82, 1992.
49. Kyritsis, AP, Yung, WKA, Bruner, J, et al: The treatment of anaplastic oligodendrogliomas and mixed gliomas. Neurosurgery 32:365–371, 1993.
50. Mason, WP, Krol, GS, and DeAngelis, LM: Low-grade oligodendroglioma responds to chemotherapy. Neurology 46:203–207, 1996.
51. Macdonald, DR, O'Brien, RA, Gilbert, JJ, and Cairncross, JG: Metastatic anaplastic oligodendroglioma. Neurology 39:1593–1596, 1989.

Chapter 11

POSTERIOR FOSSA TUMORS

Posterior fossa tumors occur most commonly in children. Brain tumors are the second most common malignancy and are the most common solid childhood tumor. Posterior fossa tumors account for more than two thirds of these brain tumors. They are, however, uncommon tumors. In the United States, there are approximately 800 posterior fossa tumors diagnosed in children each year. A total of 250 of these are medulloblastoma, and a slightly greater number are cerebellar astrocytoma. These tumors also occur in adults, predominantly young adults in their third and fourth decades of life. These tumors have the same biologic behavior in adults as they do in children, but medulloblastoma more frequently originates laterally in the cerebellar hemisphere in adults.

MEDULLOBLASTOMA (PRIMITIVE NEUROECTODERMAL TUMOR)

History and Nomenclature

Medulloblastoma, or primitive neuroectodermal tumor (PNET), was initially described in 1924 by Bailey and Cushing[1] under the designation of *spongioblastoma cerebelli*. The name was quickly changed to *medulloblastoma cerebelli* after an initial presentation at the 50th American Neurologic Association meeting of 1924, when Globus and Strauss[1] described a different tumor, spongioblastoma of the cerebrum with cellular glial differentiation. In their report on 29 cases with a median age of 7 years (range, 2 to 28 years), Bailey and Cushing[1] described a very undifferentiated small round cellular tumor arising over the fourth ventricle and projecting into the center of the cerebellum (vermis).

In 1983, Rorke[2] noted that histologically identical small round cell tumors could occur elsewhere in brain, including the cerebral cortex and pineal region, and called these tumors *PNETs*. Rorke's theory was that PNETs were derived from the subependymal matrix level, and these cells occurred in various locations in the central nervous system. PNET has been called *medulloblastoma, ependymoblastoma, neuroblastoma,* and *pineoblastoma*. Rorke[2] suggested further subdivision of PNET based on location within the CNS and histological features of cellular differentiation.

However, in the 1993 World Health Organization (WHO) classification system, the term *PNET* was limited to small round cell tumors of the cerebellum, with the capacity for divergent neuronal, astrocytic, ependymal, muscular, or melanotic differentiation.[3] It did not include neuroblastoma, pineoblastoma, or ependymoblastoma as proposed by Rorke.[2] The participants in the development of the classification system failed to embrace Rorke's definition of PNET because the cell of origin of the medulloblastoma was unknown. It was generally believed to be from the granular layer, a matrix zone for neurons, not glial cells; medulloblastomas displayed glial differentiation in addition to neuronal differentiation.[3–5] In this chapter, the term PNET is used in the more limited WHO context unless otherwise specified.

Epidemiology

Medulloblastoma is the most common primary CNS tumor of childhood, accounting for 15% to 30% of all childhood brain tumors and 30 to 40% of all childhood posterior fossa tumors.[4,6] A total of 3% to 8% percent of all tumors in the population are medulloblastomas.[6–8] Medulloblastoma occurs widely throughout the world. The only known risk factors for the development of medulloblastoma and other childhood brain tumors are radiotherapy (RT) and certain genetic conditions.[7–10]

In a Swedish study, the average annual incidence of medulloblastoma was estimated to be 7.4 per million per year, with a male:female ratio of 1.8.[10] An American study reported the male:female ratio as 1.6.[6] The peak incidence of the tumor is in the first decade of life[1,2,4] with a bimodal distribution, and there are peaks at 3 to 4 years of age and again at 8 to 9 years.[4] In adults, more than 80% of cases occur before the end of the fourth decade of life.[11,12]

Familial cases of medulloblastoma have rarely been reported in monozygotic twins and siblings.[9,13] Neurofibromatosis, Turcot's syndrome, and the nevoid basal cell carcinoma syndrome (Gorlin's syndrome) have all been associated with an increased incidence of medulloblastoma.[4] Uterine radiation during pregnancy has been reported to cause an increased incidence of medulloblastoma.[4]

Biology

Medulloblastoma is thought to arise from a primitive cell in the external granular layer of the cerebellum, but the cell of origin has never been identified.[3,4] Karyotypic analysis of 22 medulloblastomas revealed chromosome abnormalities in 19 with the most frequent structural changes, deletions, or nonreciprocal translocations. The most frequent chromosome affected was 17 in 11 cases, and an abnormality on 17q was seen in eight cases.[14] The abnormality on chromosome 17q was not specific for medulloblastomas but has also been seen in hematological malignancies and colorectal carcinoma. Other nonrandom chromosomal changes include loss of an X and 6 chromosome and trisomy 7, with frequent structural abnormalities in 5, 11, and 16.[14] In a molecular biology study using restriction fragment length polymorphism (RFLP) analysis, three of nine patients showed allelic loss on the short arm (p) of chromosome 17, the site of the p53 tumor-suppressor gene.[15] No loss of heterozygosity or rearrangements have been found in the *p53* gene in 33 patients in two series, making it unlikely that the p53 tumor-suppressor gene is implicated in the pathogenesis of medulloblastoma.[16,17] Amplification of c-*myc* and N-*myc* have been reported in medulloblastoma.[15,18]

A wild type *p53* gene has been transfected in a defective herpes simplex viral vector into a medulloblastoma cell line with a mutant *p53* gene. There was restoration of wild type *p53* expression in the cells. The gene transfer resulted in cell cycle arrest in the majority of transduced cells.[19] These results were unexpected because a *p53* mutation was not thought to be responsible for medulloblastoma.

Cell kinetic labeling studies of medulloblastoma have been performed with tritiated thymidine, with a range of 8% to 14.4%, and bromodeoxyuridine (BUdR) with a range of 6% to 20%.[20,21] (^{18}F)-2-fluoro-2-deoxyglucose positron emission tomography (PET-FDG) studies in five patients with medulloblastoma had a mean uptake of FDG of 4.8 on a qualitative scale of 5, with 4 being equal to and 5 greater than parietal gray matter.[22] The uptake of medulloblastomas was greater than brainstem gliomas or pilocytic astrocytomas. Monoclonal antibodies have been developed against the transferrin receptor and the T-199 antigen in medulloblastoma cell lines. However, no expression of the transferrin receptor occurred on the medulloblastoma cell line when implanted in nude mice, rendering the antibody useless in vivo.[23,24]

Pathology

Medulloblastoma is a malignant, embryonal tumor. It is usually a pinkish-gray mass, with a capsule infiltrated by small blood vessels. It is composed of densely packed, small, round to oval or carrot-shaped nuclei with scanty cytoplasm (see Fig. 1–16). Medulloblastoma cells form Homer Wright pseudorosettes by surrounding fibrils that protrude from the cells.[25]

Neuronal differentiation is common with positive immunohistochemical staining for synaptophysin and neurofilament protein.[3] Astrocytic differentiation occurs less frequently, and ependymal, melanotic, or rhabdomyoblastic differentiation occurs rarely. Tumors can be immunostained for glial fibrillary acidic protein (GFAP) when there is no histological astrocytic differentiation. The biologic behavior is grade IV. The desmoplastic medulloblastoma is a variant containing reticulin fibers alternating with reticulin-free areas where there is often cellular differentiation. This also has a grade IV biologic behavior but has a slightly better prognosis than other medulloblastomas.[3]

Histologically, medulloblastoma can resemble other "small blue cell tumors," such as ependymoblastoma, rhabdomyosarcoma, hemangiopericytoma, lymphoma, and small cell carcinoma, and it is differentiated by location and immunohistochemistry with neuronal and glial markers.[25,26]

Clinical Symptoms

Medulloblastoma arises most commonly from the cerebellar vermis in children.[4] In at least two thirds of children, the tumor originates in the vermis.[5,26] In adults, the tumor more frequently originates laterally in the cerebellar hemispheres in 45% to 70% of cases.[5,6,12,26–28] In childhood midline tumors, the symptoms are caused by medulloblastoma growing into the fourth ventricle, blocking the egress of CSF, and producing hydrocephalus and increased intracranial pressure. The symptom duration in children is often less than 4 months.[29] Symptoms and signs that are present in almost 90% of children at diagnosis include headache, lethargy, nausea, vomiting (particularly in the morning), and papilledema.[4,29] Truncal unsteadiness is also an early sign in children, often followed by appendicular ataxia. Diplopia is caused by pressure on the sixth nerve as it courses under the petroclival ligament, the direct infiltration of brainstem by medulloblastoma, subarachnoid spread of tumor to the sixth nerve, or a diffuse increase in intracranial pressure. If the tumor invades the meninges at the level of the foramen magnum or if there is cerebellar tonsil herniation from increased intracranial pressure, nuchal rigidity and a head tilt may result.[4]

Very young children with open sutures often present with nonspecific signs, such as anorexia, failure to thrive, irritability, developmental delay, or expanding head size. The typical signs of increased intracranial pressure may also occur.[4,29] In two series of childhood brain tumors, one covering the first 12 months of life and the second covering the first 24 months, medulloblastoma was the second most frequent tumor in both series (astrocytoma was the most frequent). It accounted for 27% of tumors in the first series and 22% in the second series.[30,31]

In adults, the tumor is more likely to arise laterally with headache, nausea, and vomiting in approximately 40% of cases[6,28] and truncal or appendicular ataxia in 25%.[28] Seventh and eighth cranial nerve palsies are present in cerebellopontine angle medulloblastomas, and the patient is frequently thought to have an acoustic neuroma.[12]

The tumor may present apoplectically with intratumoral hemorrhage, and acute leptomeningeal dissemination occurs at presentation in approximately 33% of children[4] and 31% of adults.[28] Localized or radicular back pain may occur secondary to spinal leptomeningeal dissemination at any time. Subarachnoid deposits are often asymptomatic in medulloblastoma.[4]

Differential Diagnosis

No clinical symptom or sign is pathognomonic for medulloblastoma. In clinical presentation, signs and symptoms overlap considerably with those of other common posterior fossa tumors of childhood—juvenile pilocytic astrocytoma or low-grade astrocytoma [LGA], brainstem glioma, ependymoma, dermoid cysts, pineal and suprasellar tumors—which frequently produce obstructive hydrocephalus and the symptoms associated with increased intracranial pressure (Table 11–1).[32]

Cerebellar astrocytoma occurs as frequently as medulloblastoma but is symptomatic for a longer period of time, between 6 months and 2 years.[4,29] Cerebellar astrocytoma presents more frequently with limb and truncal ataxia, and symptoms associated with increased intracranial pressure are often present at diagnosis.[29] Brainstem glioma presents with progressive cranial nerve, cerebellar, and pyramidal tract findings, which are often bilateral because of the infiltrative nature of the neoplasm. The duration of symptoms varies depending on the biologic behavior of the brainstem astrocytoma. Ependymoma may have an identical clinical presentation to medulloblastoma, but the symptom duration is somewhat longer (i.e., 6 to 12 months), and cranial nerve deficits are present more frequently.[4,29]

Table 11–1. **Differential Diagnosis of Posterior Fossa Tumors**

Medulloblastoma
Cerebellar astrocytoma
Pilocytic
Low grade
Brainstem glioma
Ependymoma
Pineal region tumors
Suprasellar tumors
Choroid plexus papilloma
Dermoid and epidermoid cysts
Metastatic tumors
Nonmalignant processes
Anticonvulsant and drug toxicity
Metabolic disease
Viral encephalitis and postviral cerebellar syndrome
Brain abscess
Demyelinating disease
Brainstem arteriovenous malformation

Dermoid and epidermoid cysts are slowly growing and developmental in origin. Dermoid cysts occur in the fourth ventricle in children and present with hydrocephalus. Epidermoid cysts occur laterally in the cerebellopontine angle, with symptoms of hearing loss, tinnitus, and appendicular ataxia. They can be distinguished from other neoplasms by their imaging characteristics. They are cystic, often have a high lipid content, and rarely enhance with contrast. Dermoid cysts may be heterogeneous on imaging studies because of dermal appendages. They do not produce brain edema. A pineal region tumor can be distinguished by vertical gaze and pupillary abnormalities. Patients with suprasellar tumors present with increased intracranial pressure and will frequently have visual field deficits, diabetes insipidus, or precocious puberty.[33]

Nonmalignant conditions that may be confused with medulloblastoma include anticonvulsant toxicity, drug ingestion, postviral cerebellar ataxia, and brain abscess. Metastatic tumor occurs rarely in children.[4] For further help in differential diagnosis, an imaging study should be performed.

Diagnostic Workup

The current diagnostic imaging procedure of choice in the evaluation of a posterior fossa mass is cranial magnetic resonance imaging (MRI) with T_1-weighted images, with and without contrast, and T_2-weighted images. Sagittal and axial T_1-weighted images are obtained before contrast administration, and sagittal, axial and coronal T_1-weighted images are obtained after contrast administration. Axial and coronal T_2-weighted images are needed. Computed tomography (CT), with and without contrast, is an acceptable alternative. MRI is superior to CT because the multiplanar images provide improved relational anatomy of tumor to surrounding normal structures. MRI has increased sensitivity to detect meningeal enhancement, both intracranially and intraspinally. MRI and CT both detect obstructive hydrocephalus. Obstructive hydrocephalus is present in 80% of cases at the time of diagnosis.[4,29]

On T_1-weighted MRI, medulloblastoma is seen as hypointense or isotense with mild to moderate homogeneous or heterogeneous patchy enhancement (Fig. 11–1). On T_2-weighted images, the tumors varied from hypointense to hyperintense.[26,27,34] On CT scans, medulloblastomas are hypodense or isodense without contrast and enhance homogeneously or heterogeneously after contrast.[4,26,29]

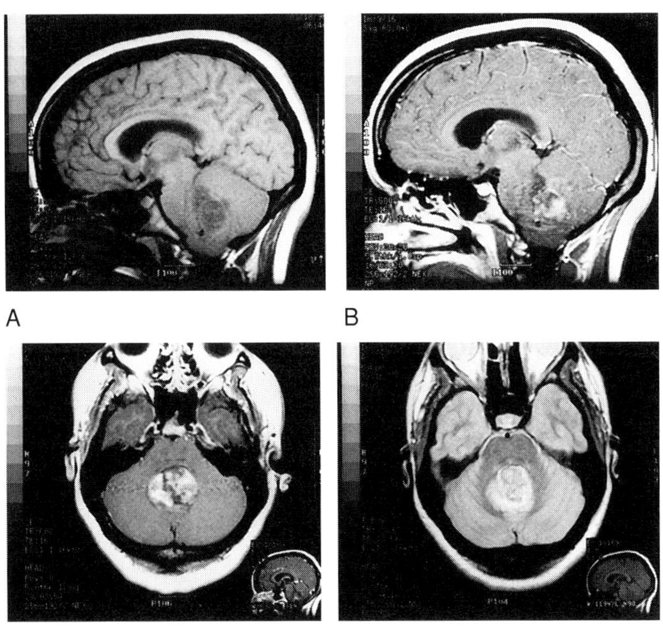

Figure 11–1. Medulloblastoma: T_1-weighted sagittal MRI. *(A)* Precontrast showing large hypointense abnormality filling the fourth ventricle, with *(B and C)* heterogeneous contrast enhancement after gadolinium, and *(D)* axial T_2-weighted MRI notes variability in signal from isointense to hyperintense.

If the patient is stable before surgery or in the immediate postoperative period, spinal MRI with and without gadolinium is important for staging of disease. CSF cytology may show evidence of spinal fluid dissemination when MRI scans show negative results. CSF polyamine monitoring of putrescine levels predicts spinal tumor recurrence in medulloblastoma but has not been incorporated into clinical practice.[35] Routine bone scan and bone marrow screening have not been studied prospectively and should be used only in children younger than 3 years of age, with the highest risk of extraneural dissemination.[4]

Medulloblastomas are staged postoperatively by criteria developed by Chang and colleagues[36] on the basis of preoperative imaging and the surgeons intraoperative view of tumor extent, and scored from T_1 through T_4 (Table 11–2). T_1 is the least aggressive tumor, less than 3 cm in diameter, that is limited to the vermis, the roof of the fourth ventricle, or less frequently, the cerebellar hemispheres. T_4 is the most aggressive medulloblastoma arising from the floor of the fourth ventricle and extending to the midbrain or upper cervical cord. T_1 and T_2 tumors are classified as "good risk" and have a better prognosis than T_3 and T_4 tumors, classified as "poor risk." Tumors are also graded according to the degree of metastases from M_0, which is no evidence of metastases ("good risk") to M_2 to M_4, in which there are varying extent of metastases ("poor risk") (Table 11–3). Medulloblastomas are also staged histopathologically from 0 to 3 in each of four categories in order to develop a histopathological tumor score (range, 0 to 12) to predict survival. The four categories include (1) the number of mitoses per high-power field, (2) the degree of necrosis, (3) the extent of cellular cytoplasmic processes, and (4) desmoplasia.[37] Desmoplasia was considered a good prognostic factor. The 5-year survival rate with a tumor score of 5 or less was 81% compared with 41% with a tumor score of 5 or more.[37]

Treatment

SYMPTOMATIC

A total of 80% of children with medulloblastoma present with hydrocephalus.[4] The patient is usually stable, and the hydrocephalus can be treated conservatively with corticosteroids. If the patient is deteriorating neurologically, is lethargic, or has severe headaches, an external temporary ventriculostomy may be needed. The ventriculostomy should drain slowly at no

Table 11–2. **Medulloblastoma Staging Location**

Stage	Description
T_1	Tumor <3 cm in diameter and limited to the classic midline position to the vermis, the roof of the fourth ventricle, and less frequently to the cerebellar hemispheres.
T_2	Tumor ≥3 cm in diameter, further invading one adjacent structure or partially filling the fourth ventricle.
T_{3a}	Tumor further invading two adjacent structures or completely filling the fourth ventricle with extension into the aqueduct of Sylvius, foramen of Magendiae, or foramina of Luschka, thus producing marked internal hydrocephalus.
T_{3b}	Tumor arising from the floor of the fourth ventricle or brain stem and filling the fourth ventricle.
T_4	Tumor further spreading through the aqueduct of Sylvius to involve the third ventricle or midbrain, or tumor extending to the upper cervical cord.

Adapted from Chang et al,[36] pp 1351–1352, with permission.

Table 11–3. **Medulloblastoma Staging Metastases**

Stage	Description
M_0	No evidence of gross subarachnoid or hematogenous metastasis.
M_1	Microscopic tumor cells found in cerebrospinal fluid.
M_2	Gross nodular seedings demonstrated in the cerebellar, cerebral subarachnoid space, or in the third or later ventricles.
M_3	Gross nodular seeding in spinal subarachnoid space.
M_4	Metastasis outside the cerebrospinal axis.

Adapted from Chang et al,[36] p 1352, with permission.

greater than 3 to 5 cc per hour to avoid too-rapid tumor decompression, with upward herniation of the tumor and vermis through the tentorium.[38] If hydrocephalus persists after decompression of the ventricular system, or if decompression is not possible, a shunting procedure is necessary. This decision is complicated by the presence of a ventriculostomy. Between 40% and 60% of patients with a temporary ventriculostomy require a permanent CSF shunting procedure. The shunting procedure does not seem to increase the incidence of systemic metastases.[38,39] Ventricular-peritoneal shunts occasionally become infected and require treatment with antibiotics or more commonly, system removal. Shunts also have to be revised as a young child grows to adulthood.

SURGERY

Surgery is the initial step in treatment, and gross total resection is the goal. It is attainable in 75% of patients. The preferred surgical position for craniotomy is the prone position, with the incision in the midline for vermian masses. A detailed description of the procedure was written by Berger and colleagues.[38] The extent of resection was not statistically correlated with survival in some studies,[40,41] but in others gross total resection significantly improved survival.[42–44] In studies without statistical significance, the trend was toward increased survival, with increase in operation from biopsy to gross total resection.[40,41] Surgery is the initial management step in the treatment of medulloblastoma and must be followed with craniospinal RT with a local RT boost to the primary tumor site, with or without chemotherapy.[4,29]

RADIATION THERAPY

Craniospinal RT and a local boost to the primary posterior fossa site is the treatment of choice for medulloblastoma for patients older than 3 years of age. Local control and survival are greater when the boost to the posterior fossa is in excess of 5000 cGy.[45,46] The standard treatment dose to the posterior fossa is now 5000 to 5580 cGy delivered over 5 to 7 weeks.[4,29,39,41,47] Other areas of bulky tumor are also treated with this radiation dose.[29]

The optimal dose for craniospinal RT is still uncertain. Craniospinal RT is technically difficult to deliver with the patient immobilized in the prone position. Particular attention must be given to difficult to radiate areas such as the cribiform plate, temporal tip, and sacral tip. If these sites are inadequately treated, site-specific recurrence is more likely.[48] The standard dose is 3600 cGy to treat the entire subarachnoid space. In two studies, one uncontrolled[49] and the other randomized,[50] lowering the craniospinal RT dose to 2400 to 2500 cGy was associated with a higher rate of leptomeningeal recurrence. Whether 30 Gy or continued use of 36 Gy is optimal, craniospinal RT dose needs to be established. Preliminary data from patients treated at 30 Gy suggest a higher rate of leptomeningeal relapse.[49]

Children younger than 7 years of age with primary CNS tumors treated with

Table 11–4. **Medulloblastoma: Chemotherapy on Recurrence**

Drug	Dose	Patients	Response CR + PR (%)	Median Duration of Response	Toxicity
Procarbazine[59]	100 mg/m² d1–14 or d 8–21	17	5 (29)	45 weeks	Myelosuppression
CCNU	75 mg/m² d1				
Vincristine	1.4 mg/m² d1,8 Q 4–6 wk				
		INDUCTION			
Vincristine[60]	2 mg/m² IV	5	5 (100)	28 months	Mild peripheral neuropathy, myelosuppression, emesis, mucosal ulcerations
MTX	12 mg/m² IT				
Dexamethasone	8 mg/m² weekly × 5				
IV MTX	500 mg/m² over 24 hr × 3, Q 3 wk				
		MAINTENANCE			
BCNU	100 mg/m² IV				
Vincristine	2 mg/m² IV monthly for 2 yr				
Procarbazine[61]	61 mg/m² d8–21	36	NA	100 weeks (median survival)	—
CCNU	61 mg/m² d1				
Vincristine	1.4 mg/m² d8, 29 Q 6 wk				
Vincristine[62]	3 mg/m²	5	At least 4 (80)	6+months	Myelosuppression, abdominal pain
Adriamycin	45 mg/m² for 3 d Q month				
Carboplatin[63]	210 mg/m²/wk Q 3 wk	14	6 (43)	10+months	Thrombocytopenia
Melphalan[64]	45 mg/m² Q 4 wk	12	3 (25)	3+months	Myelosuppression

Continued on following page

Table 11–4.—*continued*

Drug	Dose	Patients	Response CR + PR(%)	Median Duration of Response	Toxicity
CCNU[65]	100 mg/m^2	7	4 (57)	24 months	Myelosuppression, high-frequency hearing loss, decreased renal function
Cisplatin	90 mg/m^2				
Vincristine	1.5 mg/m^2 Q 6 wk				
Carboplatin[66]	560 mg/m^2 IV Q 4 wk	26	2 (8)	NA	Myelosuppression
Iproplatin	270 mg/m^2 IV Q 4 wk	14	1 (7)	NA	
Carboplatin[67]	560 mg/m^2 IV mg/m^2 IV at 4-wk intervals	19	5 (32)	7.5 months	Hearing loss, myelosuppression
Carboplatin[68]	500 mg/m^2/d × 3d	28	12 (no progression)	Median 19 months	3 toxic deaths (11%)
Thiotepa	300 mg/m^2/d × 3d	(16 medulloblastoma + 12 PNET)	13 (recurred)	Median 5 months	
Etoposide	250 mg/m^2/d × 3d				
Bone marrow rescue	mg/m^2/d × 3d				
Cisplatin[97]	60 mg/m^2/d × 2d Q 4 wk	12	3 (25)	3 months	Ototoxicity, myelosuppression, seizures
Cyclophosphamide[145]	80 mg/kg Q 4 wk	8	8 (100)	5.5 months	Myelosuppression
PCNU[147]	100–125 mg/m^2 IV Q 6–7 wk	5	0 (0)	—	Myelosuppression

CR = complete response; d = day; NA = not available; PR = partial response.

craniospinal RT were compared with similarly treated children younger than 3 years of age. After treatment, the children younger than 3 years of age had significantly lower IQ scores than those treated later in life. Performance IQ scores were more affected than verbal IQ scores for children of all ages.[52,53] Therefore, the standard treatment in children younger than 3 years of age is to defer all RT and instead use multiagent chemotherapy.[54,55]

In adults treated with surgery and craniospinal RT with a local tumor boost, the 5- and 10-year survival rates were 46% for each.[11] The 5-year survival in a second series was approximately 66%.[6]

CHEMOTHERAPY

Adjuvant

Children younger than 3 years of age were treated after surgery with a multiagent chemotherapy regimen, alternating two 28-day cycles of cyclophosphamide, and vincristine with one 28-day cycle of cisplatin (CDDP) and etoposide. Treatment continued for 24 months if the child was younger than 2 years of age at diagnosis and for 12 months if the child was older than 2 years of age. If there was disease progression initially or following chemotherapy completion, at age 3 craniospinal RT with a primary site boost was delivered. Chemotherapy was used to delay or possibly spare the developing brain RT and its neurocognitive complications. The progression-free survival rate from the multiagent regimen was 42% at 1 year and 34% at 2 years; total survival was 72% at 1 year and 46% at 2 years.[55]

For "high-risk" patients older than 3 years of age, chemotherapy also appears to be of benefit. In a randomized prospective trial, the Pediatric Oncology Group found a statistically significant increase in 5-year survival (74% versus 56%) in the group that received nitrogen mustard, procarbazine, vincristine and prednisone in addition to craniospinal RT.[56] Packer and colleagues[51,57,58] have evaluated multiagent chemotherapy in "poor-risk" patients with weekly adjuvant vincristine during craniospinal RT followed 6 weeks later with eight 6-week cycles of vincristine, CDDP, and 1-(2-chloroethyl)-3-cyclohexyl-1-nitrosourea (CCNU). The 5-year progression-free survival rate was 85%.[51] These dramatic results substantiate the role of chemotherapy in "poor-risk" patients.

The role of multiagent chemotherapy in "standard- or good-risk" patients is yet to be defined. The outcome in "poor-risk" patients is equal to or better than that attained with craniospinal RT alone in "standard-risk" patients. Logic appears to favor the use of chemotherapy in "standard-risk" patients. It is possible that chemotherapy could be combined with a craniospinal RT dose lower than 3600 cGy, decreasing CNS toxicity in "standard risk" children and achieving equal or better disease control and survival.[51] In adults treated with surgery, craniospinal RT with a local primary site boost, and vincristine and CCNU, the 5- and 10-year survival rate was 76%.[12]

Chemotherapy on Recurrence

Multiple different chemotherapy regimens have been used to treat medulloblastoma when it recurs, with response rates of 7% to 100% (Table 11–4).[59–67] Aggressive high-dose chemotherapy with CDDP, thiotepa, etoposide, and autologous marrow rescue has been used to treat 23 patients with recurrent medulloblastoma, supratentorial and spinal PNET[2], and pineoblastoma. A total of 43% of patients were without progression, for a median of 19 months. There were three therapy-related deaths.[68] Intrathecal monoclonal antibodies raised against medulloblastoma and labeled with Iodine-131 (^{131}I) have also been used to treat 15 patients with medulloblastoma subarachnoid dissemination, with 4 complete response and 1 partial response.[69]

Prognosis and Complications

PROGNOSIS

Five-year survival for patients with medulloblastoma has traditionally been between

30% and 70%.[37,40,42,44–46] The recent reports in "poor-risk" patients treated with adjuvant methotrexate, vincristine, procarbazine, and prednisone (MOPP) chemotherapy with a 74% 5-year survival rate, or adjuvant with CDDP, CCNU, and vincristine with an 83% 5-year survival rate, are very encouraging.[51,56–58]

Prognostic factors (Table 11–5) included age at diagnosis, extent of surgical resection, extent of local disease (T_1 to T_4), and metastatic involvement (M_0 to M_4). Age younger than 4 years was an unfavorable prognostic factor, with a greater incidence of metastatic disease at presentation.[40,70] Age was also a significant factor in late cognitive and learning problems after RT.[52] Children younger than 7 years of age at diagnosis had a decline in full-scale IQ of 25 points 2 years after treatment.[52] Children younger than 3 years of age had a decline in IQ of 34 to 37 points. Extent of surgical resection was positively correlated with survival in three series; in two other series, the extensive resection cohort had a nonsignificant improvement.[40–44] Patients with T_1 to T_2 disease have a significantly better 5-year survival (82% to 87%) than those with T_3 to T_4 (40% to 46%).[37,44] Patients with metastases (M_1 to M_4) had significantly poorer survival than those without metastases (M_0).[40,42]

In an immunohistochemical study of PNET, tumors that expressed GFAP had a 6.7-fold greater risk of relapse than did tumors that did not express GFAP or neurofilament protein. Tumors that expressed GFAP in clumps or sheets of cells were associated with a 3.0-fold increased risk of relapse, regardles of neurofilament expression.[71]

Table 11–5. **Medulloblastoma: Favorable Prognostic Factors**

Favorable Prognostic Factors	Reference
Age > 4 years	40, 70
Stages T_1, T_2	37, 74
Stage M_0	40, 42
Extent of resection	40–44
No GFAP staining	71

COMPLICATIONS

Leptomeningeal spread of tumor (M_1 to M_3) is present in approximately 30% of patients at diagnosis.[72] At diagnosis or postoperatively, all patients should have a staging evaluation that includes complete spinal MRI with gadolinium and CSF cytology. A total of 48 patients were followed who had no leptomeningeal disease at presentation. Leptomeningeal disease was the initial relapse in two patients (4%) without leptomeningeal disease at presentation and occurred simultaneously with local relapse in seven patients (15%). Thirteen patients (27%) had local relapse, 24 (50%) remained disease-free, and two (4%) did not achieve remission.[72] Leptomenigeal dissemination was more common in children younger than 5 years of age.

Systemic metastases occur in approximately 5% of medulloblastomas. Bone metastases are the most common sites, occurring in 90% of cases. Nearly 60% of patients had CNS recurrence at the time of the extraneural spread. At autopsy, extensive involvement of the lymph nodes and liver was often found.[73]

After use of RT and chemotherapy for medulloblastoma, endocrinopathy is common, with deficient growth hormone responses on provocative tests in 85% of cases, abnormalities in thyroid-stimulating hormone secretion in 69% and abnormalities in gonadotrophins in a significant percentage.[74] In an epidemiologic study, Farwell and colleagues[75] concluded that the occurrence of a medulloblastoma in childhood was a risk factor for the development of CNS tumors in relatives.

EPENDYMOMA

History and Nomenclature

Virchow[76] published the first description of an ependymoma in Germany in the 1860s during the American Civil War. In 1924, Bailey[77] first classified ependymomas as glial tumors, and in 1926, Bailey and Cushing[78] developed their histological classification of brain tumors with the cell of origin, a primitive spongioblast, developing into the ependymal spongioblast and ependymoblastoma. The more differentiated tumor was the ependymoma. Ependymomas and ependymoblastomas represented 4% of tumors in the Bailey and Cushing[78] series. In 1935, Kernohan and Fletcher-Kernohan[79] studied 108 cases of ependymoma; 54 were in the cranial cavity, and of these, 32 were in the fourth ventricle. The other 54 were located in the spine, with 30 intramedullary. Of the latter 54, 22 were in the thoracic and 6 in the cervical region of the spinal cord, and 23 were myxopapillary filum terminale ependymomas. Kernohan and Fletcher-Kernohan[79] reinforced Bailey and Cushing's concept that this neoplasm was distinct from a choroid plexus papilloma, which also derived from ependymal cells. Kernohan and Fletcher-Kernohan[79] classified the tumors according to histological cell type: epithelial, myxopapillary, and cellular. They noted that anaplastic ependymomas tended to be cellular and had a shorter duration of symptoms, although benign ependymomas could also be cellular.

Epidemiology

Ependymomas account for 2% to 6% of all intracranial tumors.[78,80] In children, ependymomas are the third most common intracranial neoplasm, accounting for 6% to 12% of intracranial tumors.[81–84] In children younger than 3 years of age, 30% of all intracranial neoplasms are ependymomas. The average annual incidence rate is estimated to be 1.9 per million per year.[10] Approximately one third of ependymomas can be pathologically classified as ependymoblastomas.[83] Whereas a total of 60% to 66% of ependymomas are located infratentorially, ependymoblastomas are more frequently located supratentorially.[81,83,84] The mean age at diagnosis for ependymomas was 5.6 years and ependymoblastomas, 5.0 years. The male to female ratio was 0.8 to 1.0.[83] A total of 40% to 70% of all spinal intramedullary and intradural tumors were ependymomas. Both spinal types are treated surgically, and a cure of spinal myxopapillary ependymoma is often effected with gross total resection.[80] Ependymomas have been associated with the Li-Fraumeni syndrome.[85]

Biology

Ependyma is the cellular lining of the ventricles of the brain, the central canal of the spinal cord, and vestiges of ependyma remain in the filum terminale in the coccygeal region after closure of the neural tube.[3,79,86] The function of the ependyma is not known.[86] Karyotypic and molecular biologic analysis has shown a loss of genetic information on chromosome 22.[87] In a single ependymoma studied with karyotypic analysis, there was a deletion abnormality of the short arm of chromosome 1.[14] In a single case studied with FDG-PET, the tumor could not be identified.[22]

Pathology

Ependymomas occur in any portion of the ventricular system or central canal of the spinal cord.[3,79,80,82,86] They have a predilection for the floor of the fourth ventricle.[79] When Kernohan and Fletcher-Kernohan[79] examined the anterior and posterior medullary velum of the fourth ventricles of patients with ependymomas, disorganization of the ependymal cells was present, predominately in the anterior medullary velum. In addition, and ependymal cells had migrated, singly or in groups, from their normal location into surrounding structures. The cellular ependymal disorganization may provide the substrate for tumor development.

Whereas ependymomas projecting into the fourth ventricle or foramina of Luschka tend to be soft and papillary, those in the cerebellar hemisphere are firm.[3] Infiltration of adjacent brain structures is limited. Microscopically, the tumor has small round neoplastic ependymal cells with occasional mitoses, nuclear atypia, and even necrosis.[3] The tumor is organized into ependymal rosettes and perivascular pseudorosettes (see Fig. 1–10). GFAP, if expressed, is usually in the radiating cell processes of the pseudorosette.[3]

The three cellular variants of ependymoma are clear cell, cellular, and papillary, resembling a choroid plexus papilloma.[3,79] The tumor has a grade II biologic behavior.

The histopathological changes that predict a more aggressive anaplastic ependymoma with grade III behavior have recently been described.[3,88] These changes include high cellularity, marked mitotic activity, nuclear atypia, and prominent endothelial proliferation. Rarely, the tumor transforms into a glioblastoma multiforme.

Clinical Symptoms

The most common initial symptoms in 21 patients with infratentorial ependymoma were nausea, vomiting, and headache. At diagnosis, patients had many more symptoms (Table 11–6).[80] In children younger than 2 years of age, 80% had vomiting, 60% had irritability, 50% had lethargy, 30% had gait disturbance, and 20% had a feeding problem. In children older than 2 years of age, 80% had vomiting, 68% had headache, 28% had gait disturbance, and none had lethargy or irritability.[81]

The common presenting signs in children younger than 2 years of age were increased head circumference and stiff neck in 50%, with papilledema in 40% and truncal ataxia in 20%.[81] In children older than 2 years of age, more than 70% had papilledema, and approximately 50% had truncal ataxia or nystagmus, with 30% limb ataxia, sixth nerve palsy, and brainstem signs.[81]

Differential Diagnosis

The differential diagnosis in children includes medulloblastoma, juvenile pilocytic astrocytoma, LGA of the cerebellum, brainstem glioma, pineal region tumor, suprasellar tumor, choroid plexus papilloma, and dermoid and epidermoid cyst. All of these tumors frequently present with the symptoms and signs associated with increased intracranial pressure.[29] In adults, meningioma and metastases to the posterior fossa must be considered.[89] The symptoms of ependymoma and medulloblastoma are likely to be identical, but ependymoma usually has a longer symptom duration (6 to 12 months versus 4 months).[29] Brainstem tumors typically present with crossed cranial nerve and long tract signs or bilateral cranial nerve and long tract signs.[29] Juvenile pilocytic astrocytoma and LGA present with a slower onset of symptoms similar to ependymoma, but with more frequent limb ataxia. On imaging studies, juvenile pilocytic astrocytoma is more often cystic with an enhancing nodule. LGAs of the cerebellum usually do not enhance with contrast.

Patients with pineal tumors present with pupillary and vertical gaze difficulties, and those with suprasellar tumors present frequently with an endocrinopathy. Choroid

Table 11–6. **Ependymoma: Initial Symptoms and Symptoms at Diagnosis in 21 Cases**

Initial Symptoms (% of patients)		Symptoms at Diagnosis (% of patients)
29	Nausea and vomiting	100
33	Headache	86
14	Increased head circumference	14
9	Dizziness	43
5	Diplopia	48
5	Unsteady gait	48
5	Hemiparesis	9

Adapted from Rawlings et al,[80] p 272, with permission.

plexus tumor, dermoid and epidermoid cysts, and meningioma are best differentiated by their MRI characteristics.

Diagnostic Workup

MRI is the current imaging procedure of choice in the evaluation of posterior fossa masses. Sagittal and axial T_1-weighted images are obtained before contrast administration, and sagittal, axial, and coronal T_1-weighted images are obtained after contrast administration. T_2-weighted axial and coronal images are needed. CT with and without contrast is an acceptable alternative. Ependymomas are typically hypointense or isointense on precontrast T_1-weighted images, and they enhance with contrast. The T_1 signal may be heterogeneous. On T_2-weighted images, they are hyperintense and well demarcated from surrounding brain.[89] On precontrast CT scans, they are seen as isodense or hyperdense, often with mixed signal, and enhance heterogeneously before contrast administration. They have calcification in 50% of cases.

Hydrocephalus is extremely common on either MRI or CT images. The incidence of calcification is higher in ependymomas, than medulloblastomas, brainstem gliomas, or other posterior fossa tumors. The MRI signal characteristics do not help distinguish ependymoma from medulloblastoma (Fig. 11–2). The intraventricular location of ependymoma with extension out the foramina of Luschka may distinguish it from medulloblastoma, but both tumors present as fourth ventricular masses.

Although the incidence of spinal dissemination is lower than that in medulloblastoma, all patients should be staged with CSF cytology and spinal MRI, either preoperatively if stable or in the postoperative setting.[90]

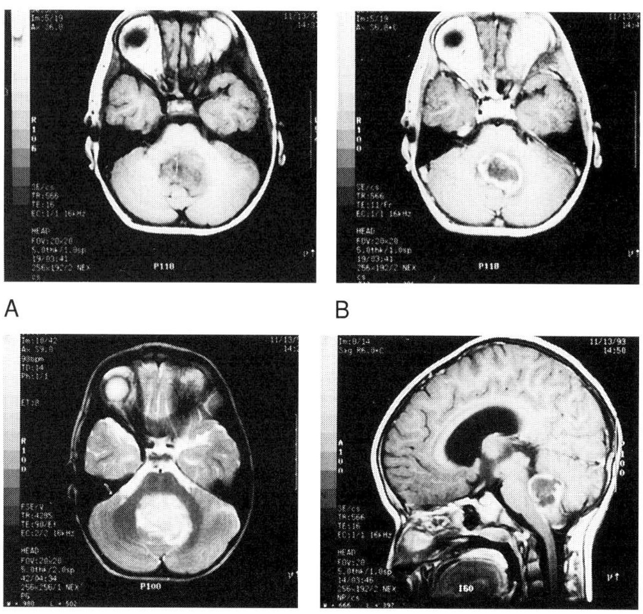

A B C D

Figure 11–2. Ependymoma: T_1-weighted axial MRI. *(A)* Precontrast hypointense signal in fourth ventricle and *(B and D)* postcontrast T_1-weighted MRI in axial and sagittal planes with heterogeneous contrast enhancement filling fourth ventricle similar to medulloblastoma. *(C)* T_2-weighted MRI with mild edema extending around mass. *(D)* Hydrocephalus produced by fourth ventricular obstruction.

Treatment

SYMPTOMATIC

Hydrocephalus is seen in the majority of patients on presentation.[81,86] Preoperative shunting is rarely necessary. Sudden decompression can be dangerous because of either upward herniation through the tentorium or shift in the infratentorial compartment producing brainstem compression or hemorrhage into the tumor.[86,91] The hydrocephalus is best treated with corticosteroids, osmotic diuretics, and hyperventilation.[86,91] If the patient is deteriorating despite treatment, a ventriculostomy is optimally performed intraoperatively through a burr hole. The management of the ventriculostomy and the decision to shunt are discussed in the symptomatic treatment of medulloblastoma.

SURGERY

The goals of surgery are gross total removal of tumor and re-establishment of normal CSF flow.[91] The patient is placed in the prone position with the neck flexed, and a midline incision is made similar to that used in medulloblastoma. A suboccipital craniectomy including the foramen magnum and the arch of C1 is then performed. A detailed description of the surgical procedure is discussed by Duncan and Hoffman.[91] In all cases, surgical resection is the first step in a combined treatment program and is most often followed with RT. If the CSF pathways cannot be decompressed or if hydrocephalus persists despite adequate decompression, ventriculoperitoneal shunting is necessary.[86] The 5-year survival rate for patients treated with surgery alone was 33% for infratentorial and 15% for supratentorial tumors.[92]

RADIATION THERAPY

Patients with infratentorial or supratentorial ependymomas should be treated with focal field RT with a total dose of 5000 to 5500 cGy.[93,95] In patients with infratentorial ependymoma, RT produced a 5-year progression-free survival rate of 58% in patients with gross total resection or more than 90% resection versus 30% for those who had only biopsy or partial resection.[93] Similar results were seen in other series and for patients with supratentorial ependymoma[93,80,81,94] Patients with anaplastic infratentorial or anaplastic supratentorial lesions adjacent to CSF pathways are best treated with craniospinal RT and a focal boost to the primary site because of the risk of leptomeningeal dissemination.[93,95] Anaplastic supratentorial lesions at a distance from CSF pathways, are treated with whole brain radiation therapy (WBRT) and a local boost to the primary site.[93] When patients with benign or anaplastic ependymomas are grouped according to whether they received prophylactic craniospinal RT or not, there was no decrease in incidence in leptomeningeal dissemination in the craniospinal RT group in either the benign or malignant ependymomas.[96] These results raise the question of the value of using craniospinal RT in anaplastic ependymomas adjacent to CSF spaces.

In children younger than 3 years of age with ependymoma, RT is deferred as in those with medulloblastoma. These patients are instead treated with a multiagent chemotherapy regimen.

CHEMOTHERAPY

Adjuvant

Sutton and colleagues[93] have treated all patients with newly diagnosed ependymomas and anaplastic ependymomas with multiagent chemotherapy, identical to the regimen described for medulloblastomas.[51,57,58] Adjuvant vincristine is administered weekly with RT, and then 6 weeks after the completion of RT, a planned regimen of eight 6-week cycles of vincristine, CDDP, and CCNU is begun. The 5-year progression-free survival rate with infratentorial ependymomas was 40%. Patients who were treated with a similar regimen without CDDP had the same outcome. The addition of RT and multiagent chemotherapy has not produced a significant increase in survival for patients with infratentorial ependymal tumors compared with a 33% 5-year survival rate for those with ependymomas with surgery alone.[92] Clearly, more effective chemotherapy drugs are needed to treat ependymoma. Chemotherapy regimens will have to be individualized for ependymomas or possibly chemotherapy will prove to be ineffective.

Chemotherapy on Recurrence

Chemotherapy has also been used after tumor recurrence (Table 11–7).[66,67,97] The three trials involved the platinum compounds carboplatin or CDDP. CDDP had a response rate of 50% and a median response duration of 4 months.[66,67,97] Carboplatin had a response rate of 12% to 14% and a median duration of response of 11.5 months in one of these two trials.

Prognosis and Complications

PROGNOSIS

The 5-year survival rate for patients treated with surgery alone was 33% for infratentorial and 15% for supratentorial tumors.[92] In patients with posterior fossa ependymoma, the addition of RT, with or without multiagent chemotherapy, produced a 5-year progression-free survival rate of 58% in patients with gross total resection or more than 90% resection. The 5-year progression-free survival rate was 30% for patients who had only biopsy or partial resection.[93] Similar results were seen with supratentorial ependymoma[93] and in other series,[80,81,94] reaffirming the importance of extent of resection for extended survival.

Age younger than 4 years is a predictor of poor outcome.[81,84,93,98] Histopathologically, the presence of calcium has been correlated with a poorer prognosis.[99] The histological degree of malignancy has been correlated with survival in some series[81,98] but not in others.[84,93]

COMPLICATIONS

Ependymomas almost always recur at the primary tumor site, and recurrence is earlier after subtotal resection than after gross total resection.[80,81,84,86,93–95] Leptomeningeal dissemination was found in 8.4% of anaplastic ependymomas and 4.5% of benign ependymomas.[96] The incidence was greater for infratentorial tumors than for supratentorial tumors. Spinal seeding occurred in 9.5% of cases with failure at the primary site and only 3.3% of cases when local control was maintained.[96] Prophylactic craniospinal RT did not decrease the incidence of leptomeningeal dissemination.[96] Craniospinal RT is now given routinely only to patients with infratentorial anaplastic ependymomas, with the highest risk of dissemina-

Table 11–7. **Ependymoma: Chemotherapy on Recurrence**

Drug	Dose	Patients	Response CR + PR (%)	Median Duration of Response	Toxicity
Carboplatin[66]	560 mg/m^2 q 4 wk	17	2 (12)	NA	Myelosuppression
Iproplatin[66]	270 mg/m^2 q 4 wk	7	0 (0)	0	Myelosuppression
Carboplatin[67]	560 mg/m^2 q 4 wk	14	2 (14)	11.5 + months	Ototoxicity, myelosuppression
Cisplatin[97]	60 mg/m^2/d × 2d q 4 wks	8	4 (50)	4 months	Ototoxicity, renal toxicity, myelosuppression

NA = Not available.

tion, but its efficacy has not been well documented.

BRAINSTEM GLIOMAS

History and Nomenclature

In 1930, Buckley[100] reviewed 1737 pathological specimens from operations by Cushing and found 25 pontine tumors, predominately gliomas. This is an underestimate of the true incidence of brainstem gliomas because of the difficulty in biopsy and removal of brainstem tumors. Gibbs[101] noted that brainstem tumors are more common in children, and he estimated the incidence in adults to be only 10% of that in children. White[102] reported the first adult series of brainstem gliomas in 1960, which included 44 cases over 31 years and a median age of 42 years.

In 1985, Epstein[103] suggested a classification system based on whether tumors were intrinsic, exophytic, or disseminated. In the intrinsic category, brainstem gliomas were subcategorized as diffuse, focal, or cervicomedullary, and within the exophytic category, by anatomic location of exophytic growth. Brainstem tumors have recently been classified with MRI according to site, longitudinal extent, growth (focal or diffuse), brainstem enlargement, exophytic growth, axial extent, contrast enhancement, presence or absence of cysts, hydrocephalus, hemorrhage, or necrosis.[104] Pontine tumors were found to have a worse prognosis than midbrain or medullary tumors. The greater the brainstem enlargement and the more diffuse the process, the worse the prognosis.[104]

Epidemiology

Brainstem gliomas account for between 10% and 20% of pediatric CNS neoplasms,[105–108] and 75% occur before the age of 20 years.[105–108] The peak prevalence is in the latter half of the first decade of life, and there is no gender preference.[106] The prevalence in the adult population is 1% to 2% of adult tumors.[101,102] The overwhelming majority of cases are sporadic, but a familial case has been reported.[107,108]

Biology

Cytogenetic studies with karyotypic analysis have been rare because of the small amount of material available from brainstem biopsies. In a single patient, trisomy of chromosome 1 was found, with translocation of the extra copy of chromosome 1 on to the distal end of chromosome 7.[109]

Jenkins and colleagues[110] thought the chromosomal changes in brainstem glioma should be identical to those in astrocytomas elsewhere in the brain. Molecular biologic analysis using RFLP in seven brainstem gliomas found that four of seven tumors lost the short arm of chromosome 17, including the *p53* gene. The *p53* gene was mutated in five cases, which resulted in base changes in two patients and a stop codon in a third patient. Four of seven cases had allelic loss of chromosome 10, and none had epidermal growth factor receptor (EGFR) amplification.[111] In another study, eight of 13 patients with pontine glioma had *p53* gene mutations, which often resulted in a missense mutation with amino acid substitution.[112] These changes appear similar to the spectrum of changes seen with astrocytoma in the cerebral hemispheres (see Chapter 2). There are no series of BUdR or Ki-67 proliferative labeling index studies in brainstem glioma.

Pathology

Brainstem gliomas present with diffuse infiltrative expansion of the brainstem in 75% of cases.[102,105,106] They also present focally within the brainstem, grow exophytically from the tectal plate or dorsal pons into the floor of the fourth ventricle or from the ventral midbrain and pons into the premesencephalic or prepontine cisterns. They may grow laterally into the cerebellopontine angle.[102,106] In children, 75% to 80% of brainstem gliomas occur in the pons, 15% to 20% in the medulla, and 10% in the midbrain.[105–108] In adults, 56% of tumors occur in the pons, 30% in the medulla, and 12% in the midbrain.[107] On macroscopic examination, the brainstem is swollen or deformed. The tumor pushes through existing structures with little tissue destruction and grows both longitudinally within the brainstem and axially. It may invade the cerebral hemispheres or cervical cord, and if it expands dorsally in the brainstem, it may produce obstructive hydrocephalus.[105,106]

The majority of childhood and adult brainstem gliomas are of astrocytic differentiation and look identical to astrocytic tumors elsewhere.[102,105–108] A small percentage of brainstem gliomas are pilocytic, with rare histological diagnoses including oligodendroglioma, mixed glioma, ganglioglioma, and ependymoblastoma.[105] The tumors are usually low-grade fibrillary astrocytomas, that would be classified with a Grade II biologic behavior, by 1993 WHO criteria. They grow as other LGAs do, infiltrating between and along nerve fiber fascicles and along the pial-limiting membrane.[107,113] Alternatively, they may grow in a focal pattern with identical histology as in the diffuse growth pattern. Tumors involving the medulla and cervical cord and those in the midbrain are more often LGA. High-grade fibrillary astrocytomas (i.e., anaplastic astrocytoma and glioblastoma multiforme) also occur and are more common in the pons. The extent of infiltration and invasiveness is greater, and they destroy surrounding normal brain just as in supratentorial malignant gliomas.[107]

Clinical Symptoms

Brainstem gliomas manifest with the insidious onset of gait abnormalities and cranial nerve abnormalities, particularly diplopia, pyramidal tract signs, and headache (Table 11–8).[102,105–108,114,115] The evolution of symptoms occurs over 2 to 10 months (median, 4 to 5 months) and depends on the location of the tumor and the tumor biology. Gait disturbance occurs in 40% to 80% of patients and is due to either pyramidal tract or cerebellar pathway abnormalities. The most common symptoms referable to cranial nerves are diplopia and facial weakness, but almost any cranial nerve or combination of cranial nerves may be involved. Focal weakness is a pyramidal tract sign that can be unilateral or bilateral; when bilateral, it is usually asymmetric. Headache is due to either obstruction of the aqueduct of Sylvius or fourth ventricle from dorsal brainstem expansion or traction on the surrounding meninges or basilar artery.

Table 11–8. **Brainstem Glioma: Presenting Symptoms in Four Series (Two Children and Two Adults)**

	Children		***Adults***	
	Halperin et al[127] (n = 38)	**Eifel et al[130] (n = 79)**	**White et al[102] (n = 44)**	**Grigsby et al[115] (n = 136)**
Presenting Symptoms	**% of cases**		**% of cases**	
Gait disturbance	63	48	77	58
Diplopia	NR	NR	70	91
Focal weakness	37	34	59	57
Headache	42	49	52	54
Vomiting	24	33	30	30
Facial numbness	11	NR	14	49
Facial weakness	39	NR	11	90
Personality changes	NR	10	20	NR

NR = Not reported.

Other common symptoms include dysarthria, focal numbness, dysphagia, nausea, vomiting, hearing loss, vertigo, tinnitus, and personality change.[102,106,107,114] Dorsal midbrain gliomas can produce a Parinaud's syndrome with pupillary and vertical gaze abnormalities. Dysarthria and dysphagia often portend a particularly difficult clinical course.[106] Facial myokymia and hemifacial spasms are rare presenting signs of brainstem gliomas.[107] Seizures occur in less than 5% of patients. Brainstem gliomas can affect central autonomic control centers within the reticular system of the pons and medulla, with respiratory symptoms of apnea, hypoventilation or hyperventilation, and autonomic symptoms of orthostatic hypotension or syncope.[102,107,116]

At diagnosis, the most common neurologic signs in approximately 75% of patients include seventh nerve palsy, nystagmus (usually horizontal), cerebellar signs, motor weakness, hyperreflexia, and unilateral or bilateral extensor plantar response.[102]

Differential Diagnosis

The differential diagnosis of infiltrative brainstem disease is limited to a few diseases. Medulloblastoma, ependymoma, and medulloepithelioma are primary neoplasms that rarely arise within the brainstem. In adults, metastatic spread to the brainstem must be considered.[107] Non-neoplastic infectious considerations affecting the brainstem include an acute viral brainstem encephalitis, a postviral autoimmune encephalitis, brainstem abscess, tuberculoma, and cysticercosis.[105–108] Encephalitis can usually be distinguished by a lymphocytic pleocytosis on CSF examination. MRI images should help distinguish brainstem and glioma from abscess, cysticercosis, or tuberculoma. TB skin testing and serum hemagglutinin tests for cysticercosis are helpful.[105] In children, metabolic abnormalities such as Kearns-Sayre syndrome may be confused with brainstem glioma.[106] Demyelinating disease (i.e., multiple sclerosis [MS]) can be particularly difficult to differentiate from brainstem gliomas because it presents with multifocal brainstem signs and symptoms and can have an insidious or fulminant course. A search for a second lesion in MS with clinical examination, visual- or somatosensory-evoked response studies, MRI, or CSF examination may help. In the era before CT, MRI, and brainstem biopsy, the misdiagnosis of MS as brainstem glioma accounted for many of the infiltrative brainstem processes reported as long-term survivors. Lastly, arteriovenous malformation of the brainstem can become symptomatic because of expansion or hemorrhage. MRI should help clarify the diagnosis: hemorrhage, calcification, and contrast enhancement occur more frequently than in brainstem gliomas.

Although CT or MRI usually help discriminate between brainstem glioma and other disease processes, 17% of 33 patients thought to have a brainstem tumor preoperatively had non-neoplastic lesions on biopsy, usually an arteriovenous malformation.[117] In a second similar study of 71 patients after brainstem biopsy, 19.4% had diagnoses other than brainstem glioma.[118] The diagnoses were nonspecific chronic inflammation (four patients), granulomatous inflammation (two patients), epidermoid cyst (two patients), brain abscess (two patients), and encephalitis (one patient).

Diagnostic Workup

MRI is the diagnostic procedure of choice.[105–108] Scans are best acquired with thin 3-mm cuts, with sagittal and axial T_1-weighted images before contrast administration and sagittal, coronal and axial T_1-weighted images after contrast administration. T_2-weighted axial and coronal images are needed.[106] On MRI scans, brainstem gliomas are seen to most frequently originate in the pons with diffuse enlargement, but they can originate anywhere in the brainstem.[105–108] Brainstem glioma signals are usually hypointense when compared with normal white matter on T_1-weighted images, and they are hyperintense on T_2-weighted images. Typically, low-grade brainstem tumors do not enhance after contrast administration. Hydrocephalus is present in only 25% to 30% of cases, less than in medulloblastomas and ependymomas.[107] Cystic changes occur in 10% of cases.[107] Higher-grade brainstem tumors are more likely to enhance after gadolinium and have signs of necrosis. Other imaging features favoring aggressive biologic behavior are subpial or subependymal extension and ill-defined tumor margins.[105] At postmortem examination, brainstem gliomas have little edema; therefore, the T_2-weighted abnormality is thought to reflect the spatial extent of the tumor.[106] The great majority of brainstem tumors are infiltrative and diffuse. They infiltrate axially within a brainstem segment and spread longitudinally into the thalamus, cerebellar peduncle, cerebellum, and upper cervical spinal cord (Fig. 11–3). Focal tumors are smaller and frequently grow exophytically into the subarachnoid cisterns around the

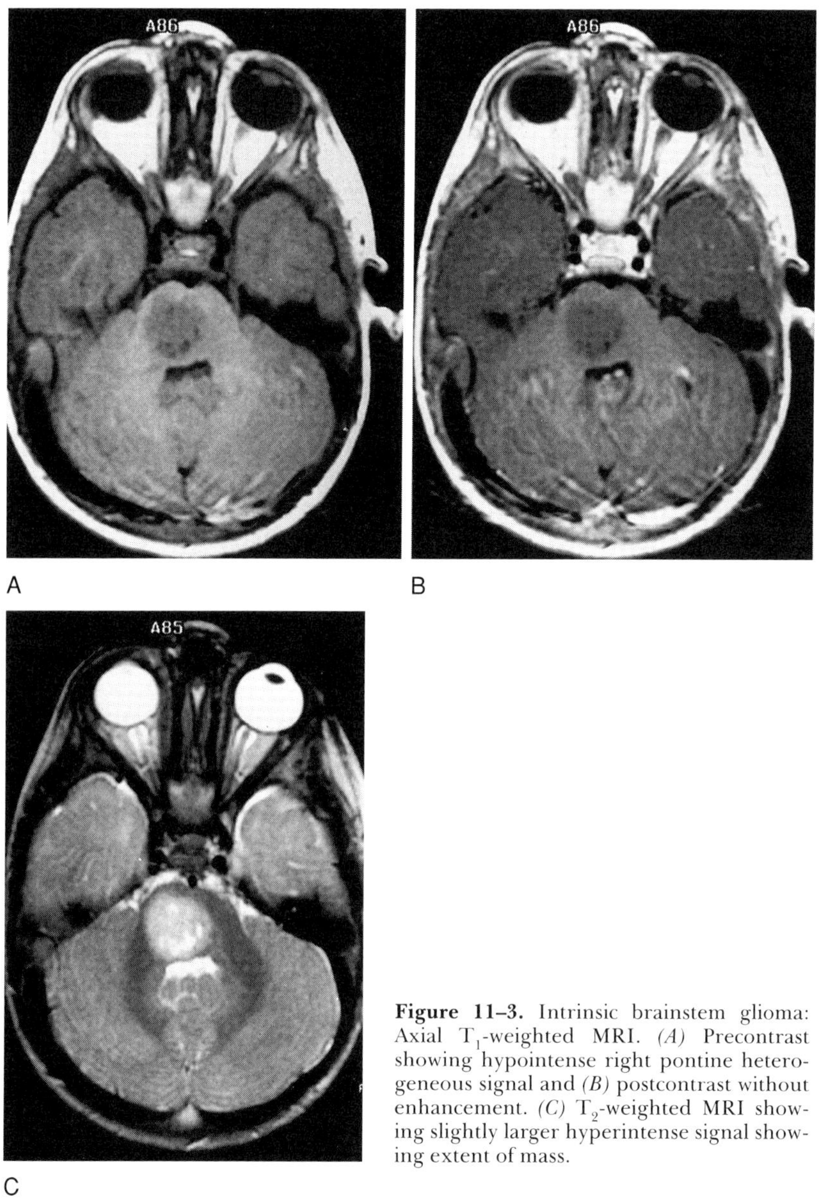

Figure 11–3. Intrinsic brainstem glioma: Axial T_1-weighted MRI. *(A)* Precontrast showing hypointense right pontine heterogeneous signal and *(B)* postcontrast without enhancement. *(C)* T_2-weighted MRI showing slightly larger hyperintense signal showing extent of mass.

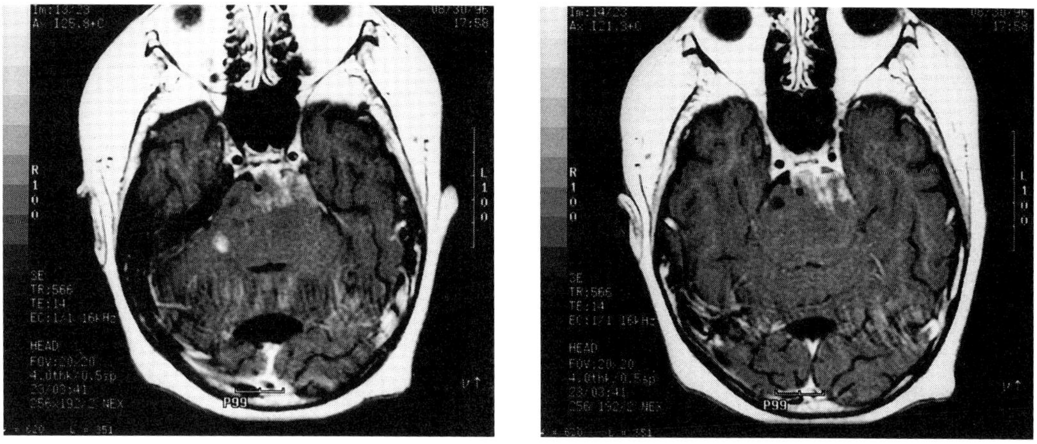

A B

Figure 11–4. Intrinsic brainstem glioma: Axial MRI. *(A and B)* Postcontrast showing ventrally exophytic, contrast-enhancing tumor encasing the basilar artery. There are small hypointense cystic regions, and *(A)* the enhancement is multifocal.

brainstem and may encase the basilar artery or grow into the cerebellopontine angle (Fig. 11–4). The exophytic portion often enhances with contrast (Fig. 11–5).[106,107]

CT detects the great majority of brainstem gliomas but is not as sensitive as MRI and does not provide the same level of anatomic detail. Small focal lesions that do not deform the fourth ventricle and exophytic tumor in the basal cisterns may not be detected. Bone- and beam-hardening artifacts in the posterior fossa may obscure tumors, particularly at the cervicomedullary junction. On CT scans, the tumor usually appears hypodense or iso-

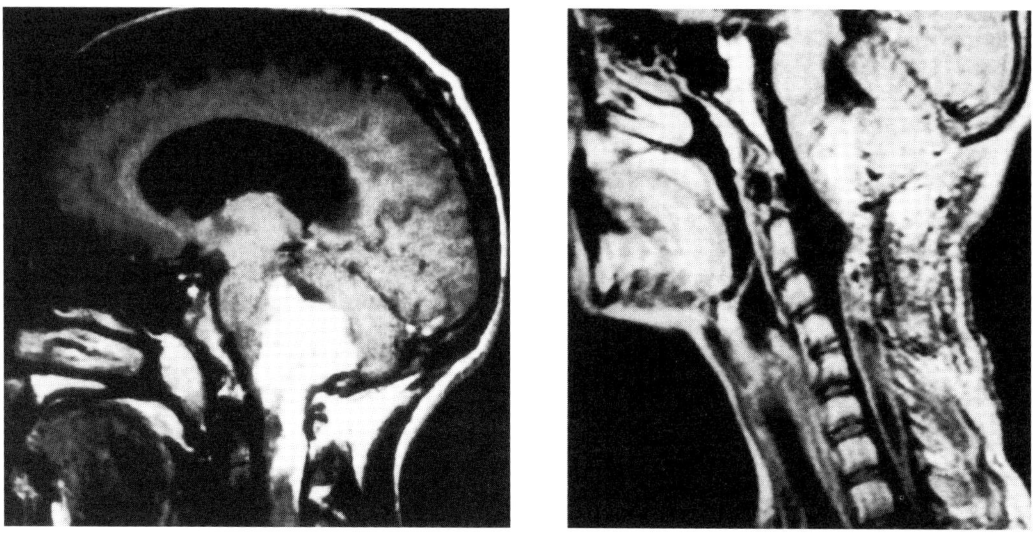

A B

Figure 11–5. Dorsally exophytic cervicomedullary glioma: Preoperative sagittal T_1-weighted MRI. *(A)* Postcontrast infusion with large dorsally exophytic cervicomedullary contrast enhancing mass filling the fourth ventricle producing hydrocephalus. *(B)* Postoperative sagittal T_1-weighted MRI showing partial resection of a significant portion of the dorsal exophytic component, with the anterior part of the fourth ventricle now visible. (From Robertson et al.,[123] p 1081, with permission.)

dense and typically does not enhance. Calcification is seen in 10% to 15% of cases.

CSF examination is rarely needed for positive diagnosis, but it may provide information about infectious or demyelinating differential diagnoses. Brainstem auditory-evoked potentials are not useful diagnostically but may be used during surgery for brainstem monitoring or to assess eighth nerve involvement in young patients.[106,107]

Treatment

SYMPTOMATIC

Hydrocephalus occurs in 25% to 30% of patients and should be treated initially with corticosteroids. If there is no response or if the patient is deteriorating, a ventriculoperitoneal shunt may be needed, particularly if surgery cannot restore the patency of the CSF pathways through removal of a dorsally exophytic mass or cyst drainage.[119]

SURGERY

Stereotactic Biopsy

The four aims of surgery in brainstem gliomas are to: (1) obtain a tissue diagnosis, (2) remove as much exophytic tumor as possible, (3) drain cysts, and (4) restore patency to the CSF pathways. Controversy exists over whether tissue diagnosis is needed in a patient with a diffuse, nonenhancing pontine abnormality that enlarges the brainstem. Reasons physicians may be reluctant to perform biopsy include (1) the operative morbidity and mortality are high, (2) the biopsy may be nondiagnostic, (3) the treatment will be the same regardless of the grade of the tumor, and (4) MRI establishes the diagnosis with certainty.[120] If 17% to 19% of patients with suspected brainstem glioma have nonmalignant pathology, a strong argument can be made for stereotactic biopsy, whenever safe.[117,118,120] However, the complications of brainstem stereotactic biopsy were significant in one series, in which one patient (3%) died, two (6%) had significant neurological morbidity, and five (15%) developed acute hydrocephalus.[117] In other series,[118–121] the complication rate was low.

In the series of Stroink and colleagues,[119] patients with a predominantly diffuse or solid intrinsic masses had more than a 50% rate of nondiagnostic biopsies. Biopsies were successfully obtained for all cystic tumors in the series of Stroink and associates[119] and Hood and McKeever.[121] The guidelines for stereotactic biopsy in brainstem gliomas will continue to evolve over time, but a biopsy should be obtained if it can be performed safely and if there is a reasonable doubt about diagnosis. In summary, diffuse infiltrative pontine abnormalities that expand the brainstem have a high yield of nondiagnostic biopsies, a small likelihood of an alternative diagnosis, a high complication rate, and can probably be treated with RT without biopsy.

Surgical Resection

Epstein and Wisoff[122] concluded that patients with diffuse tumors of the brainstem could not be treated with surgical resection. The authors thought that surgery was indicated for focal cystic and cervicomedullary lesions.[122] Intra-axial cervicomedullary tumors were resected in 17 children. In 11 children without previous therapy, the 4-year progression-free survival rate was 70%, and total survival was 100%. Fifteen of the 17 patients had low-grade glial tumors, and two had anaplastic astrocytomas.[123]

Surgery is beneficial in exophytic lesions, particularly dorsal exophytic lesions.[124–127] Pollack[125] and Khatib[126] and their colleagues reported on the successful radical but subtotal resection of tumors that arise from the dorsum of the medullary portion of the brainstem in young children and fill the fourth ventricle. The tumors were juvenile pilocytic astrocytomas in one series[125] and were predominantly grade I and II astrocytomas in the other study.[126] Thirteen of 17 patients in one study have not had disease progression with a median follow-up of 113 months. Two patients were treated with RT.[125] In a second study of 12 patients, the progression-free survival rate was 67%, and total survival was 100%. Three patients received RT.[126] Following surgery, patients were observed postoperatively; 25% showed tumor progression and were treated with reoperation, RT, or both. No operative morbidity was found in the two series, but neurological deficits frequently worsened transiently, and five of 30 patients developed new deficits. Pierre-Khan and colleagues[124] expanded the indications for surgery to exophytic tumor in any brainstem location. The operative mortality in this series was high at 16% and was still 10% after introduction of the Cavitron Ultrasonic Aspirator (Cavitron, Boulder, Colorado). Pathology was benign in 47 patients (including those with pilocytic astrocytomas), malignant in 22, and of uncertain grade in eight. The 5-year survival rate of the 63 patients who survived surgery was 55%, and the 10-year survival rate was 49%. Patients who had a subtotal resection received RT.[124]

RADIATION THERAPY

RT is the primary treatment modality for the majority of patients with brainstem gliomas, particularly those with diffuse and infiltrative tumors. Brainstem glioma is a focal disease, and the majority of postradiation recurrences occur in the original tumor bed. In one study, 22 of 25 patients (88%) recurred totally within field, with two of 25 (8%) both inside and outside field. Therefore, patients should be treated with focal field irradiation.[127] A total of 38 patients with brainstem glioma (100% of those biopsied were malignant glioma) were treated with RT (23 focal and 14 WBRT). The 5-year survival rate was 39%. Kim and colleagues[128] treated 80 patients with brainstem gliomas (39% of those biopsied were glioblastoma multiforme) with RT. When doses of at least 5000 cGy were used, the 3-year survival rate was 40%, and the 5-year survival rate was 35%. There were no 4-year survivors for patients treated with less than 5000 cGy.[127] Shibamoto and associates[129] treated 79 patients (61% of those biopsied were high-grade astrocytoma), and there was a 5-year survival rate of 17%. In another study of 79 patients (malignancy percentage unknown), the 5-year survival rate was 50%, and the 10-year survival rate was 41%.[130] Patients with thalamic and midbrain tumors fared better than those with pontine and medullary tumors.

Hyperfractionated twice-daily RT in a cumulative dose of between 6400 cGy and 7200 cGy has been used to treat brainstem gliomas in at least three single-institution studies. A multi-institution trial has also been reported.[131–134] The median survival time has varied between 10 and 17 months in these trials, with the 5-year survival rate ranging from less than 7 to 37%. The trial with the longest median survival and greatest 5-year survival rate had a relatively low percentage (45%) of malignant biopsied lesions. In summary, hyperfractionated RT has shown no increase in 5-year survival over focal conventionally fractionated RT.

Interstitial brachytherapy with Iodine-125 (^{125}I) or Iridium-192 (^{192}Ir) has been used to treat 89 patients with brainstem gliomas, 55 of which were predominantly in the midbrain.[135] A total of 61% of patients had pilocytic astrocytomas, and the others had LGAs. The median survival was estimated to be approximately 18 months.

Stereotactic radiosurgery (SR), in a dose of 1400 to 3500 cGy, has been used to treat seven patients with midbrain low-grade tectal gliomas. Five tumors progressively shrank, and all patients were alive at a median follow-up of 6 years. Patients treated at higher doses developed radiation necrosis and progression of deficits.[136] Midbrain tectal gliomas are thought to be relatively benign. In a recent series of midbrain tectal gliomas, 12 children presented with hydrocephalus, and all were treated with ventriculoperitoneal shunts. No patient received further therapy until disease progression. Three patients progressed and were treated with RT alone or RT and chemotherapy. The median progression-free survival was 24 months, and the median survival was 50 months.[137] The utility of adjuvant interstitial brachytherapy or SR in this setting is questioned.

CHEMOTHERAPY

Adjuvant Chemotherapy

A Children's Cancer Group Study[138] randomized 74 children with brainstem gliomas to RT or RT and adjuvant chemotherapy with CCNU, vincristine, and prednisone. There was no difference between treatments, and there was a 5-year median survival rate of 20%. An increased risk of infection was associated with chemotherapy treatment.[138] A total of 37 patients with brainstem gliomas were treated either adjuvantly (n = 13) or on recurrence (n = 24), with a nitrosourea, procarbazine, or a combination of both, sometimes including vincristine.[139] The median survival for a subset of the 37 patients who received all their care at the parent institution, including all adjuvant and half the recurrent patients, was 44 weeks with a 5-year survival of 8%. In summary, no benefit has been seen with adjuvant chemotherapy.

Chemotherapy on Recurrence

Thirteen patients with brainstem gliomas were treated with a combination of 5-fluorouracil (5-FU), CCNU, hydroxyurea, and 6-mercaptopurine, with 4 CR + PR (30%) and a median duration of response of 12 weeks. An additional five patients had SD with a median duration of response of 25 weeks for these nine patients and a median survival of 27 weeks. Four patients survived more than 1 year after chemotherapy (Table 11–9).[106,140] Chamberlain and colleagues[141] used oral etoposide to treat 12 patients with recurrent brainstem glioma after RT, and nitrosourea-based chemotherapy failure. One patient had a CR, 3 PR, and 2 SD, with a median duration of response of 8 months.[141]

Platinum compounds have been used to treat brainstem gliomas. CDDP has been used in two trials, with 1 PR in nine patients.[142,143] In four clinical trials with carboplatin, 51 brainstem glioma patients were treated, with 4 PR (8%).[63,66,67,144] Among the 51 patients, an infant with a recurrent brainstem glioma had a 39+ month CR with carboplatin.[144] Iproplatin was also used in 14 patients, with no responses.[66]

Two other alkylating agents have been used with minor success to treat brainstem gliomas. Cyclophosphamide produced a PR in four of five (80%) patients with recurrent brainstem gliomas.[145] In a subsequent trial, six patients with brainstem gliomas were treated with marrow ablative doses of cyclophosphamide and thiotepa with autologous bone marrow rescue followed by adjuvant hyperfractionated RT to 75.6 Gy. In five evaluable patients, there was 1 PR (16%) and 1 (16%) minor response.[146] 1-(2-chloroethyl)-2-(2,6-dioxo-3-piperidyl)-nitrosourea was used to treat 17 patients with brainstem gliomas, with 3 PR (17.6%).[147] Tamoxifen was used to treat four children with intrinsic brainstem gliomas and one with cervicomedullary glioma, with four objective responses for a duration of 6 to 30 months.[148]

In summary, chemotherapy for recurrent brainstem gliomas has consisted of predominantly small, single-agent chemotherapy trials, with response rates (CR + PR) of 0% to 33%. A single small trial of cyclophosphamide reported in 1981 had an 80% response rate, but when higher doses of the same agent were used with adjuvant hyperfractionated RT to 75.6 Gy, there was a more typical 20% response rate.[145] The most promising results appear to be with oral tamoxifen or etoposide.

Adjuvant Immunotherapy

A total of 32 patients with diffuse intrinsic brainstem glioma were treated with 7200 cGy hypofractionated RT and recombinant β-interferon 3 times per week during and 8 weeks following RT.[149] The safe interferon starting dose was 100×10^6 IU/m^2. The median time to progression was 5 months with a median survival of 9 months, suggesting that recombinant β-interferon did not improve survival.

Prognosis and Complications

PROGNOSIS

The 5-year survival rate for brainstem gliomas treated with focal RT in clinical

Table 11–9. **Brainstem Glioma: Chemotherapy on Recurrence**

Drug	Dose	Patients	Response CR + PR (%)	Median Duration of Response	Toxicity
Carboplatin[63]	210 mg/m²/wk × 4	8	1 (12)	5 months	Myelosuppression
Carboplatin[66]	560 mg/m² IV q 4 wks	21	1 (5)	NA	Myelosuppression
Iproplatin[66]	270 mg/m² IV q 4 wks	14	0 (0)	0	Myelosuppression
Carboplatin[67]	560 mg/m² IV q 4 wks	19	1 (5)	33 + months	Myelosuppression
5-FU[140]	1 g/m²/d x d × dl-3	13	4 (31)	3 mo; four 1-y survivors	Myelosuppression, nausea, vomiting
CCNU	100 mg/m² on day 8				
Hydroxyurea	400 mg/m² q 6 hrs d21–23				
6-mercaptopurine	100 mg/m² PO or 6 h, d28–30, q 8 wk × 6				
Etoposide[141]	50 mg/m²/d × 21d q 5 wk	12	6 (50)	8 mo	No toxicity
Cisplatin[142]	60 mg/m² IV × 2	5	0 (0)	0	Myelosuppression, ototoxicity, renal toxicity
Cisplatin[143]	120 mg/m² IV × 1d q 3–4 wk	6	1 (16)	4 mo	Myelosuppression, ototoxicity, renal toxicity
Carboplatin[144]	560 mg/m² IV q 4 wks	1 (cervicomedullary)	1 (100)	39 + months	No toxicity
Cyclophosphamide[145]	80 mg/kg q 4 wks	5	4 (80)	9 mo	Myelosuppression
Cyclophosphamide[145]	750–975 mg/m²/d × 4d	7	1 (14)	12.5 mo (median survival)	One toxic death
Thiotepa	250–300 mg/m²/d × 4				
Bone marrow rescue					
PCNU[147]	100–125 mg/m² IV q 6–7 wks	17	3 (18)	NA	Myelosuppression
Tamoxifen[148]	80 mg/m² PO daily	4	3 (75)	6–30 mo range	Amenorrhea, abdominal cramps

NA = not available; PO—orally.

trials has varied between 17% and 50%.[127–130] Clinical trials with a smaller percentage of high-grade gliomas generally have a more prolonged survival. Hyperfractionated RT has not increased the survival rate.[131–134] The chemotherapy response rate at tumor recurrence has been less than 50% in all trials but one; therefore, median survival has not been significantly affected.[138–147]

A significant prognostic variable for survival is tumor location. In a univariate analysis of survival of thalamic/midbrain (TM) versus pons/medulla (PM) brainstem tumors, the 5-year survival rate was 73% for TM and 38% for PM.[115] In a second study, the 5-year survival rate for TM was 73% compared with 28% for PM ($p = .016$).[127] Epstein[103] classified brainstem tumors in two different three-tiered classification systems; the most recent system includes cervicomedullary, focal medullary or dorsally exophytic medullary, and diffuse pontine.[103,150] On histological examination, the pathology of cervicomedullary tumors was 91% low-grade glioma. Patients with dorsally exophytic and focal medullary pathology were 75% low-grade glioma, and those with diffuse pontine glioma were 100% anaplastic astrocytomas.[150] Cervicomedullary tumors have a 4-year progression-free survival rate of 70% and a total survival of 100% in newly treated patients with partial or gross total removal alone.[123]

In two series, dorsally exophytic medullary tumor was resected with no effort to remove intrinsic brainstem tumor.[125,126] Pathology was low grade in 29 of 30 tumors.[125,126] Thirteen of 17 patients in one study did not have disease progression, with a median follow-up of 113 months.[125] In the second study of 12 patients, the 2-year progression-free survival rate was 67%, and total survival was 100%.[126] Dorsally exophytic midbrain tectal tumors have been treated with interstitial brachytherapy and SR.[135,136] However, when patients were treated with only ventriculoperitoneal shunting, they had a progression-free survival of more than 24 months and a total survival of more than 50 months.[137]

Six cases of facial nerve nucleus pontine tumor presented with facial weakness or dizziness. Five biopsies revealed pilocytic astrocytoma, and these patients were treated with focal RT. Four of the five patients had CR, and one had PR. No patient had disease progression, with five of the patients followed up with for more than 4 years.[151]

Patients with cervicomedullary tumors, dorsally exophytic medullary or midbrain tumors, and focal pontine tumors frequently have benign pathology and a high proportion of juvenile pilocytic astrocytomas. Surgical shunting is the best treatment for tectal tumors; combined biopsy and focal RT is effective for focal pontine tumors, and maximum surgical resection is reserved for dorsally exophytic medullary and cervicomedullary tumors.

A retrospective MRI study of 87 patients with brainstem glioma reported three favorable prognostic variables: a midbrain or medullary location, mild or no brainstem enlargement, and focal disease.[104] Age at diagnosis, duration of symptoms, and clinical findings were not significant.[104]

The histological grade of tumor was significant, with increased anaplasia associated with a poorer prognosis.[115,120,129] Increased symptom duration prior to diagnosis was associated with increased survival in some series.[115,127,132]

A review of prognostic factors shows that location and pathology are important. Why are all the dorsal tumors low grade and frequently pilocytic? The answer is unknown.

COMPLICATIONS

Hydrocephalus is common in midbrain tectal plate tumors, approaching 100% on presentation.[137] It is much less common in other locations and has an incidence of 25% to 30%.[107] It should be treated initially with corticosteroids, although with midbrain lesions, a CSF diversion procedure will likely be needed.[140]

Leptomeningeal spread of brainstem tumor occurs in 10% to 30% of cases. Clinically, leptomeningeal spread presents with cerebral, cranial, and spinal nerve symptoms,[105–107,152] and is associated with a poor prognosis. Rarely, brainstem tumors metastasize outside the CNS, usually with previous meningeal dissemination.

Common sites of extraneural metastatic spread include the lungs, pleura, and lymph nodes.[107] Aspiration pneumonia occurs with dysphagia secondary to progressive, diffuse, intrinsic, lower brainstem tumors.[153]

CEREBELLAR PILOCYTIC ASTROCYTOMAS

See Chapter 9.

CHOROID PLEXUS PAPILLOMAS

Choroid plexus papillomas are rare lesions of the CNS, accounting for 0.4% to 0.6% of all tumors.[5,154] The prevalence in children is between 2% and 4% of all tumors.[154] They are located predominantly in the lateral ventricles in children and the fourth ventricle in adults.[5,155] The median age in most series is 12 months,[156,157] with the range in adults from 21 to 60 years of age.[158,159]

Choroid plexus papilloma is a benign tumor with grade I biologic behavior. Grossly, it is an irregular pinkish-gray mass that expands and obstructs the ventricular system. Microscopically, it consists of columnar and cuboidal cells resting on a basement membrane, which surrounds papilla of connective tissue containing blood vessels. Choroid plexus carcinoma is the malignant form of papilloma with grade III biologic behavior. Microscopically, there is a loss of papillae with significant mitotic activity in the cuboidal and columnar cells. These tumors have a tendency to seed the CSF.[3] They account for 20% to 30% of all choroid plexus tumors.[160]

The clinical symptoms in both children and adults are usually caused by increased intracranial pressure. The hydrocephalus is due to both overproduction of CSF and obstruction of CSF flow. In young children, frequent presenting symptoms are increased head circumference, failure to thrive, and lethargy.[161] In adults, the most common symptom is headache, and other symptoms are a manifestation of the posterior fossa location of the tumor.[158,159]

The differential diagnosis includes ependymoma, dorsally exophytic brainstem glioma, and dermoid cyst. The younger median age of choroid plexus papilloma and its tendency to occur in the third ventricle are helpful in distinguishing it from the ependymoma, which more frequently occurs in the fourth ventricle.[5,155] Dorsally exophytic brainstem tumors occur early in life but occur in the fourth ventricle.[125,126] Dermoid cyst can be distinguished on MRI or CT images. In adults, the differential diagnosis is choroid plexus papilloma and metastatic tumor to the choroid plexus.

MRI is the diagnostic procedure of choice because of the superior anatomical localization of tumor relative to surrounding structures and its ability to visualize feeding blood vessels. On T_1-weighted images, these tumors are seen as smooth or lobulated and heterogeneous, with intermediate signal intensity. Signal voids of feeding blood vessels are often seen (Fig. 11–6). Contrast enhancement is markedly homogeneous. Signal is mixed on the T_2-

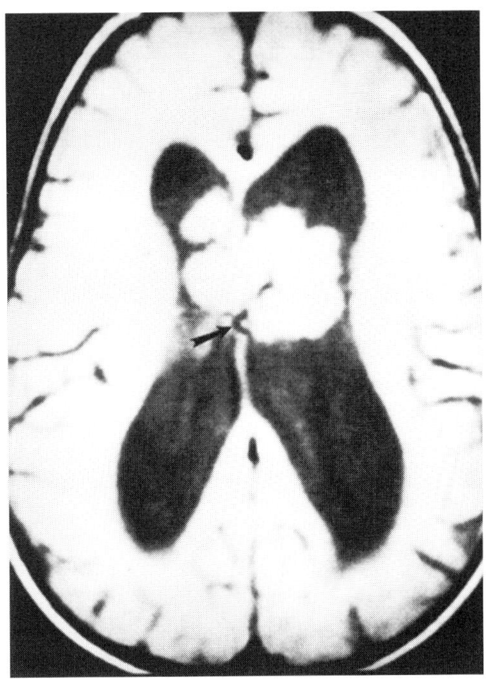

Figure 11–6. Choroid plexus papilloma. Axial CT scan with large contrast enhancing papillary tumor partially filling the body of both lateral ventricles. Note flow void at the arrow entering the tumor.

weighted images, with areas of necrosis and edema having increased signal.[162] On CT, the mass is smooth or lobulated, and is isodense or hyperdense when compared with normal brain. The increased density is due to its vascularity. It enhances with contrast.[162] Occasionally, preoperative angiography is needed to obtain a more definitive location of vascular structures.

The goal of surgery is gross total resection and management of the hydrocephalus.[154] Surgery is difficult because of the size of the tumor, the vascularity of the tumor, and the location of the tumor intraventricularly. Children have a small blood volume, and blood loss can be large. Removal of a choroid plexus tumor most often treats the hydrocephalus, but 20% of patients may require a ventriculoperitoneal shunt. Gross total surgical resection frequently cures choroid plexus papillomas and should also be the goal in choroid plexus carcinomas.

In children younger than 3 years of age who have subtotally resected or recurrent choroid plexus carcinomas, multiagent chemotherapy, identical to the protocol for medulloblastomas, should be used.[54,55,57] Children older than 6 years of age and adults with choroid plexus carcinomas should receive RT after gross total or subtotal resection.[156,159,163] Craniospinal RT may be considered because of the risk of spinal dissemination.[163,164] The role of chemotherapy for children older than age 3 years and adults with choroid plexus carcinoma is uncertain, but given the chemosensitivity of the carcinoma, it is reasonable to recommend multiagent chemotherapy for adults and children with recurrent or residual disease after RT or patients with disseminated disease.[160,164] Surgery should also be strongly considered at recurrence.[153]

DERMOID AND EPIDERMOID CYSTS

Dermoid and epidermoid cysts are commonly referred to as *dysontogenetic processes* along with Rathke's cleft cysts, craniopharyngiomas, germinomas, and nongerminomatous germ cell tumors. Dermoids and epidermoid cysts are developmental in origin.[165] They are caused by incomplete cleavage of neural from cutaneous ectoderm during the third to fifth week of gestation, when the neural tube closes.[166] Epidermoid cysts have been induced iatrogenically by lumbar puncture, percutaneous cranial subdural aspiration, and myelomeningocele repair.[167,168] Dermoid and epidermoid cysts are each estimated to account for approximately 1% of CNS tumors.[5]

Pathologically, both cysts are lined by squamous epithelium. The dermoid has a thicker wall and contains dermal appendages, such as hair follicles and adnexae.[3] Dermoid cysts occur in the midline of the fourth ventricle, between the cerebellar hemispheres, in the skull, spinal dura, and cauda equina. Intracranial dermoid cysts frequently communicate with the skin surface, usually at the occiput or the lumbar spine.[169] Epidermoid cyst more often occur laterally in the cerebellopontine angle around the pons, within the temporal lobe, in the diploe, and in the spinal canal.[3,25] Macroscopically, epidermoid cysts are thin-walled and pearly, and are also called *cholesteatoma* or *pearly tumors*.[3]

Dermoid and epidermoid cysts grow slowly and displace or surround neural structures insidiously over several years.[170] Patients with posterior fossa cerebellopontine angle epidermoid cysts present most commonly with decreased hearing, tinnitus, headache, gait disturbance, and diplopia.[171,172] Dermoid and epidermoid cysts of the fourth ventricle present with headache, truncal ataxia, internuclear ophthalmoplegia, cranial nerve palsies, facial numbness, and increased intracranial pressure.[170–173]

The differential diagnoses of fourth ventricular dermoid cysts include ependymoma, dorsally exophytic brainstem glioma, choroid plexus papilloma, epidermoid cyst, and metastatic carcinoma. The differential diagnoses of a cerebellopontine-angle epidermoid cyst includes acoustic neuroma, meningioma, hemangioblastoma, and medulloblastoma.[170]

The appearances of dermoid and epidermoid cysts on MRI images are usually characteristic and allow differentiation from other posterior fossa mass lesions, but not necessarily each other.[174] Epidermoid cysts are cystic and produce a variable signal on T_1-weighted images, depending on lipid content. If lipid content is low, the signal is hypointense; if lipid content is high, the signal is hyperintense. Epidermoid cysts do not enhance. On T_2-weighted images, the signal is hyperintense.[175] Dermoid cyst gives a high signal on T_1-weighted images in regions of fat and a variable signal where there is a combination of lipid, muscle, bone, or teeth (Fig. 11–7). On T_2-weighted signal, they are hyperintense. They rarely enhance.

CT of epidermoid cyst shows a cystic, nonenhancing, hypodense lesion, with the density of the fluid in the cyst between CSF and brain. The cyst wall may be thinly calcified. Dermoid cyst tends to have thicker cyst walls and lower cyst fluid density, and they more commonly demonstrate calcification.[176] Dermoid cysts rarely enhance, and there is no brain reaction to either dermoid or epidermoid cysts.[171]

The procedure of choice is gross total surgical removal with microsurgical excision of the total cyst wall at first operation.[171,177–179] Small accessible cysts should be removed intact. If complete removal is impossible, the cyst contents should be emptied with subtotal resection of the cyst wall.[179] To minimize the risk of aseptic meningitis, cyst wall contents should not be spread. These cysts adhere to neural structures and seldom have a clean plane for dissection from cranial nerves and blood vessels. Yasargil and colleagues[171] have reported gross total removal of large cerebellopontine angle epidermoids. Recurrence may take years because of the slow growth rate, so it is important not to damage neural structures in the removal. The most frequent surgical complications are aseptic meningitis and cranial nerve palsies.[171] Recurrent aseptic meningitis can occur from sponta-

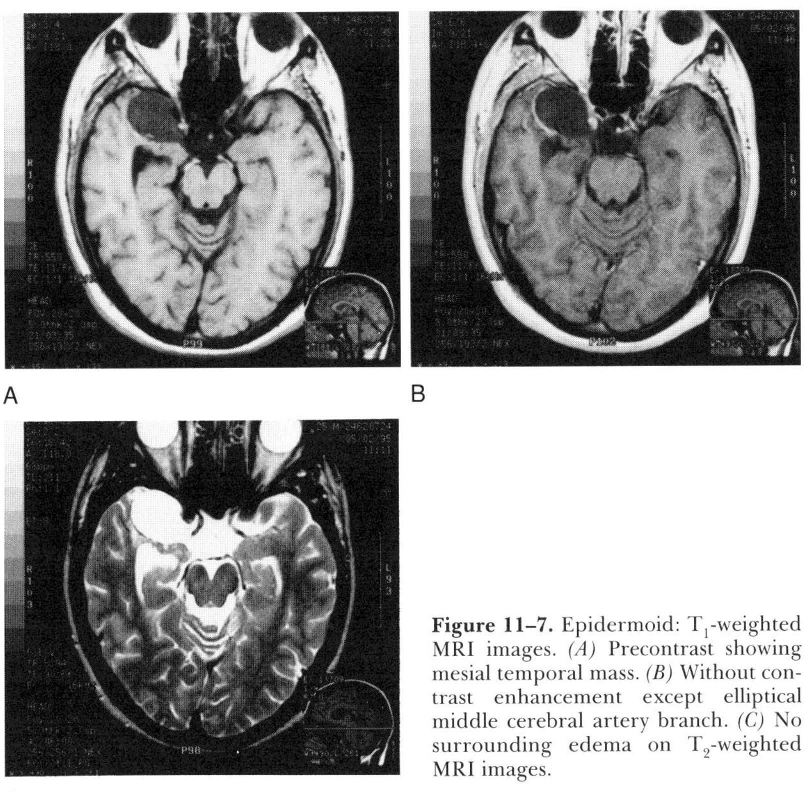

Figure 11–7. Epidermoid: T_1-weighted MRI images. *(A)* Precontrast showing mesial temporal mass. *(B)* Without contrast enhancement except elliptical middle cerebral artery branch. *(C)* No surrounding edema on T_2-weighted MRI images.

neous rupture of dermoid and epidermoid cysts.[180,181]

SUBEPENDYMOMA

Subependymomas are benign tumors that develop in the ventricular walls, particularly in the fourth ventricle, and protrude into the CSF space.[3,25] They are composed of nests of round ependymal cells with glial fibrillary processes admixed with fibrillary astrocytes. They have a grade I biologic behavior. Microcysts, calcification, hemosiderin deposits from previous hemorrhage, and vascular hyalinization are frequently seen.[3] Subependymoma may be mixed with ependymoma and has grade II biologic behavior.

They present in the ventricle as well-delineated single or multiple nodules and are most often asymptomatic. In adults, they may grow slowly into the fourth ventricle, and they present with obstructive hydrocephalus and the symptoms associated with increased intracranial pressure. The treatment for subependymoma is surgical resection.[182]

CHAPTER SUMMARY

Posterior fossa tumors are intimately related to the fourth ventricle. They frequently present with obstructive hydrocephalus and the symptoms associated with increased intracranial pressure. Medulloblastoma arises in the roof of the fourth ventricle and grows into the cerebellar vermis and the roof of the fourth ventricle, presenting with symptoms associated with obstructive hydrocephalus in up to 90% of children. Ependymoma takes origin from the lining of the ventricle and fills the ventricle, producing obstructive hydrocephalus at presentation in more than 80% of children. Brainstem glioma arises in the basement of the fourth ventricle, and when they grow dorsally and exophytically or symmetrically expand in size, they produce obstructive hydrocephalus. This occurs in 30% of patients. Cerebellar astrocytoma (see Chapter 9) is most frequently pilocytic. It originates laterally in the cerebellar hemisphere, often with appendicular cerebellar signs. As the tumor and cyst grow, the patient often presents with obstructive hydrocephalus. Choroid plexus papilloma takes origin in the ventricle and presents with hydrocephalus, not only by obstruction of CSF flow, but also by increased production of CSF. Posterior fossa dermoid cyst grows in the fourth ventricle with outflow obstruction and presents with the symptoms associated with increased intracranial pressure. Lastly, subependymoma, when symptomatic, grows into the fourth ventricle, producing obstructive hydrocephalus.

MRI has provided the clinician with superb anatomical detail of posterior fossa tumors and their anatomical relationship to normal structure. Microsurgical techniques have fostered gross total tumor removal and frequent cure of pilocytic astrocytoma, choroid plexus papilloma, dermoid and epidermoid cysts, and subependymoma. Extent of surgical resection has been correlated with survival in both medulloblastoma and ependymoma. Surgical biopsy of pontine glioma continues to be a controversial area, but cervicomedullary and dorsally exophytic medullary gliomas, both of which are usually pilocytic, may be cured with surgery.

Craniospinal RT with a posterior fossa boost has increased survival for patients with medulloblastoma. Focal RT has improved outcome in ependymoma and brainstem glioma. Multiagent adjuvant chemotherapy with vincristine, CDDP, and CCNU has significantly improved the survival of "poor-risk" patients with medulloblastoma, but not ependymoma. Treatment must be individualized for ependymoma.

REFERENCES

1. Bailey, P, and Cushing, H: Medulloblastoma cerebelli. A common type of midcerebellar glioma of childhood. Arch Neuro Psychiatr 14: 192–224, 1924.
2. Rorke, LB: The cerebellar medulloblastoma and its relationship to primitive neuroectoder-

mal tumors. J Neuropathol Exp Neurol 42:15, 1983.
3. Kleihues, P, Burger, PC, and Scheithauer, BW: Histological Typing of Tumours of the Central Nervous System, Second Edition. World Health Organization, Springer-Verlag, 1993.
4. Packer, RJ: Medulloblastoma. In Gilman S, Goldstein G, Waxman S (eds): Neurobase. Arbor Publishing Corporation, San Diego, 1998.
5. Russell, DS, and Rubinstein, LJ: Pathology of Tumours of the Nervous System, Ed. 4. The Williams and Wilkins Company, Baltimore, 1977, pp 244–255.
6. Hubbard, JL, Scheithauer, BW, Kispert, DB, et al: Adult cerebellar medulloblastomas: the pathological, radiographic, and clinical disease spectrum. J Neurosurg 70:536–544, 1989.
7. Helseth, A, and Mork, SJ: Neoplasms of the central nervous system in Norway. III. Epidemiological characteristics of intracranial gliomas according to histology. APMIS 97:547–555, 1989.
8. Chi, JG, and Khang, SK: Central nervous system tumors among Koreans. A statistical study of 697 cases. J Korean Medical Science 4:77–90, 1989.
9. Kuijten, RR, and Bunin, GR: Risk factors for childhood brain tumors. Cancer Epidemiology Biomarkers Prevention 2:277–288, 1993.
10. Lannering, B, Markey, I, and Nordborg, C: Brain tumors in childhood and adolescence in West Sweden 1970–1984. Epidemiology and survival. Cancer 66:604–609, 1990.
11. Kopelson, G, Linggood, RM, and Kleinman, GM: Medulloblastoma in adults: improved survival with supervoltage radiation therapy. Cancer 49:1334–1337, 1982.
12. Bloom, HJG, and Bessell, EM: Medulloblastoma in adults: a review of 47 patients treated between 1952 and 1981. Int J Radiat Oncol Biol Phys 18:763–772, 1990.
13. Tijssen, CC: Genetic factors and family studies in medulloblastoma. In Zeltzer, PM, and Pochedly, C (eds) Medulloblastomas in Children: New Concepts in Tumor Biology, Diagnosis and Treatment. Praeger, New York, 1986, pp 61–75.
14. Biegel, JA, Rorke, LB, Packer, RJ, et al: Isochromosome 17q in primitive neuroectodermal tumors of the central nervous system. Genes Chrom Cancer 1:139–147, 1989.
15. Raffel, C, Gilles, FE, and Weinberg, KI: Reduction to homozygosity and gene amplification in central nervous system primitive neuroectodermal tumors of childhood. Cancer Res 50:587–591, 1990.
16. Saylors, RL, Sidransky, D, Friedman, HS, et al: Infrequent p53 gene mutations in medulloblastomas. Cancer Res 51:4721–4723, 1991.
17. Raffel, C, Thomas, GA, Tishler, DM, et al: Absence of p53 mutations in childhood central nervous system primitive neuroectodermal tumors. Neurosurgery 33:301–306, 1993.
18. Tomlinson, FH, Jenkins, RB, Scheithauer, BW, et al: Aggressive medulloblastoma with high-level N-*myc* amplification. Mayo Clin Proc 69:359–365, 1994.
19. Rosenfeld, MR, Meneses, P, Dalmau, J, et al: Gene transfer of wild-type p53 results in restoration of tumor-suppressor function in a medulloblastoma cell line. Neurology 45:1533–1539, 1995.
20. Hoshino, T, Kobayashi, S, Townsend, JJ, and Wilson, CB: A cell kinetic study on medulloblastomas. Cancer 55:1711–1713, 1985.
21. Murovic, JA, Nagashima, T, Hoshino, T, et al: Pediatric central nervous system tumors: a cell kinetic study with bromodeoxyuridine. Neurosurgery 19:900–904, 1986.
22. Hoffman, JM, Hanson, MW, Friedman, HS, et al: FDG-PET in pediatric posterior fossa brain tumors. J Computer Assisted Tomography 16:62–68, 1992.
23. Wen, DY, Hall, WA, Conrad, J, et al: In vitro and in vivo variation in transferrin receptor expression on a human medulloblastoma cell line. Neurosurgery 36:1158–1164, 1995.
24. Feickert, H-J, Pietsch, T, Hadam, MR, et al: Monoclonal antibody T-199 directed against human medulloblastoma: characterization of a new antigenic system expressed on neuroectodermal tumors and natural killer cells. Cancer Res 49:4338–4343, 1989.
25. McKeever, PE, and Blaivas, M: The brain, spinal cord, and meninges. In Sternberg, SS (ed) Diagnostic Surgical Pathology, Second Edition. Raven Press Ltd., New York, 1994, pp 409–492.
26. Becker, RL, Becker, AD, and Sobel, DF: Adult medulloblastoma: review of 13 cases with emphasis on MRI. Neuroradiology 37:104–108, 1995.
27. Koci, TM, Chiang, F, Mehringer, CM, et al: Adult cerebellar medulloblastoma: imaging features with emphasis on MR findings. AJNR 14:929–939, 1993.
28. Peterson, K, and Walker, RW: Medulloblastoma/primitive neuroectodermal tumor in 45 adults. Neurology 45:440–442, 1995.
29. Packer, RJ, and Finlay, JL: Medulloblastoma: presentation, diagnosis and management. Oncology 2:35–44, 1988.
30. Haddad, SF, Menezes, AH, Bell, WE, et al: Brain tumors occurring before 1 year of age: a retrospective review of 22 cases in an 11-year period (1977–1987). Neurosurgery 29:8–13, 1991.
31. Tomita, T, and McLone, DG: Brain tumors during the first twenty-four months of life. Neurosurgery 17:913–919, 1985.
32. Pollack, IF: Brain tumors in children. N Engl J Med 331(22):1500–1507, 1994.
33. Packer, RJ: Chiasmatic Gliomas. In Gilman, S, Goldstein, G, and Waxman, S (eds): Neurobase. Arbor Publishing Corporation, San Diego, 1995.
34. Zimmerman, RA, Gusnard, DA, and Bilaniuk, LB: Gadolinium DTPA enhanced MR evaluation of pediatric brain tumors. In Packer, RJ, Bleyer, WA, and Pochedly, C (eds): Pediatric Neuro-oncology. New Trends in Clinical

Research. Harwood Publishing, Philadelphia, 1992, pp 42–76.
35. Marton, LJ, Edwards, MS, Levin, VA, et al: CSF polyamines: a new and important means of monitoring patients with medulloblastoma. Cancer 47:757–760, 1981.
36. Chang, CH, Housepian, EM, and Herbert, C Jr: An operative staging system and a megavoltage radiotherapeutic technic for cerebellar medulloblastomas. Radiology 93:1351–1359, 1969.
37. Kopelson, G, Linggood, RM, and Kleinman, GM: Medulloblastoma. The identification of prognostic subgroups and implications for multimodality management. Cancer 51:312–319, 1983.
38. Berger, MS, Magrassi, L, and Geyer, R: Medulloblastoma and primitive neuroectodermal tumors. Kaye, AH, Laws, ER Jr (eds): Brain Tumors. An Encyclopedic Approach. Churchill Livingstone, New York, 1995, pp 561–574.
39. Tarbell, NJ, Loeffler, JS, Silver, B, et al: The change in patterns of relapse in medulloblastoma. Cancer 68:1600–1604, 1991.
40. Evans, AE, Jenkin, RDT, Sposto, R, et al: The treatment of medulloblastoma. Results of a prospective randomized trial of radiation therapy with and without CCNU, vincristine, and prednisone. J Neurosurg 72:572–582, 1990.
41. Raimondi, AJ, and and Tomita, T: The advantage of total resection of medulloblastoma and disadvantages of whole brain postoperative radiation therapy. Child's Brain 5:585–590, 1979.
42. Garton, GR, Schomberg, PJ, Scheithauer, BW, et al: Medulloblastoma: Prognostic factors and outcome of treatment: Review of the Mayo Clinic experience. Mayo Clin Proc 65:1077–1086, 1990.
43. Tomita, T, and McLone, DG: Medulloblastoma in childhood: results of radical resection and low-dose neuraxis radiation therapy. J Neurosurg 64:238–242, 1986.
44. Jenkin, D, Goddard, K, Armstrong, D, et al: Posterior fossa medulloblastoma in childhood: treatment results and a proposal for a new staging system. Int J Radiat Oncol Biol Phys 19: 265–274, 1990.
45. Hershatter, BW, Halperin, EC, and Cox, EB: Medulloblastoma: The Duke University Medical Center experience. Int J Radiat Oncol Biol Phys 12:1771–1777, 1986.
46. Hughes, EN, Shillito, J, Sallan, SE, et al: Medulloblastoma at the Joint Center for Radiation Therapy between 1968 and 1984. The influence of radiation dose on the patterns of failure and survival. Cancer 61:1992–1998, 1988.
47. Allen, JC, Bloom, J, Ertel, I, et al: Brain tumors in children: current cooperative and institutional chemotherapy trials in newly diagnosed and recurrent disease. Seminars in Oncology 13:110–122, 1986.
48. Dunbar, SF, Barnes, PD, and Tarbell, NJ: Radiologic determination of the caudal border of the spinal field in cranial spinal irradiation. Int J Radiat Oncol Biol Phys 26:669–673, 1993.
49. Prados, MD, Wara, WM, Edwards, MSB, and Cogen, PH: Hyperfractionated craniospinal radiation therapy for primitive neuroectodermal tumors: early results of a pilot study. Int J Radiat Oncol Biol Phys 28:431–438, 1993.
50. Deutsch, M, Thomas, P, Boyett, J, et al: Low stage medulloblastoma: a Childrens Cancer Study Group (CCSG) and Pediatric Oncology Group (POG) randomized study of standard vs reduced neuraxis irradiation. Proc Amer Soc Clin Oncol 10:124(Abstract 363), 1991.
51. Packer, RJ, Sutton, LN, Elterman, R, et al: Outcome for children with medulloblastoma treated with radiation and cisplatin, CCNU, and vincristine chemotherapy. J Neurosurg 81: 690–698, 1994.
52. Packer, RJ, Sutton, LN, Atkins, TE, et al: A prospective study of cognitive function in children receiving whole-brain radiotherapy and chemotherapy: 2-year results. J Neurosurg 70: 707–713, 1989.
53. Johnson, DL, McCabe, MA, Nicholson, HS, et al: Quality of long-term survival in young children with medulloblastoma. J Neurosurg 80: 1004–1010, 1994.
54. Duffner, PK, and Cohen, ME: Treatment of brain tumors in babies and very young children. Pediat Neurosci 12:304–310, 1985–1986.
55. Duffner, PK, Horowitz, ME, Krischer, JP, et al: Postoperative chemotherapy and delayed radiation in children less than three years of age with malignant brain tumors. N Engl J Med 328: 1725–1731, 1993.
56. Krischer, JP, Ragab, AH, Kun, L, et al: Nitrogen mustard, vincristine, procarbazine, and prednisone as adjuvant chemotherapy in the treatment of medulloblastoma. J Neurosurg 74:905–909, 1991.
57. Packer, RJ, Siegel, KR, Sutton, LN, et al: Efficacy of adjuvant chemotherapy for patients with poor-risk medulloblastoma: a preliminary report. Ann Neurol 24:503–508, 1988.
58. Packer, RJ, Sutton, LN, Goldwein, JW, et al: Improved survival with the use of adjuvant chemotherapy in the treatment of medulloblastoma. J Neurosurg 74:433–440, 1991.
59. Crafts, DC, Levin, VA, Edwards, MS, et al: Chemotherapy of recurrent medulloblastoma with combined procarbazine, CCNU, and vincristine. J Neurosurg 49:589–592, 1978.
60. Duffner, PK, Cohen, ME, Thomas, PRM, et al: Combination chemotherapy in recurrent medulloblastoma. Cancer 43:41–45, 1979.
61. Levin, VA, Vestnys, PS, Edwards, MS, et al: Improvement in survival produced by sequential therapies in the treatment of recurrent medulloblastoma. Cancer 51:1364–1370, 1983.
62. Walker, RW, Allen, JC, Jennings, MT, and Helson, L: Continuous infusion vincristine and adriamycin in the treatment of recurrent childhood brain tumors. Ann Neurol 22:448(Abstract 132), 1987.
63. Allen, JC, Walker, R, Luks, E, et al: Carboplatin and recurrent childhood brain tumors. J Clin Oncol 5:459–463, 1987.

64. Friedman, HS, Schold, SC Jr, and Mahaley, MS Jr, et al: Phase II treatment of medulloblastoma and pineoblastoma with melphalan: Clinical therapy based on experimental models of human medulloblastoma. J Clin Oncol 7:904–911, 1989.
65. Lefkowitz, IB, Packer, RJ, Siegel, KR, et al: Results of treatment of children with recurrent medulloblastoma/primitive neuroectodermal tumors with lomustine, cisplatin, and vincristine. Cancer 65:412–417, 1990.
66. Friedman, HS, Krischer, JP, Burger, P, et al: Treatment of children with progressive or recurrent brain tumors with carboplatin or iproplatin: a Pediatric Oncology Group randomized phase II study. J Clin Oncol 10:249–256, 1992.
67. Gaynon, PS, Ettinger, LJ, Baum, ES, et al: Carboplatin in childhood brain tumors. A Children's Cancer Study Group phase II trial. Cancer 66:2465–2469, 1990.
68. Finlay, J, Garvin, J, Allen, J, et al: High-dose chemotherapy (HDCx) with autologous marrow rescue (ABMR) in patients with recurrent medulloblastoma (MB)/primitive neuroectodermal tumors (PNET). Proc Amer Soc Clin Oncol 13:176(Abstract 493), 1994.
69. Friedman, HS, and Oakes, WJ: New therapeutic options in the management of childhood brain tumors. Oncology 6:27–36, 1992.
70. Allen, JC, and Epstein, F: Medulloblastoma and other primary malignant neuroectodermal tumors of the CNS. The effect of patients' age and extent of disease on prognosis. J Neurosurg 57: 446–451, 1982.
71. Janss, AJ, Yachnis, AT, Silber, JH, et al: Glial differentiation predicts poor clinical outcome in primitive neuroectodermal brain tumors. Ann Neurol 39:481–489, 1996.
72. Packer, RJ, Siegel, KR, Sutton, LN, et al: Leptomeningeal dissemination of primary central nervous system tumors of childhood. Ann Neurol 18:217–221, 1985.
73. Kleinman, GM, Hochberg, FH, and Richardson, EP: Systemic metastases from medulloblastoma: Report of two cases and review of the literature. Cancer 48:2296–2309, 1981.
74. Pasqualini, T, Diez, B, Domene, H, et al: Long-term endocrine sequaleae after surgery, radiotherapy, and chemotherapy in children with medulloblastoma.
75. Farwell, J, and Flannery, JT: Cancer in relatives of children with central-nervous-system neoplasms. 311:749–753, 1984.
76. Virchow, R: Die krankhaften Gerschwülste. Berlin, Hirschwald, 1863–1865.
77. Bailey, P: A study of tumors arising from ependymal cells. Arch Neurol Psychiat 11:1–27, 1924.
78. Bailey, P, and Cushing, H. A Classification of the Tumors of the Glioma Group on a Histogenetic Basis with a Correlated Study of Prognosis. JP Lippincott Company, Philadelphia, 1926.
79. Kernohan, JW, and Fletcher-Kernohan, EM: Ependymomas: A study of 109 cases. Res Publ Assoc Res Nerv Ment Dis 16:182–209, 1937.
80. Rawlings, CE III, Giangaspero, F, Burger, PC, and Bullard, DE: Ependymomas: A clinicopathologic study. Surgical Neurol 29:271–281, 1988.
81. Nazar, GB, Hoffman, HJ, Becker, LE, et al: Infratentorial ependymomas in childhood: prognostic factors and treatment. J Neurosurg 72: 408–417, 1990.
82. West, CR, Bruce, DA, and Duffner, PK: Ependymomas: Factors in clinical and diagnostic staging. Cancer 56:1812–1816, 1985.
83. Dohrmann, GJ, Farwell, JR, and Flannery, JT: Ependymomas and ependymoblastomas in children. J Neurosurg 45:273–283, 1976.
84. Goldwein, JW, Leahy, JM, Packer, RJ, et al: Intracranial ependymomas in children. Int J Radiat Oncol Biol Phys 19:1497–1502, 1990.
85. Metzger, AK, Sheffield, VC, Duyk, G, et al: Identification of a germ-line mutation in the p53 gene in a patient with an intracranial ependymoma. Proc Natl Acad Sci 88:7825– 7829, 1991.
86. Marsh, WR, and Laws, ER Jr: Intracranial ependymomas. Prog Exp Tumor Res 30:175–180, 1987.
87. Bigner, SH, Mark, J, and Bigner, DD: Cytogenetics of human brain tumors. Cancer Genet Cytogenet 47:141–154, 1990.
88. Burger, PC, and Fuller, GN: Pathology: Trends and pitfalls in histologic diagnosis, immunopathology, and applications of oncogene research. Neurologic Clinics 9:249–271, 1991.
89. Spoto, GP, Press, GA, Hesselink, JR, and Solomon, M: Intracranial ependymoma and subependymoma: MR manifestations. AJNR 11:83–91, 1990.
90. Goldwein, JW, Corn, BW, Finlay, JL, et al: Is craniospinal irradiation required to cure children with malignant (anaplastic) intracranial ependymomas? Cancer 67:2766–2771, 1991.
91. Duncan, JA III, and Hoffman, HJ: Intracranial ependymomas. In Kaye, AH, and Laws, ER Jr (eds): Brain Tumors. An Encyclopedic Approach. Churchill Livingstone, New York, 1995, pp 493–504.
92. Ringertz, N, and Reymond, A: Ependymomas and choroid plexus papillomas. J Neuropath Exper Neurol 8:355–380, 1949.
93. Sutton, LN, Goldwein, J, Perilongo, G, et al: Prognostic factors in childhood ependymomas. Pediatr Neurosurg 16:57–65,1990–91.
94. Rousseau, P, Habrand, JL, Sarrazin, D, et al: Treatment of intracranial ependymomas of children: Review of a 15-year experience. Int J Radiat Oncol Biol Phys 28:381–386, 1993.
95. Wallner, KE, Wara, WM, Sheline, GE, and Davis, RL: Intracranial ependymomas: Results of treatment with partial or whole brain irradiation without spinal irradiation. Int J Radiat Oncol Biol Phys 12:1937–1941, 1986.
96. Vanuytsel, L, and Brada, M: The role of prophylactic spinal irradiation in localized intracranial ependymoma. Int J Radiat Oncol Biol Phys 21:825–830, 1991.
97. Bertolone, SJ, Baum, ES, Krivit, W, and Hammond, GD: A phase II study of cisplatin therapy

in recurrent childhood brain tumors: A report from the Childrens Cancer Study Group. J Neurooncol 7:5–11, 1989.
98. Papadopoulos, DP, Giri, S, and Evans, RG: Prognostic factors and management of intracranial ependymomas. Anticancer Research 10: 689–692, 1990.
99. Rorke, LB: Relationship of morphology of ependymoma in children to prognosis. Prog Exp Tumor Res 30:170–174, 1987.
100. Buckley, RC: Pontine gliomas. A pathologic study and classification of twenty-five cases. Arch Pathol 9:799–819, 1930.
101. Gibbs, FA: Frequency with which tumors in various parts of the brain produce certain symptoms. Arch Neurol Psychiat 28:969–989, 1932.
102. White, HH: Brain stem tumors occuring in adults. Neurology 13:292–300, 1963.
103. Epstein, F: A staging system for brain stem gliomas. Cancer 56:1804–1806, 1985.
104. Barkovich, AJ, Krischer, J, Kun, LE, et al: Brain stem gliomas: a classification system based on magnetic resonance imaging. Pediatr Neurosurg 16:73–83, 1990–91.
105. Maria, BL, Rehder, K, Eskin, TA, et al: Brainstem glioma: I. Pathology, clinical features, and therapy. J Child Neurol 8:112–128, 1993.
106. Packer, RJ, Nicholson, HS, Vezina, LG, and Johnson, DL: Brainstem gliomas. Neurosurg Clin N Am 3:863–879, 1992.
107. Newton, HB: Brainstem gliomas in adults. In Gilman S, Goldstein G, Waxman S (eds): Neurobase. Arbor Publishing Corporation, San Diego, 1996.
108. Schianchi,P, and Kraus-Ruppert, R: Familial brain tumors: rhombencephalon-astrocytoma grade I in father and son. Acta Neuropathol (Berl) 52:153–155, 1980.
109. Sawyer, JR, Roloson, GJ, Hobson, EA, et al: Trisomy for chromosome 1q in a pontine astrocytoma. Cancer Genet Cytogenet 47:101–106, 1990.
110. Jenkins, RB, Kimmel, DW, Moertel, CA, et al: A cytogenetic study of 53 human gliomas. Cancer Genet Cytogenet 39:253–279, 1989.
111. von Deimling, A, von Ammon, K, Schoenfeld, D, et al: Subsets of glioblastoma multiforme defined by molecular genetic analysis. Brain Pathol 3:19–26, 1993.
112. Zhang, S, Feng, X, Koga, H, et al: p53 gene mutations in pontine gliomas of juvenile onset. Biochem Biophys Res Com 196:851–857, 1993.
113. Coons, SW, and Johnson, PC: Pathology of primary intracranial malignant neoplasms. In Morantz, RA, and Walsh, JW (eds): Brain Tumors: A Comprehensive Text. Marcell Dekker, New York, 1994, pp 45–108.
114. Tokuriki, Y, Handa, H, Yamashita, J, et al: Brainstem glioma: an analysis of 85 cases. Acta Neurochir (Wien) 79:67–73, 1986.
115. Grigsby, PW, Thomas, PR, Schwartz, HG, and Fineberg, BB: Multivariate analysis of prognostic factors in pediatric and adult thalamic and brainstem tumors. Int J Radiat Oncol Biol Phys 16:649–655, 1989.
116. Rodriguez, M, Baele, PL, Marsh, HM, and Okazaki, H: Central neurogenic hyperventilation in an awake patient with brainstem astrocytoma. Ann Neurol 11:625–628, 1982.
117. Frank, F, Fabrizi, AP, Frank-Ricci, R, et al: Stereotactic biopsy and treatment of brain stem lesions: combined study of 33 cases. Acta Neurochir Suppl (Wien) 42:177–181, 1988.
118. Rajshekhar, V, and Changy, MJ: Computerized tomography-guided stereotactic surgery for brainstem masses: A risk-benefit analysis in 71 patients. J Neurosurg 82:976–981, 1995.
119. Stroink, AR, Hoffman, HJ, Hendrick, EB, and Humphreys, RP: Diagnosis and management of pediatric brain-stem gliomas. J Neurosurg 65: 745–750, 1986.
120. Albright, AL, Price, RA, and Guthkelch, AN: Brain stem gliomas of children: A clinicopathological study. Cancer 52:2313–2319, 1983.
121. Hood, TW, and McKeever, PE: Stereotactic management of cystic gliomas of the brain stem. Neurosurgery 24:373–378, 1989.
122. Epstein, F, and Wisoff, JH: Intrinsic brainstem tumors in childhood: surgical indications. J Neurooncol 6:309–317, 1988.
123. Robertson, PL, Allen, JC, Abbott, IR, et al: Cervicomedullary tumors in children: A distinct subset of brainstem gliomas. Neurology 44: 1798–1803, 1994.
124. Pierre-Kahn, A, Hirsch, J-F, Vinchon, M, et al: Surgical management of brain-stem tumors in children: results and statistical analysis of 75 cases. J Neurosurg 79:845–852, 1993.
125. Pollack, IF, Hoffman, HJ, Humphreys, RP, and Becker, L: The long-term outcome after surgical treatment of dorsally exophytic brain-stem gliomas. J Neurosurg 78:859–863, 1993.
126. Khatib, ZA, Heideman, RL, Kovnar, EH, et al: Predominance of pilocytic histology in dorsally exophytic brain stem tumors. Pediatr Neurosurg 20:2–10, 1994.
127. Halperin, EC: Pediatric brain stem tumors: patterns of treatment failure and their implications for radiotherapy. Int J Radiat Oncol Biol Phys 11:1293–1298, 1985.
128. Kim, TH, Chin, HW, Pollan, S, et al: Radiotherapy of primary brain stem tumors. Int J Radiat Oncol Biol Phys 6:51–57, 1980.
129. Shibamoto, Y, Takahashi, M, Dokoh, S, et al: Radiation therapy for brain stem tumor with special reference to CT feature and prognosis correlations. Int J Radiat Oncol Biol Phys 17: 71–76, 1989.
130. Eifel, PJ, Cassady, JR, and Belli, JA: Radiation therapy of tumors of the brainstem and midbrain in children: experience of the Joint Center for Radiation Therapy and Children's Hospital Medical Center (1971–1981). Int J Radiat Oncol Biol Phys 13:847–852, 1987.
131. Packer, RJ, Littman, PA, and Sposto, RM, et al: Results of a pilot study of hyperfractionated radiation therapy for children with brain stem gliomas. Int J Radiat Oncol Biol Phys 13:1647– 1651, 1987.
132. Shrieve, DC, Wara, WM, Edwards, MSB, et al: Hyperfractionated radiation therapy for

gliomas of the brainstem in children and in adults. Int J Radiat Oncol Biol Phys 24:599–610, 1992.

133. Packer, RJ, Allen, JC, Goldwein, JL, et al: Hyperfractionated radiotherapy for children with brainstem gliomas: A pilot study using 7,200 cGy. Ann Neurol 27:167–173, 1990.

134. Freeman, CR, Krischer, JP, Sanford, RA, et al: Final results of a study of escalating doses of hyperfractionated radiotherapy in brain stem tumors in children: A Pediatric Oncology Group study. Int J Radiat Oncol Biol Phys 27:197–206, 1993.

135. Mundinger, F, Braus, DF, Krauss, JK, Birg, W: Long-term outcome of 89 low-grade brain-stem gliomas after interstitial radiation therapy. J Neurosurg 75:740–746, 1991.

136. Kihlström, L, Lindquist, C, Lindquist, M, and Karlsson, B: Stereotactic radiosurgery for tectal low-grade gliomas. Acta Neurochir Suppl (Wien) 62:55–57, 1994.

137. Squires, LA, Allen, JC, Abbott, R, and Epstein, FJ: Focal tectal tumors: management and prognosis. Neurology 44:953–956, 1994.

138. Jenkin, RDT, Boesel, C, Ertel, I, et al: Brainstem tumors in childhood: a prospective randomized trial of irradiation with and without adjuvant CCNU, VCR, and prednisone. J Neurosurg 66:227–233, 1987.

139. Fulton, DS, Levin, VA, Wara, WM, et al: Chemotherapy of pediatric brain-stem tumors. J Neurosurg 54:721–725, 1981.

140. Rodriguez, LA, Prados, M, Fulton, D, et al: Treatment of recurrent brain stem gliomas and other central nervous system tumors with 5-fluorouracil, CCNU, hydroxyurea, and 6-mercaptopurine. Neurosurgery 22:691–693, 1988.

141. Chamberlain, MC: Recurrent brainstem gliomas treated with oral VP-16. J Neurooncol 15:133–139, 1993.

142. Sexauer, CL, Khan, AB, Burger, PC, et al: Cisplatin in recurrent pediatric brain tumors: A POG phase II study. A Pediatric Oncology Group study. Cancer 56:1497–1501, 1985.

143. Walker, RW, and Allen, JC: Treatment of recurrent primary intracranial childhood tumors with cis-diamminedichloroplatinum. Ann Neurol 14:371–372, 1983.

144. Zeltzer, PM, Epport, K, Nelson, MD Jr, et al: Prolonged response to carboplatin in an infant with brain stem glioma. Cancer 67:43–47, 1991.

145. Allen, JC, and Helson, L: High dose cyclophosphamide chemotherapy for recurrent CNS tumors in children. J Neurosurg 55:749–756, 1981.

146. Kedar, A, Maria, BL, Graham-Pole, J, et al: High dose chemotherapy with marrow reinfusion and hypefractionated irradiation for children with brain stem glioma. Proc Amer Soc Clin Oncol 13:177 (Abstract 498), 1994.

147. Allen, JC, Hancock, C, Walker, R, and Tan, C: PCNU and recurrent childhood brain tumors. J Neurooncol 5:241–244, 1987.

148. Pons, M, Hetherington, M, Massey, V, et al: Preliminary results: recurrent intrinsic brainstem gliomas of childhood respond to tamoxifen. Ann Neurol 36:514 (Abstract 499), 1994.

149. Packer, RJ, Prados, M, Phillips, P, et al: Treatment of children with newly diagnosed brain stem gliomas with intravenous recombinant b-interferon and hyperfractionated radiation therapy. A Childrens Cancer Group Phase I/II Study. Cancer 77:2150–2156, 1996.

150. Epstein, FJ, and Farmer, J-P: Brain-stem glioma growth patterns. J Neurosurg 78:408–412, 1993.

151. Edwards, MSB, Wara, WM, Ciricillo, SF, and Barkovich, AJ: Focal brain-stem astrocytomas causing symptoms of involvement of the facial nerve nucleus: Long-term survival in six pediatric cases. J Neurosurg 80:20–25, 1994.

152. Packer, RJ, Allen, JC, and Ghavimi, F: Meningeal gliomatosis secondary to brain stem glioma. Proc Annu Meet Amer Soc Clin Oncol 1:177, 1982.

153. Newton, HB, Newton, C, Pearl, D, and Davidson, T: Swallowing assessment in primary brain tumor patients with dysphagia. Neurol 44: 1927–1932, 1994.

154. Scott, RM, and Knightly, J: Choroid plexus papilloma. In Kaye, AH, and Laws, ER Jr (eds): Brain Tumors. An Encyclopedic Approach. Churchill Livingstone, New York, 1995, pp 505–524.

155. Burger, PC, Scheithauer, BW, and Vogel, FS: Brain tumors. In Burger, PC, Scheithauer, BW, and Vogel, FS (eds): Surgical Pathology of the Nervous System and Its Coverings, Third Edition. Churchill Livingstone, New York, 1991, pp 289–296.

156. Matson, DD, and Crofton, FDL: Papilloma of the choroid plexus in childhood. J Neurosurg 17:1002–1027, 1960.

157. Pasual-Castroviejo, I, Villarejo, F, Perez-Higueras, A, et al: Childhood choroid plexus neoplasms. A study of 14 cases less than 2 years old. Eur J Pediatr 140:51–56, 1983.

158. Boyd, MC, and Steinbok, P: Choroid plexus tumors: problems in diagnosis and management. J Neurosurg 66:800–805, 1987.

159. Bohm, E, and Strang, R: Choroid plexus papillomas. J Neurosurg 18:493–500, 1961.

160. Allen, J, Wisoff, J, Helson, L, et al: Choroid plexus carcinomaL: Responses to chemotherapy alone in newly diagnosed young children. J Neurooncol 12:69–74, 1992.

161. Lena, G, Genitori, L, Molina, J, et al: Choroid plexus tumors in children: Review of 24 cases. Acta Neurochir (Wien) 106:68–72, 1990.

162. Coates, TL, Hinshaw, DB Jr, Peckman, N, et al: Pediatric choroid plexus neoplasms: MR, CT, and pathologic correlation. Radiology 173:81–88, 1989.

163. Palazzi, M, Di Marco, A, Campostrini, F, et al: The role of radiotherapy in management of choroid plexus neoplasms. Tumori 75:463–469, 1989.

164. Packer, RJ, Perilongo, G, Johnson, D, et al: Choroid plexus carcinoma of childhood. Cancer 69:580–585, 1992.

165. Niikawa, S, Yamada, H, Sakai, N, et al: Distribution of cellular carbohydrate moieties in human dysontogenetic brain tumors, especially in craniopharyngioma and epidermoid/dermoid. Acta Neuropathol 85:71–78, 1992.
166. Conley, FK: Epidermoid and dermoid tumors. Clinical features and surgical management. In Wilkins, RH, and Rengachary, SS (eds): Neurosurgery, Vol. 1. McGraw-Hill, New York, 1985, pp 668–673.
167. Baxter, JW, and Netsky, MG: Epidermoid and dermoid tumors: Pathology. In Wilkins, RH, and Rengachary, SS (eds): Neurosurgery, Vol 1. McGraw-Hill, New York, 1985, pp 665–661.
168. Storrs, BB: Are dermoid and epidermoid tumors preventable complications of myelomeningocele repair? Pediatr Neurosurg 20: 160–162, 1994.
169. Goffin, J, Plets, C, Van Calenbergh, F, et al: Posterior fossa dermoid cyst associated with dermal fistula: report of 2 cases and review of the literature. Childs Nerv Syst 9:179–181, 1993.
170. Grant, R: Dermoid and epidermoid tumors. In Gilman S, Goldstein G, Waxman S (eds): Neurobase. Arbor Publishing Corporation, San Diego, 1995.
171. Yasargil, MG, Abernathey, CD, and Sarioglu, AC: Microneurosurgical treatment of intracranial dermoid and epidermoid tumors. Neurosurgery 24:561–567, 1989.
172. Yamakawa, K, Shitara, N, Genka, S, et al: Clinical course and surgical prognosis of 33 cases of intracranial epidermoid tumors. Neurosurgery 24:568–573, 1989.
173. Lunardi, P, Missori, P, Gagliardi, FM, and Fortuna, A: Epidermoid tumors of the 4th ventricle: report of seven cases. Neurosurgery 27: 532–534, 1990.
174. Ishikawa, M, Kikuchi, H, and Asato, R: Magnetic resonance imaging of the intracranial epidermoid. Acta Neurochir (Wien) 101:108–111, 1989.
175. Tampieri, D, Melanson, D, and Ethier, R: MR imaging of epidermoid cysts. AJNR 10:351–356, 1989.
176. Olson, JJ, Beck, DW, Crawford, SC, and Menezes, AH: Comparative evaluation of intracranial epidermod tumors with computed tomography and magnetic resonance imaging. Neurosurgery 21:357–360, 1987.
177. Altschuler, EM, Jungreis, CA, Sekhar, LN, et al: Operative treatment of intracranial epidermoid cysts and cholesterol granulomas: Report of 21 cases. Neurosurgery 26:606–613, 1990.
178. Fonari, M, Solero, CL, Lasio, G, et al: Surgical treatment of intracranial dermoid and epidermoid cysts in children. Childs Nerv Syst 6: 66–70, 1990.
179. Lunardi, P, Missori, P, Innocenzi, G, et al: Long-term results of surgical treatment of cerebello-pontine angle epidermoids. Acta Neurochir (Wien) 103:105–108, 1990.
180. Becker, WJ, Watters, GV, de Chadarevian, J-P, and Vanasse, M: Recurrent aseptic meningitis secondary to intracranial epidermoids. Can J Neurol Sci 11:387–389, 1984.
181. Achard, J-M, Lallement, P-Y, and Veyssier, P: Recurrent aseptic meningitis secondary to intracranial epidermoid cyst and Mollaret's meningitis: Two distinct entities or a single disease? A case report and a nosologic discussion. Am J Med 89:807–810, 1990.
182. Jooma, R, Torrens, MJ, Bradshaw, J, and Brownell, B: Subependymomas of the fourth ventricle. Surgical treatment in 12 cases. J Neurosurg 62:508–512, 1985.

Chapter 12

PRIMARY CENTRAL NERVOUS SYSTEM LYMPHOMA

HISTORY AND NOMENCLATURE

Bailey[1] first described primary central nervous system lymphoma (PCNSL) in 1929 and called it a "perithelial or perivascular sarcoma of leptomeningeal origin." One of Bailey's cases was reviewed by another pathologist, who said it resembled a lymphosarcoma, or malignant lymphoma. In the ensuing years, a variety of synonyms have been used to describe this lymphoid reticuloendothelial neoplasm: reticulum cell sarcoma, microgliomatosis, adventitial sarcoma, histiocytic sarcoma, reticuloendothelial sarcoma, malignant lymphoma, malignant reticuloendotheliosis, reticulohistiocytic encephalitis, atypical granulomatous encephalitis, and lymphoproliferative disorder.[2,3] The controversy over the tumor's name was largely a semantic one, with Europeans believing that the reticulum cell was a primitive cell, with origin in microglia, and Americans equating the reticulum cell with the histiocyte, macrophage, or microglia of the reticuloendothelial system.[4] In 1974, Henry and colleagues[2] concluded that the histological patterns observed in this central nervous system (CNS) tumor were analogous to tumors arising in the reticuloendothelial system of other organs. Modern immunologic techniques with lymphocytic markers have confirmed that most PCNSLs are composed of neoplastic B lymphocytes.[5]

EPIDEMIOLOGY

PCNSL is a rare CNS neoplasm, accounting for approximately 1% to 2% of primary brain tumors.[6,7] The incidence of PCNSL has been increasing in the United States in both the immunocompetent and the immunocompromised populations.[5–8] The National Cancer Institute, Surveillance, Epidemiology, and End Results (SEER) program looked at the incidence of primary brain lymphoma in two time periods, 1973 to 1975 and 1982 to 1984, excluding from analysis unmarried men at high risk for acquired immunodeficiency syndrome (AIDS). They found an increase from 2.7 cases per ten million from 1973 to 1975 to 7.5 cases per ten million from 1982 to 1984. The increase in incidence was observed in persons both younger and older than age 60. The time periods analyzed are largely before the

AIDS epidemic but do incorporate the discovery and widespread implementation of computed tomography (CT) diagnostic radiology, particularly in the 1982 to 1984 period.[7] On re-analysis of SEER program data, and with the addition of the 1984 to 1988 time interval, there was a continued further increase in incidence rate of PCNSL, greater than the increase in systemic nodal non-Hodgkin's lymphoma.[8] Ocular lymphoma also increased in incidence from the time interval of 1974 to 1978 to the 1984 to 1988 time interval; it increased by 140%.[8] Between 1985 and 1989, 15.4% of all immunocompetent patients with primary brain tumors were diagnosed with PCNSL at the Memorial Sloan-Kettering Cancer Center.[9]

It was estimated that by the early 1990s PCNSL would become a far more common neurological neoplasm because of the increased incidence in the immunocompetent population, but more importantly, because of the increased incidence in AIDS. Three percent of AIDS patients will develop PCNSL, either before or during the course of their illness.[5] AIDS treatment and the treatment of opportunistic infections in patients with AIDS has improved, with the result that AIDS patients are living longer. This has been associated with an increased incidence of lymphoma, including brain lymphoma.[10,11] The calculated risk of lymphoma in the AIDS population is 1000 times that of the general population, with an estimated 600 new cases per year.[5,12] In addition to AIDS patients, organ transplantation recipients and patients with the some inherited disorders—Wiskoff-Aldrich syndrome, severe combined immunodeficiency, and X-linked immunodeficiency—are all at increased risk for developing PCNSL.

Kidney transplant recipients had a 350 times higher risk of developing reticulum cell sarcoma than the general population with, 2.2 cases per 1000 transplants; 50% of these were located intracranially, and most occurred in the first year after transplantation.[5,13] After heart transplantation, the risk is still higher, with three cases in 182 organ recipients.[5,14,15] PCNSL induced by immunosuppressive treatment after heart transplantation has regressed after the immunosuppressive treatment is stopped. In the Wiskoff-Aldrich syndrome, lymphoma is common, and 25% of these are PCNSLs. PCNSL is caused by uncontrolled Epstein-Barr virus (EBV) infection in the X-linked immunodeficiency syndrome.[15]

BIOLOGY

EBV has an important etiologic role in the development of PCNSL, in AIDS, and in other immunocompromised populations. The EBV genome has been detected in the tumor tissue of a high proportion of patients with AIDS-related PCNSL. The EBV genome has not been found in tumors of immunocompetent patients with PCNSL.[16–20] Two hypotheses exist for the pathogenesis of EBV-related PCNSL. The first hypothesis is that most adults have an acute EBV infection at a young age, and after the infection, a population of B lymphocytes is immortalized by the virus. A second event then attracts the B lymphocytes into the brain and transforms these cells. T lymphocytes normally control the proliferation of this B-lymphocyte population. However, T lymphocytes are not capable of suppressing B lymphocyte growth with the development of PCNSL in patients with an immunocompromised surveillance system.[3,5] The second hypothesis is that B lymphocytes are transformed at a systemic site and develop antigenic binding sites for and migrate to the CNS.[5] These EBV-induced lymphomas probably develop in the brain in increased frequency because it is an immunologically privileged site. EBV is unlikely to play a role in the development of PCNSL in the immunocompetent individual. The mechanisms that cause B- or T-cell proliferation in the immunocompetent population are unknown.

PATHOLOGY

The macroscopic appearance of PCNSL is variable: whereas some of the tumors distinct, well-defined masses, others are a diffuse infiltration of normal appearing brain.[6] The cut surface may be homogeneous, gray and granular, or variegated, with foci of necrosis and hemorrhage. The tumors lack cysts, which are commonly seen in malignant astrocytomas. The lesions are solitary in 60% of cases and have a predilection for periventricular locations.[5,6] Lymphomas are typically deeper seated than metastatic carcinomas. The multiplicity of lesions in 40% of patients leads to frequent bilaterality. In 68 immunocompetent patients with 109 lesions, 70 were in the cerebrum, 21 in the brainstem, 14 in the cerebellum, and four in the spinal cord.[2]

The majority of PCNSL is cerebral in location; however, the primary site may be ocular,[21–24] spinal,[25–27] or leptomeningeal.[28] The intraparenchymal location of most PCNSLs contrasts markedly with the typically meningeal location of systemic lymphoma metastatic to the CNS.[29,30] The vast majority of PCNSL are B-cell lymphomas, although T-cell lymphomas are being identified with increasing frequency.[6,29] They appear to occur in a younger male population.[6]

The accurate pathologic identification of PCNSL requires differentiation from primitive neuroectodermal tumors (PNET) and undifferentiated small cell carcinoma, small cell neoplasms that closely resemble PCNSL.[30] Whereas PCNSL characteristically invades the vascular wall glioma, carcinoma and PNET produce endothelial proliferation and desmoplasia. This can be distinguished with histological stains.[30] Immunohistochemistry with B- and T-cell markers also helps.[6,29,30]

The majority of PCNSLs can be classified histologically according to the International Working Classification of lymphoma.[5,31] The large cell immunoblastic group accounted for approximately 40% of all tumors, followed by small cleaved (18%), large noncleaved (15%), and large noncleaved and not otherwise specified (9%).[5] PCNSL often grows initially in the adventitia of blood vessels and then infiltrates diffusely into normal brain.[5] Reactive gliosis may surround and intermix with the infiltrating lymphoma, making distinction from an astrocytic neoplasm difficult. Glial markers may be positive.[30] The vasculature in all lymphomas has a characteristic increase in perivascular reticulin.[6,29]

AIDS-related PCNSL is distinctive pathologically, having a higher incidence of multifocal lesions. These lesions are typically more diffuse and are large cell immunoblastic or small cell cleaved. The tumors are more often hemorrhagic and necrotic than in non-AIDS cases and are often found with other infectious CNS processes.

The pathologic characterization of PCNSL includes the application of a panel of monoclonal antibodies, which may be particularly helpful in interpretation of small stereotactic biopsies.[6] The B-cell origin of PCNSL can be proven in formalin fixed paraffin-embedded tissue by monoclonal antibody staining with CD20 and MB2. Cytoplasmic or cell surface staining for immunoglobulin (Ig) confirms the B-cell nature of the neoplasm. T-cell markers used in paraffin-embedded tissue include CD45RO, CD43, and anti-CD3.[6] Genotypic analysis is valuable in establishing the monoclonal nature of B- or T-cell lymphomas by looking for gene rearrangements of the Ig heavy- and light-chain genes or the T-cell receptor gene. Needle biopsy material should be sufficient for these molecular biological techniques.[6]

CLINICAL SYMPTOMS

PCNSL peak incidence is in the sixth and seventh decades of life in immunocompetent hosts[2–6] and in the fourth decade of life in the AIDS population.[32] The tumor affects patients of all ages, including children.[2,3,5–7] The male-to-female ratio in PCNSL cohorts varies from 1:1[4] to 3:1.[2] In the AIDS population, 90% of patients with PCNSL are male, reflecting the distribution and duration of AIDS in the population.

PCNSL arises in the CNS, which is usually thought to be devoid of reticuloendothelial tissue.[15] It most commonly arises in the brain,[2] but can arise alone in the eye,[21–24] spinal cord,[25–27] or leptomeninges[28] (Table 12–1). Multiple sites occur often during the course of the disease.

The great majority of patients present with symptoms of a subacute expanding intracranial tumor, with an average duration of symptoms prior to diagnosis of 2 weeks to 2.5 months (Table 12–2).[2,3] Neurological dysfunction often progresses rapidly because PCNSL is a rapidly dividing neoplasm with a high labeling index. Cognitive changes are the most frequent presenting symptom (36%) because of the deep frontal lobe location and bilaterality of many of these tumors. During the course of PCNSL, more than two thirds of patients develop cognitive changes.[3,5] Headaches are also common initially, and 22% have headaches at onset and more than 50% have them during their illness.,[3,5] Other common presenting symptoms include cerebellar signs (31%), seizures (20%), motor dysfunction (17%), and visual changes (12%).[5] Rarely, patients also present with primary central neurogenic hyperventilation as the initial symptom.[33,34]

Ocular lymphoma is lymphoma restricted to the globe, usually involving the vitreous, retina, and choroid.[23,24] It is distinct from orbital lymphoma, an extranodal site of systemic lymphoma, involving the adnexal structures of the eye, including the lacrimal gland, eyelid, and conjunctiva.[22] Ocular lymphoma can present in patients before (50% to 77%), concurrent with (25%), or following the development of PCNSL (25%).[24] Visual symptoms are nonspecific (i.e, visual blurring or floaters) and are most often diagnosed as "uveitis" or "vitreitis."[23,24] Eye pain occurs rarely. The pace of disease is often slower for patients with initial ocular symptomatology; however, more than 90% develop CNS disease in 1 to 84 months (mean, 23 months).[21–24] The ocular involvement is bilateral in 67% to 81% of cases.[21–24] In patients in whom ocular and CNS disease were diagnosed concurrently, two thirds had asymptomatic disease, diagnosed by slit-lamp examination.[21–24]

Table 12–1. **Sites of Central Nervous System Presentation**

Brain
Cerebral hemispheres
Cerebellum
Brainstem
Spinal cord
Leptomeninges
Eye

Table 12–2. **Presenting Symptoms of PCNSL**

Symptom	Approximate % of Patients*
Cognitive changes	35
Headache	20
Cerebellar signs	30
Seizures	20
Motor dysfunction	15
Visual disturbances	10

*May have more than one presenting symptom.

Spinal lymphoma is an intramedullary spinal cord expansile mass that resents most often as a painless myelopathy and produces motor, sensory, and often sphincter disturbances.[25–27] Spinal lymphoma can present concurrently with brain or leptomeningeal lymphoma.[26] Primary leptomeningeal lymphoma presents most commonly with lumbosacral polyradiculopathy (33%), and/or signs of cerebral meningeal involvement (i.e., cranial nerve abnormalities [33%], headache [33%], and confusion [25%]).[28] It accounts for approximately 7% of all cases of PCNSL.[28] It must be differentiated from the much more common involvement of the leptomeninges in systemic lymphoma.[29,30] Meningeal disease rarely precedes the diagnosis of systemic lymphoma, but when it does, systemic lymphoma usually develops within 4 months.[28] Primary leptomeningeal lymphoma is suspected or diagnosed by magnetic resonance imaging (MRI), showing hydrocephalus or meningeal enhancement, cerebrospinal fluid (CSF) examination with increased cell count, positive cytology and immunostain results, or positive biopsy results of an affected meningeal area.

DIFFERENTIAL DIAGNOSIS

The most common presentation of PCNSL is with cerebral symptoms, attributable to single or multiple intracranial masses (>95%).[2,3,5] The lesions are single in approximately 60% of cases, and when multiple, are often bilateral. The tumors are located both supratentorially (65%) and infratentorially (30%), most often deep in the brain in a periventricular location.[2,29] The clinical symptoms of cognitive change, headaches, cerebellar or motor dysfunction, seizures, and visual changes, suggests to the physician the need for an imaging study.[3,5] MRI is the procedure of choice, but CT is an acceptable alternative.[3]

On imaging studies, there are certain imaging features that strongly point to the diagnosis of PCNSL and should prompt physicians to modify presurgical and surgical management to optimize the likelihood of making the correct diagnosis. Imaging characteristics are distinctly different in immunocompetent and immunocompromised patients.

In immunocompetent patients, PCNSL is isodense or hyperdense on precontrast CT scans. MRI is isointense or hyperintense on precontrast T_1-weighted images. CT and MRI images show marked uniform enhancement in the majority of patients (Fig. 12–1). The precontrast hyperintense signal on T_1 MRI or hyperdensity on CT is thought to be due to a high nuclear-to-cytoplasmic ratio. In approximately 10% of patients, PCNSL presents as a nonenhancing mass on CT or MRI.[35] After contrast administration, there is most often dense and homogeneous enhancement and variable edema (see Fig. 12–1).[36] Occasionally, there is heterogeneous contrast enhancement, which is more typical in immunocompromised patients with PCNSL (Fig. 12–2). Dense and homogeneous enhancement seen on CT and MRI in PCNSL are atypical in malignant gliomas, brain abscesses, and brain metastases, in which ring or serpiginous enhancement is likely. A multiplicity of lesions is atypical for malignant gliomas but is seen frequently with brain metastases or abscesses. Another clinical factor confounding differential diagnosis is that 15% of patients with PCNSL have a history of prior malignancy, including systemic lymphoma.[37] A malignancy history makes it more likely that a new brain lesion or lesions would be attributed to metastatic disease. In patients with prior malignancy, PCNSL developed a median of 10 years after initial tumor diagnosis and a median of 6 years after treatment completion.[37] Typically, PCNSL does not have the massive edema on imaging studies that is usu-

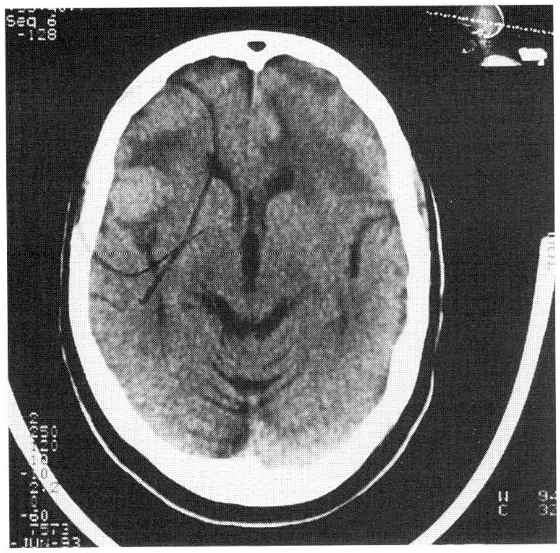

A

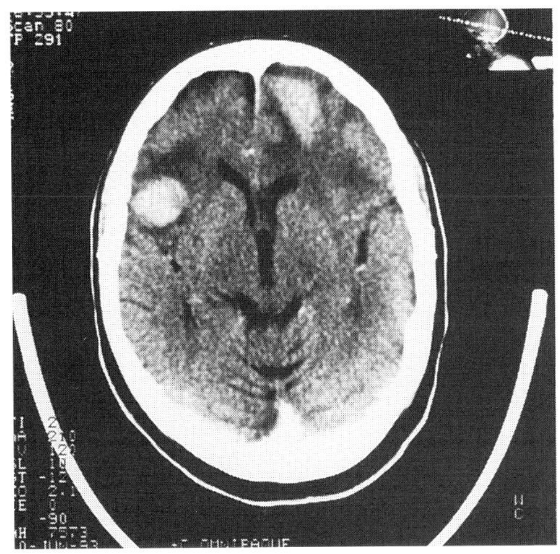

B

Figure 12–1. PCNSL in immunocompetent patient. *(A)* CT with right frontal hyperdense and left frontal isodense abnormality. *(B)* Both enhance homogeneously with contrast and have surrounding hypodense edema.

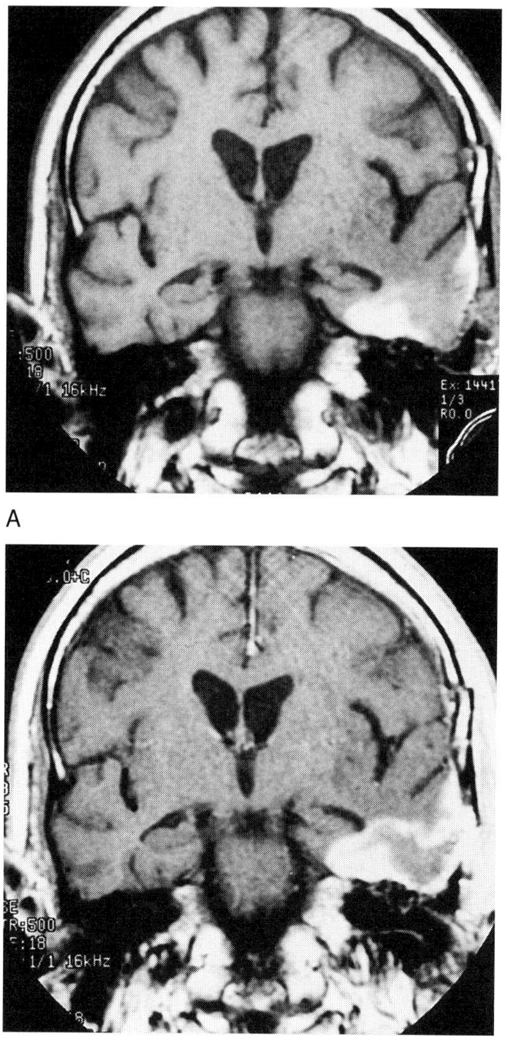

A

B

Figure 12–2. PCNSL in immunocompetent patient. *(A)* Precontrast T_1-weighted MRI with hyperintense signal left mesial temporal lobe with enhancement, and *(B)* with postcontrast heterogeneous enhancement.

ally seen with brain metastases or abscesses. If PCNSL is suspected from evaluation of imaging studies, the use of steroids and the surgical approach should be carefully examined.[2,3,38]

Steroids are cytolytic for PCNSL, often leading to prompt tumor regression and a nondiagnostic stereotactic biopsy.[3,39,40] Steroids are used in almost all combination chemotherapy regimens for systemic lymphoma because of their cytolytic effect. In patients suspected of having PCNSL, steroids should only be used to treat cerebral edema when there is a significant risk of cerebral herniation. Following steroid use, neurosurgical biopsy is often nondiagnostic or the tissue is necrotic, delaying diagnosis. After nondiagnostic biopsy, steroid therapy should be discontinued, and the patient should be observed for the return of symptoms and imaging abnormalities with serial scans. When the lesion(s) returns, it should be biopsied promptly. The cytolytic effect of steroids is not diagnostic of PCNSL and can occur in multiple sclerosis or sarcoidosis. Therefore, stereotactic biopsy is needed before treatment can proceed.

If the imaging abnormality is typical for PCNSL, stereotactic biopsy is the surgical procedure of choice. Large surgical resection does not improve outcome and may, in fact, produce unnecessary surgical complications, particularly in deep-seated periventricular lesions.[2,3,38,41,42]

In immunocompromised AIDS patients who present with cerebral symptoms, the differential diagnosis is more complicated and the imaging picture less precise. In AIDS patients no radiological features allow distinction among PCNSL, toxoplasmosis, and other CNS infections. Multifocal lesions occur in 63% of patients with AIDS-related PCNSL. Multifocality is more common in immunocompromised than immunocompetent patients. MRI abnormalities are hypointense before contrast administration and enhance in a ring-like fashion in 19% to 59% of cases (Fig. 12–3).[43] CT lesions are usually hypodense precontrast and enhance inhomogenously in a ring-like pattern.[32] The ring enhancement and deep periventricular location make PCNSL indistinguishable, clinically and radiographically, from toxoplasmosis. In fact, the two disease processes may coexist in the same patient. Diagnostic workup should include a lumbar puncture and toxoplasmosis serology. The CSF of immunocompromised patients with AIDS-related PCNSL has EBV DNA in 100% of cases, which may be diagnostic of cerebral lymphoma.[44]

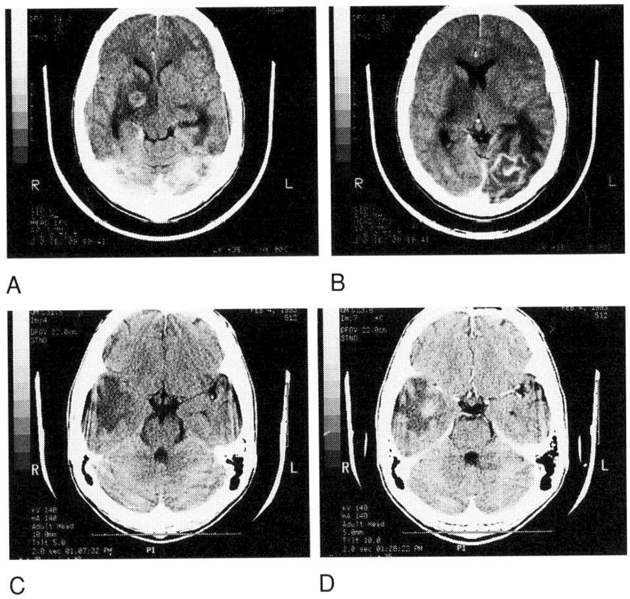

Figure 12–3. AIDS-related toxoplasmosis and PCNSL: A 26-year-old man with AIDS presented in August 1990 with increasing headaches. CT postcontrast showed *(A)* a deep right internal capsule ring-like contrast-enhancing mass and *(B)* a second left occipital serpiginously enhancing abnormality with excessive surrounding hypodense edema. He was treated presumptively for toxoplasmosis with pyrimethamine and sulfadiazine and then monthly pentamidine with clearing of headaches and resolution of enhancement. In late January 1993 he had increasing occipital headaches. *(C)* CT precontrast revealed a right temporal hypodensity with *(D)* medial contrast enhancement. Right temporal stereotactic biopsy revealed a B cell lymphoma.

DIAGNOSTIC WORKUP

Contrast-enhanced cranial MRI is the diagnostic procedure of choice when a patient presents with symptoms of an expanding intracranial mass.[3,45] Similarly, if the symptoms are of a painless myelopathy, contrast-enhanced spinal MRI is the most appropriate procedure. If the patient is suspected of having PCNSL and the intracranial pressure is not considered significantly elevated, a lumbar puncture should be obtained for evaluation of protein, glucose, cell count, differential, cultures, india ink preparation, and cytology. A positive cytology may obviate the need for a stereotactic biopsy. At the time of diagnosis, patients with PCNSL often have asymptomatic lymphomatous leptomeningeal involvement.[3,42] The exact frequency of involvement has been debated. Balmaceda and colleagues[46] examined the CSF of 86 patients with PCNSL at diagnosis and 42 at recurrence. The incidence of leptomeningeal tumor was 42% at diagnosis and 41% at recurrence.[43] If a lumbar puncture is not possible preoperatively or was not performed preoperatively, it should be part of the staging evaluation postoperatively (Table 12–3). An ocular slit lamp is required to look for asymptomatic ocular lymphoma; vitrectomy represents an alternative diagnostic route for tissue when the vitreous is involved.[23,24] Multiple vitrectomies may be necessary.[23]

Debate continues concerning the extent of systemic staging necessary when a patient presents with PCNSL. O'Neill and colleagues[47] carried out a retrospective study of 128 patients with PCNSL to examine whether staging was necessary to exclude stage IV non-Hodgkin's lymphoma. Five patients (3.9%) fulfilled the criteria for PCNSL but were also found at diagnosis to have occult non-Hodgkin's lymphoma. The systemic disease sites

Table 12–3. **Staging Evaluation in PCNSL**

Immunocompetent
Cranial MRI with contrast
Lumbar puncture with cytology
Ophthalmologic slit-lamp examination
Abdominal and pelvic CT
Bone marrow examination
Spinal MRI with contrast (if spinal symptoms)
Immunocompromised
All of the foregoing procedures
Chest radiograph or CT
Consider CSF for EBV genome

CSF = cerebrospinal fluid;
CT = computed tomography;
EBV = Epstein-Barr virus;
MRI = magnetic resonance imaging;
PCNSL = primary central nervous system lymphoma.

were bone marrow (one patient), abdominal (three patients), and colon (one patient).[47] Current recommendations are in flux with some clinicians including abdominal and pelvic CT's and bone marrow examination to rule out systemic disease before proceeding with treatment.

In immunocompromised patients, all of the aforementioned examinations are necessary; in addition, a chest radiograph or CT is recommended.[45] If the chest examination reveals an abnormality, it may provide a diagnostic clue about the intracerebral process.

TREATMENT

Surgery

Conventional therapy for PCNSL includes stereotactic biopsy followed by WBRT. Maximum surgical resection, the treatment of choice for malignant gliomas, is not of benefit for PCNSL.[2,3]

Radiation Therapy

Radiotherapy (RT) generally results in clinical and radiographic improvement; there is a complete response in approximately 50% of patients.[48,49] Most patients are treated to the whole brain with a coned-down boost to a cumulative radiation dose in excess of 5000 cGy. Berry and Simpson[50] found median survival to be better for patients who received more than 5000 cGy. However, despite significant responses in an overwhelming majority of patients, the durability of response and survival are poor. The range of median survival in RT trials is from 5.5 to 42 months.[48,49] The 5-year survival rate is less than 5%.[4,51] The poor stability of response and survival has prompted the addition of adjuvant chemotherapy to RT for the treatment of PCNSL.

The principal treatment of ocular lymphoma, when present, is RT in a dose of approximately 3600 cGy.[23,24] Treatment of isolated ocular lymphoma is controversial with ocular radiation alone; some investigators recommend concurrent cranial radiation because of the high incidence of cranial relapse.[52] This has not received widespread acceptance because of the potential toxicity of brain irradiation. Both eyes should be irradiated because the disease is bilateral in more than 80% of patients.[24] The length of remission varies from months to years after ocular irradiation.[24,47] If the patient has an ocular recurrence after WBRT for PCNSL, ocular radiation can be tailored to the previous RT ports.[47]

Craniospinal RT is generally not used to treat asymptomatic leptomeningeal disease in patients with PCNSL. Patients are treated with high-dose systemic chemotherapy, with or without IT methotrexate (MTX) chemotherapy. Patients with primary leptomeningeal lymphoma are generally treated with craniospinal radiation and IT MTX chemotherapy.[28] Spinal lymphoma is generally treated with local RT, with or without adjuvant chemotherapy.[25,27]

In AIDS-related PCNSL treated with RT, six of 10 patients had a complete response (CR) and one partial response (PR). The median survival was 5.5 months. Two patients with a CR died of opportunistic infections, two of disease relapse, and two had ongoing response for more than 8 and 14 months.[53]

Chemotherapy

Patients treated with intra-arterial (IA) MTX chemotherapy after osmotic blood-brain barrier disruption (BBBD) and the addition of multiagent adjuvant chemotherapy to RT appear to have prolonged disease-free survival (Table 12–4).[54,55] DeAngelis[3] emphasizes that the drugs used or the method of drug delivery must be capable of penetrating the blood-brain barrier (BBB) for effective chemotherapy. Neuwelt and colleagues[54] treated patients with PCNSL with monthly cycles of IA osmotic BBBD with mannitol followed by IA MTX. Patients received oral procarbazine and dexamethasone for 14 days on each cycle after the disruption procedure. The median survival in 17 patients treated adjuvantly was 44.5 months. Patients were treated with RT only if drug failure occurred. Cognitive function was preserved for patients maintaining a CR after IA osmotic BBBD. This suggests the neurological sequelae seen with many combined-modality regimens is not due to disease but instead is secondary to treatment toxicity from a combination of RT and systemic and IT therapy. When IA osmotic BBBD with MTX was used on tumor recurrence, the median survival was only 17.8 months.

DeAngelis and colleagues[55] treated 31 patients with multiagent chemotherapy before and after RT. Initially, an intraventricular reservoir was placed, and patients were treated with six doses of intrathecal (IT) MTX and two weekly cycles of intravenous (IV) MTX. RT followed to a dose of 4000 cGy whole brain over 4 weeks, and a 1440 cGy coned down boost to the tumor bed. Following a pause, patients received two monthly cycles of high-dose cytosine arabinoside (HAraC). Patients treated adjuvantly had a median time to recurrence of 41 months and median survival of 42.5 months. Patients treated on recurrence had an increase in median survival to 41 months, but when this was compared with a historical control group with a 21-month median survival, the difference was not significant.[55] Cher and colleagues[56] treated 19 patients with high-dose MTX (3.5 to 8.0 gm/m^2) every 10 to 21 days for three cycles of induction therapy, followed by maintenance MTX chemotherapy. WBRT was deferred until progressive disease. Response duration was 11 to 52 months in the first eight patients.

IV combination chemotherapy regimens for PCNSL, which include cyclophosphamide and adriamycin and mimic those used successfully in systemic lymphoma, have been ineffective or less effective because of poor BBB penetration.[57–62] Patients with PCNSL have also been treated adjuvantly, after RT and hydroxyurea, with PCV chemotherapy. The median survival in 16 patients was 41 months.[63,64] Patients unable to receive chemotherapy before RT, should most likely receive PCV chemotherapy after RT because it does not potentiate radiation toxicity.[47] Patients older than 50 years of age with PCNSL have a greater incidence of neurological sequelae after combined RT and chemotherapy. Thirteen patients older than age 50 were treated with only multiagent chemotherapy without RT. Chemotherapy drugs included procarbazine and MTX in all patients. Ten patients had a CR, and two had a PR. The median survival of the 10 patients with a diagnosis of PCNSL was 30.5 months.[65] The results were comparable to combined RT and chemotherapy results in patients older than 50 years of age.[55]

Ocular lymphoma can be treated at relapse with HAraC in a dose of 3 gm/m^2. It is one of the few drugs able to penetrate the vitreous.[66] Its role as an adjuvant therapy with RT for ocular lymphoma is not defined. HAraC has been used in multiagent chemotherapy regimens for the adjuvant treatment of PCNSL.[55,67]

Asymptomatic leptomeningeal disease is usually treated with high-dose systemic chemotherapy, with or without IT chemotherapy. IT chemotherapy increases the risk of diffuse leukoencephalopathy, and patients should have a CSF flow study with a radioactive tracer injected intrathecally after reservoir place-

Table 12–4. **Chemotherapy Trials for PCNSL**

Trial	Number of Patients	Treatment (In Order of Treatment)	Radiation Therapy (Dose)	Median Survival (Mo)
Neuwelt et al[54] (1991)	17	IA osmotic BBBD + MTX, oral procarbazine, and dexamethasone, monthly × 12	On drug failure only	44.5
DeAngelis et al[55] (1992)	31	IT MTX × 6, IV MTX × 2, RT, HAraC × 2	40 Gy WBRT + 14.4 Gy boost	42.5
Cher et al[56] (1996)	19	IV MTX (3.5–8.0 g/m2) 3 or greater cycles + CHOD (four patients)	On drug failure only	≅12+
Lachance et al[57] (1994)	6	CHOP × 4, RT	45 Gy WBRT + 10 Gy boost + 30 Gy spinal axis	8.5
Rosenthal et al[58] (1993)	6	RT, CHOP for 3 weeks, IT MTX (1 patient)	45 Gy WBRT + 10 Gy boost or 50.4 Gy if multiple lesions	25+
Shibamoto et al[59] (1990)	10	RT; cyclophosphamide, doxorubicin, vincristine, prednisolone q 14 days × 4–6	30–40 WBRT+ boost to 50–60 Gy	8/10 alive >(16 mo) 3 > 5 yy
Brada et al[60] (1990)	10	MACOP-B for 6–12 weeks, RT	30–40 Gy WBRT + boost to 55 Gy ± 30 Gy spinal axis	14

Continued on following page

ment and before chemotherapy instillation.[68] If CSF flow is obstructed, IT chemotherapy should be deferred and RT or systemic chemotherapy delivered. A CSF flow study can be repeated following these treatments and a decision made regarding IT chemotherapy.[61] Patients with primary leptomeningeal lymphoma are generally treated with IT MTX and craniospinal radiation.[28] Insufficient information is present to define the role of systemic chemotherapy in leptomeningeal lymphoma.

Ten immuncompromised patients with AIDS-related PCNSL have been treated with chemotherapy, usually consisting of MTX, thiotepa, and procarbazine. Four of seven assessable patients had a CR before RT, and six of seven had a CR after RT. Median survival was 3.5 months for the 10 treated patients and 7 months for the eight patients who completed therapy.[43] Four AIDS patients with PCNSL were treated with RT and hydroxyurea followed by PCV chemotherapy, with a median survival after tumor diagnosis of 13.5 months (range, 11 to 16 months).[68]

In summary, a combination of RT and adjuvant chemotherapy that passes an intact BBB appears to increase patient survival in immunocompetent patients and may have a positive effect in immunocompromised hosts with AIDS-related PCNSL.

Table 12–4.—*continued*

Trial	Number of Patients	Treatment (In Order of Treatment)	Radiation Therapy (Dose)	Median Survival (Mo)
Liang et al[61] (1993)	9	Two patients: CHOP, RT ± IT MTX 7 patients: RT, IT MTX, CHOP	36 Gy WBRT + 18-Gy boost	30
O'Neill et al[62] (1995)	46	CHOP × 2, RT, HAraC × 2	50.4 Gy WBRT	11.25
Chamberlain and Levin[64] (1992)	16	RT (hydroxyurea), PCV × 1–6	55–62 Gy WBRT	41
McLaughlin et al[67] (1988)	3	Cisplatin, HAraC, dexamethasone ± RT, monthly × 1–3	30.6 Gy WBRT	18+

BBBD = blood-brain barrier disruption;
CHOP = cyclophosphamide, doxorubicin, vincristine, prednisone;
CHOD = cyclophosphamide, doxorubicin, vincristine, decadron;
HAraC = high dose cytosine arabinoside;
IA = intra-arterial;
IT = intrathecal;
IV = intravenous;
MACOP-B = cyclophosphamide, doxorubicin weekly alternating with either MTX and vincristine or bleomycin and vincristine, together with oral prednisone;
MTX = methotrexate;
PCNSL = primary central nervous system lymphoma;
PCV = procarbazine, CCNU, vincristine;
RT = radiation therapy;
WBRT = whole brain radiation therapy.

PROGNOSIS AND COMPLICATIONS

Prognosis

Immunocompetent patients with PCNSL treated with RT have a median survival of 12 to 24 months in most series.[48,49] The best adjuvant chemotherapy that crosses the BBB increases median survival to approximately 40 months.[54,55,64] Patients with AIDS respond to radiation and chemotherapy, but survival is usually short, with a median survival of 3.5 to 13.5 months.[43,69]

Prognostic factors, which have been significantly associated with decreased survival in patients with PCNSL treated with RT alone or RT plus chemotherapy include age older than 60 years at diagnosis, focal neurological deficit, ependymal contact of tumor, and first-degree relatives with cancer.[49,70]

Complications

PCNSL recurs locally in more than 90% of patients, with 7% having solely distant metastases. Distant metastases have been reported to occur in the testes; supraclavicular, abdominal, and inguinal nodes; and multiple organs.[49,71,72] Primary leptomeningeal lymphoma has been reported to remit spontaneously for 7 months before recurring on other spinal nerve roots.[73]

CHAPTER SUMMARY

PCNSL is most often a rapidly growing B-cell lymphomatous neoplasm. The incidence of PCNSL is increasing in both immunocompetent and immunocompromised populations. PCNSL presents typically with signs and symptoms of cranial involvement, its most common primary site of neurological disease. Other sites of disease include the leptomeninges, eye, and intramedullary spinal. These sites may present as the primary site, occur with cranial disease, or develop at recurrence. After diagnosis of PCNSL, staging is necessary and should include lumbar puncture; ophthalmologic slit-lamp examination; review of HIV status; bone marrow, abdominal, and pelvic CT; and spinal MRI if spinal symptoms are present. In immunocompetent patients, the addition of chemotherapy that passes the BBB to RT appears to create increased median survival. The median survival was increased from 12 to 24 months with radiation alone, to approximately 40 months with the addition of chemotherapy. The treatment of immunocompromised patients with AIDS-related PCNSL is less clear.

REFERENCES

1. Bailey, P: Intracranial sarcomatous tumors of leptomeningeal origin. Arch Surg 18:1359–1402, 1929.
2. Henry, JM, Heffner, RR Jr, Dillard, SH, et al: Primary malignant lymphomas of the central nervous system. Cancer 34:1293–1302, 1974.
3. DeAngelis, LM: Primary central nervous system lymphoma. In Gilman, S, Goldstein, G, and Waxman, S (eds): Neurobase. Arbor Publishing Corporation, San Diego, 1998.
4. Littman, P, and Wang, CC: Reticulum cell sarcoma of the brain. A review of the literature and a study of 19 cases. Cancer 35:1412–1420, 1975.
5. Hochberg, FH, and Miller, DC: Primary central nervous system lymphoma. J Neurosurg 68:835–853, 1988.
6. Grant, JW, and Isaacson, PG: Primary central nervous system lymphoma. Brain Pathology 2: 97–109, 1992.
7. Eby, NL, Grufferman, S, Flannelly, CM, et al: Increasing incidence of primary brain lymphoma in the US. Cancer 62:2461–2465, 1988.
8. Devesa, SS, and Fears, T: Non-Hodgkin's lymphoma time trends: United States and international data. Cancer Res 52(Suppl):5432s-5440s, 1992.
9. DeAngelis, LM: Primary central nervous system lymphoma: A new clinical challenge. Neurology 41:619–621, 1991.
10. Gail, MH, Pluda, JM, and Rabkin, CS, et al: Projections of the incidence of non-Hodgkin's lymphoma related to acquired immunodeficiency syndrome. J Natl Cancer Inst 83:695–701, 1991.
11. Pluda, JM, Yarchoan, R, Jaffe, ES, et al: Development of non-Hodgkin lymphoma in a cohort of patients with severe human immunodeficiency virus (HIV) infection on long-term antiretroviral therapy. Ann Intern Med 113:276–282, 1990.
12. Beral, V, Peterman, T, Berkelman, R, and Jaffe, H: AIDS-associated non-Hodkin lymphoma. Lancet 337:805–809, 1991.
13. Hoover, R, and Fraumeni, JF Jr: Risk of cancer in renal-transplant recipients. Lancet 2(820):55–57, 1973.
14. Weintraub, J, and Warnke, RA: Lymphoma in cardiac allotransplant recipients: Clinical and histological features and immunological phenotypes. Transplantation 33:347–351, 1982.
15. Velasquez, WS: Primary central nervous system lymphoma. J Neurooncol 20:177–185, 1994.
16. Rosenberg, NL, Hochberg, FH, Miller, G, and Kleinschmidt-DeMasters, BK: Primary central nervous system lymphoma related to Epstein-Barr virus in a patient with acquired immune deficiency syndrome. Ann Neurol 20:98–102, 1986.
17. Bashir, RM, Harris, NL, Hochberg, FH,and Singer, RM: Detection of Epstein-Barr virus in CNS lymphomas by in-situ hybridization. Neurology 39:813–817, 1989.
18. DeAngelis, LM, Wong, E, Rosenblum, M,and Furneaux, H: Epstein-Barr virus in acquired immune deficiency syndrome (AIDS) and non-AIDS primary central nervous system lymphoma. Cancer 70:1607–1611, 1992.
19. Paulus, W, Jellinger, K, Hallas, C, et al: Human herpesvirus-6 and Epstein-Barr virus genome in primary cerebral lymphomas. Neurology 43: 1591–1593, 1993.
20. Bashir, R, Luka, J, Cheloha, K, et al: Expression of Epstein-Barr virus proteins in primary CNS lymphoma in AIDS patients. Neurology 43: 2358–2362, 1993.
21. Rockwood, EJ, Zakov, ZN, and Bay, JW: Combined malignant lymphoma of the eye and CNS (reticulum-cell sarcoma). J Neurosurg 61:369–374, 1984.
22. Trudeau, M, Shepherd, FA, Blackstein, ME, et al: Intraocular lymphoma: Report of three cases and review of the literature. Am J Clin Oncol 11(2):126–130, 1988.
23. Char, DH, Ljung, BM, Miller, T, and Phillips, T: Primary intraocular lymphoma (ocular reticulum cell sarcoma) diagnosis and management. Ophthalmology 95:625–630, 1988.
24. Peterson, K, Gordon, KB, Heinemann, M-H, and DeAngelis, LM: The clinical spectrum of ocular lymphoma. Cancer 72:843–849, 1993.
25. Hautzer, NW, Aiyesimoju, A, and Robitaille, Y: "Primary" spinal intramedullary lymphomas: A review. Ann Neurol 14:62–66, 1983.

26. Nelson, KD, Binkovitz, LA, and Lyons, MK: Primary lymphoma of the spinal cord. Mayo Clin Proc 68:1097–1098, 1993.
27. Schild, SE, Wharen, RE, Menke, DM, et al: Primary lymphoma of the spinal cord. Mayo Clin Proc 70:256–260, 1995.
28. Lachance, DH, O'Neill, BP, Macdonald, DR, et al: Primary leptomeningeal lymphoma: Report of 9 cases, diagnosis with immunocytochemical analysis, and review of the literature. Neurology 41:95–100, 1991.
29. Kleihues, P, Burger, PC, and Scheithauer, BW: Histological Typing of Tumours of the Central Nervous System, Second Edition. World Health Organization, Springer-Verlag, Berlin, 1993.
30. McKeever, PE, and Blaivas, M: The brain, spinal cord, and meninges. In Sternberg, SS (ed): Diagnostic Surgical Pathology, Second Edition. Raven Press Ltd, New York, pp 409–492, 1994.
31. The Non-Hodgkin's Lymphoma Pathologic Classification Project: The National Cancer Institute sponsored study of classifications of non-Hodgkin's lymphomas: Summary and description of a working formulation for clinical usage. Cancer 49:2112–2135, 1982.
32. Baumgartner, JE, Rachlin, JR, Beckstead, JH, et al: Primary central nervous system lymphomas: Natural history and response to radiation therapy in 55 patients with acquired immunodeficiency syndrome. J Neurosurg 73:206–211, 1990.
33. Pauzner, R, Mouallem, M, Sadeh, M, et al: High incidence of primary cerebral lymphoma in tumor-induced central neurogenic hyperventilation. Arch Neurol 46:510–512, 1989.
34. Krendel, DA, Pilch, JF, and Stahl, RL: Central hyperventilation in primary CNS lymphoma: Evidence implicating CSF lactic acid. Neurology 41:1156–1157, 1991.
35. DeAngelis, LM: Cerebral lymphoma presenting as a nonenhancing lesion on computed tomographic/magnetic resonance scan. Ann Neurol 33:308–311, 1993.
36. Mendenhall, NP, Thar, TL, Agee, OF, et al: Primary lymphoma of the central nervous system. Computerized tomography scan characteristics and treatment results for 12 cases. Cancer 52: 1993–2000, 1983.
37. DeAngelis, LM: Primary central nervous system lymphoma is a secondary malignancy. Cancer 67: 1431–1435, 1991.
38. O'Neill, BP, Kelly, PJ, Earle, JD, et al: Computer-assisted stereotaxic biopsy for the diagnosis of primary central nervous system lymphoma. Neurology 37:1160–1164, 1987.
39. Singh, A, Strobos, RJ, Singh, BM, et al: Steroid-induced remissions in CNS lymphoma. Neurology 32:1267–1271, 1982.
40. Geppert, M, Ostertag, CB, Seitz, G, and Kiessling, M: Glucocorticoid therapy obscures the diagnosis of cerebral lymphoma. Acta Neuropathol 80:629–634, 1990.
41. Hochberg, FH, Loeffler, JS, and Prados, M: The therapy of primary brain lymphoma. J Neurooncol 10:191–201, 1991.
42. DeAngelis, LM, Yahalom, J, Heinemann, M-H, et al: Primary CNS lymphoma: Combined treatment with chemotherapy and radiotherapy. Neurology 40:80–86, 1990.
43. Forsyth, PA, Yahalom, J, and DeAngelis, LM: Combined-modality therapy in the treatment of primary central nervous system lymphoma in AIDS. Neurology 44:1473–1479, 1994.
44. Cinque, P, Brytting, M, Vago, L, et al: Epstein-Barr virus DNA in cerebrospinal fluid from patients with AIDS-related primary lymphoma of the central nervous system. Lancet 342:398–401, 1993.
45. DeAngelis, LM: Current management of primary central nervous system lymphoma. Oncology 9(1):63–71, 1995.
46. Balmaceda, C, Graynor, JJ, Sun, M, et al: Leptomeningeal tumor in primary central nervous system lymphoma: Recognition, significance, and implications. Ann Neurol 38:202–209, 1995.
47. O'Neill, BP, Dinapoli, RP, Kurtin, PJ, and Habermann, TM: Occult systemic non-Hodgkin's lymphoma (NHL) in patients initially diagnosed as primary central nervous system lymphoma (PCNSL): How much staging is enough? J Neurooncol 25:67–71, 1995.
48. Leibel, SA, and Sheline, GE: Radiation therapy for neoplasms of the brain. J Neurosurg 66:1–22, 1987.
49. Nelson, DF, Martz, KL, Bonner, H, et al: Non-Hodgkin's lymphoma of the brain: Can high dose, large volume radiation therapy improve survival? Report on a prospective trial by the Radiation Therapy Oncology Group (RTOG): RTOG 8315. Int J Radiat Oncol Biol Phys 23: 9–17, 1992.
50. Berry, MP, and Simpson, WJ: Radiation therapy in the management of primary malignant lymphoma of the brain. Int J Radiat Oncol Biol Phys 7:55–59, 1981.
51. Murray, K, Kun, L, and Cox, J: Primary malignant lymphoma of the central nervous system. Results of treatment of 11 cases and review of the literature. J Neurosurg 65:600–607, 1986.
52. Buettner, H, and Bolling, JP: Intravitreal large-cell lymphoma. Mayo Clin Proc 68:1011–1015, 1993.
53. Formenti, SC, Gill, PS, Lean, E, et al: Primary central nervous system lymphoma in AIDS. Results of radiation therapy. Cancer 63:1101–1107, 1989.
54. Neuwelt, EA, Goldman, DL, Dahlborg, SA, et al: Primary CNS lymphoma treated with osmotic blood-brain barrier disruption: Prolonged survival and preservation of cognitive function. J Clin Oncol 9:1580–1590, 1991.
55. DeAngelis, LM, Yahalom, J, Thaler, HT, and Kher, U: Combined modality therapy for primary CNS lymphoma. J Clin Oncol 10:635–643, 1992.
56. Cher, L, Glass, J, Harsh, GR, and Hochberg, FH: Therapy of primary CNS lymphoma with methotrexate-based chemotherapy and deferred radiotherapy: Preliminary results. Neurology 46: 1757–1759, 1996.
57. Lachance, DH, Brizel, DM, Gockerman, JP, et al: Cyclophosphamide, doxorubicin, vincristine,

and prednisone for primary central nervous system lymphoma: Short-duration response and multifocal intracerebral recurrence preceding radiotherapy. Neurology 44:1721–1727, 1994.
58. Rosenthal, MA, Sheridan, WP, Green, MD, et al: Primary cerebral lymphoma: An argument for the use of adjunctive systemic chemotherapy. Aust NZ J Surg 63:30–32, 1993.
59. Shibamoto, Y, Tsutsui, K, Dodo, Y, et al: Improved survival rate in primary intracranial lymphoma treated by high-dose radiation and systemic vincristine-doxorubicin-cyclophosphamide-prednisolone chemotherapy. Cancer 65:1907–1912, 1990.
60. Brada, M, Dearnaley, D, Horwich, A, and Bloom, HJG: Management of primary cerebral lymphoma with initial chemotherapy: Preliminary results and comparison with patients treated with radiotherapy alone. Int J Radiat Oncol Biol Phys 18:787–792, 1990.
61. Liang, BC, Grant, R, Junck, L, et al: Primary central nervous system lymphoma: Treatment with multiagent systemic and intrathecal chemotherapy with radiation therapy. Int J Oncology 3:1001–1004, 1993.
62. O'Neil, BP, O'Fallon, JR, Earle, JD, et al: Primary central nervous system non-Hodgkin's lymphoma: Survival advantages with combined initial therapy? Int J Radiat Oncol Biol Phys 33: 663–673, 1995.
63. Chamberlain, MC, and Levin, VA: Adjuvant chemotherapy for primary lymphoma of the central nervous system. Arch Neurol 47:1113–1116, 1990.
64. Chamberlain, MC, and Levin, VA: Primary central nervous system lymphoma: a role for adjuvant chemotherapy. J Neurooncol 14:271–275, 1992.
65. Freilich, RJ, Delattre, J-Y, Monjour, A, and DeAngelis, LM: Chemotherapy without radiation therapy as initial treatment for primary CNS lymphoma in older patients. Neurology 46:435–439, 1996.
66. Strauchen, JA, Dalton, J, and Friedman, AH: Chemotherapy in the management of intraocular lymphoma. Cancer 63:1918–1921, 1989.
67. McLaughlin, P, Velasquez, WS, Redman, JR, et al: Chemotherapy with dexamethasone, high-dose cytarabine, and cisplatin for parenchymal brain lymphoma. J Natl Cancer Inst 80:1408–1412, 1988.
68. Chamberlain, MC: Current concepts in leptomeningeal metastasis. Current Opinion in Oncology 4:533–539, 1992.
69. Chamberlain, MC: Long survival in patients with acquired immune deficiency syndrome-related primary central nervous system lymphoma. Cancer 73:1728–1730, 1994.
70. Tomlinson, FH, Kurtin, PJ, Suman ,VJ, et al: Primary intracerebral malignant lymphoma: a clinicopathological study of 89 patients. J Neurosurg 82:558–566, 1995.
71. Loeffler, JS, Ervin, TJ, Mauch, P, et al: Primary lymphomas of the central nervous system: Patterns of failure and factors that influence survival. J Clin Oncol 3:490–494, 1985.
72. Brown, MT, McClendon, RE, and Gockerman, JP: Primary central nervous system lymphoma with systemic metastasis: Case report and review. J Neurooncol 23:207–221, 1995.
73. Galetta, SL, Sergott, RC, Wells, GB, et al: Spontaneous remission of a third-nerve palsy in meningeal lymphoma. Ann Neurol 32:100–102, 1992.

Chapter 13

PITUITARY AND PINEAL REGION TUMORS

This chapter details the diagnosis and treatment of a variety of tumors occurring in the regions of the sella and of the pineal gland. Although many of the tumors are benign, those that appear in the region of the sella are very different from those found only slightly more posteriorly in the region of the pineal gland.

PITUITARY TUMORS

History and Nomenclature

The existence of the pituitary gland has been recognized since before the time of Artistotle. From the second until the seventeenth century, it was believed that the pituitary secreted mucus produced by the brain. Rathke described the embryology of the pituitary in 1838,[1] and Marie described the clinical syndrome of acromegaly in 1886,[2] but it was Minkowski in 1887[3] who first linked the symptoms of acromegaly to a dysfunction of the pituitary gland. Benda[4] and Fränkel and colleagues[5] recognized that acromegaly was caused by a hyperfunction of the pituitary. It was not until 1962 that a radioimmunoassay for growth hormone (GH) became available to finally prove that the proliferation of GH-secreting cells in pituitary adenomas produced acromegaly.

Babinski[6] and Fröhlich[7] described the clinical condition of hypopituitarism and related it to the lack of pituitary function. Cushing[8] described the condition of hypercortisolism and linked it to a basophil adenoma of the pituitary in 1932. In 1958, Nelson and associates[9] described the effects of excessive adrenocorticotrophin hormone (ACTH) production from a pituitary tumor after bilateral adrenalectomies. In 1954, Forbes and coworkers[10] described the syndrome of amenorrhea-galactorrhea and related it to a pituitary adenoma. The radioimmunoassay for prolactin was not developed until 1971. Since the rare thyroid-stimulating hormone (TSH)–secreting tumor was described in 1969, many tumors previously thought to be "null cell" or non-hormone–producing have been shown to contain cells producing follicle-stimulating hormone (FSH), luteinizing hormone (LH), or glycoprotein subunits.

Sir Victor Horsley performed the first craniotomy for a pituitary tumor in 1889, and Schloffer performed the first transnasal approach in 1907. Cushing began using the transsphenoidal route in 1909 but eventually reverted back to the transcranial route in the late 1920s because he found it more versatile. Guiot[11] repopularized the transsphenoidal route in the mid-1950s, and Hardy[12] introduced the microscope and selective microadenomectomy in 1962.

Epidemiology

Pituitary adenomas represent 10% of all intracranial neoplasms and present clinically in women at a rate of 70 per million and in men at a rate of 28 per million.[13] Pituitary tumors are found in 6% to 22% of adults during unselected autopsies.

Biology

Pituitary adenomas are benign epithelial tumors originating from cells of the adenohypophysis. Certain types of cell lines may predominate, such as corticotrophs (Cushing's disease), somatotrophs (acromegaly), mammotrophs (prolactinoma), or the rare TSH-secreting tumor. These tumors are endocrinologically active and result in the associated clinical syndromes. The number of true null-cell adenomas is shrinking as more tumors are being identified by immmunostaining to contain cells secreting FSH, LH or the α subunit of these glycoproteins. Only 36 cases of true pituitary carcinoma have been reported this century.

The etiology of pituitary adenomas in humans is unknown. Investigators have demonstrated that mammosomatotroph adenomas can be induced in mice by sustained stimulation with GH-releasing hormone (GHRH). Thus it is suggested that continued hormonal stimulation may play a role in tumorigenesis, perhaps by promoting cell replication.[14,15]

Currently, because no known risk factors for pituitary adenomas exist, no prevention is available. Patients with known macroadenomas should avoid pregnancy because adenomas enlarge during pregnancy and may cause impairment of vision.

Pathology

The typical light microscopic picture of a pituitary adenoma is a sea of normal-appearing adenohypophyseal cells with marked loss of the normal acinar stromal pattern. Immunostaining reliably identifies the specific types of secretory cells, and use of electron microscopic evaluation adds information about the size and type of secretory granules, the cellular synthetic activity, and the unique features of adenoma subtypes. Sophisticated molecular biological analysis including in situ hybridization has added another important level to the understanding of the basic biology of pituitary tumors.[16]

Clinical Syndromes

Patients with pituitary adenomas may present with symptoms and signs related to mass effect on the pituitary and its surrounding structures or to hypersecretion of hormones by the tumor. Tumors are generally larger than 1 cm before they produce symptoms related to compression. As a tumor enlarges, it may cause loss of function of the pituitary, usually manifested by a decrease in the secretion of hormones from the adenohypophysis. This may result in a loss of TSH and subsequent hypothyroidism. A decrease in ACTH results in development of Addison's disease, and a decrease in LH and FSH causes amenorrhea. A decline in GH is noted clinically in children only by a decrease in normal growth progress. The one exception to this pattern is that generalized pituitary compression may cause a rise in prolactin because the prolactin-inhibitory factor (i.e., dopamine) from the hypothalamus may be compromised by the compression. Generalized intrasellar compression rarely causes a loss of anti-diuretic hormone (neurohypophyseal) and diabetes insipidus. However, patients with lesions originating in the region of the pituitary stalk often present with early signs of diabetes insipidus. Symptoms related to loss of pituitary function are usually insidious in onset, with the exception of a sudden hemorrhage within the sella, or so called "pituitary apoplexy." Such hemorrhages are usually associated with the presence of a pituitary adenoma.

When mass lesions in the region of the pituitary enlarge, they may also compress or invade nearby structures, causing a number of neurological symptoms. As tumors grow laterally from the sella, they encounter the contents of the cavernous sinus. These include the third, fourth, sixth and first two divisions of the fifth cranial nerves as well as the internal carotid artery. Compression of cranial nerves III, IV, or VI causes diplopia, and compression of cranial nerve V causes ipsilateral facial numbness. Invasion or constriction of the carotid may result in carotid occlusion, which in rare cases may lead to cerebral infarction. Growth of a tumor in the relatively unrestricted upward direction is much more common than lateral or inferior growth and often results in compression of the optic chiasm with resultant loss of vision, typically a bitemporal visual field cut. Extensive upward intracranial growth may result in hypothalamic compression, compression of the third ventricle causing hydrocephalus, or both. Rarely, intracranial extension can result in cortical irritation and associated seizures. Downward growth of tumors into the sphenoid sinus is common and most often causes no clinical symptoms or signs.

The syndromes associated with hypersecretion of pituitary hormones by "functional" pituitary tumors include Cushing's disease (from ACTH hypersecretion), acromegaly (from GH hypersecretion), hyperprolactenemia (from prolactin hypersecretion), and Nelson's syndrome (from ACTH hypersecretion after adrenalectomy). Rare cases of TSH-secreting adenomas have been documented.

Although the diagnosis of Cushing's disease is often reached after physical examination by an astute physician, the physical manifestations are not always obvious, and often the precise cause of hypercortisolism is difficult to ascertain even with detailed endocrine and imaging tests. Patients with Cushing's disease usually have central obesity, hypertension, hirsutism, fatigue, easy bruisability, abdominal stria, "moon" facies, dorsal fat pad, and often depression or other mental changes. Less common abnormalities include headache, osteoporosis, diabetes mellitus, galactorrhea, edema, and amenorrhea. Often a patient presents without the classic "Cushingoid" appearance and only complains of severe fatigue or depression. The etiology of hypercortisolism (Cushing's syndrome) is an ACTH-secreting pituitary adenoma (Cushing's disease) in up to 80% of cases, with the remainder due either to an adrenocortical tumor or an ectoptic neoplasm secreting ACTH, corticotropin releasing factor CRF, or both. Pituitary-dependent hypercortisolism is much more common in women (80%) and an ectopic etiology more common in men (80%).

As with Cushing's syndrome, the diagnosis of acromegaly may be reached clinically when patients present with advanced stages of the disease. However, the obvious enlargement of facial features and acral enlargement may be subtle and the presenting symptoms may be nonspecific headaches, fatigue, arthralgias, decreased libido, or amenorrhea. Patients often have hypertension, diabetes mellitus, and early onset of atherosclerotic cardiovascular disease. It is critical that this disease be diagnosed and treated because the mortality rate is 50% greater than expected in the normal population at each decade over the age of 40 years. With rare exceptions, the cause of acromegaly is a GH-secreting pituitary adenoma. As with other functioning adenomas, the tumors may be very small or large and invasive. Patients with larger tumors may, of course, present with visual loss. Rarely elevated GH levels are secondary to GH-releasing hormone produced by an ectopic tumor.

Because 60% to 70% of prolactin-secreting pituitary adenomas are microadenomas, most patients present with endocrine symptoms as opposed to local mass effects. In women, hyperprolactinemia usually causes amenorrhea and often galactorrhea, and thus young women more often seek early medical evaluation. However, in men, this early warning sign is not available, so they almost invariably present with macroadenomas, usually causing loss of libido, infertility, or loss of vision. It should be kept in mind that the finding of amenorrhea or galactorrhea associated with an elevated prolactin level does not always indicate the presence of a pituitary tumor. Other possible causes of hyperprolactinemia include renal failure, hypothyroidism, or the use of various drugs (Table 13–1). Compression on the pituitary stalk by any type of mass lesion invariably results in the increased secretion of prolactin.

In 1958, Nelson and colleagues[9] identified a syndrome of progressive hyperpigmentation, visual field loss, and amenorrhea associated with elevated ACTH levels related to a functional pituitary adenoma in a patient who had undergone bilateral adrenalectomy for hypercortisolism. Today this syndrome generally represents a missed diagnosis of Cushing's disease that has been treated with adrenalectomy. Often these tumors are aggressive or frankly malignant.

Table 13–1 **Causes of Hyperprolactinemia**

Pituitary disease
Prolactinoma
GH secreting adenoma
Pituitary stalk section
Empty sella syndrome
Hypothalamic disease
Tumors
Sarcoidosis
Irradiation
Hypothyroidism
Chronic renal failure
Hepatic disease
Drugs
Phenothiazines
Tricyclic antidepressants
Estrogen
Opiates
Reserpine
Verapamil
Others
Pregnancy
Stress

Diagnostic Workup

IMAGING

Modern computerized imaging technology now provides us with remarkably detailed multiplanar images of the pituitary and parasellar structures. Magnetic resonance imaging (MRI) has evolved to be the first choice for diagnostic imaging and is often the only test needed to reach a therapeutic decision. MRI, with intravenous infusion of a paramagnetic substance such as gadolinium, demonstrates intrasellar tumors as small as 5 mm in size and shows the growth pattern of larger tumors (Figure 13–1). MRI reveals the extent of suprasellar and sphenoid sinus extension, as well as lateral extension into the cavernous sinuses (Figure 13–2). Cysts and hemorrhage can be differentiated, as can blood flowing within an aneurysm.

Computed tomography (CT) scanning shows calcification better than MRI and therefore is often helpful in imaging a craniopharyngioma. At present, angiography is performed only if an aneurysm is suspected or if a lesion is so large that occlusion or compression of the internal carotid artery is in question. Giant aneurysms can generally be ruled out with high-resolution MRI scanning.

GENERAL ENDOCRINE

The extent of the endocrine evaluation of a patient with a pituitary lesion depends on the urgency of the situation and whether or not a hypersecretion state is suspected. Pituitary endocrine evaluation should include the following baseline values: prolactin, GH, LH, FSH, testosterone (male), estrogen (female), cortisol, ACTH,

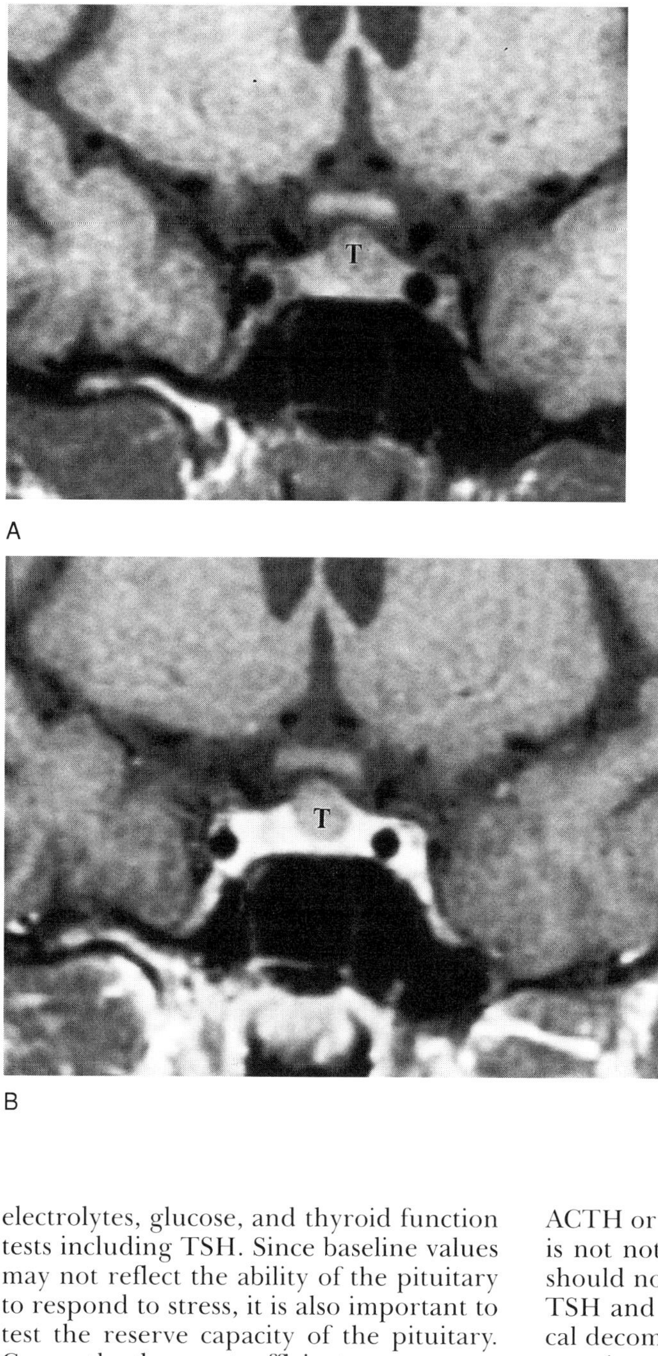

Figure 13–1. Coronal MRI of pituitary microadenoma. *(A)* Nonenhanced MRI showing tumor (T) is nearly isointense with the surrounding pituitary. *(B)* After gadolinium the pituitary enhances and the tumor remains less intense.

electrolytes, glucose, and thyroid function tests including TSH. Since baseline values may not reflect the ability of the pituitary to respond to stress, it is also important to test the reserve capacity of the pituitary. Currently the most efficient way to test this is with insulin-induced hypoglycemia combined with thyrotropin-releasing hormone (TRH). In patients with normal pituitary function, this causes an increase in cortisol level to more than 20 μg/100 mL and an increase in GH level to more than 10 ng/mL. In patients with compromise of ACTH or GH production, such a response is not noted. The administration of TRH should normally cause an increase in both TSH and prolactin levels. If urgent surgical decompression is indicated, the abovementioned baseline values are obtained and the patient is prepared for surgery with sufficient hydrocortisone to cover the possibility of inadequate cortisol reserve. If diabetes insipidus is supected, urine-specific gravity and serum sodium should be checked and a careful evaluation of fluid intake and output done.

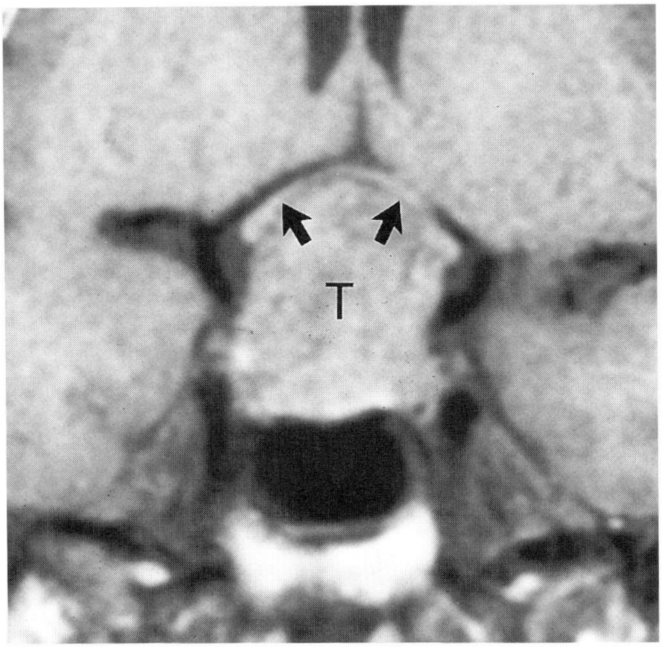

A

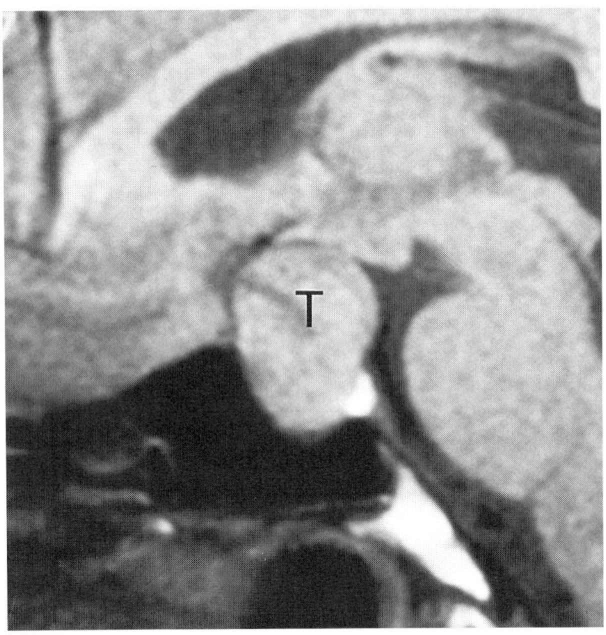

B

Figure 13–2. Nonenhanced MRI of pituitary macroadenoma. *(A)* Coronal view showing suprasellar extension of the tumor (T) with elevation of the optic chiasm (arrows). *(B)* Midsagittal view demonstrating the intrasellar and suprasellar extent of the tumor (T).

CUSHING'S DISEASE

Because up to 60% of patients with a pituitary source of their hypercortisolism have nondiagnostic imaging studies, the diagnosis often relies completely on endocrine testing. Multiple measurements of cortisol and ACTH levels to evaluate the diurnal pattern are important but often misleading. They are mainly of value when clearly elevated.

Urinary-free cortisol in a 24-hour urine collection is an extremely important and reliable measurement because it accurately reflects the hypercortisolemia in patients with Cushing's disease over an entire day. This test is not entirely specific for Cushing's disease: values are elevated in certain cases of depression or alcoholism but are not elevated in those with obesity.

If the overnight screening test for dexamethasone (1 mg at 10 PM) yields cortisol of less than 5 mcg/dl at 8 am, then true hypercortisolism is rarely present. Generally patients with a pituitary etiology of hypercortisolism do not suppress with the low-dose dexamethasone test (0.5 mg q 6 hours × 8 doses) but do suppress with the higher dose (2 mg q 6 hours × 8 doses). There are exceptions, however, with both of these tests. Patients with adrenal or ectopic etiologies classically do not suppress with either dose of dexamethasone. When metyrapone is given, an increase in serum 11-deoxycortisol (or urinary 17-hydroxycortisol) levels is seen in normal individuals and in patients with Cushing's disease. Unfortunately, this increase in 11-deoxycortisol does not absolutely rule out an adrenal or ectopic lesion.

The most specific diagnostic test is measurement of ACTH levels in both inferior petrosal sinuses by transfemoral catheterization along with measurement of simultaneous peripheral blood levels. This provides very convincing evidence for the existence of an ACTH-secreting pituitary tumor and even the laterality of the tumor.[17] Along with this intensive endocrine workup, CT scanning of the adrenal glands and chest should be carried out to look for adrenal or lung tumors.

ACROMEGALY

The endocrine diagnosis rests largely on serum GH levels because 90% of patients have levels greater than 10 ng/mL. Normally, the GH level in a resting nonstressed patient is less than 5 ng/mL, but both normal individuals and patients with acromegaly may have levels between 5 and 10 mg/mL. Somatomedin-C, or insulinlike growth factor 1 (IGF-1), which mediates the effect of GH on peripheral tissues, should also be measured in all situations. When the diagnosis is suspected but consistantly elevated GH levels are not obtained, the glucose suppression test is the most useful diagnostic procedure. In normal patients, the GH level will decrease to well below 5 ng/mL 1 to 2 hours after the oral administration of 100 gm of glucose. This suppression is not seen with GH-secreting adenomas, and often a paradoxical rise in GH is observed. The cause of acromegaly is usually a GH-secreting pituitary adenoma, but rarely elevated GH levels are secondary to GH-releasing hormone produced by an ectopic tumor.

PROLACTINOMAS

A serum prolactin level greater than 200 ng/mL almost invariably indicates the presence of a prolactinoma, but levels lower than this may be caused by micro-prolactinomas. Other etiologies for hyperprolactinemia must be ruled out with levels below 200 ng/mL. The size of pituitary adenomas correlates with the degree of prolactin elevation. No reliable provocative tests exist to differentiate prolactinomas from other causes of hyperprolactinemia.

Differential Diagnosis

The differential diagnosis of intrasellar and parasellar masses is extensive and fortunately includes mainly benign lesions (Table 13–2). Craniopharyngiomas are the next most common parasellar tumor, and although they are usually more suprasellar in location, they may be exclusively intrasellar. They are more common in children, but up to one third occur in adults. They are usually, but not always, cystic and are calcified in 70% of children and 40% in adults. Meningiomas are also generally more suprasellar and enhance very strongly with CT and MRI. Rarely they are exclusively intrasellar and are impossible to differentiate from an adenoma. Germinomas, or "ectopic pinealomas," generally involve the pituitary stalk, and patients who have them usually present with diabetes insipidus. As a general principle, if a patient presents with diabetes insipidus, one should think of a lesion other than a pituitary adenoma. Metastatic malignancies, commonly lung and breast, may be found in the pituitary, with 70%

Table 13–2 **Differential Diagnosis of Intrasellar and Parasellar Lesions**

- Tumors
  - Pituitary adenoma
  - Craniopharyngioma
  - Meningioma
  - Lymphoma
  - Chordoma
  - Granular cell tumor (choristoma)
  - Neuroma (arising from CN V)
  - Metastatic
  - Optic nerve glioma
  - Epidermoid
  - Dermoid
  - Infundibuloma
  - Hypothalamic glioma
- Cysts
  - Rathke's cleft cyst
  - Pituitary cyst
- Inflammatory and granulomatous lesions
  - Bacterial abscess
  - Sarcoidosis
  - Eosinophilic granuloma (histiocytosis-X)
  - Tuberculosis
  - Mycoses
  - Granulomatous hypophysitis
- Aneurysm
- Hamartoma
- Empty sella syndrome
- Pituitary apoplexy

residing in the posterior pituitary. Optic nerve gliomas and hypothalamic gliomas may occasionally be confused with pituitary adenomas, as the rare granular cell tumor (choristoma) can be. Dermoids and epidermoids may occur in an intrasellar location, and fifth nerve neuromas may compress the sella as well.

Rathke's cysts are benign congenital remnants that occur within the sella and can cause headaches and loss of pituitary function by compression. Inflammatory and granulomatous processes, including bacterial abscesses, may occur within the sella. Sarcoidosis may invade the pituitary or its stalk as can the granulomas associated with histiocytosis X. Hamartomas may involve the pituitary stalk and hypothalamus and are impossible to differentiate from invasive gliomas on imaging studies. Aneurysms, usually from the internal carotid arteries, but occasionally from the basilar artery, may appear within the sella and must be ruled out preoperatively with MRI or angiography.

Pituitary apoplexy only rarely causes symptoms but may cause an emergent situation. Infarction or hemorrhage, usually within a pituitary adenoma, causes sudden intrasellar expansion with severe headache and rapid loss of pituitary function resulting in hypotension. Sudden loss of vision may occur, and cranial nerve palsies may develop. Treatment in severe cases involves the administration of steroids and surgical decompression of the sella.

Treatment

The management of pituitary adenomas includes medical treatment, surgery, radiation therapy (RT) and, in some cases, simply following the lesion with serial imaging studies. Since the management is different for each subtype of tumor, these are discussed by subtype.

NONFUNCTIONAL ADENOMAS

Because patients with nonfunctioning adenomas usually present with the effects of a mass lesion, these tumors are rarely microadenomas. No drugs that affect nonfunctioning adenomas are available, so most of these tumors are initially treated surgically, and almost all can be approached transsphenoidally. The goals of surgery include (1) establishment of a diagnosis, (2) decompression of surrounding structures, and (3) attempt at gross total removal of tumor tissue.

The first goal is usually accomplished easily, and although most tumors turn out to be adenomas, surprise diagnostic findings are not unusual. The second goal, decompression, is also usually accomplished readily, since most tumors are soft and easily decompressed. Less than 5% of adenomas are fibrous, making decompression difficult. Evidence for this decompression is demonstrated by the consistent finding that 75% to 80% of patients with visual field loss show recovery after transsphenoidal decompression.[18]

The third goal of total tumor resection is much more difficult to accomplish with macroadenomas. Most macroadenomas (88% to 94%) invade at least the dura, and many have gross invasion of surrounding structures.[19] This invasion makes complete surgical resection impossible; therefore, these patients need to be followed up with indefinitely with high-quality imaging to look for signs of tumor progression or recurrence. Whereas it was common practice in the past to give postoperative radiation to all patients with macroadenomas, with today's high-resolution imaging most patients can be watched for tumor progression, with focal radiation reserved for situations of definite progression.

CUSHING'S DISEASE

After it has been established that the etiology of a patient's hypercortisolism is a pituitary lesion, the treatment of choice is transsphenoidal exploration of the pituitary. No satisfactory long-term medical treatment of Cushing's disease exists (see farther on). Because only 40% to 50% of such patients have positive imaging study results, many of them require a careful systematic exploration of the sellar contents by an experienced pituitary surgeon. Microadenomas secreting ACTH may be very small and are often located deep within the gland itself. If a tumor is not evident upon opening the dura and examining all surfaces of the pituitary, then incisions must be made into the gland and an internal exploration carried out. These tumors are usually in one lateral aspect of the pituitary, and the choice of which side to explore first may be guided by the results of the preoperative petrosal sinus sampling for ACTH levels as described earlier.

If no tumor is identified, then a decision must be made as to whether to resect all or only a portion of the gland. If the endocrine evidence is convincing for a pituitary origin and the patient has no desire to have children, then total hypophysectomy is warranted. If the petrosal sinus sampling clearly indicates laterality of the ACTH secretion, then an appropriate hemi-resection of the gland is carried out.

The author's experience as well as the experience of others has demonstrated that in about 75% of patients explored microadenoma is found to be the source of ACTH secretion.[20] The postoperative remission rate in these patients is 88% to 96%, and the long-term recurrence rate appears to be no more than 5%.[21–24]

Approximately 10% to 20% of patients explored have macroadenomas, and the postoperative remission rates in the patients have been reported to be from 33% to 61%. Many of these patients receive postoperative RT, which provides remission in some of the surgical failures.

Patients who fail to remit with both surgery and radiation require either a surgical adrenalectomy or attempts at medical management of hypercortisolism. In a small percentage of patients who have undergone adrenalectomy, the pituitary tumor continues to grow and secrete ACTH, thus producing Nelson's syndrome. Of the various drugs that have shown some efficacy in suppressing cortisol levels, none has proven effective and reliable in the long run. These drugs suppress ACTH secretion, act primarily on the adrenal gland to suppress the production of cortisol, or act to block cortisol receptors. Drugs that suppress ACTH secretion include cyproheptadine, bromocriptine, sodium valproate, and octreotide. Those that suppress cortisol production include mitotane, metyrapone, ketoconazole, aminoglutethimide, and etomidate. We have little experience with drugs acting to block glucocorticoid receptors, which include RU 486 and nivazol. We occasionally use mitotane and ketoconazole preoperatively or postoperatively to treat patients with highly active Cushing's disease who are awaiting the effects of RT.

ACROMEGALY

Like Cushing's disease, acromegaly is a condition that ultimately threatens the life of the patient. For this reason, it must be treated aggressively, even at the expense of normal pituitary function. Over the past two decades, various medical and surgical therapies, as well as RTs have evolved that have proven effectiveness in lowering GH levels. No one treatment is uniformly effective, and often a combination of treatments is necessary. The goals of treatment are to lower the circulating GH and IGF-1 levels to within a normal range and to reduce the size of a mass lesion that is causing symptoms by compression.

Unfortunately, only 20% to 34% of GH-secreting tumors are microadenomas, thus making microsurgical tumor resection less effective than in Cushing's disease. When a microadenoma is selectively removed transsphenoidally, endocrine remission may be expected in 65% to 90% of cases.[25] When a macroadenoma is resected, immediate postoperative remission is reported in 30% to 79% of cases. The rate of remission is adversely affected by higher preoperative GH levels and larger invasive tumors. Preoperative treatment of macroadenomas with somatostatin analogue may improve postoperative remission rates.[26]

RT has proven moderately effective either as a primary mode of treatment or to augment partial surgical resection. Proton-beam heavy-particle therapy has been used by Kliman and associates[27] in 510 patients, 428 of whom have been followed for between 1 and 20 years. Analysis of these patients reveals that there is a progressive fall in GH levels beginning immediately after treatment and continuing for up to 20 years. At 2 years, 47.5% of patients have a GH level less than 10 ng/mL, and at 4, 10, and 20 years the rate is 65%, 87.5% and 97.5%, respectively. If a GH level of less than 5 ng/mL is considered a "cure," then 75% of patients have been cured at 10 years and 92.5% of patients at 20 years.

Conventional RT provides comparable results (10-year post-treatment levels: <10 ng/mL in 81% and <5 ng/mL in 69%).[28] However, a recent review of our own patients, showed that with an average 6.8 year follow-up, only two of 36 patients radiated (45 to 50 Gy) after surgical failure attained normalization of their IGF-1 levels.[29] The remaining 34 patients had persistently elevated IGF-1 levels (219 $\pm$ 26% of upper normal limit) despite plasma GH levels averaging 4.6 $\pm$ 1.1 μg/L.

Bromocriptine, a dopamine agonist, has been demonstrated to lower GH levels in up to 71% of patients, but unfortunately GH levels of less than 10 ng/mL have been achieved in only 14% of patients. A somatostatin analog has recently been used to treat GH-secreting adenomas and has significantly reduced GH and insulinlike growth factor levels in most patients. This treatment, however, provides only minimal tumor shrinkage, and GH levels increase again immediately after stopping the drug. This drug may prove to be useful as a preoperative treatment or in surgical failures.[26] The recurrence of GH-secreting tumors appears to be only 4% in cases in which surgery normalized the GH and IGF-1 and less than 1% if radiation has normalized these values.

PROLACTINOMAS

Prolactin-secreting adenomas are the most common functioning pituitary tumors, but they remain the most controversial with regard to treatment. The controversy exists because, unlike ACTH- or GH-secreting adenomas, there is a reasonably effective medical treatment available in the form of dopamine agonists.

The goal in treating a patient with a prolactin *macroadenoma* is to decompress the optic pathways and to reduce the prolactin levels to a normal level. Surgery is effective in improving vision in 80% of cases, but vision has also been reported to improve for patients treated with bromocriptine. The ability of surgery to reduce prolactin levels to normal has generally been disappointing. The uniform finding of various investigators is that the ability to normalize prolactin is greatly reduced if the prolactin level is greater than 200 ng/mL or the tumor size is more than 10 mm.

Treatment of macroadenomas with bromocriptine reduces prolactin levels significantly in almost all patients and to normal ranges in more than 46%. In 90% of patients, the size of the tumor is decreased to some degree and dramatically in many (Figure 13–3). If significant tumor regression is not documented after bromocriptine therapy, then surgery should be performed. If a large invasive tumor is encountered and cannot be grossly totally removed, then postoperative RT is recommended.

In a study of a mixture of prolactin-secreting and nonfunctioning macroadenomas, Sheline and colleagues have shown that the recurrence rate is 21% at 10 years after RT plus surgery, 29% with RT alone,

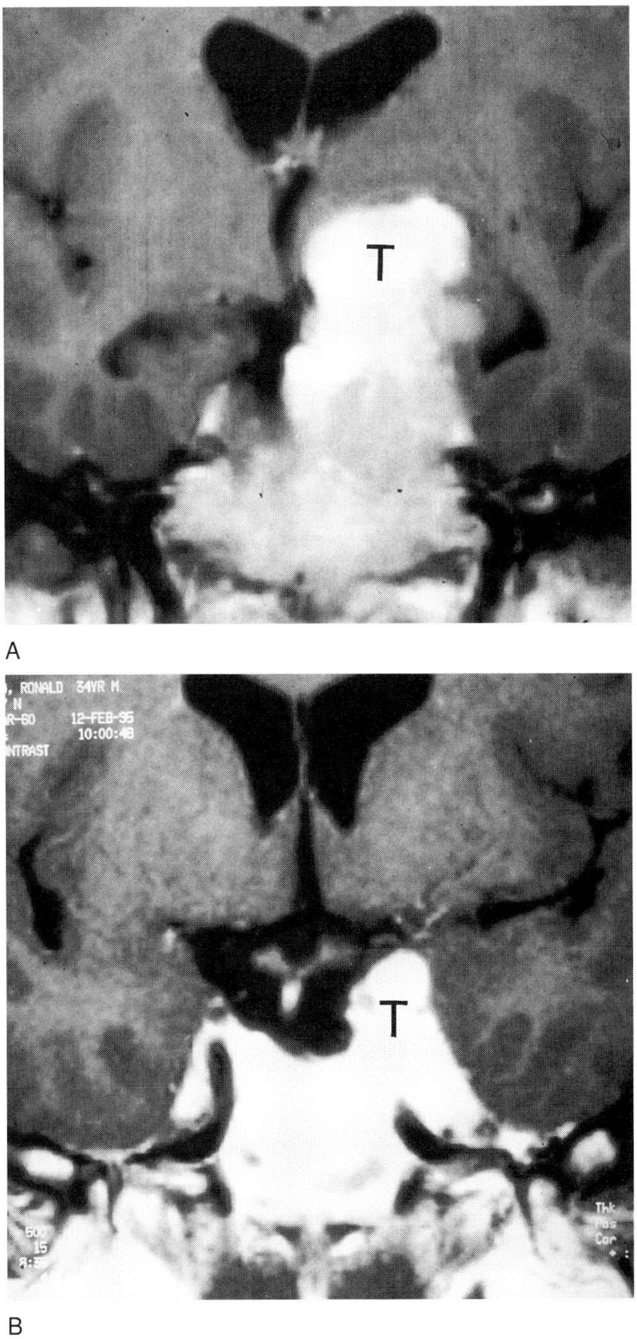

Figure 13–3. Gadolinium-enhanced coronal MRI of macroprolactinoma. *(A)* Massive suprasellar extension of tumor (T). *(B)* Marked reduction in tumor (T) after treatment with bromocriptine for three months.

and 91% with surgery alone.[30] If the tumor is grossly removed but remission not achieved, then bromocriptine is used alone postoperatively. Careful follow-up with CT or MRI scanning is required for the lifetime of the patient because rapid tumor growth may occur. The recurrence rate of macroadenomas is from 25% to 75% by 5 years, so adjunctive therapy is clearly indicated if the postoperative prolactin level begins to increase.

The surgical treatment of prolactin *microadenomas* results in postoperative remission for a much higher percentage of patients. Remission rates range from 50% to 88% with better results when the preoperative prolactin level is less than 100 ng/mL. Primary medical treatment with bromocriptine is also a safe and effective treatment, but the medication may have side effects and may lessen the chance of cure from surgical resection of tumor by causing fibrosis. The recurrence rate for patients initially in remission after microsurgical tumor removal has been somewhat disappointing compared with results in other functioning tumors. Recurrences range from 17% to 24% and have uniformly been found to be higher for patients with postoperative prolactin levels in the upper end of the normal range.[31]

RT does not play a role currently in the treatment of microadenomas unless they recur in an aggressive manner. The author's current approach to prolactin-secreting microadenomas that can be visualized on imaging studies is to explain carefully the medical and surgical options to the patient. Surgery is offered as a primary option because it allows the possibility of long-term remission without continued medical therapy. In the final analysis, patients must make an educated choice between primary medical or surgical treatment.

Prognosis and Complications

Prognosis is related to the size and cell type of the tumor. With nonfunctional macroadenomas, visual field deficits can be improved in 80% of patients with surgery, and in more than 95% of cases the growth of the tumor can be controlled over the lifetime of the patient with a surgical resection and RT as needed.

The prognosis for patients with Cushing's disease is poor unless ACTH and cortisol levels can be normalized. This can be accomplished by pituitary surgery alone in 93% of microadenomas and 50% of macroadenomas.[18] Radiation, adrenalectomy, and/or medical therapy is needed for surgical failures.

The prognosis for patients with acromegaly is likewise grim unless GH and IGF-1 levels can be normalized. This can be accomplished in 85% of microadenomas and 40% of macroadenomas by surgery alone but may be acheivable in patients with a combination of RT and medical treatment.[24]

The prognosis for patients with prolactinomas is generally better than that for those with Cushing's disease or acromegaly because they do not have the systemic problems associated with these conditions. Over 95% of patients with prolactinomas are controlled with the available treatments of bromocriptine, surgery, and RT.

PINEAL REGION TUMORS

History and Nomenclature

Although tumors in the pineal region were recognized as early as the seventeenth and eighteenth centuries, it was Krabbe in 1916 who coined the term "pinealoma" for these tumors. The first operative approaches were performed subtentorially by Horsley in 1910 and Krause in 1913,[32] followed in 1921 by Dandy's posterior transcallosal approach.[33]

The classification and nomenclature of pineal region tumors are complicated and have evolved over the past eight decades. The most significant advance came with the recognition that the most commonly occuring tumors (originally called "pinealomas of the two-cell type") are of germ cell origin rather than from the pineal parenchyma. Thus pineal region tumors are principally divided into either "germ cell tumors" (germinomas, choriocarcinomas, embryonal carcinomas, endodermal sinus tumors, teratomas) or "pinealomas" (pineocytomas, pineoblastomas). The specifics of the current classification are discussed in the pathology section farther on.

Epidemiology

Pineal region tumors represent 0.5% to 1.6% of brain tumors in most areas of the world. However, in Japan, nearly 4% of intracranial tumors are in the pineal region. An increase in germinomas accounts for this disproportionate number of pineal tumors. The various types of tumors in the pineal region are not familial but obviously may have an ethnic preponderance.

Biology

Germ cell tumors occur in young people with a predilection for males (the male-to-female ratio is 2.24: 1). More than 70% of germ cell origin pineal region tumors occur between the ages of 10 and 21 years, with a peak incidence of age 11 years. Choriocarcinomas tend to occur in somewhat younger children (peak age, 8 years), and teratomas have two incidence peaks with most occurring at an average age of 5 but 20% occurring between ages 16 and 18 years.[34] No familial trait for germ cell tumors is known to exist.

Pineal cell tumors present somewhat later than germ cell tumors but still in young adults. The average age of patients with pineocytomas is 32 years; it is age 22 years for pineoblastomas.[35] No familial characteristic for pineal cell tumors is known other than when pineoblastomas occur as part of a childhood syndrome known as "trilateral retinoblastoma." Patients with this syndrome have bilateral retinoblastomas and a pineoblastoma.[36]

Pathology

Pineal region tumors are of germ cell origin 80% of the time and arise from the pineal parenchyma in 20% of instances. Germinomas comprise 65% of the germ cell tumors and are made up of a mixture of large round cells with glycogen-laden cytoplasm and numerous small lymphocytes.[34] Germinomas are histologically indistinguishable from the seminoma of the testicle and the dysgerminoma of the ovary. Nongerminomatous germ cell tumors include teratomas, embryonal carcinomas, endodermal sinus (yolk sac) tumors, and choriocarcinomas.

Teratomas comprise 18% of germ cell tumors and by definition contain cells arising from ectoderm, mesoderm, and endoderm. Teratomas may contain histologically mature tissue such as bone, respiratory, or nervous tissue or may be immature and poorly differentiated. The immature types tend to be more aggressive and potentially malignant. The remaining germ cell tumors (embryonal carcinomas, endodermal sinus [yolk sac] tumors, and choriocarcinomas) are much less common and are generally quite malignant. Together these constitute 17% of germ cell tumors. Many germ cell tumors are a mixture of the various subtypes. For example, the combination of a teratoma and an embryonal cell carcinoma is called a *teratocarcinoma*.

Tumors arising from pineal parenchyma are either pineocytomas or pineoblastomas. Pineocytomas are better differentiated and more benign than pineoblastomas and may show astrocytic or neuronal differentiation. Pineoblastomas are malignant tumors, are usually seen in children or young adults, and are similar histologically to the primitive neuroectodermal tumors such as medulloblastomas, retinoblastomas, and neuroblastomas.

Other tumors that may occur in the pineal region include astrocytomas and other glial tumors, benign pineal cysts, meningiomas, dermoids, epidermoids, metastases, and aneurysms of the vein of Galen.

Clinical Syndromes

Tumors in the pineal region commonly result in hydrocephalus from compression of the aqueduct of Sylvius or from anterior growth with obstruction of the third ventricle itself. Tumors may compress the quadrigeminal plate causing Parinaud's syndrome with loss of upward gaze. Compression of the inferior colliculi may cause hyperacusis and loss of hearing. With larger tumors, invasion of the thalamus and internal capsule may cause hemihypesthesia and hemiparesis. Invasion of the hypothalamus may cause somnolence, weight gain, or temperature fluctuations.

Diagnostic Workup

MRI has rapidly become the imaging study of choice for differentiating lesions in the pineal region (Table 13–3). Solid and cystic tumors can be precisely defined and the degree of hydrocephalus assessed (Figure 13–4). CT scanning may be helpful if the presence of calcification is useful in formulating a treatment plan. Calcification and fat may be present in teratomas, but germinomas and pineocytomas may also be calcified. Gliomas are usually noncalcified, enhancing, and show a variable degree of invasion into brain surrounding the third ventricle. If a vein of Galen aneurysm is suspected, angiography is the definitive diagnostic study. A meningioma is very sharply marginated, strongly enhancing, and usually attached to the tentorial edge.

Table 13–3 **Differential Diagnosis of Pineal Region Lesions**

Tumors
- Pineal parenchyma origin
  - Pineocytoma
  - Pineoblastoma
- Germ cell origin
  - Germinoma
  - Nongerminomatous germ cell tumors
    - Teratoma
    - Embryonal cell carcinoma
    - Teratocarcinoma
    - Endodermal sinus (yolk sac) tumor
    - Choriocarcinoma
- Glioma
- Meningioma
- Metastatic tumor

Cysts
- Benign cyst
- Cystic glioma

Vein of Galen aneurysm

The other mode of prebiopsy diagnosis involves tumor markers. α-Fetoprotein (α-FP) and β-human chorionic gonadotropin (β-HCG) are produced by certain tumors in the pineal region. α-FP is normally produced in the fetal yolk sac and is not measurable in the normal adult blood or cerebrospinal fluid (CSF). β-HCG is normally produced in the placenta and is elevated in the mother's blood during pregnancy.

Germinomas generally are nonsecretory, but they produce low levels of β-HCG up to 10% of the time and rarely α-FP. Choriocarcinomas usually secrete β-HCG and endodermal sinus (i.e., yolk sac) tumors generally secrete α-FP. Most embryonal cell carcinomas produce one or both markers. Pure teratomas usually do not produce a marker. It is important to sample both blood and CSF (when safe) to look for markers because it is impossible to predict which will be more positive in a specific situation.

Overall, tumor markers are more useful as a measure of response to therapy than they are as a diagnostic tool. Only an elevated α-FP (occurring in only 7.5% of pineal tumors) is statistically specific, indicating the presence of either an embryonal cell or an endodermal sinus tumor. The absolute level of the tumor marker is also a prognosticator for survival.[37]

When CSF is sent for marker analysis, it should also be analyzed for cytology because 10% of malignant germ cell tumors have CSF seeding.[35] However, negative CSF cytology results do not rule out the presence of dissemination throughout the central nervous system pathways.

Treatment

Unless very specific tumor markers or positive cytology results are seen, a specific diagnosis must be established; therefore, surgery, either in the form of a stereotactic biopsy or an open procedure, is generally needed as an initial step in

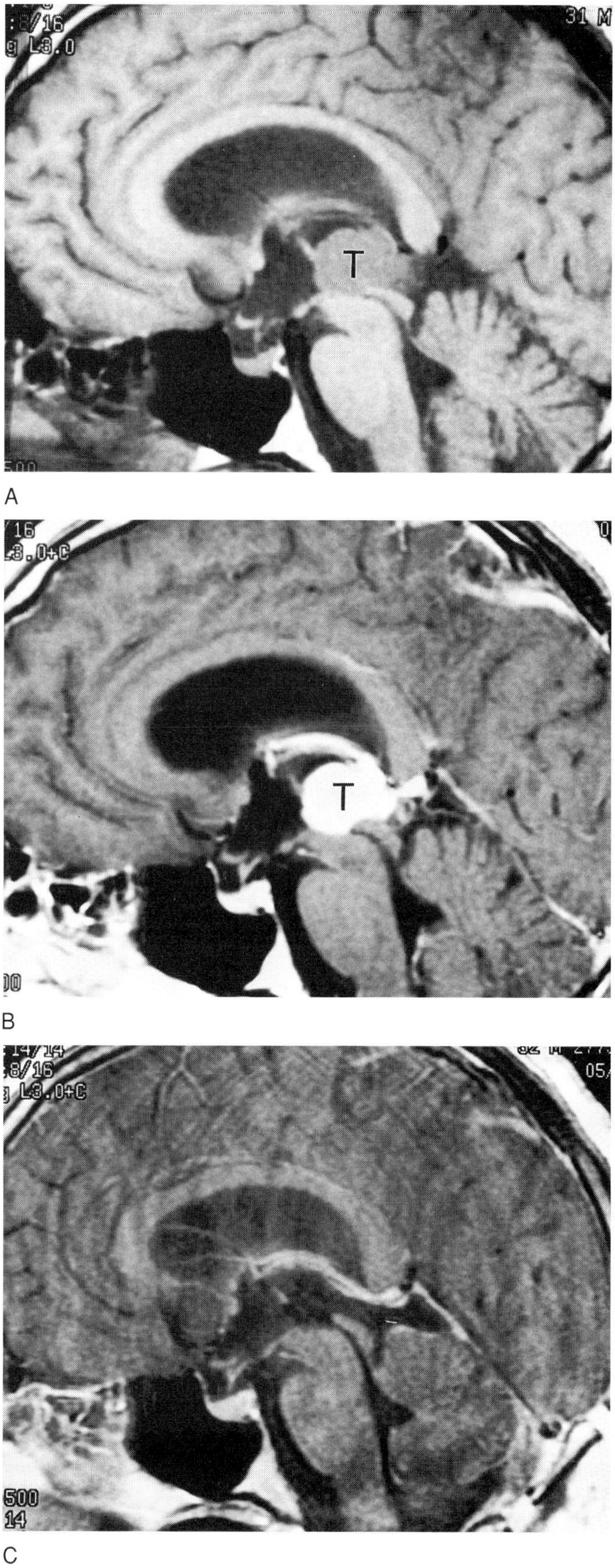

Figure 13–4. Midsagittal MRI of pineocytoma. *(A)* Isointense pineocytoma tumor (T) is noted compressing the cerebral aqueduct. *(B)* Same view after gadolinium demonstrating tumor enhancement (T). *(C)* Same enhanced view after surgical removal of tumor via the subtentorial supracerebellar route.

treatment. RT is usually indicated for malignant or incompletely resected germ cell tumors and for pineal cell tumors. Chemotherapy may be helpful in malignant nongerminomatous germ cell tumors and in recurrent or metastatic germinomas.

SURGERY

Open surgical approaches to the pineal region remain multiple and have evolved and developed over the past 75 years. In 1921, Dandy[31] popularized the parietal interhemispheric transcallosal approach to the pineal region. This has now largely been abandoned because it requires considerable retraction and often results in a visual disconnection syndrome. The posterior fossa supracerebellar subtentorial approach was first described by Krause[38] in 1926 and brought into modern surgical prominence by Stein[39] in 1971. This midline approach for a midline tumor allows a pathway below most of the large venous structures overlying the tumor.

An occipital-transtentorial approach first described by Foerster[32] in 1928 and modified by Poppen[40] in 1966 is satisfactory for tumors with prominent supratentorial extension, but it involves a greater risk of a visual field deficit and makes it difficult for the surgeon to deal with the overlying venous structures.

Although in general an aggressive surgical resection is desirable, a stereotactic biopsy may be the best option in selected cases. The drawbacks of sterotactic biopsy in this area include (1) deep location with the tumor often surrounded by large venous structures, (2) potential sampling error because these are often mixed cell types, and (3) risk of bleeding from a very vascular tumor such as a pineoblastoma. Indications for a stereotactic biopsy include patients with poor medical risk and those with extensive unresectable tumors. Stereotactic biopsy can be carried out with a precoronal or parietal entry using standard techniques.

If hydrocephalus is present, it is often advisable to perform a ventricular shunt procedure before direct surgery on the lesion.

RADIATION THERAPY

Because pineal region germinomas are extremely radiosensitive, external-beam RT offers an important yet controversial role in the treatment of these tumors. On the nonsurgical end of this controversy is an approach that involves a "test dose" of 20 Gy to a pineal region tumor that is consistent with a germinoma on imaging studies. If the tumor shrinks dramatically, then a total of 40 Gy is given to the entire brain with a boost of 15 Gy to the tumor.

The other end of the surgical spectrum is an aggressive direct maximal surgical resection with radiation given only to patients with obvious residual tumor. This approach may be most appropriate in young children in whom RT has greater risk of causing brain injury.

An intermediate approach involves a stereotactic biopsy followed by radiation if a germinoma is confirmed. Spinal radiation is reserved for patients with MRI-confirmed spinal seeding.

All malignant nongerminomatous germ cell tumors should be radiated; all pineoblastomas and most pineocytomas should also be radiated. If a pineal cell tumor is histologically benign and completely excised, RT may be withheld. Again, spinal radiation should be given if there is MRI evidence of seeding. Approximately 10% of pineal tumors seed to the spinal canal.

CHEMOTHERAPY

Because germinomas are so radiosensitive, chemotherapy is generally only used for recurrent or metastatic lesions. Experience is limited, indicating that initial treatment with chemotherapy may allow a reduced dose of radiation to be given effectively. Drugs used to treat germinomas include bleomycin, cisplatin, vinblastine, etoposide, and cyclophosphamide.[37]

Nongerminomatous malignant germ cell tumors should be treated with chemotherapy as well as RT, but the prognosis remains poor. Recently, cisplatin and etoposide have been used in combination rather than the more traditional triad of cisplatin, vinblastine, and bleomycin.[37]

Evidence that chemotherapy plays a role in the treatment of pineal cell tumors is not convincing. Given the poor prognosis of patients with recurrent or disseminated pineal cell tumors, use of a variety of agents, including bleomycin, cisplatin, vinblastine, etoposide and cyclophosphamide, lomustine, methotrexate, and actinomycin D, has been attempted.

Prognosis and Complications

Patients with pineal region germinomas have a 75% to 80% 5-year survival rate and a 69% 10-year survival rate with a combination of surgery and RT. Patients with malignant nongerminomatous germ cell tumors have a much worse prognosis and rarely survive past 2 years. The immature teratomas have a slightly better prognosis at 25% survival for 5 years.

Patients with pineocytomas have a 5-year survival rate of approximately 75%, but the diagnosis of pineoblastoma carries a worse prognosis.

Complications ultimately related to having a pineal region tumors are numerous and may be related to ventricular shunting, surgical biopsy, surgical resection, RT, or chemotherapy. In general, the fewer the treatment modalities and the smaller the area of radiation, the fewer the complications.

REFERENCES

1. Rathke, H: Ueger die Entstehung der Glandula pituitaria. Arch Anat Physiol Wissensch Med 482–485, 1838.
2. Marie, P: Sur deux cas d'acromégalie: hypertrophie sungulière non congénitale des extrémieies supérieures, inferieures et céphalique. Rev Med [Paris] 6:297–333, 1886.
3. Minkowski, O: Ueber einen Fall von Akromegalie. Berl Klin Wochenschr 24:371–374, 1887.
4. Benda, GM: Beiträge zur normalen und pathologischen Histologie der menschlichen Hypophysis cerebri. Berl Klin Wochenschr 36:1205–1210, 1900.
5. Fränkel, A, Stadelmann, E, and Benda, C: Klinische und anatomische Breiträge zur Lehre von der Akromegalie. Dtsch Med Wochenschr 27: 513–517, 1901.
6. Babinski, J: Tumeur du corps pituitaire sans acromégalie et avec arrêt de dévelopement des organes génitaux. Rev Neurol [Paris] 8:531–533, 1900.
7. Fröhlich, A: Ein Fall von Tumor der Hypophysis cerebri ohne Akromegalie. Wein Klin Rundschau 15:883–906, 1901.
8. Cushing, H. The basophil adenomas of the pituitary body and their clinical manifestations [pituitary basophilism]. Bull Johns Hopkins Hosp 50:137–195, 1932.
9. Nelson, DH, Meakin, JW, Dealy, JB, et al: ACTH-producing tumor of the pituitary gland. N Engl J Med 259:161–164, 1958.
10. Forbes, AP, Henneman, PH, Griswold, GC, and Albright, F: Syndrome characterized by galactorrhea, amenorrhea and low urinary FSH: Comparison with acromegaly and normal lactation. J Clin Endocrinol Metab 14:265–271, 1954.
11. Guiot, G, Bouche, J, Hertzog, E, Demailly, P. Deux formes atypiques des adénomes hypophysaires. Indications idéales de la voie d'abord transsphénoidale. Gazette Medicale de France 69:13–33, 1962.
12. Hardy, J. Transsphenoidal microsurgery of the normal and pathological pituitary. Clinical Neurosurgery 16:185–216, 1969.
13. Annegers, JF, Coulam, CB, Abbour, CF, et al: Pituitary adenomas in Olmsted county, Minnesota, 1935–1977. Mayo Clin Proc 53:641–643, 1978.
14. Asa, SL: The role of hypothalamic hormones in the pathogenesis of pituitary adenomas. Path Res Pract 187:581–583, 1991.
15. Faglia, G: Epidemiology and pathogenesis of pituitary adenomas. Acta Endocrinol 129, suppl 1:1–4, 1993.
16. Lloyd, RV: Molecular biological analysis of pituitary disorders. In: Lloyd, RV (ed): Surgical pathology of the pituitary gland. WB Saunders, Philadelphia, 1993, pp 85–93.
17. Oldfield, EH, Chrousos, GP, Schulte, HM, et al: Preoperative lateralization of ACTH-secreting pituitary microadenomas by bilateral and simultaneous inferior petrosal venous sinus sampling. N Engl J Med 312:100–103, 1985.
18. Ebersold, MJ, Quast, LM, Laws, ER, et al: Long-term results in transsphenoidal removal of nonfunctioning pituitary adenomas. J Neurosurg 64: 713–719, 1986.
19. Selman, WR, Laws, ER, Scheithauer, BW, and Carpenter, SM: The occurence of dural invasion in pituitary adenomas. J Neurosurg 64:402–407, 1986.
20. Chandler, WF, Schteingart, DE, Lloyd, RV, and McKeever, PE: Surgical treatment of Cushing's disease. J Neurosurg 66:204–212, 1987.
21. Hardy, J: Cushing's disease: 50 years later. Can J Neurol Sci 9:375–380, 1982.
22. Salassa, RM, Laws, ER, Carpenter, PC, and Northcutt, RC: Cushing's disease: 50 years later. Am Clin Climatol Assoc (transactions) 94:122–129, 1982.
23. Kuwayama, A, and Kageyama, N: Current management of Cushing's disease. Part II. Contemp Neurosurgery 7:1–6, 1985.
24. Boggan, JE, Tyrrell, JB, and Wilson, CB: Transsphenoidal microsurgical management of Cushing's disease. J Neurosurg 59:195–200, 1983.

25. Laws, ER: Neurosurgical management of acromegaly. In: Cooper, PR (ed): Contemporary diagnosis and management of pituitary adenomas. American Association of Neurological Surgeons, Park Ridge, IL, 1991, pp 53–59.
26. Barkan, AL, Lloyd, RV, Chandler, WF, et al: Preoperative treatment of acromegaly with long-acting sondostatin: Shrinkage of invasive pituitary macroadenomas and improved surgical remission rate. J Clin Endocrinol Metab 67:1040–1048, 1988.
27. Kliman, B, Kjellberg, RN, Swisher, B, and Butler, W: Proton beam therapy acromegaly: a 20 year experience. In: Black, PM, Zervas, NT, Ridgeway, EC, and Martin, JB (eds): Secretory Tumors of the Pituitary Gland. Raven Press, New York, 1984, pp 191–211.
28. Bloom, B, and Kramer, S: Conventional radiation therapy in the management of acromegaly. In: Black, PM, Zervas, NT, Ridgeway, EC, and Martin, JB, (eds): Secretory Tumors of the Pituitary Gland. Raven Press, New York, 1984, pp 179–190.
29. Barkan, AL, Halasz, I, Dornfeld, KJ, et al: Pituitary irradiation is ineffective in normalizing plasma insulin-like growth factor I in patients with acromegaly. J Clin Endocrinol Metab 82(10): 3187–191, 1997.
30. Sheline, GE, Grossman, A, Jones, AE, and Besser, GM: Radiation therapy for prolactinomas. In: Black, PM, Zervas, NT, Ridgeway, EC, and Martin, JB (eds): Secretory Tumors of the Pituitary Gland. Raven Press, New York, 1984, pp 93–108.
31. Charpentier, G, dePlunkett, T, Jedynak, P, et al: Surgical treatment of prolactinomas: Short and long term results, prognostic factors. Hormone Res 22:222–227, 1985.
32. Zulch, KJ: Reflections on the surgery of the pineal gland (a glimpse into the past). Neurosurg Rev 4:159–162, 1981.
33. Dandy, WE: An operation for the removal of pineal tumors. Surg Gynecol Obstet 33:112–119, 1921.
34. Jennings, M, Gelman, R, and Hochberg, F: Intracranial germ cell tumors: natural history and pathogenesis. J Neurosurg 63:155–167, 1985.
35. Bruce, JN, Connolly, EZ, and Stein, BM: Pineal cell and germ cell tumors. In: Kaye, AH, and Laws, ER (eds): Brain Tumors, Churchill Livingstone, Edinburgh, 1995, pp 725–755.
36. Bader, JL, Meadows, AT, Zimmerman, LE, et al: Bilateral retinoblastoma with ectopic intracranial retinoblastoma : Trilateral retinoblastoma. Cancer Genet Cytogenics 5:201–213, 1982.
37. Sawaya, R, Hawley, DK, Tobler, WD, et al: Pineal and third ventricle tumors. In: Youmans, JR (ed): Neurological Surgery, WB Saunders, Philadelphia, 1990, pp 3171–3203.
38. Krause, F: Operative freilegung der vierhugel, mebst beobachtungen uber hirndruck und dekompression. Zbl Chir 53:2812–2819, 1926.
39. Stein, MB: The infratentorial supracerebellar approach to pineal lesions. J Neurosurg 35:197–202, 1971.
40. Poppen, JL: The right occipital approach to a pinealoma. J Neurosurg 25:706–710, 1966.

Chapter 14

EXTRA-AXIAL BRAIN TUMORS

ACOUSTIC NEURINOMA

History and Nomenclature

Acoustic neurinomas (i.e., acoustic schwannoma and vestibular schwannoma) are benign posterior fossa tumors of Schwann cell origin. They originate from the vestibular branches of the eighth cranial nerve, most commonly in the internal auditory canal, distal to where Schwann (peripheral) cells have replaced oligodendroglial (central) cells. This transition zone is variable in location and explains why some tumors arise within the internal auditory canal and others within the cerebellopontine angle.[1]

Cruveilhier[2] reported in 1842 the clinical and pathological features of a 26-year-old patient who died from an acoustic neurinoma. Two distinct histological patterns of architecture were described by Antoni[3] in 1920, and Murray and Stout[4] recognized the Schwann cell as the cell of origin in 1940. Surgical approaches to the tumor had a mortality rate of 85% in Henschen's[5] 1910 series. By 1932, with improvements in surgical and anesthetic technique, Cushing[6] reported a mortality rate of 4%. The operating microscope and middle fossa and translabyrinthine surgical approaches have further lowered mortality. As surgical techniques have matured, the priority has shifted to preservation of hearing and other cranial nerve functions.

Epidemiology

A total of 6% to 8% of all intracranial tumors are acoustic neurinomas. They account for more than 75% of the tumors in the cerebellopontine angle.[6] Five percent are bilateral and are almost always associated with neurofibromatosis II (NF2). A total of 2000 to 3000 new tumors are discovered per year in the United States.[7] At autopsy, asymptomatic tumors were identified in 0.8% to 2.7% of cases.[8] The most common decades for presentation of sporadic acoustic neurinomas are the fifth and sixth decades of life.[1] There is a slight female preponderance of cases in most series.

Biology

The most common karyotypic abnormality in acoustic neurinomas is partial or complete monosomy of chromosome 22.[9–16] This has been demonstrated in both sporadic acoustic neurinomas, those associated with NF2, and in sporadic spinal and peripheral neurinomas. Many tumors have normal karyotypes, and others are composed of a mosaic of normal and abnormal cells.[10] Karyotypic abnormalities have also been seen less commonly on chromosomes 6 and 9.[11,14,16]

Molecular genetic analysis of chromosome 22 in sporadic acoustic neurinomas, with restriction fragment-length polymorphism (RFLP) analysis, found loss of part of the chromosome in 44% of 16 cases with informative loci.[17] Other studies have localized the loss of genetic material to the region of chromosome 22 between the CRYB2A and the MB loci.[15] The loss has been attributed to a partial deletion or mitotic recombination.[18]

NF2 is an inherited genetic disease with the clinical marker bilateral acoustic neurinomas. Bilateral acoustic neurinomas are diagnostic of NF2; however, they are not fully penetrant. The disorder is due to a loss of genetic material on chromosome 22 in the region of 22q12 and linked to the marker D22S1.[19] The genetic difference between NF2 and sporadic acoustic neurinomas is that the defect is present in both the tumor and the patient's germ line in NF2 and only in the tumor in the sporadic disease. Whereas in sporadic acoustic neurinomas mutations of both alleles of the NF2 gene must occur in at least a single Schwann cell, in NF2 a single mutation will produce the tumors.

A candidate gene was identified by positional cloning and called *merlin* or *schwannomin*.[20–22] Two independent families had nonoverlapping deletions. The gene encodes a protein of 595 residues and has high homology to the band 4.1 superfamily, a protein family linking cytoskeletal components to the cell membrane.[23] This gene is thought to be a tumor-suppressor gene with the loss of function leading to the development of tumors.

Pathology

Acoustic neurinomas are discrete, firm, encapsulated tumors that press on and distort brain. They arise from the vestibular portion of the eighth nerve at the variable point where glial nerve sheaths are transitioned to Schwann cells and fibroblasts.[1] This usually occurs in the internal auditory canal but may occur in the cerebellopontine angle. Microscopically, the tumor is composed of two different histological patterns called *Antoni A* and *Antoni B* (see Fig. 1–18A and B). Antoni A tissue consists of compact, elongated groups of spindle-shaped cells and their nuclei (see Fig. 1–18A). Antoni B tissue has a less compact and cellular structure with marked lipidization (see Fig. 1–18B). Tumor cells show immunoreactivity for S-100 protein and leu 7 antigen.[24] Vessels are usually hyalinized and surrounded by hemosiderin deposits. Acoustic neurinomas have a grade I biologic behavior, and axons of the parent nerve may be stretched over the tumor rather than entwined within the tumor. Malignant acoustic neurinomas are rare and may occur de novo or after previous surgical resection. The latter is extremely rare. Histologically, the tumor resembles a neurofibrosarcoma,[24] and in the 1993 World Health Organization (WHO) classification is thought more commonly to arise from malignant transformation of a neurofibroma. The biologic behavior is grade III to IV.

Clinical Symptoms

The symptoms of patients with acoustic neurinoma can be categorized into three groups: (1) otologic, (2) focal neurological deficits, and (3) generalized neurological deficits.[25] Unilateral hearing loss is the most common presenting symptom in acoustic neurinomas (98%), with high frequency hearing and speech discrimination most affected.[26,27] The loss of speech discrimination is often more severe than pure tone thresholds would explain, with less than half of patients with acoustic neurinoma having good speech discrimination.[28] Occasionally, patients have sudden hearing loss that may result from compressive occlusion of the internal auditory artery. Less than 5% of patients with acoustic neurinoma have normal hearing. This occurs more often when there is a small tumor in the cerebellopontine angle with no intracanalicular component.[29] Tinnitus (70%) and dysequilibrium (67%) are also common presenting symptoms, with less frequent symptoms of headache (32%), facial numbness (29%), facial weakness (10%), diplopia (10%), otalgia (9%), nausea and vomiting (9%), and change of taste (6%).[25]

The mode of presentation depends on the size of the tumor and whether the early symptom of hearing loss has been minimized. If hearing loss is minimized or not perceived, the patient may go years before developing other symptoms as the tumor grows into the cerebellopontine angle. Unilateral tinnitus may rarely be the only symptom. When it is present alone or with other symptoms, it is usually constant with a wide variety of sounds perceived. Dysequilibrium may be described as dizziness or vertigo. Over the past three decades, with the advent of computed tomography (CT) and magnetic resonance imaging (MRI), the percentage of small tumors diagnosed has increased; therefore, fewer tumors present with focal and generalized neurological symptoms.[27,29]

Differential Diagnosis

Acoustic neurinomas are by far the most common tumor in the cerebellopontine angle, accounting for 78% of the tumors.[6,30] The differential diagnosis of other cerebellopontine angle tumors include meningioma (6%), epidermoid cyst (6%), exophytic glioma (6%), arachnoid cyst, other neurinomas, metastasis, choroid plexus papilloma, glomus jugulare tumor, hemangioblastoma, lymphoma and lipoma, and primary bone tumors.[30–32] Meningiomas can be difficult to distinguish from acoustic neurinomas, but they more typically arise from the arachnoidal cap cells at the anterior or superior lip of the internal auditory canal with resultant facial paralysis and facial numbness or neuralgia more often early in the course. Meningiomas typically are not centered on and do not extend into the internal auditory canal, and they homogeneously enhance. They have a dural tail that is absent in acoustic neurinomas.[33] Neurinomas of the fifth, seventh, ninth, and tenth cranial nerves can also grow to involve the cerebellopontine angle. Facial neurinomas that arise in the region of the internal auditory canal are particularly difficult to distinguish preoperatively. Neurinomas may also arise from branches of the seventh (chorda tympani), ninth (Jacobsen's), or tenth (Arnold's) cranial nerves in the petrous temporal bone.[34]

Diagnostic Workup

The diagnostic evaluation usually begins with a standard audiogram including speech-discrimination testing (Fig. 14–1A). Brainstem auditory evoked responses (BAERs) and acoustic reflex threshold testing are other important diagnostic tests of auditory function. In acoustic neurinomas, BAERs have a 94% to 96% detection rate, an 8% false-positive rate, and a 4% false-negative rate when CT is used as the "gold standard."[8] Recent prospective and retrospective studies have questioned the sensitivity of BAER in the era of MRI diagnosis.[35–37] The typical finding is a delay in the absolute latency of wave V or an increased interval between waves I and V (Fig. 14–1B). The acoustic reflex and its decay are based on the fact that a loud sound causes a reflex contraction of the stapedius muscle.[26] It has a higher percentage of false-positives than BAER.[28] The typical audiometry profile for an acoustic neurinoma is unilateral sensorineural hearing loss with speech discrimination poorer than expected for

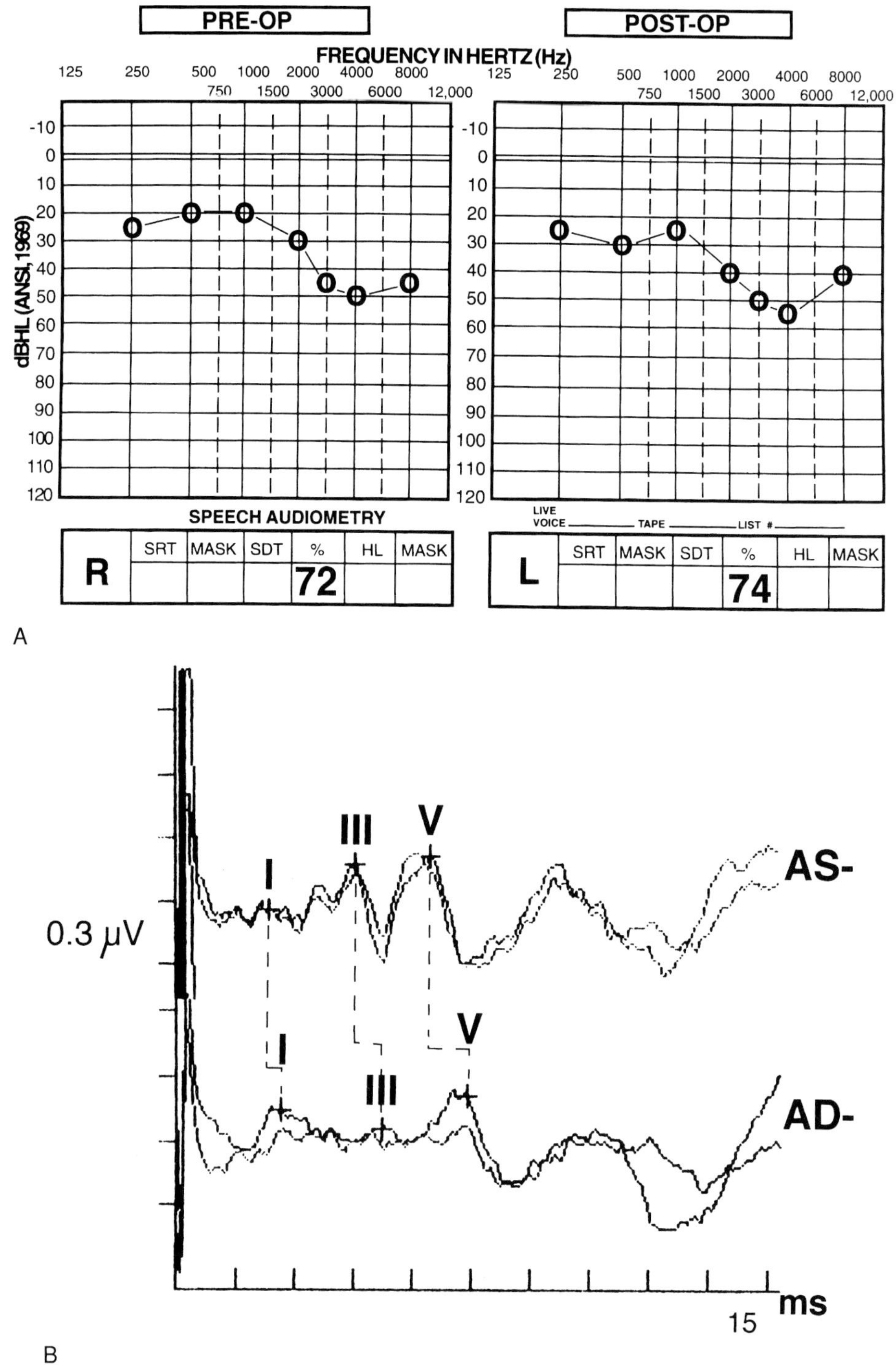

Figure 14–1. A 50-year-old man with progressive hearing loss in the right ear. He denied facial numbness or weakness or difficulty with his balance. Neurologic exam was normal except for decreased finger rub in the right ear. *(A)* Audiogram preoperatively shows moderate high-frequency hearing loss from 3000 to 8000 Hz. Speech discrimination score was 72%. (Courtesy of Paul Kileny, PhD, Department of Otorhinolaryngology, University of Michigan Medical School, Ann Arbor, MI). *(B)* Brainstem auditory evoked response: There was a delay in the absolute latency of wave V (7.38 ms) and an increase in I-V interval (4.74 ms). The patient underwent a suboccipital craniectomy with tumor resection to preserve hearing and a) postoperative hearing is functionally unchanged. (Courtesy of Paul Kileny, PhD, Department of Otorhinolaryngology, University of Michigan Medical School, Ann Arbor, MI).

the pure tone loss, an absent acoustic reflex or positive decay, and a delayed BAER.

MRI is the diagnostic procedure of choice, particularly for the detection of small intracanalicular tumors. However, due to its expense, the National Institutes of Health Consensus Statement did not recommend it as a screening tool; instead, it recommended that MRI should be reserved for patients whose history, examination, and audiometry results are suggestive of tumor.[7] Others think that a single MRI scan is the most cost-effective screening procedure.[38] Acoustic neurinomas are hypointense (66%) or isointense with brain on noncontrast T_1-weighted images. On T_1-weighted MRI, two thirds of these tumors enhance homogeneously and one third heterogeneously with gadolinium. On T_2-weighted images, the tumor is often not visible and isointense with cerebrospinal fluid (CSF) or is hyperintense (Fig. 14–2).[33,39] Gadolinium allows the detection of small lesions of 2 to 3 mm.[40]

Contrast-enhanced CT with 5-mm axial slices through the posterior fossa is also an excellent diagnostic test and is superb for delineation of bone anatomy. To diagnose small intracanalicular tumors, the center of the internal auditory meatus must be included. The most typical appearance is of a hypodense lesion with homogeneous contrast enhancement. Posterior fossa beam hardening artifact arising from the petrous temporal bones limits definition of soft tissue structures.

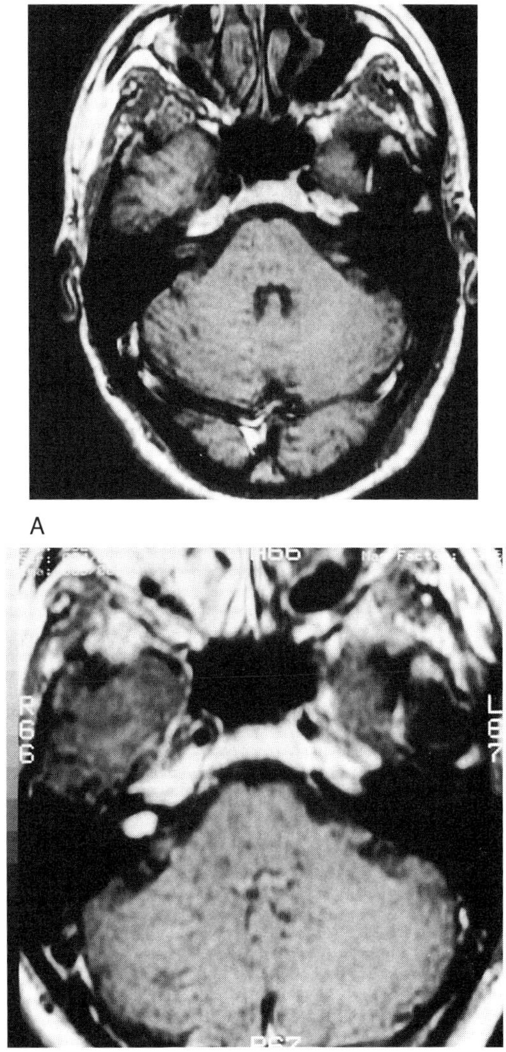

Figure 14–2. Acoustic neurinoma: A 50-year-old man with gradual loss of hearing in the right ear. *(A)* T_1-weighted noncontrast MRI reveals an acoustic neurinoma, less than 1 cm in diameter, that is intracanalicular. *(B)* It enhances homogeneously with gadolinium.

Treatment and Prognosis

Early surgery is the treatment of choice for most patients with an acoustic neurinoma. However, modern imaging techniques have shown that the rate of growth of acoustic neurinomas varies widely. These tumors are usually slow growing, with growth varying from no growth in 40% of patients treated conservatively to less than 2 mm in diameter per year in 78% of patients.[7,41–47] In one study, the growth rate in the first year after diagnosis was predictive of subsequent growth,[43] and in other studies slow or absent growth during the 18 months to 3 years after discovery was predictive of minimal future growth.[42,44]

Slow growth or no growth at all may be reason to follow these tumors when they are small or asymptomatic, when the patient is a poor surgical risk or is elderly, or when, in patients with NF2 bilateral tumors are present and hearing is preserved. Patients younger than 60 tended to present with larger tumors than patients older than 60.[47] The majority of acoustic neuromas are not calcified, but there are rare reports of calcification on CT scanning.[48] Some investigators have found the growth rate to be slower in the elderly, but others have not.[42,49] In a patient with a small or asymptomatic presumed acoustic neurinoma, watchful waiting with careful MRI follow-up at frequent intervals to determine whether the tumor is growing is an acceptable alternative to surgery.

Surgery is the treatment of choice in younger patients and patients with symptomatic tumors larger than 2.5 cm in size. Surgical morbidity and mortality is increased when the tumor is larger than 2.5 cm. Whether to perform a complete or subtotal resection is decided on an individual basis and is based on tumor size and location, patient age and health, preoperative hearing, and facial nerve function. The operative mortality has decreased significantly over the years, with preservation of facial nerve function the primary goal of surgery. Hearing preservation is usually attempted in cases with good preoperative hearing and small (<1.5 cm) tumors. Minimal or no chance exists to preserve hearing in tumors larger than 1.5 cm.[7,50,51]

Normal preoperative BAER and intraoperative BAER monitoring are reported to increase the likelihood of hearing preservation.[52,53] If hearing is preserved postoperatively, the prognosis for functional hearing is improved, but hearing may still deteriorate suddenly.[54] Intraoperative facial nerve electrophysiologic monitoring is a routine part of surgery.[7] The stimulation threshold at the end of the procedure is thought to be a good predictor of long-term function.[55] The size of the tumor is also important: whereas 92% of tumors smaller than 2 cm have preservation of facial nerve function at 1 month postoperatively, only 52% of tumors larger than 3 cm had facial nerve function.

Surgery is generally performed by a combined team of neurosurgeons and otorhinolaryngologists with neurophysiologists performing the electrophysiologic monitoring. Three basic surgical approaches to these cerebellopontine angle tumors are (1) posterior fossa suboccipital craniectomy, (2) translabyrinthine, and (3) subtemporal approach through the middle cranial fossa. Consensus about the best surgical approach for a given tumor is not always achievable. A combination of approaches may be used.

The posterior fossa approach is indicated when tumors are very large and preservation of hearing is desirable. The approach is a standard neurosurgical procedure with cerebellar retraction that provides a large opening and does not destroy the hearing apparatus. In a large series,[56] hearing was preserved in 13.4%, facial nerve function in 86.3%, and gross total resection achieved in greater than 97%.

The translabyrinthine approach destroys the hearing apparatus and is therefore indicated for patients without useful hearing or when preservation is unlikely. This approach involves no cerebellar retraction and permits identification of the facial nerve both proximal and distal to tumor, which enhances the ability to preserve it. House and Hitselberger,[57] studying more than 1600 patients, found more than 86% facial nerve function, 99% gross total removal, and 1.75% mortality.[58]

The middle fossa approach is used for hearing preservation for tumors confined to the internal auditory canal or extending less than 5 mm into the cerebellopontine angle.[59,60] The limitations of this approach are poor posterior fossa access, increased chance of facial nerve injury (because the nerve lies above the tumor), and potential trauma to the temporal lobe. It may be indicated to preserve hearing in an only-hearing ear. Intracapsular subtotal resection may be indicated to preserve hearing for patients with NF2 and bilateral tumors, or in the elderly. After subtotal resection, further tumor growth may not occur. Long-term MRI follow-up is needed after subtotal resection. Postsurgical management should include the availability of facial nerve reconstruction, prosthetic hearing devices, and vestibular rehabilitation.

Radiosurgery has been used as an alternative to surgery in the management of acoustic neurinomas less than 3 cm in diameter. In a series of 20 patients with tumors less than 3 cm, 12 patients had tumor stabilization, and seven had shrinkage. Useful hearing was observed in 100% of patients postoperatively, 50% at 6 months, and 45% at both 1 and 2 years. Facial nerve function was preserved in 90% of patients, and 75% had normal trigeminal nerve function.[61] The tumor control rate has been 91% to 95%, with new or worsened fifth and seventh cranial nerve function of 15% to 23%.[62,63]

Patients with NF2 who have bilateral acoustic neurinomas represent a much more complex management problem; the major treatment objective is to preserve hearing. Most surgeons favor removing the tumor in the poorer-hearing ear first. If hearing is lost after the first operation, the options for the second ear include waiting until hearing is lost, and intracapsular subtotal resection, gross total removal, or stereotactic radiosurgery if the tumor is less than 3 cm. Patients and their families should learn to use sign language as early as possible in their course of disease. Recently, an auditory brainstem implant that electrically stimulates neurons of the cochlear nucleus has been used for rehabilitation of patients with NF2 after bilateral tumor resection with results that compare favorably to those with single-channel cochlear implants.

Chemotherapy has no documented efficacy in the management of patients with acoustic neurinomas.[28]

Complications

The most common complication of acoustic neurinoma surgery other than cranial nerve palsies is CSF leakage from the operative site or middle ear. The usual incidence in most series is 10% to 15%.[39,56,60,64,65] If CSF leakage does occur, additional sutures or lumbar-drain insertion should be attempted initially, but approximately 75% will need re-exploration. Meningitis (5%) may also occur and is related to CSF leakage, communication of the eustachian tube with the operative site, and the long duration of the operation.[62]

Hearing loss may occur permanently secondary to the surgery or be a transient complication. If the hearing loss is permanent, implanted otologic devices may be used to stimulate the cochlear nerve (if it is intact) or possibly the brainstem if the cochlear nerve is damaged.[66,67]

Paralysis of the facial nerve occurs frequently after acoustic neurinoma surgery secondary to surgical trauma. Postoperative exposure keratitis and secondary infection are considerable risks, and treatment should begin with adequate lubrication, shielding by day, and patching the eye at night. Facial nerve repair can be done at the initial operation if the nerve is cut or by hypoglossal facial nerve anastomosis; there is a good outcome in 65% of patients when using either approach.[28] Diplopia may occur secondary to trauma to the sixth nerve or direct injury to the brainstem. The eye can be patched.

MENINGIOMAS

History and Nomenclature

In 1922, Cushing[68] first used the term *meningioma* to describe a tumor originating from the meninges. In 1938, Cushing and Eisenhardt,[69] in a classic monograph, described a classification system for these tumors. In this monograph, meningiomas were classified by their sites of origin. This system is still used today. The common sites of origin and incidence rates are shown in Table 14–1.[69–71] Meningiomas were also divided into nine morphologic types, with seven of these further divided into subtypes. These morphologic subtypes were subsequently found to have no prognostic significance.

The 1993 WHO pathological classification system subdivides meningioma into 11 histological subtypes. The first three subtypes are meningothelial, fibrous, or transitional. These terms refer to the predominant histological background, with transitional a combination of the other two histological subtypes. The other eight histological variants often occur in a background of meningothelial or fibrous cells.[24] This classification system is not

Table 14–1. **Location of Meningioma and Site-Specific Symptoms**

Tumor Location	Relative Incidence (%)	Site-Specific Symptoms
Convexity	34.7	Headaches, seizures, motor and sensory deficits
Parasagittal	22.3	*Anterior:* chronic headaches, memory and behavior changes *Middle:* motor and sensory deficits *Posterior:* homonymous hemianopsia *All:* venous occlusion
Sphenoid ridge	17.1	*Medial:* visual loss, third, fourth, sixth cranial nerve palsies *Lateral:* headaches, seizures, motor and sensory deficits
Lateral ventricle	5.2	Headaches, seizures, hydrocephalus
Tentorium	3.6	Ataxia, headaches, visual loss, diplopia
Cerebellar convexity	4.7	Headaches, ataxia, dizziness, facial pain, dysarthria
Tuberculum sellae	3.6	Visual loss, headaches, optic atrophy, noncongruent homonymous hemianopsia
Optic nerve sheath	2.1	Visual loss
Cerebellopontine angle	2.1	Hearing loss, headaches, ataxia, dizziness, tinnitus, facial palsy
Olfactory groove	3.1	Anosmia, Foster-Kennedy syndrome, headaches
Foramen magnum	0.52	Nuchal and occipital pain, emesis, ataxia, dysphagia, motor and sensory deficits
Clivus	0.5	Headaches, emesis, ataxia, motor and sensory deficits
Other	0.5	—

prognostically significant, and it is used to correctly identify these tumors as meningiomas.

Meningiomas are also classified as benign, atypical, or malignant. Atypical meningiomas have frequent mitoses, increased cellularity, and high nuclear cytoplasmic ratios. Malignant meningiomas possess to a greater degree the histological features of atypical meningioma and have conspicuous necrosis. Some authors think that brain invasion is the most definite characteristic of malignancy, which can be seen without a malignant histological phenotype.[24]

Epidemiology

Meningiomas represent approximately 20% of all symptomatic intracranial tumors.[72] Meningiomas occur at a rate of 7.8 per 100,000 per year, and only 25% of these (or two per 100,000 per year) are symptomatic on presentation.[73] The majority of meningiomas are incidental findings on imaging studies or found at autopsy. The male-to-female ratio was 1 to 1.8 for all meningiomas and 1 to 2.3 for symptomatic meningiomas.[73] The incidence of meningiomas increases with age, reaching its peak at age 85 years. However, in one epidemiological study, the incidence of symptomatic meningiomas remains relatively unchanged between 40 and 90 years of age. Most other studies report a steady increase in incidence rate of meningiomas after age 20.[69–71]

Some reports show that meningiomas may occur intracranially and spinally in association with breast carcinoma.[74,75] Other investigators dispute this association.[76,77]

Biology

Chromosomal abnormalities may be important in the pathogenesis of sporadic meningiomas. Sporadic meningiomas were examined for loss of heterozygosity (LOH) on chromosome 22 in the region of the NF2 gene because of the almost 50% incidence of meningiomas in NF2. Sixty-one percent of patients (14/23) had a LOH in at least one locus on chromosome 22. Somatic abnormalities of the NF2 gene on the long arm of chromosome 22 were seen in 8 tumors.[78] The same locus has been found to have chromosomal abnormalities in sporadic acoustic neurinomas. Chromosomal abnormalities and NF2 gene mutations were seen in meningotheliomatous, fibroblastic, and transitional histological patterns.

Meningiomas express both estrogen and progesterone female sex hormone receptors.[79–84] The expression of the progesterone receptor is seen in a greater percentage of meningiomas than the estrogen receptor, and the percentage of meningioma cells expressing the progesterone receptor is generally greater in any tumor.[79–81,83,84] Progesterone-receptor mRNA staining was nuclear and was functional using transfection techniques.[81] The expression of receptor proteins was not linked to histological type of meningioma.[80,81] The presence of progesterone receptors is the scientific basis for the clinical trial with the antiprogestational agent RU-486.[85]

Meningiomas also express receptors for platelet-derived growth factor (PDGF).[80,81,86,87] PDGF receptor (PDGFR) type BB was found in 100% of meningiomas in one study, and 95% of these tumors were PDGF positive.[80] Conditioned medium from meningiomas grown in vitro contained proteins related to the B chain of PGDF and stimulated the proliferation of meningioma cells. This was blocked by a neutralizing antibody against PDGFR-BB.[86,87] In one study, statistical analysis showed an inverse correlation between progesterone-receptor staining and features of malignancy.[88] Epidermal growth factor receptor (EGFR) has been discovered in nearly 100% of meningioma specimens in tissue culture, with increased meningioma DNA synthesis after exogenous epidermal growth factor (EGF) is added.[89–91] A high incidence of somatostatin receptors has also been found, the significance of which is unknown.[91]

The etiology of the majority of meningiomas is unknown. Radiation is the only definite causative factor, with an increased incidence of meningiomas in children radiated with as little as 10 Gy for tinea capitis.[92,93] Moderate radiation doses between 10 and 20 Gy, large doses greater than 20 Gy, and most often those greater than 40 Gy also produce an increased rate of meningiomas.[93,94] In 10 patients, most treated with more than 40 Gy, the median time to meningioma development was 20 years after the radiation.[94] Little prospective evidence exists to indicate that head trauma plays an etiologic role in the development of meningiomas. In a prospective study of nearly 3000 patients with head injury, no increased incidence was found.[95]

Multiple meningiomas are uncommon, representing 1.1% of all meningiomas.[96] Multiple meningiomas from each of four patients were studied with polymerase chain reaction for X-chromosome inactivation to determine if the multiple tumors of each patient came from the same clonal population. In each patient, the same X chromosome was inactivated, suggesting that the tumors originated from a single progenitor cell.[97]

Pathology

Meningiomas originate from the arachnoidal cap cell, a meningothelial cell in the arachnoidal membrane. They generally arise in areas where arachnoidal villi are numerous.[24] Meningiomas are classified as benign, atypical, or malignant. Benign meningiomas are not encapsulated and grow invaginating but remaining demarcated from brain. They grow with fingerlike projections and penetrate surrounding mesenchymal tissue, including bone. They may produce both an osteoblastic and lytic reaction.[24] Meningiomas immunostain with vimentin, desmoplakin, and epithelial membrane antigen. They have a grade 1 biologic behavior. Meningiomas grow in three primary histological patterns: (1) meningothelial, (2) fibroblastic, or (3) transitional (a combination of meningothelial and fibrous). Meningothelial meningiomas consist of lobules of cells with oval pale nuclei, with chromatin marginated around the nucleus. The cell has an ill-defined cellular membrane, and nuclear and cytoplasmic invaginations often produce pseudoinclusions (see Fig. 1–19A).[24] Fibroblastic meningiomas have parallel interlacing bundles of spindle shaped cells with abundant collagen and reticulin between cells (see Fig. 1–19B). Whorl formation and psammoma bodies are infrequent in these two histological pattern types. Transitional meningiomas have a mixed pattern of both meningothelial and fibroblastic features. They more often contain whorls or psammoma bodies. The other eight meningioma subtypes are psammomatous (see Fig. 1–19C), angiomatous, microcystic, secretory, clear cell, chordoid, lymphoplasmacyte-rich, and metaplastic. The prognosis is independent of histology.

Atypical meningiomas have several of the features of malignancy, including frequent mitoses, increased cellularity, increased nuclear-to-cytoplasmic ratio or prominent nucleoli, sheetlike growth, and geographic necrosis. Nuclear atypia or invasion of bone alone does not meet the criteria for atypical meningioma. The biologic behavior is grade II. Malignant meningiomas have further increases in mitoses and cellularity with conspicuous necrosis. Some pathologists think that a meningioma should be called malignant only when there is frank brain invasion. The biologic behavior is grade III.[24] Atypical and malignant meningiomas have a much higher recurrence rate after resection than do benign meningiomas. Recurrence rates were 6.9% for benign meningiomas, 34.6% for atypical meningiomas, and 72.7% for malignant meningiomas.[98]

Papillary meningiomas have a histological pattern of meningioma that is associated with a more aggressive behavior with frequent recurrence after resection, brain invasion, and metastases. They have a grade II or III biologic behavior.[24] The cells resemble meningothelial cells. Their cell processes terminate in papilla on blood vessels with tapering of their processes to form pseudorosettes. Hemangiopericytoma is an aggressive mesenchymally derived tumor with oval nuclei that have scant cytoplasm. There is dense intercellular reticulin staining. Tumor cells can be fibroblastic, myxoid, or pericytic. These tumors, in contrast to meningiomas, do not stain with epithelial membrane antigen. They have a grade II or III biologic behavior and need to be distinguished from benign meningiomas because of their high rate of recurrence (68.2%) and metastases.[24,98]

Meningioma mitotic labeling index has been measured with bromodeoxyuridine (BUdR), Ki-67, MIB1, and silver colloid nucleolar organizer region.[86,99–101] In all of these studies, lower labeling activity has been associated with a decreased risk of recurrence.

Clinical Symptoms

The clinical symptoms of a meningioma are determined by its anatomic site (see Table 14–1). A total of 85% to 90% of meningiomas are located supratentorially. Meningiomas are rare in children; when they do occur, they are more often aggressive and located in the posterior fossa or intraventricularly. The most common presenting symptoms for meningiomas are headache (36%), change in mental status (21%), and paresis (22%). The most common exam results are paresis (33%), normal examination (27%), and memory impairment (16.5%).[70] The site-specific symptoms are of much greater significance and are shown in Table 14–1.

Parasagittal meningiomas can occur anywhere along the anterior or posterior course of the falx, with symptoms dependent on the location. Anterior parasagittal tumors produce headaches, memory loss, and personality changes. Tumors located in the middle of the falx produce motor and sensory deficit, and those located posteriorly produce homonymous hemianopsia. Anterior tumors may obstruct CSF outflow at the foramen of Monro, and obstruction of the sagittal sinus by posterior tumors can produce a sagittal sinus syndrome. The symptoms of sphenoid ridge meningiomas depend on the medial to lateral location along the sphenoid ridge. The medial tumors originate from near the anterior clinoid process with unilateral visual loss early, and they invade the cavernous sinus with attendant cranial nerve deficits. The lateral tumors displace the frontal and temporal lobes while growing in the Sylvian fissure and produce headache, seizures, and motor and speech deficits.

In one large series,[70] malignant meningiomas were located exclusively in the convexity, parasagittal, or tuberculum sellae locations.

Differential Diagnosis

The differential diagnosis depends entirely on the suspected anatomic location of the meningioma. No single symptom is diagnostic of a meningioma. Benign meningiomas grow very slowly over years and produce symptoms when they encroach on critical structures. These symptoms evolve gradually in contrast to the typical rapid symptom development in anaplastic astrocytoma, anaplastic oligodendroglioma, glioblastoma multiforme, metastases, primary central nervous system lymphoma, and medulloblastoma. Malignant meningiomas, which represent approximately 10% of meningiomas, may have a more rapid symptom development.

Diagnostic Workup

The diagnostic procedure of choice for meningioma is a gadolinium-enhanced MRI scan. On T_1-weighted images prior to gadolinium enhancement, 65% of tumors were isointense and 35% hypointense when compared with gray matter of brain.[102] On T_2-weighted images, 47% were isointense with gray matter, 35% hyperintense, and 18% hypointense. In one series,[102] fibroblastic and transitional meningiomas were found more often to be hypointense, and meningothelial and angioblastic meningiomas were hyperintense relative to brain gray matter. On T_1-weighted images with gadolinium enhancement, these tumors typically enhance diffusely and homogeneously (Fig. 14–3). The dural tail of a meningioma can be visualized and can be used to guide the surgeon in extent of resection. MRI also provides the ability to image vascular and neural distortion and invasion of blood vessels, particularly in the optic nerve, tuberculum sellae, and medial sphenoid ridge, and this may guide the neurosurgeon (Fig. 14–4). Postoperatively, MRI is useful to monitor for residual tumor requiring either further monitoring or additional treatment.[103]

CT scans can show all but the smallest meningiomas, and they are particularly useful to document the extent of bony involvement. Before contrast administration, the tumor is hypodense to slightly hyperdense compared with brain gray matter. Calcification is present in 29% of benign meningiomas and rarely present in malignant meningiomas.[70] Calcification can vary from punctate areas to dense calcification of the whole tumor. Homogeneous contrast enhancement occurs in 72% of benign and 36% of malignant meningiomas. Benign and malignant meningiomas can both have peritumoral edema, but it is more common and most often greater in extent in malignant meningiomas.[70]

Magnetic resonance angiography has largely replaced arterial angiography and has the ability to detect the patency of venous sinuses. In large tumors that may be

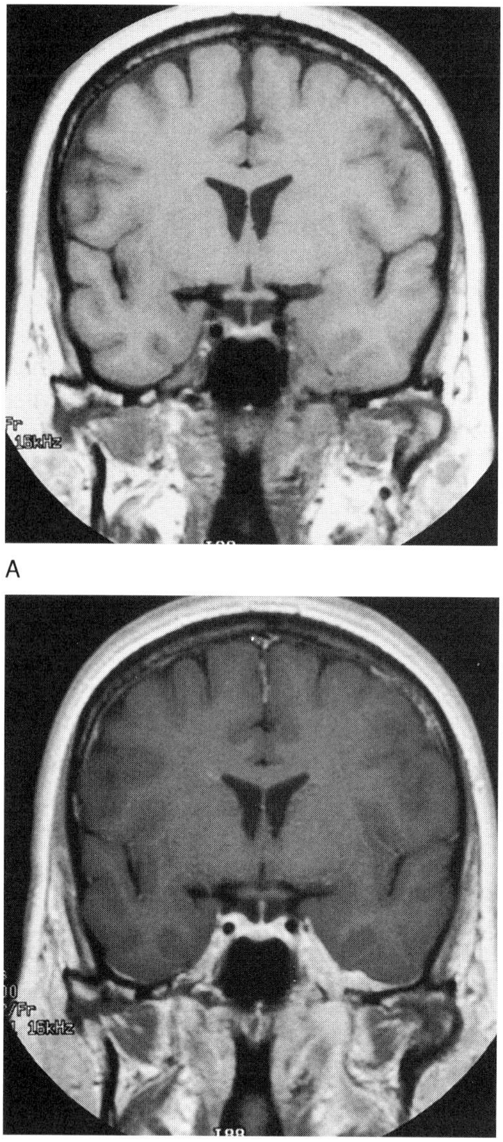

A

B

Figure 14–3. A 52-year-old woman with a long history of headaches that are increasing in severity and more constant in the left face and retro-orbital region. Neurologic exam is normal. T_1-weighted MRI prior to gadolinium shows *(A)* a mass medial to the temporal lobe extending medially to the cavernous sinus. *(B)* Postgadolinium, it extends inferiorly and medially to the left internal carotid artery and encases it (not shown). It extends laterally enplaque inferior to the temporal lobe. It was felt to be a meningioma on the basis of its imaging characteristics and not surgically resectable. Radiation therapy was recommended.

candidates for preoperative embolization, arterial angiography is necessary for delineation of the tumor blood supply. Tumor embolization may reduce vascularity and decrease operative bleeding.

Treatment

ASYMPTOMATIC TUMORS

In a recent epidemiologic study, only 25% of meningiomas were symptomatic. A total of 75% of the meningiomas were found incidentally on imaging study or at postmortem.[73] Asymptomatic meningiomas averaging 2.15 cm (range, 0.5 to 5.0 cm) were followed for an average of 32 months, and none of 57 patients became symptomatic during the follow-up period. Forty-five patients had follow-up imaging studies, and 35 of these patients showed no growth with an average follow-up of 29 months. Ten patients showed growth ranging from 0.2 cm over 15 years to 1 cm over 12 months, with an average growth of 0.24 cm per year. The authors concluded that patients with asymptomatic meningiomas can be followed with noninvasive imaging studies at intervals and only require operation if there is significant growth or the patient becomes symptomatic or is likely to become symptomatic.[104]

SURGERY

Surgery is the treatment of choice for symptomatic meningiomas. Preoperative management includes the administration of anticonvulsants and dexamethasone. If significant brain edema is present, dexamethasone should be given for 1 to 2 weeks before surgery. The primary aim is gross total resection, with improvement or preservation of neurological function. At the time of initial surgery, a layer of arachnoid membrane separates the tumor from the brain parenchyma, cranial nerves, and blood vessels. When the neurosurgeon stays within that plane during the resection, the chances of damage to neural and vascular structures are reduced.[72] Debulking the tumor from the inside often allows

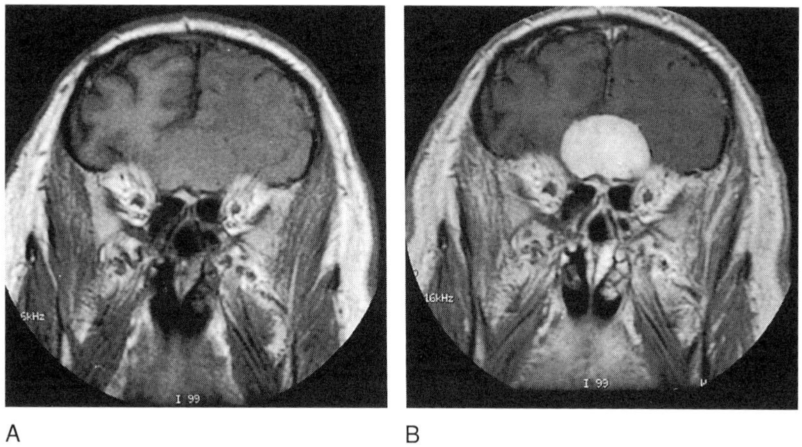

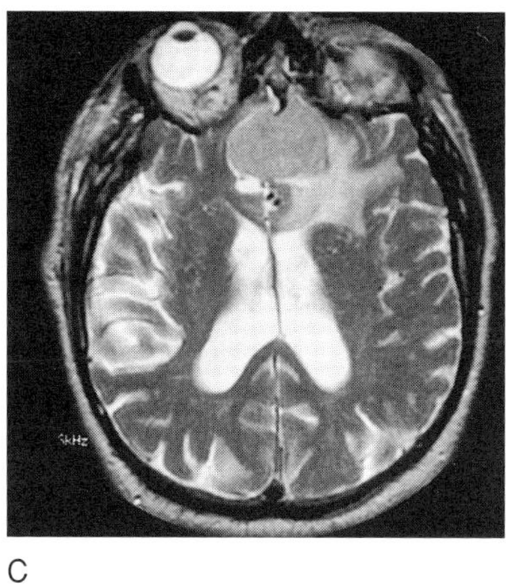

Figure 14–4. A 78-year-old man with asymptomatic subfrontal meningioma. After 3–4 years he developed slight difficulty walking, greater with the right leg. *(A)* Coronal T_1-weighted MRI shows an isointense bilateral subfrontal mass that *(B)* enhances homogeneously and diffusely with gadolinium. *(C)* Axial T_2-weighted MRI shows a mildly hyperintense mass with significant hyperintense signal extending into the white matter of the left frontal lobe.

collapse of the tumor with continued visualization of the arachnoidal membrane. After meningioma removal, the involved dura and bone must be removed. CT scans with bone windows will allow imaging of hyperostotic bone that should be removed.[72] Tuberculum sellae meningiomas are difficult to remove because the tumor stretches the optic nerves, and distinction between tumor and optic nerves is obscured. These tumors may involve both optic nerves. Medial sphenoid ridge meningiomas (i.e., parasellar) are difficult to remove completely because they invade the cavernous sinus or extend along the clivus. Parasagittal meningiomas often cannot be removed completely when they invade the sagittal sinus posteriorly.

The recurrence rate for meningiomas is dependent on the length of follow-up. Recurrence rates in one series were reported at 5% at 5 years, 10% at 10 years, and 32% at 15 years.[105] Progression of disease after subtotal resection at 5, 10, and 15 years was 37%, 55%, and 91%, respectively.

EXTERNAL-BEAM RADIATION THERAPY

External-beam radiation therapy (RT) has been used for the treatment of meningiomas when only a subtotal resection can be performed. The median treatment dose was 54 Gy for both benign and malignant meningiomas, with the upper end of the dose range to 59 Gy for benign meningiomas and 69 Gy for malignant meningiomas. The 5-year progression-free survival rate for patients with benign meningiomas was 98% when CT or MRI was used for treatment planning. The 5-year progression-free survival rate for malignant meningiomas was slightly less than 50%. Morbidity was 3.6% with two patients developing cerebral radiation necrosis and three patients developing visual loss.[106] In optic nerve, tuberculum sellae, and medial sphenoid ridge meningiomas, the risk of damage to optic nerves is greater after RT because of their proximity to the radiated field. In another series[107] following subtotal resection, irradiated patients had a 32% progression rate versus 60% in nonirradiated patients. The median time to recurrence in the irradiated group was 125 months versus 66 months in the nonirradiated group. The 10-year survival rate of patients with 38 inoperable meningiomas after RT was 46%, with 38% of patients having an improvement in neurological performance.[108] After gross total resection, patients with malignant meningiomas should also be considered for RT. Patients with recurrent benign meningiomas should be considered for RT on recurrence or after reresection.[109,110] Patients with benign meningiomas who received RT after reresection had a local control rate of 89% versus 30% with surgery alone.[110]

STEREOTACTIC RADIOSURGERY

The role of stereotactic radiosurgery and the dose to be used in the treatment of meningiomas is evolving. Fifty patients were treated for 52 meningiomas after failure of previous surgery (n=36) or at presentation with symptomatic meningiomas (n=16).[111] For tumors in the region of the optic pathways, the optic nerve dose was less than 9 Gy. The actuarial tumor control rate at 24 months was 96%. None of the 16 patients treated initially with stereotactic radiosurgery have progressed, but follow-up time is limited. In the 24 patients with a 1- to 3-year follow-up period, 54% of patients had a decrease in tumor size and 38% were stable. In the two patients with tumor growth, the growth was outside the treated field.[111] Three patients developed temporary new focal neurological deficits (n=2) or cranial nerve palsies (n=2) 3 to 12 months after radiosurgery with subsequent improvement of the neurological deficits. A larger group of 94 patients with benign meningiomas had a 4-year tumor-control rate of 92%.[112] In a series of recurrent cavernous sinus meningiomas, tumor control was obtained in all 34 patients with 56% of patients having tumor shrinkage. The median follow-up period was 26 months.[113] The exact role of this treatment modality will be decided with future studies.

INTERSTITIAL BRACHYTHERAPY

Thirteen base-of-skull meningiomas were initially treated with high-activity iodine-125 seeds with nine of 11 patients without calcification having a complete response and the two with calcification a partial response.[114] How these results compare with stereotactic radiosurgery or with new base of skull surgery techniques has not been determined.

CHEMOTHERAPY

Chemotherapy has no role in the initial treatment of benign meningiomas. Hydroxyurea (20 mg/kg/d) has been reported to produce dramatic slow MRI cytoreduction in four patients with recurrent benign to malignant meningiomas after prior surgical and RT failure. This agent was used clinically after experimental data showed that hydroxyurea inhibited growth of meningioma cells in culture and in nude mice implanted with meningioma.[115] Multiagent cyclophosphamide, adriamycin, and vincristine has been used adjuvantly in the treatment of malignant meningiomas after surgery and RT. The median time to tumor progression was 4.6 years, with two patients having radiographic responses on MRI when compared with their prechemotherapy scans. The role of chemotherapy in the treatment of malignant meningioma is still to be defined.[116]

HORMONAL THERAPY

Tamoxifen (40 mg/m^2 twice daily for 4 days and then 10 mg twice daily), an antiestrogen, was used to treat 19 patients with unresectable or refractory meningiomas with progression in 10 patients, temporary disease stabilization in six, and minor response in three.[117]

The antiprogestational agent RU-486 (200 mg daily) has been used to treat recurrent benign meningiomas after failure of surgery and RT. Five of 14 patients treated with long-term RU-486 had tumor regression (amount not specified), and three had disease progression.[85] Three patients had symptomatic improvement. A double-blind, placebo-controlled trial is in progress.

IMMUNOTHERAPY

Six recurrent, unresectable, malignant meningiomas were treated with interferon-α-2b subcutaneously continuously for 5 days a week, with four patients having disease stabilization and one partial response for 6 to 14 months.[118]

Prognosis and Complications

The prognosis for meningiomas after gross total resection depends on the histology. In a single series of 1799 meningioma specimens from 1582 patients followed for an estimated average of 13 years, 93.1% of benign meningiomas, 65.4% of atypical meningiomas, and 27.3% of malignant meningiomas were cured by surgery.[98] A study from Finland[119] found the recurrence rate for benign meningiomas to be higher, with 19% recurring at 20 years. After subtotal resection of meningioma, RT decreases recurrence rate from 60% with surgery alone to 32% with RT, with a longer time to recurrence in the radiated group.[107]

Metastasis from meningioma is uncommon. Benign meningiomas have very rarely been reported to metastasize to the lungs and other organs.[120] Malignant meningiomas metastasize rarely, but more commonly, the lungs are the most common site followed by the abdominal viscera, bones, and lymph nodes.[121] Breast, lung, squamous cell carcinomas, and lymphoma metastasize to meningioma.[122]

SKULL-BASE TUMORS

Skull-base tumors are benign and malignant tumors of the cranial base. They arise intradurally (i.e., acoustic neurinoma, meningioma), extradurally above the cranial base (i.e., pituitary adenoma, esthesioneuroblastoma), in the basicranium itself (i.e., chordoma, chondrosarcoma), or below the cranium originating in the paranasal sinuses, infratemporal fossa, parapharyngeal spaces, and middle ear (i.e., squamous cell carcinoma, adenoid cystic carcinoma, nasopharyngeal carcinoma, angiofibroma, glomus tumors).[123,124]

The skull base is an anatomically complex region with the spinal cord, arteries, and veins supplying the brain and virtually all cranial nerves exiting through the area.[123,125,126] In the past, the removal of benign and malignant tumors at the base of the brain was limited by surgical access and a high risk of neurological damage. Two important advances in skull-base surgery have been the development of interdisciplinary surgical approaches and improved radiological techniques. The multidisciplinary team involves neurosurgery, otolaryngology or head and neck surgery, plastic or reconstructive surgery, neuroradiology, neurophysiology, and neuroanesthesiology. Accurate determination of the extent of the tumor with the use of CT (including bone windows) and MRI scans allows preoperative surgical planning.[123,125,126] Three-dimensional frameless stereotaxy with the use of thin slices provide elegant three-dimensional anatomy. The imaging data is then correlated with the operative approach with fiducial markers placed on the scalp or natural bony landmarks. After the data has been correlated with operative head position, a series of images can be generated for a simulated approach and localization during surgery.[127,128]

This technology is particularly appropriate for skull-base surgery because tumors attached to bony structures do not move significantly during the operation. Intraoperatively, this system aids the surgeon in localizing tumor, finding small pockets of residual tumor, and locating critical neural and vascular structures in the operative field. New anesthetics, air drills, the operating microscope, surgical lasers, and electrophysiologic monitoring of cranial nerves have all made surgery safer in the past 15 years. Postoperative rehabilitation of speech and swallowing has become more sophisticated. RT and chemotherapy have produced better control of residual malignant skull-base tumors and uncontrolled or recurrent benign tumors.[123,126]

Anatomically, the skull base includes the frontal bone, ethmoid bone, rostrum, lesser and greater wings of the sphenoid, petrous, and tympanic portions of the temporal bone (excluding the squama), clivus, dorsum sella, and the occipital bone to the midline (Fig. 14–5).[129,130] The intracranial surface of the skull base is divided into the anterior, middle, and posterior cranial fossa.[129] A bicoronal scalp incision is used to access the anterior cranial base. This may be extended to the preauricular regions or the neck (Fig. 14–6). A bifrontal craniotomy is then used to gain access to the anterior cranial fossa. The anterior cranial fossa is formed by the frontal, ethmoid, and sphenoid bones (Fig. 14–7). Extracranially, it is neighbored inferiorly by the paranasal sinuses. Most neoplasms in the anterior cranial fossa are paranasal sinus tumors. The olfactory nerves pass through the cribriform plate, and the optic nerve foramina form the posterior border of the anterior cranial fossa.

The middle cranial fossa is formed by the body of the sphenoid bone and the squamous and petrous parts of the temporal bone. The middle fossa is most often approached extradurally from the infratemporal fossa. The extent of the surgical incision is determined by the anatomic area to be approached. For tumors involving the infralabyrinth and apical components of the temporal bone, a lateral approach through the petrous temporal bone is performed with the incision inferior and surrounding the lower ear ("type A"). For tumors involving the clivus, the incision is carried anteriorly and superiorly to the temporal bone and a temporal or frontotemporal craniotomy is performed ("type B"). The sellar or parasellar and infratemporal region is operated on through a wider incision with removal of the zygomatic arch and the lateral orbital rim ("type C") (Fig. 14–8).[123,131] These

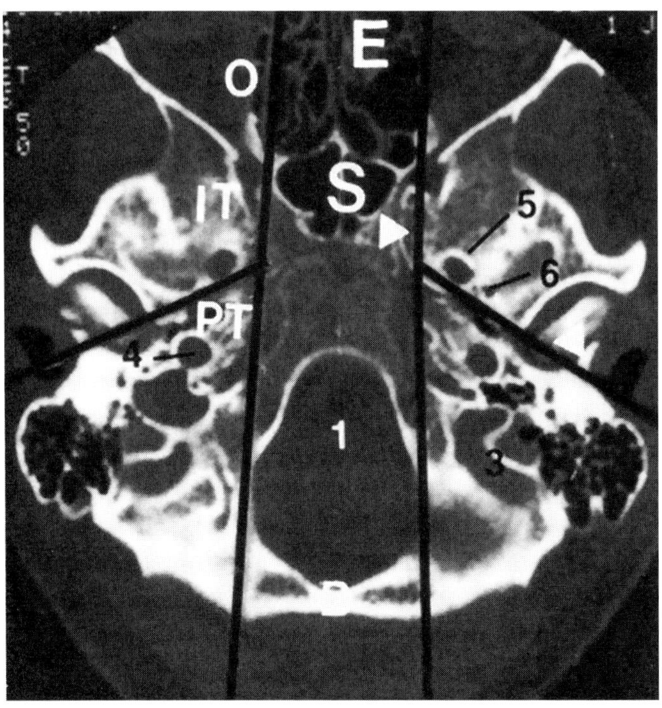

Figure 14–5. Axial CT with bone window settings obtained at the level of the foramen magnum (1), *(A)* anterior and posterior to the foramen magnum lies the midline compartment. The foramen lacerum (4) lies in the lateral, petrotemporal compartment (PT). The foramen ovale (5) and foramen spinosum (6) both lie in the lateral infratemporal compartment (IT). Sphenoid (S) and ethmoid sinuses (E) and medial orbital wall (O) are also shown. Medial pterygoid plate and glenoid fossa = arrowheads. Basiocciput =B. (From Rodas and Greenberg,[130] p 128, with permission.)

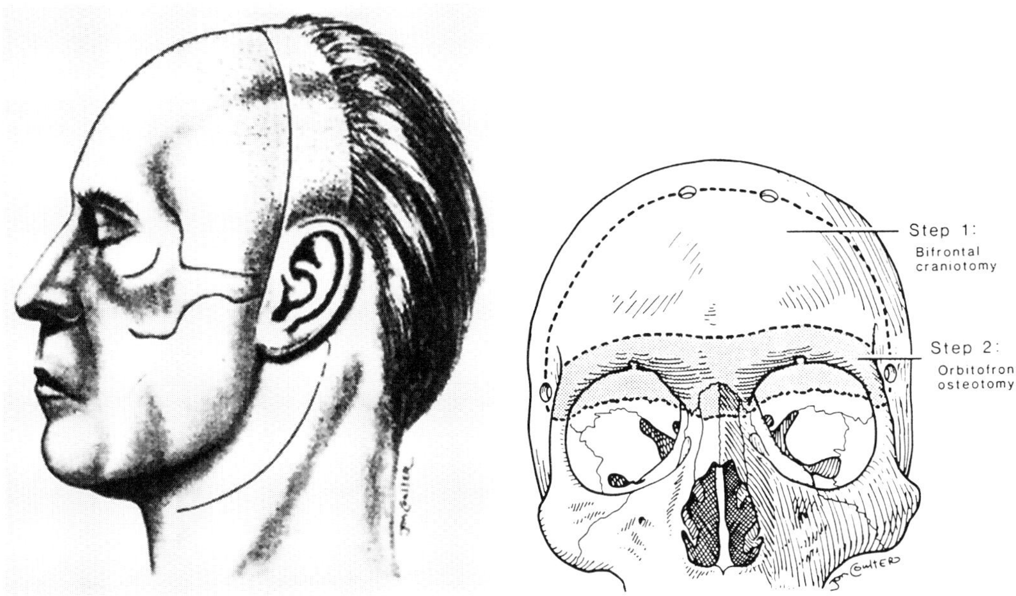

A B

Figure 14–6. *(A)* A bicoronal scalp excision is employed to access the anterior cranial skull base. This may be extended into the left preauricular regions as necessary for increased lateral exposure as seen in this figure and Fig. 14–8. (From Sekhar LN, Janecka IP, Jones NF: Subtemporal, infratemporal and basal subfrontal approach to extensive cranial base tumors. Acta Neurochir 92:83, 1988, p 84, with permission) *(B)* Following scalp incision a bifrontal craniotomy is performed. Additional segments of the superior orbital rims and superior orbital walls are removed to increase intraoperative exposure and minimize frontal lobe retraction. (From Snyderman et al.,[123] p 253, with permission).

may be combined with anterior cranial or posterior fossa surgical procedures. Neural and vascular structures are extensive in the middle cranial fossa.

The posterior cranial fossa is formed by the occipital, sphenoid, and petrous temporal bones. The clivus is formed by the basilar part of the occipital bone and the posterior part of the sphenoid bone.[123] The occiput and clivus are sometimes called the *central skull base*.[132] The anatomic openings include the foramen mag-

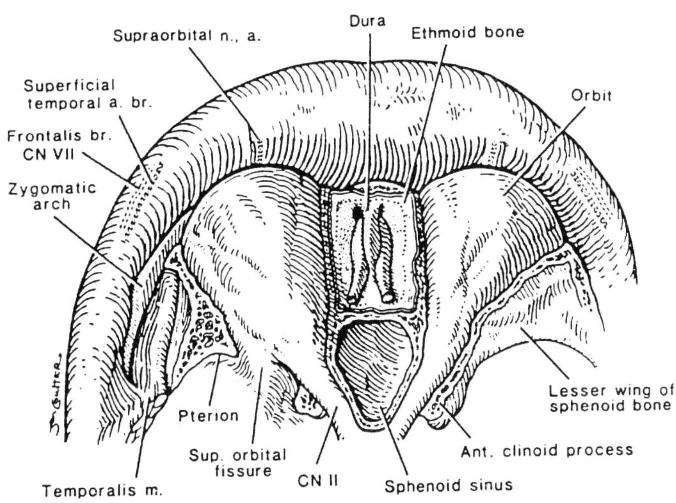

Figure 14–7. Schematic intracranial view of anterior skull base structures following retraction of the frontal lobes and exposure of the optic nerves. Tumor can be resected from this exposure in anterior skull base. (From Snyderman et al.,[123] p 254, with permission).

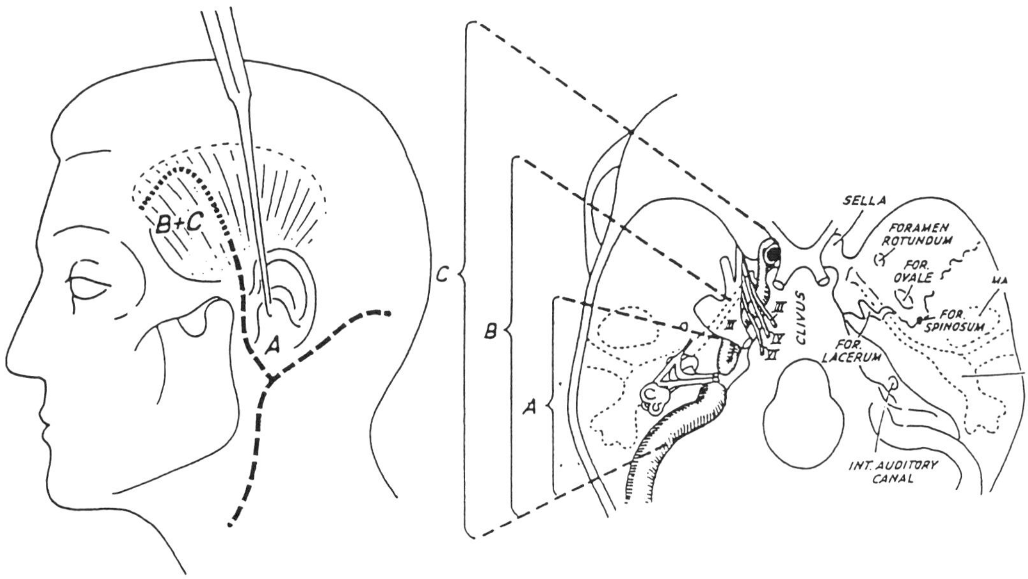

Figure 14–8. The three types of approach to the infratemporal fossa and respective skin incisions. Type A gives access to the infralabyrinthin and apical compartments of the temporal bone. Type B to the clivus, and Type C to the parasellar region. (From Fisch,[131] pp 952–953, with permission).

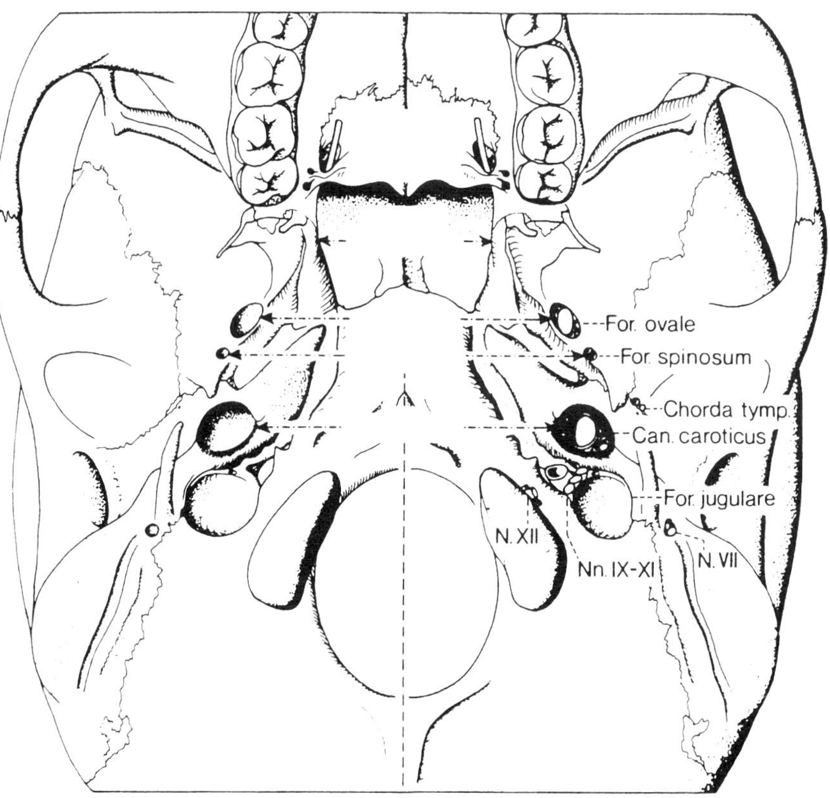

Figure 14–9. Foramina in the inferior skull base. (From Sekhar LN and Janecka IP: Surgery of Cranial Base Tumors. Raven Press, New York, 1993, p 112, with permission.)

num, internal auditory meatus, vestibular aqueduct, jugular foramen, and hypoglossal canal (Fig. 14–9). The changing relationships of the facial, auditory, and vestibular nerves are important surgically as they course through the petrous temporal bone. The contents of the jugular foramen include the internal jugular vein, inferior petrosal sinus, and ninth to eleventh cranial nerves. Cerebellopontine angle and temporal bone lesions may be approached with a retromastoid or retrosigmoid approach, which enables preservation of hearing.[123]

The key elements of skull-base surgery include a basal approach to minimize brain retraction, adequate tumor exposure, proximal and distal internal carotid artery control, and reconstruction of the cranial nerves, vasculature, and bony base to prevent CSF leakage. Technical descriptions of both classical and contemporary surgical approaches to skull-base lesions are beyond the scope of this chapter. The reader is referred to the works of Snyderman and coworkers,[123] Fisch,[131] Sekhar and associates,[133] and Derome.[134]

CT and MRI have facilitated the development of new surgical approaches to the skull base.[131] The imaging techniques are complementary. CT provides images of the dense bone cortex and the trabeculae and marrow of the bone cavity. Bone is easily distinguished from tumor, muscle, and fat. Noncontrast CT scans do not distinguish tumor from other soft tissues. Contrast-enhanced CT scans demonstrate the different vascularity in tumor and adjacent tissues. Whereas CT requires contrast infusion to visualize blood vessels, blood flowing through the internal carotid artery can be visualized using routine spin-echo MRI pulse sequences.[132] Both CT and MRI image the blood vessels at the base of the brain. MRI provides greater soft tissue differentiation between tumor and brain, particularly when the tumor involves the meninges.

Tumor involvement of the carotid artery may prevent complete removal. Balloon occlusion of the internal carotid artery decreases collateral flow to determine if it is safe to sacrifice the carotid artery or whether a bypass graft is needed.[123,132] During the procedure, a balloon-tipped catheter is advanced into the internal carotid artery. The patient is then transferred to a CT scanner and inhales xenon gas in the nonoccluded and balloon-occluded state that mimics carotid occlusion. The xenon gas is transferred to the bloodstream and the xenon blood flow can be compared in the occluded and nonoccluded states. If blood flow is more than 35 cc per 100 g of brain tissue, the patient will usually tolerate the internal carotid occlusion.[123,132]

In conclusion, multidisciplinary surgical collaboration and new imaging techniques with computer integration make the surgical approach to the base of the skull more effective and safer. The surgical morbidity rate with the most skilled surgical team is 2%, and significant morbidity occurs in 33% of patients. This includes surgical morbidity in 21% and medical complications in 12%, with 75% of the medical complications pulmonary. The most common surgical complications were seizure (3.6%), CSF leakage (3.6%), infection (2.4%), pneumocephalus (2.3%), flap necrosis (2.3%), and vascular event (1.7%).[135]

Chordoma and Chondrosarcoma

CHORDOMA

Chordomas take origin from notochordal remnants located in adults in the bones of the skull and the nucleus pulposus of intervertebral discs. The sphenoccipital bone is the site of approximately one third of chordomas, and in this region they occur in the sellar, parasellar, clivus, nasopharynx, and foramen magnum. Grossly, they are lobulated, gelatinous, grayish, semitranslucent tumors that start in the extradural space and with growth infiltrate bone and dura.[136,137] They are locally invasive tumors that stretch and displace cranial nerves. They frequently recur after both surgery and RT, and they metastasize. Pathologically, the chordoma has a lobular arrangement of mucus containing physalliferous cells (see Fig. 1–25) and large amounts of extracellular mucus.

Many tumors contain a significant chondroid component that resembles hyaline cartilage interspersed with groups of chordoma cells.[136] Patients with chondroid chordomas have a significantly better prognosis: they have an average survival of 16 years.[123] Chordomas immunostain with the epithelial markers cytokeratin and epithelial membrane antigen and the oncofetal markers, carcinoembryonic antigen, and α-fetoprotein.[138] They may show signs of malignancy with nuclear pleomorphism and mitoses.

The most common clinical symptoms are headache and cranial nerve palsies. The most common cranial nerve deficit is the sixth nerve in more than 50% of cases. When the clivus is involved, the lower cranial nerves (eighth to twelfth) may become involved or there may be symptoms referable to the cerebellum or pons. They are most common in the third to fifth decades of life, with men being affected twice as often as women in many series.[136,139] Chordomas most often appear isodense with brain on noncontrast CT and with invariable but heterogeneous enhancement after contrast. CT scans with bone windows show the margins of bony destruction. Calcification may be present in up to 45% of cases.[139,140] T_1-weighted MRI precontrast show a hypointense tumor in 75% of cases, which enhances heterogeneously. On T_2-weighted MRI the tumor is hyperintense and readily distinguishable from surrounding structures (Fig. 14–10).[140–142]

Surgical excision is the treatment of choice, although total excision may not be possible because of the extensive infiltration. After surgery, RT is given. In a 1973 series, nontreated chordomas had a survival of 0.9 years; surgery alone, 1.5 years; RT alone, 4.8 years; and surgery and radiation together, 5.2 years.[136] Proton-beam radiation and charged-particle radiation with three-dimensional treatment planning have been evaluated in clinical trials with a 5-year local disease control rate of 76% for proton-beam radiation and 62% for charged-particle radiation.[143,144] Interstitial brachytherapy has been used in approximately 12 patients for locally recurrent tumors after previous radiation with response durations from 1 to 52 months.[145,146]

Chemotherapy has not played an effective role in the treatment of chordomas. Cyclophosphamide, actinomycin D, dacarbazine, methotrexate, carboplatin, and cisplatin have been given as single agents without response. Cyclophosphamide, vincristine, doxorubicin, and dacarbazine have been used in combination without response.[147] Approximately 30% of the tumors ultimately metastasize.

CHONDROSARCOMAS

Chondrosarcomas are extradural tumors that originate from either embryonal rests of cartilaginous skull matrix or from malignant change of fibroblasts.[137] They grow slowly in a pattern similar to that of chordomas, with frequent recurrences. They metastasize in approximately 15% of cases.[124] Pathologically, chondrosarcomas contain large cartilaginous cells in a chondroid matrix. More malignant tumors have increased nuclear pleomorphism and mitoses and less chondroid matrix. They do not express epithelial or oncofetal markers.[148] The clinical symptomatology and radiological appearance of chondrosarcomas are similar to and not differentiable from those of chordomas, although they tend to be situated somewhat more laterally in the parasellar region. Chondrosarcomas affect men twice as frequently as women, and their incidence peaks between ages 30 and 50 years.[123,124] Most chondrosarcomas are in the parasellar region of the middle cranial fossa and are difficult to resect completely.[124] The tumors are not radiosensitive or chemosensitive. The prognosis is related to the histological grade, with a 5-year survival rate of approximately 50% for all patients with chondrosarcoma.[123]

Glomus Tumors

Glomus tumors arise from specialized neural crest cells associated with autonomic ganglia in the temporal bone called *glomus bodies.*[124,125] Glomus tumors are the

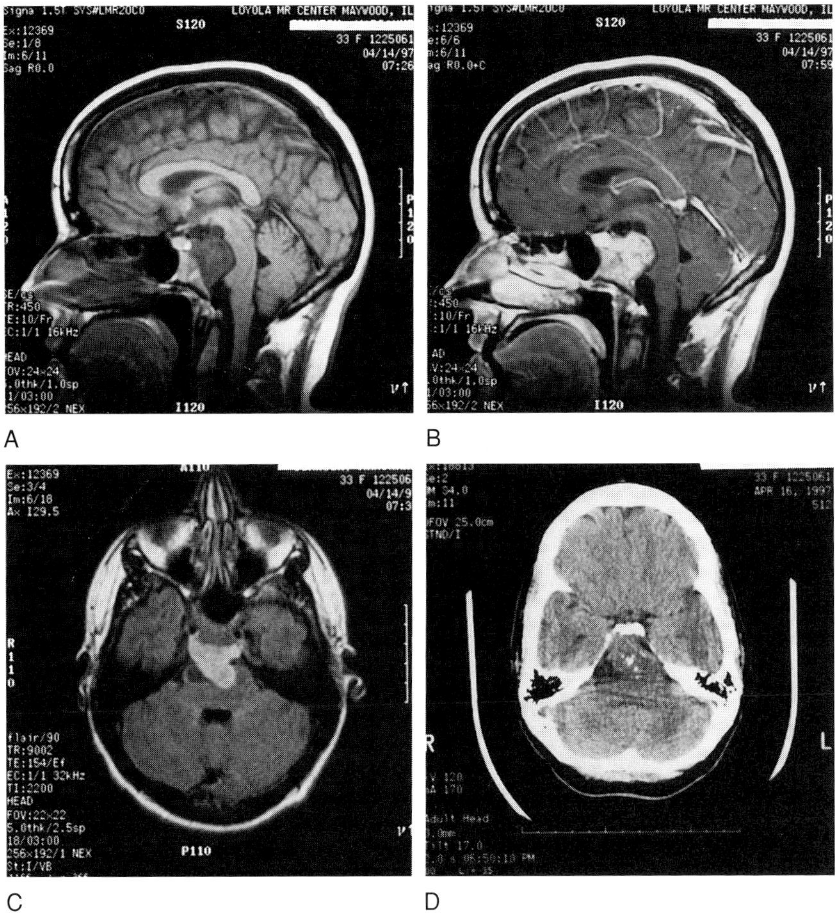

Figure 14–10. Chordoma. A 33-year-old woman with a 1-year history of intermittent left face pain in a V_{II} and V_{III} distribution triggered by talking, chewing or brushing teeth. The pain occurs in episodes lasting from hours to weeks and between episodes she has no neurologic symptomatology and neurologic exam is normal. *(A)* Parasagittal T_1-weighted MRI shows large clival based soft tissue mass indenting the pons. Extensive bone modeling is present. *(B)* The clivus and the mass enhance heterogeneously with gadolinium. *(C)* On axial T_2 the mass is very hyperintense with a hypointense cystic component on the right side. *(D)* Axial CT shows punctate calcification in the mass.

second most frequent neoplasms of the temporal bone, next to acoustic neurinoma and are the most common neoplasm of the middle ear. These tumors occur in two locations: (1) neurovascular tissue located in and around the dome of the jugular bulb (i.e., glomus jugulare) and (2) on the promontory of the middle ear associated with Jacobsen's nerve and the auricular branch of the vagus (i.e., glomus tympanicum).[123,125] Glomus tumors belong to a larger group of histologically similar neoplasms originating from neural crest cells in other locations, such as the carotid body tumor, adrenal gland (pheochromocytoma), and tumors of other autonomic ganglia. This larger group of neoplasms is called *paraganglioma*.[124]

Glomus jugulare tumors may occur bilaterally (1% to 2%), with a carotid body tumor (7%) or other paraganglioma. Bilaterality and multicentricity are more often associated with a familial history, probably related to a deletion in a tumor-suppressor gene.[123] Glomus tumors can be neurosecretory (1%) and have been associated with multiple endocrine neoplasia syndromes.[123,149]

Pathologically, glomus tumors are friable unencapsulated neoplasms with a surface that is gray to reddish-brown from hemorrhage and necrosis. Microscopically, they are composed of polygonal or round epithelioid cells and modified Schwann cells arranged in compact bundles (Zellballen) within a highly vascular stroma containing capillary endothelium and vascular spaces.[123,124] The cells differ from normal autonomic tissue by their pleomorphism. The typical features of malignancy—mitoses, nuclear pleomorphism, vascular and neural invasion, and necrosis—are not sufficient pathological criteria for malignancy. Only metastases, which rarely occur, establish a diagnosis of malignancy. These tumors immunostain positively with synaptophysin, chromogranin A, and neuron-specific enolase.

Patients with glomus jugulare tumors present with conductive hearing loss and pulsatile tinnitus usually after they have had considerable growth and extended into the mesotympanum. These tumors may cause deficits in the ninth through twelfth cranial nerves located near the jugular bulb, seventh from extension of tumor into the mastoid, and eighth from bony tumor erosion into the labyrinth.

Glomus tympanicum tumors cause pulsatile tinnitus, conductive hearing loss or, rarely, a bleeding mass in the external auditory canal. They may be asymptomatic and diagnosed on a routine ear examination.[125] Only if there are visible margins around a glomus tympanicum tumor viewed otoscopically can one be sure the mass has not extended upward from a glomus jugulare site of origin.[125,150]

Use of CT and MRI may likely establish a diagnosis and determine the extent of the abnormality, although MRI may overlook smaller glomus tympanicum tumors (Fig. 14–11).[123] MRI with spin-echo sequences, magnetic resonance angiography, and magnetic resonance venography have been effective in evaluating patients with pulsatile tinnitus for glomus tumors.[151] Angiography is used to confirm the diagnosis and determine whether tumor embolization may assist in decreasing blood supply before the surgical procedure. Neuroendocrine screening should be performed in all cases before surgery for glomus jugulare tumors.[123,149,150]

The treatment of choice for glomus jugulare tumors is debated; there are proponents for observation, surgery, and RT including radiosurgery.[123,125,149,150,152] Glomus tympanicum tumors can be simply and effectively managed by surgical resection.[123] Elderly or infirm asymptomatic patients with glomus jugulare tumors who are not candidates for extensive skull-base surgery should be followed up with serial imaging studies. Symptomatic elderly patients should be treated with RT with consideration given for radiosurgery. Young healthy symptomatic patients generate the most management controversy.

Surgeons who do skull-base surgery believe that all glomus tumors are resectable, but the question is at what risk of morbidity and mortality.[123,149,150,152] Surgical complications include frequent cranial nerve palsies of the seventh, ninth, tenth, and eleventh cranial nerves, meningitis, and CSF leakage.

In a series of 49 patients treated with radiation as a primary treatment modality, approximately 85% had disease control with a median follow-up of more than 10 years.[153] RT does not cure the tumor but slowly shrinks it in some cases and stabilizes it in others.[154] Radiosurgery has been performed on a small number of elderly patients with good tumor control for an average of 33 months, but longer follow-up is needed.[123] Preoperative RT is not recommended by skull-base surgeons because they feel the resulting fibrosis obscures surgical anatomy.[123,149] RT is sometimes recommended postsurgery for residual or recurrent disease.

Paranasal Sinus Carcinoma

Paranasal sinus tumors are a rare tumor group, originating mostly from the maxillary and ethmoid sinuses (60% and 16%, respectively), nasal cavity (20%), and nasal vestibule (4%).[156] These tumors are more common in males than females 1.5–3.0 to 1), with the peak age range for presentation between 45 and 65 years of age.[124,155] These cancers begin growing within one sinus or cavity and then invade bone, extending into another cavity or the base of the skull. They produce cranial nerve deficits as they grow through the skull base.

These tumors usually present with unilateral nasal obstruction, epistaxis, and

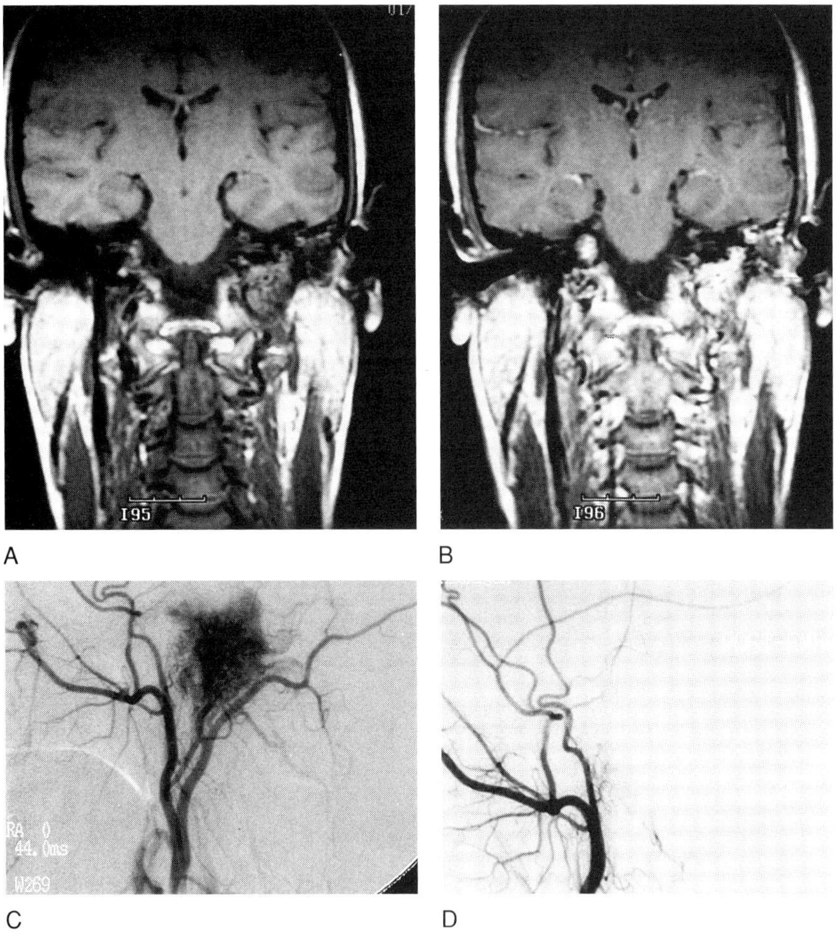

Figure 14–11. Glomus jugulare. A 37-year-old woman with a 6-month history of left hearing loss and 2-month history of pulsatile tinnitus. T_1 MRI showed *(A)* a 25×23×18 mm mass centered in an expanded left jugulare foramen with mixed signal characteristics, and *(B)* lush pathologic contrast enhancement with gadolinium. The mass extends exophytically into the middle ear and partially blocks the Eustachian tube. It extends into the basal aspect of the left sigmoid sinus, *(C)* angiogram preembolization and *(D)* postembolization. Surgery was performed postembolization on 1/27/97 with resection of a glomus jugulare tumor.

discharge. Less frequently, patients present with facial pain, facial numbness, diplopia or other visual disturbance, proptosis, cheek swelling, or anosmia if the ethmoid region is involved.[155]

MRI is the imaging procedure of choice and is able to differentiate between tumor and inspissated mucus (Fig. 14–12). CT is often unable to differentiate tumor from inspissated mucus.[155] Diagnosis requires adequate examination and positive biopsy. Initial management options include radical resection of tumor, preoperative or postoperative RT, high-dose RT, and adjuvant chemotherapy. Surgery includes radical tumor resection with modern anterior and middle cranial fossa skull-base techniques. Postoperative RT of the entire operative field to a dose between 60 and 80 Gy is recommended.[155,157] The 5-year survival of patients treated without modern skull-base techniques and 60 to 80 Gy is 56%. A significant ocular radiation complication is delayed retinal damage in a majority of patients, with unilateral or bilateral blindness in approximately 10% to 20%.[155,157]

SQUAMOUS CELL CARCINOMA

Squamous cell carcinoma (SCC) is the most common of the paranasal sinus tu-

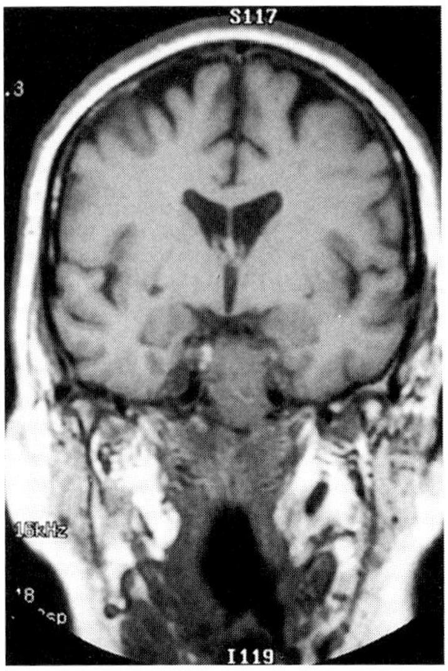

A

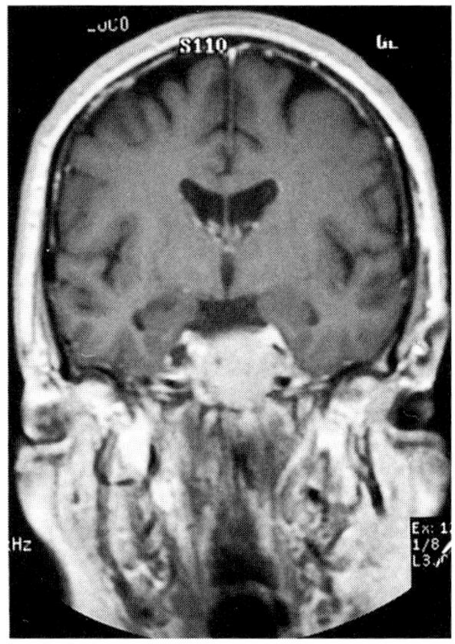

B

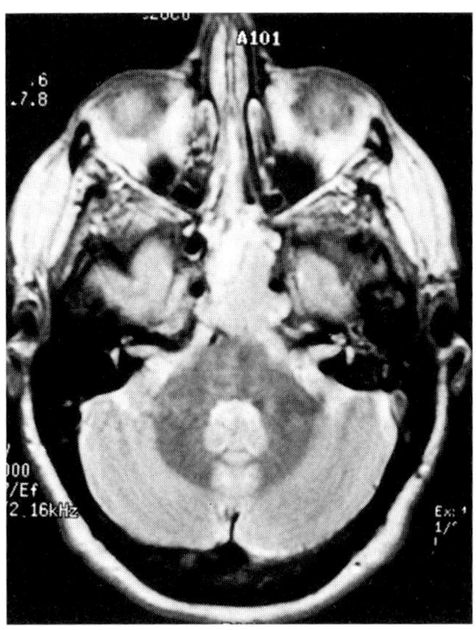

C

Figure 14–12. Squamous cell carcinoma. A 56-year-old woman who suddenly developed left temporal headaches and dilopia. Neurologic exam showed only a complete left VIth nerve palsy. Initial CT of the brain without contrast was normal, but CT of the sinus revealed a large destructive lesion of the skull base. *(A)* Coronal T_1-weighted MRI with large squamous cell carcinoma extending from nasopharnyx into sphenoid sinus and intracranially. *(B)* After gadolinium the tumor can be seen to extend laterally to surround the carotid arteries in the cavernous sinus bilaterally. The tumor enhances homogeneously and extends to the temporal lobe medially. *(C)* On T_2-weighted MRI the tumor is isointense with brain gray matter.

mors and accounts for 40% to 50% of patients in most series.[155] SCC is the most common histological type of nasopharyngeal carcinoma with other histological types including the differentiated nonkeratinizing carcinoma and undifferentiated carcinoma.[124] Microscopically, SCC demonstrates areas of keratin formation with a sheetlike structure or as epithelial pearls.[155] Occupational exposures associated with an increased incidence of these tumors are nickel refining, radium usage, mustard gas manufacturing, isopropyl alcohol manufacturing, and hydrocarbon exposure.[155] The maxillary sinus is the most common site for this tumor, and tumors in the maxillary sinus, nasal cavity, or ethmoid sinus may attain large size before patients develop symptoms.[123]

In patients with advanced nasopharyngeal carcinoma, sequential chemotherapy with three courses of 3-day, 4-hour infusion of cisplatin and 24-hour infusion of 5-fluorouracil have been sequenced with RT with impressive response. In 23 patients, 87% had a complete response with 9% a partial response.[158] In another trial of patients with advanced nasopharyngeal carcinoma, no differences were found between chemotherapy followed by RT, RT followed by chemotherapy, or RT alone.[159]

ADENOCARCINOMA

Adenocarcinoma usually originates in the upper nasal cavity or the ethmoid sinus. There are papillary and sessile forms. The tumor is rare in the general population, but there is a 1000-fold increased incidence with occupational inhalation of hardwood dusts.[155]

ADENOID CYSTIC CARCINOMA

Adenoid cystic tumors are malignant tumors that arise from salivary gland tissue in many locations in the head and neck including the parotid gland, oral cavity, nasal cavity, or paranasal sinuses.[123] Pathologically, they are composed of both microcystic pseudolumens and tubular epithelial-lined structures.[155] The peak age of presentation of these slowly growing tumors is 30 to 50 years. These tumors often spread perineurally into the foramina of the skull base and may involve bone without significant bone destruction or new bone formation. Wide surgical excision is often incomplete because of their invasive nature. These tumors are radiosensitive, and radiation should be used to delay recurrence.[123] However, they eventually progress locally and may metastasize hematogeneously. Single-agent chemotherapy with cisplatin in a dose of 80 to 100 mg/m^2 every 4 to 6 weeks, produced a 70% response rate with maximum duration of response of 18 months in the 10 treated patients. Multiagent chemotherapy with cisplatin, cyclophosphamide, and doxorubicin administered every 4 weeks produced a 38% response for a median duration of 7 months.[147]

ESTHESIONEUROBLASTOMA (OLFACTORY NEUROBLASTOMA)

Esthesioneuroblastoma is a malignant tumor of neural crest origin that develops from the olfactory mucosa.[123] Grossly, the tumor is reddish-gray and composed of nests or lobules of small round cells that are separated into nodules by septa. These tumors are graded by mitotic activity, nuclear pleomorphism, and necrosis.[124] Electron microscopy reveals neurosecretory granules, cytoplasmic neurofilaments, neurotubules, and mitochondria.[123,124] The median age at presentation is 45 years. Wide surgical excision is necessary, and RT should be used postoperatively.

ANGIOFIBROMA

Angiofibroma is a benign fibrovascular tumor that originates from a vascular nidus in the posterior lateral wall of the nasal cavity in the vicinity of the sphenopalantine ganglion.[124] Pathologically, the tumor is composed of blood vessels and fibrous stroma. The blood vessels can be capillaries, sinusoids, or larger vessels with dense, cellular stroma. These tumors occur almost exclusively in males between the ages of 10 and 20 years. Surgery with preoperative embolization is the treatment of choice. The incidence of local recurrence is 5% to 25% and should decrease with improved MRI imaging and aggressive skull-base surgical techniques. RT and chemotherapy are used only for recurrent aggressive tumors.[124]

Modern multidisciplinary skull-base surgery with CT, MRI, and frameless stereotaxy has effected gross total or more complete removal of many benign and malignant skull-base tumors. Gross total resection of chordoma, adenoid cystic carcinoma, and many nasopharyngeal carcinomas may not be possible because of their growth patterns. RT with sophisticated three-dimensional treatment planning allows the delivery of radiation to the tumor volume accurately, sparing critical structures. Heavy-particle, proton-beam, and stereotactic radiosurgery are new radiation techniques to deliver effective doses with rapid dose decrease in normal tissue. New and better chemotherapy and immunotherapy are needed.

Pituitary Adenoma

See Chapter 13.

Acoustic Neurinoma

See earlier.

Meningioma

See earlier.

REFERENCES

1. Vogel, FS: Tumors of the cerebellopontine angle: pathology. In: Wilkins, RH, and Rengachary, SS (eds). Neurosurgery. McGraw-Hill, New York, 1985, pp 694–698.
2. Cruveilhier, J: Anatomie pathologique du corps humain II, part 26. Bailliere, Paris, 1842, pp 1–8.
3. Antoni, N: Üeber Rückenmarkstumoren und Neurofibrome. Verlag von J F Bergmann, München und Wiesbaden, 1920, pp 6–115.
4. Murray, MR, and Stout, AP: Schwann cell versus fibroblast as the origin of the specific nerve sheath tumor. Observations upon normal nerve sheaths and neurilemomas in vitro. Am J Pathology 16:41–60, 1940.
5. Henschen, F: Über Geschwülste der hinteren Schädelgrube insbesondere des Kleinhirnbrückenwinkels: Klinische und anatomische Studien. Jena, Verlag von Gustav Fischer, 1910, pp 265–269.
6. Cushing, H: The surgical mortality percentages pertaining to a series of two thousand verified intracranial tumors. Standards of computation. Arch Neurol Psychiatry 27:1273–1280, 1932.
7. National Institutes of Health: Acoustic neuroma. NIH Consensus Statement 9:1–24, 1991.
8. Cox, GJ: Intracanalicular acoustic neuromas: a conservative approach. Clin Otolaryngol 18: 153–154, 1993.
9. Krone, W, Högemann, I: Cell culture studies on neurofibromatosis (von Recklinghausen). V. Monosomy 22 and other chromosomal anomalies in cultures from peripheral neurofibromas. Hum Genet 74:453–455, 1986.
10. Rey, JA, Bello, MJ, de Campos, JM, et al: Cytogenetic analysis in human neurinomas. Cancer Genet Cytogenet 28:187–188, 1987.
11. Rogatto, SR, and Casartelli, C: Cytogenetic study of human neurinomas. Cancer Genet Cytogenet 41:278, 1989.
12. Couturier, J, Delattre, O, Kujas, M, et al: Assessment of chromosome 22 anomalies in neurinomas by combined karyotype and RFLP analyses. Cancer Genet Cytogenet 45:55–62, 1990.
13. Webb, HD, and Griffin, CA: Cytogenetic study of acoustic neuroma. Cancer Genet Cytogenet 56:83–84, 1991.
14. Stenman, G, Kindblom, L-G, Johansson, M, and Angervall, L: Clonal chromosome abnormalities and in vitro growth characteristics of classical and cellular schwannomas. Cancer Genet Cytogenet 57:121–131, 1991.
15. Bijlsma, EK, Brouwer-Mladin, R, Bosch, DA, et al: Molecular characterization of chromosome 22 deletions in schwannomas. Genes Chrom Cancer 5:201–205, 1992.
16. Bello, MJ, de Campos, JM, Kusak, ME, et al: Clonal chromosome aberrations in neurinomas. Genes Chrom Cancer 6:206–211, 1993.
17. Seizinger, BR, Martuza, RL, and Gusella, JF: Loss of genes of chromosome 22 in tumorigenesis of human acoustic neuroma. Nature 322: 644–647, 1986.
18. Kaplan, J-C, Aurias, A, Julier, C, et al: Human chromosome 22. J Med Genet 24:65–78, 1987.
19. Rouleau, GA, Wertelecki, W, Haines, JL, et al: Genetic linkage of bilateral acoustic neurofibromatosis to a DNA marker on chromosome 22. Nature 329:246–248, 1987.
20. Rouleau, GA, Merel, P, Lutchman, M, et al: Alteration in a new gene encoding a putative membrane-organizing protein causes neuro-fibromatosis type 2. Nature 363:515–521, 1993.
21. Trofatter, JA, MacCollin, MM, Rutter, JL, et al: A novel moesin-, ezrin-, radixin-like gene is a candidate for the neurofibromatosis 2 tumor suppressor. Cell 72:791–800, 1993.
22. Bianchi, AB, Hara, T, Ramesh, V, et al: Mutations in transcript isoforms of the neurofibromatosis 2 gene in multiple human tumour types. Nature Genetics 6:185–192, 1994.
23. Belliveau, MJ, Lutchman, M, Claudio, JO, et al: Schwannomin: new insights into this member of the band 4.1 superfamily. Biochem Cell Biol 73:733–737, 1995.
24. Kleihues, P, Burger, PC, and Scheithauer, BW: Histological Typing of Tumours of the Central Nervous System, Ed 2. World Health Organization, Springer-Verlag, Berlin, 1993, p 30.
25. Harner, SG,and Laws, ER Jr: Clinical findings in patients with acoustic neurinoma. Mayo Clin Proc 58:721–728, 1983.
26. Kenan, PD: Tumors of the cerebellopontine angle: neurotologic aspects of diagnosis. In: Wilkins, RH, and Rengachary, SS (eds). Neurosurgery. McGraw-Hill, New York, 1985, pp 698–704.
27. Selesnick, SH, Jackler, RK, and Pitts, LW: The changing clinical presentation of acoustic tumors in the MRI era. Laryngoscope 103:431–436, 1993.
28. Macfarlane, R, and King, TT: Acoustic neurinoma (vestibular schwannoma). In: Kaye, AH, and Laws, ER Jr (eds). Brain Tumors. An Encyclopedic Approach. Churchill Livingstone, New York, 1995, pp 577–622.
29. Beck, HJ, Beatty, CW, Harner ,SG, and Ilstrup, DM: Acoustic neuromas with normal pure tone hearing levels. Otolaryngology Head Neck Surgery 94:96–103, 1986.
30. Revilla, AG: Differential diagnosis of tumors at the cerebellopontile recess. Bulletin of Johns Hopkins Hospital 83:187–212, 1948.
31. Ross, DA: Vestibular schwannomas. In: Gilman, S, Goldstein, G, and Waxman, S (eds). Neu-

robase Arbor Publishing Corporation, San Diego, 1998.
32. Yamada, S, Aiba, T, and Hara, M: Cerebellopontine angle medulloblastoma: Case report and literature review. Br J Neurosurgery 7:91–94, 1993.
33. Mulkens, TH, Parizel, PM, Martin, J-J, et al: Acoustic schwannoma: MR findings in 84 tumors. AJR Am J Roentgenol 160:395–398, 1993.
34. Amoils, CP, Lanser, MJ, and Jackler, RK: Acoustic neuroma presenting as a middle ear mass. Otolaryngol Head Neck Surg 107:478–482, 1992.
35. Ruckenstein, MJ, Cueva, RA, Morrison, DH, and Press, G: A prospective study of ABR and MRI in the screening for vestibular schwannomas. Am J Otology 17:317–320, 1996.
36. Burkey, JM, Rizer, FM, Schuring, AG, et al: Acoustic reflexes, auditory brainstem response, and MRI in the evaluation of acoustic neuromas. Laryngoscope 106:839–841, 1996.
37. Naessens, B, Gordts, F, Clement, PAR, and Buisseret, T: Re-evaluation of the ABR in the diagnosis of CPA tumors in the MRI-era. Acta Otorhinolaryngologica Belg 50:99–102, 1996.
38. Saeed, SR, Woolford, TJ, Ramsden, RT, and Lye, RH: Magnetic resonance imaging: A cost-effective first line investigation in the detection of vestibular schwannomas. Br J Neurosurg 9:497–503, 1995.
39. Brackmann, DE, and Kwartler, JA: A review of acoustic tumors: 1983–1988. Am J Otology 11:216–232, 1990.
40. Welling, DB, Glasscock, ME, Woods, CI, and Jackson, CG: Acoustic neuroma: A cost-effective approach. Otolaryngol Head Neck Surg 103:364–370, 1990.
41. Luetje, CM, Whittaker, CK, Davidson, KC, and Vergara, GG: Spontaneous acoustic tumor involution: a case report. Otolaryngol Head Neck Surg 98:95–97, 1988.
42. Valvassori, GE, and Guzman, M: Growth rate of acoustic neuromas. Am J Otology 10:174–176, 1989.
43. Bederson, JB, von Ammon, K, Wichmann, WW, and Yasargil, MG: Conservative treatment of patients with acoustic tumors. Neurosurgery 28:646–651, 1991.
44. Nedzelski, JM, Schessel, DA, Pfleiderer, A, et al: The natural history of growth of acoustic neuromas and its role in non-operative management. In: Tos, M, and Thomsen, J (eds). Proceedings of the First International Conference on Acoustic Neuroma. Kugler Publications, Amsterdam/New York, 1992, pp 149–158.
45. Rosenberg, SI, Silverstein, H, Gordon, MA, et al: A comparison of growth rates of acoustic neuromas: nonsurgical patients vs. subtotal resection. Otolaryngol Head Neck Surg 109:482–487, 1993.
46. Strasnick, B, Glasscock, ME III, Haynes, D, et al: The natural history of untreated acoustic neuromas. Laryngoscope 104:1115–1119, 1994.
47. Wiet, RJ, Zappia, JJ, Hecht, CS, and O'Connor, CA: Conservative management of patients with small acoustic tumors. Laryngoscope 105:795–800, 1995.
48. Thomsen, J, Klinken, L, and Tos, M: Calcified acoustic neurinoma. J Laryngology Otology 98:727–732, 1984.
49. Sterkers, O, El Dine, MB, Martin, N, et al: Slow versus rapid growing acoustic neuromas. In: Tos, M, and Thomsen, J (eds). Proceedings of the First International Conference on Acoustic Neuroma. Kugler Publications, Amsterdam/New York, 1992, pp 145–147.
50. Kemink, JL, LaRouere, MJ, Kileny, PR, et al: Hearing preservation following suboccipital removal of acoustic neuromas. Laryngoscope 100:597–602, 1990.
51. Shelton, C, Hitselberger, WE, House, WF, and Brackmann, DE: Hearing preservation after acoustic tumor removal: long-term results. Laryngoscope 100:115–119, 1990.
52. Koos, WT, and Perneczky, A: Suboccipital approach to acoustic neurinomas with emphasis on preservation of facial nerve and cochlear nerve function. In: Rand, RW (ed). Microneurosurgery. Ed. 3. CV Mosby Company, St. Louis, 1985, pp 335–365.
53. Fischer, G, Fischer, C, and Rémond, J: Hearing preservation in acoustic neurinoma surgery. J Neurosurg 76:910–917, 1992.
54. Arriaga, MA, Luxford, WM, Atkins, JS Jr, and Kwartler, JA: Predicting long-term facial nerve outcome after acoustic neuroma surgery. Otolaryngol Head Neck Surg 108:220–224, 1993.
55. Silverstein, H, Willcox, TO Jr, Rosenberg, SI, and Seidman, MD: Prediction of facial nerve function following acoustic neuroma resection using intraoperative facial nerve stimulation. Laryngoscope 104:539–544, 1994.
56. Ebersold, MJ, Harner, SG, Beatty, CW, et al: Current results of the retrosigmoid approach to acoustic neurinoma. J Neurosurg 76:901–909, 1992.
57. House, WF, and Hitselberger, WE: The neuro-otologist's view of the surgical management of acoustic neuromas. Clin Neurosurg 32:214–222, 1985.
58. Pellet, W, Emram, B, Cannoni, M, et al: Les résultats fonctionnels de la chirurgie des neurinomes de l'acoustique unilatéraux. Neurochirurgie 39:24–41, 1993.
59. House, WF: Surgical exposure of the internal auditory canal and its contents through the middle, cranial fossa. Laryngoscope 71:1363–1385, 1961.
60. Glasscock, ME III, Kveton, JF, Jackson, CG, et al: A systematic approach to the surgical management of acoustic neuroma. Laryngoscope 96:1088–1094, 1986.
61. Ogunrinde, OK, Lunsford, LD, Flickinger, JC, et al: Facial nerve preservation and tumor control after gamma knife radiosurgery of unilateral acoustic tumors. Skull Base Surgery 4:87–92, 1994.
62. Mendenhall, WM, Friedman, WA, Buatti, JM, and Bova, FJ: Preliminary results of linear accelerator radiosurgery for acoustic schwannomas. J Neurosurg 85:1013–1019, 1996.

63. Flickinger, JC, Kondziolka, D, Pollock, BE, and Lunsford, LD: Evolution in technique for vestibular schwannoma radiosurgery and effect on outcome. Int J Radiat Oncol Biol Phys 36:275–280, 1996.
64. House, JL, Hitselberger, WE, and House, WF: Wound closure and cerebrospinal fluid leak after translabyrinthine surgery. Am J Otology 4: 126–128, 1982.
65. Hardy, DG, Macfarlane, R, Baguley, D, and Moffat, DA: Surgery for acoustic neurinoma: An analysis of 100 translabyrinthine operations. J Neurosurg 71:799–804, 1989.
66. Waltzman, SB, Cohen, NL, Shapiro, WH, and Hoffman, RA: The prognostic value of round window electrical stimulation in cochlear implant patients. Otolaryngol Head Neck Surg 103:102–106, 1990.
67. Nelson, RA: Auditory brainstem implant. In: Tos, M, and Thomsen, J (eds). Proceedings of the First International Conference on Acoustic Neuroma. Kugler Publications, Amsterdam/New York, 1992, pp 869–872.
68. Cushing, H: The meningiomas (dural endotheliomas): Their source, and favoured seats of origin. Brain 45:282–316, 1922.
69. Cushing, H, and Eisenhardt, L: Meningiomas: Their classification, regional behaviour, life history, and surgical end results, Part One and Part Two. Hafner Publishing Company, New York, 1962.
70. Rohringer, M, Sutherland, GR, Louw, DF, and Sima, AAF: Incidence and clinicopathological features of meningioma. J Neurosurg 71:665–672, 1989.
71. MacCarty, CS, and Taylor, WF: Intracranial meningiomas: Experiences at the Mayo Clinic. Neurol Med Chir (Tokyo) 19:569–574, 1979.
72. DeMonte, F, and Al-Mefty, O: Meningiomas. In: Kaye, AH, and Laws, ER Jr (eds). Brain Tumors. An Encyclopedic Approach. Churchill Livingstone, New York, 1995, pp 675–704.
73. Radhakrishnan, K, Mokri, B, Parisi, JE, et al: The trends in incidence of primary brain tumors in the population of Rochester, Minnesota. Ann Neurol 37:67–73, 1995.
74. Schoenberg, BS, Christine, BW, and Whisnant, JP: Nervous system neoplasms and primary malignancies of other sites: The unique association between meningiomas and breast cancer. Neurology 25:705–712, 1975.
75. Knuckey, NW, Stoll, J Jr, and Epstein, MH: Intracranial and spinal meningiomas in patients with breast carcinoma: Case reports. Neurosurgery 25:112–117, 1989.
76. Burns, PE, Jha, N, and Bain, GO: Association of breast cancer with meningioma: A report of five cases. Cancer 58:1537–1539, 1986.
77. Jacobs, DH, Holmes, FF, and McFarlane, MJ: Meningiomas are not significantly associated with breast cancer. Arch Neurol 49:753–756, 1992.
78. Harada, T, Irving, RM, Xuereb, JH, et al: Molecular genetic investigation of the neurofibromatosis type 2 tumor suppressor gene in sporadic meningioma. J Neurosurg 84:847–851, 1996.
79. Blaauw, G, Koudstaal, J, Blankenstein, MA, et al: Projestin receptors in meningiomas: Comparison of cytosolic assays with immunocytochemical identification in cryostat and paraffin sections. Acta Neurochir (Wien) 134:83–87, 1995.
80. Kuratsu, J-I, Seto, H, Kochi, M, and Ushio, Y: Expression of PDGF, PDGF-receptor, EGF-receptor and sex hormone receptors on meningioma. Acta Neurochir (Wien) 131:289–293, 1994.
81. Black, P, Carroll, R, and Zhang, J: The molecular biology of hormone and growth factor receptors in meningiomas. Acta Neurochir (Suppl) 65:50–53, 1996.
82. Khalid, H, Yasunaga, A, Kishikawa, M, and Shibata, S: Immunohistochemical expression of the estrogen receptor-related antigen (ER-D5) in human intracranial tumors. Cancer 75:2571–2578, 1995.
83. Khalid, H: Immunohistochemical study of estrogen receptor-related antigen, progesterone, and estrogen receptors in human intracranial meningiomas. Cancer 74:679–685, 1994.
84. Bouillot, P, Pellissier, J-F, Devictor, B, et al: Quantitative imaging of estrogen and progesterone receptors, estrogen-regulated protein, and growth fraction: immunocytochemical assays in 52 meningiomas: Correlation with clinical and morphological data. J Neurosurg 81: 765–773, 1994.
85. Grunberg, SM, Weiss, MH, Spitz, IM, et al: Treatment of unresectable meningiomas with the antiprogesterone agent mifepristone. J Neurosurg 74:861–866, 1991.
86. Adams, EF, Todo, T, Schrell, UMH, et al: Autocrine control of human meningioma proliferation: secretion of platelet-derived growth-factor-like molecules. Int J Cancer 49:398–402, 1991.
87. Todo, T, Adams, EF, Fahlbusch, R, et al: Autocrine growth stimulation of human meningioma cells by platelet-derived growth factor. J Neurosurg 84:852–859, 1996.
88. Hsu, DW, Efird, JT, and Hedley-Whyte, ET: Progesterone and estrogen receptors in meningiomas: prognostic considerations. J Neurosurg 86:113–120, 1997.
89. Westphal, M, and Herrmann, H-D: Epidermal growth factor-receptors on cultured meningioma cells. Acta Neurochir (Wien) 83:62–66, 1986.
90. Horsfall, DJ, Goldsmith, KG, Ricciardelli, C, et al: Steroid hormone and epidermal growth factor receptors in meningiomas. Aust NZ J Surg 59:881–888, 1989.
91. Reubi, JC, Horisberger, U, Lang, W, et al: Coincidence of EGF receptors and somatostatin receptors in meningiomas but inverse, differentiation-dependent relationship in glial tumors. Am J Pathol 134:337–344, 1989.
92. Modan, B, Baidatz, D, Mart, H, et al: Radiation-induced head and neck tumours. Lancet 1:277–279, 1974.

93. Mack, EE, and Wilson, CB: Meningiomas induced by high-dose cranial irradiation. J Neurosurgery 79:28–31, 1993.
94. Harrison, MJ, Wolfe, DE, Lau, T-S, et al: Radiation-induced meningiomas: experience at the Mount Sinai Hospital and review of the literature. J Neurosurg 75:564–574, 1991.
95. Annegers, JF, Laws, ER Jr, Kurland, LT, and Grabow, JD: Head trauma and subsequent brain tumors. Neurosurgery 4:203–206, 1979.
96. Sheehy, JP, and Crockard, HA: Multiple meningiomas: a long-term review. J Neurosurg 59:1–5, 1983.
97. Larson, JJ, Tew, JM Jr, Simon, M, and Menon, AG: Evidence for clonal spread in the development of multiple meningiomas. J Neurosurg 83:705–709, 1995.
98. Maier, H, Öfner, D, Hittmair, A, et al: Classic, atypical, and anaplastic meningioma: three histopathological subtypes of clinical relevance. J Neurosurg 77:616–623, 1992.
99. Shibuya, M, Hoshino, T, Ito, S, et al: Meningiomas: clinical implications of a high proliferative potential determined by bromodeoxyuridine labeling. Neurosurgery 30:494–498, 1992.
100. Ohta, M, Iwaki, T, Kitamoto, T, et al: MIB1 staining index and scoring of histologic features in meningioma: Indicators for the prediction of biologic potential and postoperative management. Cancer 74:3176–3189, 1994.
101. Bagni, A, Botticelli, A, Martinelli, A, et al: AgNOR counts in recurrent and non-recurrent meningiomas. Histopathology 19:465–467, 1991.
102. Elster, AD, Challa, VR, Gilbert, TH, et al: Meningiomas: MR and histopathologic features. Radiology 170:857–862, 1989.
103. Newman, SA: Meningiomas: a quest for the optimum therapy. J Neurosurg 80:191–194, 1994.
104. Olivero, WC, Lister, JR, and Elwood, PW: The natural history and growth rate of asymptomatic meningiomas: a review of 60 patients. J Neurosurg 83:222–224, 1995.
105. Mirimanoff, RO, Dosoretz, DE, and Linggood, RM: Meningioma: Analysis of recurrence and progression following neurosurgical resection. J Neurosurg 62:18–24, 1985.
106. Goldsmith, BJ, Wara, WM, Wilson, CB, Larson,and DA: Postoperative irradiation for subtotally resected meningiomas. A retrospective analysis of 140 patients treated from 1967–1990. J Neurosurg 80:195–201, 1994.
107. Barbaro, NM, Gutin, PH, Wilson, CB, et al: Radiation therapy in the treatment of partially resected meningiomas. Neurosurgery 20:525–528, 1987.
108. Glaholm, J, Bloom, HJG, and Crow, JH: The role of radiotherapy in the management of intracranial meningiomas: the Royal Marsden Hospital experience with 186 patients. Int J Radiat Oncol Biol Phys 18:755–761, 1990.
109. Solan, MJ, and Kramer, S: The role of radiation therapy in the management of intracranial meningiomas. Int J Radiat Oncol Biol Phys 11:675–677, 1985.
110. Taylor, BW Jr, Marcus, RB Jr, Friedman, WA, et al: The meningioma controversy: postoperative radiation therapy. J Radiat Oncol Biol Phys 15: 299–304, 1988.
111. Kondziolka, D, Lunsford, LD, Coffey, RJ, and Flickinger, JC: Stereotactic radiosurgery of meningiomas. J Neurosurg 74:552–559, 1991.
112. Lunsford, LD: Contemporary management of meningiomas: radiation therapy as an adjuvant and radiosurgery as an alternative to surgical removal? J Neurosurg 80:187–190, 1994.
113. Duma, CM, Lunsford, LD, Kondziolka, D, et al: Stereotactic radiosurgery of cavernous sinus meningiomas as an addition or alternative to microsurgery. Neurosurgery 32:699–705, 1993.
114. Kumar, PP, Patil, AA, Leibrock, LG, et al: Brachytherapy: a viable alternative in the management of basal meningiomas. Neurosurgery 29:676–680, 1991.
115. Schrell, UMH, Rittig, MG, Anders, M, et al: Hydroxyurea for treatment of unresectable and recurrent meningiomas. II. Decrease in the size of meningiomas in patients treated with hydroxyurea. J Neurosurg 86:840–844, 1997.
116. Chamberlain, MC: Adjuvant combined modality therapy for malignant meningiomas. J Neurosurg 84:733–736, 1996.
117. Goodwin, JW, Crowley, J, Eyre, HJ, et al: A phase II evaluation of tamoxifen in unresectable or refractory meningiomas: A southwest oncology group study. J Neurooncol 15: 75–77, 1993.
118. Kaba, SE, DeMonte, F, Bruner, JM, et al: The treatment of recurrent unresectable and malignant meningiomas with interferon-alpha-2b. Neurosurgery 40:271–275, 1997.
119. Jääskeläinen, J: Seemingly complete removal of histologically benign intracranial meningioma: Late recurrence rate and factors predicting recurrence in 657 patients. A multivariate analysis. Surg Neurol 26:461–469, 1986.
120. Miller, DC, Ojemann, RG, Proppe, KH, et al: Benign metastasizing meningioma: Case report. J Neurosurg 62:763–766, 1985.
121. Rawat, B, Franchetto, AA, and Elavathil, J: Extracranial metastases of meningioma. Neuroradiology 37:38–41, 1995.
122. Doron, Y, and Gruszkiewicz, J: Metastasis of invasive carcinoma of the breast to an extradural meningioma of the cranial vault. Cancer 60: 1081–1084, 1987.
123. Snyderman, CH, Sekhar ,LN, Sen, CN, and Janecka, IP: Malignant skull base tumors. Neurosurg Clin North Am 1:243–259, 1990.
124. Barnes, L, and Kapadia, SB: The biology and pathology of selected skull base tumors. J Neurooncol 20:213–240, 1994.
125. Kemink, JL, and Graham, MD: Advances in the diagnosis and management of neoplasms of the skull base. Cancer Treat Res 22:53–82, 1984.
126. DeMonte, F: Surgery of skull base tumors. Curr Opin Oncol 7:201–206, 1995.
127. Robinson, JR Jr, Golfinos, JG, and Spetzler, RF: Skull base tumors: A critical appraisal and clinical series employing image guidance. Neurosurg Clin North Am 7:297–311, 1996.
128. McDermott, MW, and Gutin, PH: Image-guided surgery for skull base neoplasms using

the ISG viewing wand. Anatomic and technical considerations. Neurosurg Clin North Am 7: 285–295, 1996.
129. Glasscock, ME III, Miller, GW, Drake, FD, and Kanok, MM: Surgery of the skull base. Laryngoscope 88:905–923, 1978.
130. Rodas, RA, and Greenberg, HS: Dural, calvarial and skull base metastasis. In: Vinken, PJ, and Bruyn, GW (eds). Handbook of Clinical Neurology, Vol. 69 (Vecht ChJ vol ed) Neuro-Oncology, Part III. Elsevier Science B.V., Amsterdam, 1997, pp 123–134.
131. Fisch, U: Infratemporal fossa approach to tumours of the temporal bone and base of the skull. J Laryngol Otol 92:949–967, 1978.
132. Weissman, JL, and Curtin, HD: Advances in imaging. J Neurooncol 20:193–211, 1994.
133. Sekhar, LN, Ross, DA, and Sen, C: Cavernous sinus and sphenocavernous neoplasms: Anatomy and surgery. In: Sekhar, LN, and Janecka, IP (eds). Surgery of Cranial Base Tumors. Raven Press, New York, 1993, pp 521–604.
134. Derome, PJ: The transbasal approach to tumors invading the base of the skull. In: Schmidek, HH, and Sweet, WH (eds). Operative Neurosurgical Techniques. Grune and Stratton, Philadelphia, 1982, pp 357–379.
135. Janecka, IP, Sen, C, and Sekhar, LN, et al: Cranial base surgery: Results in 183 patients. J Neurooncol 20:281–289, 1994.
136. Heffelfinger, MJ, Dahlin, DC, MacCarty, CS, and Beabout, JW: Chordomas and cartilaginous tumors at the skull base. Cancer 32:410–420, 1973.
137. Gay, E, Sekhar, LN, and Wright, DC: Chordomas and chondrosarcomas of the cranial base. In: Kaye, AH, and Laws, ER Jr (eds). Brain Tumors. An Encyclopedic Approach. Churchill Livingstone, New York, 1995, pp 777–794.
138. Walass, L, and Kindblom, L-G: Fine-needle aspiration biopsy in the preoperative diagnosis of chordoma: A study of 17 cases with application of electron microscopic, histochemical, and immunocytochemical examination. Human Pathology 22:22–28, 1991.
139. Kendall, BE, and Lee, BCP: Cranial chordomas. Br J Radiology 50:687–698, 1977.
140. Sze, G, Uichanco, LS III, Brant-Zawadzki, MN, et al: Chordomas: MR imaging. Radiology 166: 187–191, 1988.
141. Bourgouin, PM, Tampieri, D, Robitaille, Y, et al: Low-grade myxoid chondrosarcoma of the base of the skull: CT, MR, and histopathology. J Comput Assist Tomogr 16:268–273, 1992.
142. Meyers, SP, Hirsch, WL, Curtin, HD, et al: Chondrosarcomas of the skull base: MR imaging features. Radiology 184:103–108, 1992.
143. Muzenrider, JE, Liebsch, NJ, and Efird, JT: Chordoma and chondrosarcoma of skull base: treatment with fractionated x-ray and proton radiotherapy. In: Johnson, JT, and Didolkar, MS (eds). Head and Neck Cancer, Volume III. Elsevier Science Publishers B.V., 1993, pp 649–654.
144. Castro, JR, Linstadt, DE, Bahary, J-P, et al: Experience in charged particle irradiation of tumors of the skull base: 1977–1992. Int J Radiat Oncol Biol Phys 29:647–655, 1994.
145. Gutin, PH, Seibel, SA, Hosobuchi, Y, et al: Brachytherapy of recurrent tumors of the skull base and spine with iodine-125 sources. Neurosurgery 20:938–945, 1987.
146. Leibel, SA, Son, YH, Harrison, L, and Gutin, PH: Principles of interstitial implantation of skull base tumors. In: Anderson, E, and Lowell, L (eds). Interstitial Brachytherapy. Raven Press, Ltd, New York, 1990, pp 85–89.
147. Jacob, HE: Chemotherapy for cranial base tumors. J Neurooncol 20:327–335, 1994.
148. Tomlinson, FH, Scheithauer, BW, Forsythe, PA, et al: Sarcomatous transformation in cranial chordoma. Neurosurgery 31:13–18, 1992.
149. Ebersoldk MF, Moritak A, Olsenk KD, and Quastk LM: Glomus jugulare tumors. In: Kaye, AH, and Laws, ER Jr (eds). Brain Tumors. An Encyclopedic Approach. Churchill Livingstone, New York, 1995, pp 795–807.
150. Jackson, CG: Section III. Diagnosis for treatment planning and treatment options. Laryngoscope 103:17–22, 1993.
151. Vogl, TJ, Juergens, M, Balzer, JO, et al: Glomus tumors of the skull base: Combined use of MR angiography and spin-echo imaging. Radiology 192:103–110, 1994.
152. Gardner, G, Cocke, EW Jr, Robertson, JH, et al: Skull base surgery for glomus jugulare tumors. Am J Otology (suppl):126–134, 1985.
153. Larner, JM, Hahn, SS, Spaulding, CA, and Constable, WC: Glomus jugulare tumors. Long-term control by radiation therapy. Cancer 69:1813–1817, 1992.
154. Brown, JS: Glomus jugulare tumors revisited: A ten-year statistical follow-up of 231 cases. Laryngoscope 95:284–288, 1985.
155. Danks, RA, and Kaye, AH: Carcinoma of the paranasal sinuses. In: Kaye, AH, and Laws, ER Jr (eds). Brain Tumors. An Encyclopedic Approach. Churchill Livingstone, New York, 1995, pp 809–824.
156. Robin, PE, Powell, DJ, and Stansbie, JM: Carcinoma of the nasal cavity and paranasal sinuses: Incidence and presentation of different histological types. Clin Otolaryngol 4:431–456, 1979.
157. Paulino, AC, Marks, JE, and Leonetti, JP: Postoperative irradiation of patients with malignant tumors of the skull base. Laryngoscope 106: 880–883, 1996.
158. Tsao, SY, and Shiu, WCT: Radiotherapy and chemotherapy for nasopharyngeal carcinoma. Ear Nose Throat J 69:272–278, 1990.
159. Dimery, IW, Legha, SS, Peters, LJ, et al: Adjuvant chemotherapy for advanced nasopharyngeal carcinoma. Cancer 60:943–949, 1987.

Chapter 15

BRAIN METASTASES

HISTORY AND NOMENCLATURE

Brain metastases are secondary deposits that arise from primary systemic cancer outside the brain and spread to involve the brain. Brain metastases can be divided into metastases to the dura, leptomeninges, and brain parenchyma. Parenchymal brain metastases are the most common symptomatic lesion, and may be single or multiple.[1] The distinction between single and multiple metastases is important for treatment. Single and multiple brain metastases refer only to the brain parenchyma and do not address the extent of systemic disease. Solitary brain metastasis are the rare occurrence of a single parenchymal brain metastasis, with no other systemic metastatic disease.[2] "Brain metastases" refers to parenchymal brain metastases, unless otherwise specified in this chapter.

In 1926, Grant[3] reported the first surgical series for treatment of brain metastases. In 1954, Chao and colleagues[4] reported on palliative radiation therapy (RT) in the treatment of brain metastases. Surgery and RT have been the mainstays of treatment for brain metastases. More recently, stereotactic radiosurgery (SR) and systemic chemotherapy have been used to treat brain metastases.

Brain metastases usually occur in patients with disseminated disease and are often thought by both the patient and physician to be the end stage of the metastatic process. Brain metastases are frightening because higher integrative function and emotional affect are or may be compromised, and these are man's highest functions. In addition, mobility and independence are often affected.[5] Although some patients have a progressive downhill course, early diagnosis and treatment with surgery and RT may produce prolonged palliation and rarely a central nervous system (CNS) cure.[6]

EPIDEMIOLOGY

The number of new cases of brain metastases in the United States is approximately 170,000 per year. This is based on the number of new cases of cancer in the United States, the number of cancer deaths, and the percentage with brain metastases at autopsy.[1] Intracranial metastases (dura, leptomeninges, and brain) occur in approximately 24% of autopsies with brain examination.[7] Parenchymal brain metastases occurred in 15% of autopsies, but the metastatic disease was solely intraparenchymal in only 9%. Dural disease occurred in 8% and was the only site in 4%. Leptomeningeal disease occurred in 8%, and was the sole site in 3%. The frequency that individual tumor types metastasize to the brain,[1,7] the number of metastases,[1,7,8] and the location of metastases vary markedly (Table 15–1).[8]

In adults, the most common tumors to metastasize to the brain, in order of prevalence, are lung, breast, gastrointestinal, genitourinary tract, and malignant melanoma.[9] Breast cancer is the the most common tumor to metastasize to brain in women, and lung cancer is the most common tumor to spread to brain in men. Whereas adenocarcinomas and small cell carcinomas of the lung metastasize to the brain frequently, squamous cell carcinoma metastasizes rarely.[10] The tumors with the highest prevalence of brain metastases at autopsy are melanoma (40% to 68%), lung (21% to 36%), breast (10% to 21%), genitourinary (10% to 21%), and gastrointestinal (3% to 6%).[7,11] In patients younger than 21 years of age, sarcomas and germ cell tumors metastasize most often to the brain.[12,13]

Computed tomography (CT) identified a single metastasis in 49% of imaged cases with brain metastases. In 51% of cases, there were multiple metastases, and 42% of the multiple metastases had two metastases.[8] Magnetic resonance imaging (MRI) reveals that two thirds to three fourths of brain metastases are multiple.[14] In autopsy series, the percentage of cases with multiple metastases ranges from 53% to 86%.[7,15–17] The percentage of multiple metastases also varies with the tumor type. On CT, pelvic and abdominal tumors had the smallest percentage of multiple metastases (31%), breast had 44%, lung had 54%, and melanoma had 59%.[8]

When the primary tumor was located in the gastrointestinal tract or pelvic area, the posterior fossa was the site of the metastases in 50% of patients.[8] Tumor spread was not believed to be through Batson's plexus because the incidence of spine metastases was lower than the incidence of intracranial metastases. Posterior fossa was involved in only 10% of the metastases from other tumors.

Table 15–1. **Prevalence of Parenchymal Brain Metastases by Primary Tumor**

Primary Tumor	Prevalence (%)*
Lung	21–36
Breast	10–21
Melanoma	40–68
Renal	10–21
Gastrointestinal	3–6
Testis	46
Sarcoma	6
Ovary	5
Lymphoma	1
Prostate	1

*When different incidence numbers are reported in different studies, the total range is given.

Adapted from DeAngelis,[5] p 157, Posner and Chernik,[7] p 583, and Sawaya and Bindal,[11] p 924, with permission.

BIOLOGY

The metastatic process consists of a series of interrelated steps beginning at the primary site. Each of the steps can be rate limiting. The major steps include: (1) initial transforming event(s) at the primary site; (2) extensive vascularization at the primary site for growth; (3) local invasion of the host stroma into thin-walled venules or lymphatics (i.e., venolymphatic spread); (4) detachment and arterial embolization of tumor cell aggregates, (5) tumor cell survival in the circulation and arrest in the capillary bed of brain; (6) tumor cell adherence to and penetration into the endothelial cell blood-brain barrier (BBB); (7) the tumor cell extravasation through the basement membrane and astrocytic foot processes; and finally (8) tumor cell proliferation within the brain parenchyma.[18]

Cells with different metastatic potential have been isolated from the same parent tumor. Metastatic brain clones may be different from the parent clone or a lung metastasis.[19] Fidler[20] demonstrated that 24 hours after entry into the circulation, less than 1% of B16-radiolabeled melanoma cells remained in the circulation, and less than 0.1% of tumor cells survived to produce metastases. A certain cell line may go preferentially to brain, and it expresses particular adhesion molecules to adhere to endothelial cells and the necessary ECM proteins to dissolve the endothelium and basement membrane.[21] The brain, as the host organ, must bind the metastatic cells and provide an environment for growth. Continued growth requires the development of a vasculature. The tumor vasculature disrupts the BBB. Disruption of the BBB often results in extensive edema, surrounding the metastases. The amount of edema does not always parallel the size of the tumor.[11]

Approximately 80% of metastases occur in the cerebral hemispheres, 15% in the cerebellum, and 5% in the brainstem, which is approximately proportional to the relative weight and blood flow of these areas.[8] The hematogenous spread of metastatic cancer to the brain is almost always through the lung, with the lung either as a primary or secondary site.[1,2] All blood flow initially passes through the lung from the heart, and the lung acts as a filter for tumor cells.

The growth rate of metastatic brain tumors has been measured with an IV infusion of the S-phase labeling index marker bromodeoxyuridine (BUdR) immediately prior to surgical excision. Thirteen patients had a mean S-phase labeling index of 13.3%, with a standard deviation of 7%. All tumors had a labeling index greater than 5%, and moderately differentiated and poorly differentiated adenocarcinomas had a higher labeling index than well-differentiated adenocarcinomas. The labeling index of metastatic tumors was higher than that of primary tumors with a similar pathology, suggesting that metastatic tumors grow faster than primary tumors.[22]

PATHOLOGY

Parenchymal brain metastases grow rapidly as spherical masses and have a clearly demarcated boundary with normal brain tissue (Fig. 15–1). Occasionally, metastatic tumor infiltrates the surrounding brain, which is more common with colon, epidermoid carcinoma, or small cell lung tumors.[23,24] Metastases to the cerebral hemispheres preferentially localize to watershed regions of the brain. The watershed regions of brain account for 29% of the cerebral hemispheric area and contain 37% of the metastases.[8] The majority of tumor emboli are transported arterially, and tend to lodge in the narrowing capillaries of the superficial arteries at the gray-white junction (Fig. 15–2).[8]

Microscopically, the histology of the metastasis most often resembles the pathology of tissue of origin, but occasionally may be so dedifferentiated that it can only be labeled as metastatic neoplasm. This is particular problem when the brain metastasis is the presenting sign of malignancy (unknown primary).[25] Small cell carcinoma is often difficult to distinguish histologically from primary central nervous system lymphoma (PCNSL) and from primitive neuroectodermal tumors (PNET). Most often, the small cell neoplasm has a rim of epithelial cytoplasm and cohesive nonfibrillar cells, which distinguish it from PCNSL or PNET. The small cell neoplasm also immunostains with epithelial membrane antigen or cytokeratin.[24]

CLINICAL SYMPTOMS

Brain metastases are usually symptomatic; more than two thirds of patients have symptoms during life.[1,2,9] The symptoms and signs of metastases to the brain are from (1) local neuronal damage and mass

Table 15–2. **Brain Metastases Incidence of Symptoms and Signs at Diagnosis**[9,27–33]

Sympton or Sign	Incidence (%)*
Headache	25–57
Focal weakness	26–75
Mental and behavioral	22–77
Focal sensory changes	2–28
Seizures	6–21
Ataxia	5–24
Aphasia	1–19
Visual field cut	1–21

*When different incidence numbers are reported in different studies, the total range is given.

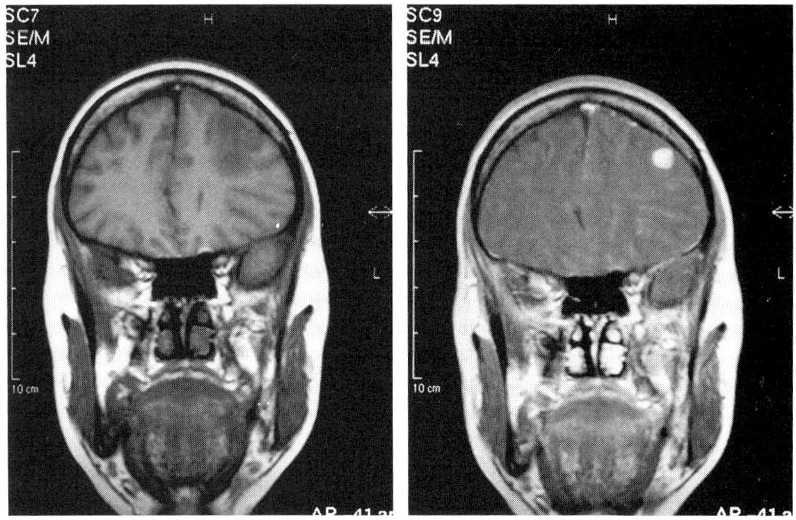

A B

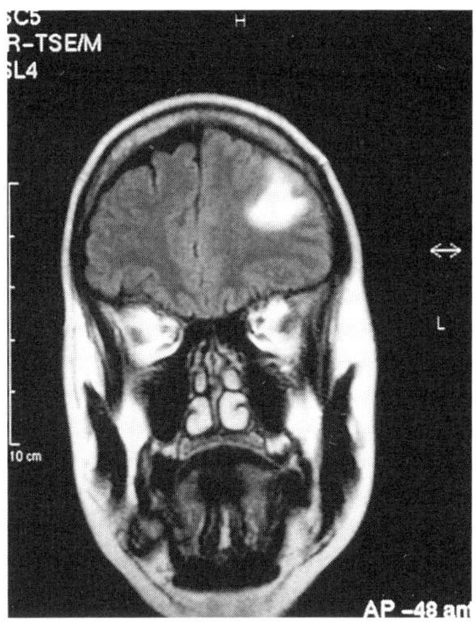

C

Figure 15–1. Single brain metastasis. *(A)* T_1-weighted MRI with hypointense signal left frontal lobe involving gray and white matter. *(B)* After gadolinium there is homogeneous enhancement at the junction of gray and white matter. A sharp demarcation is present between metastatic tumor and surrounding brain. *(C)* On T_2-weighted MRI note the large amount of vasogenic edema extending deeply into the white matter, in comparison to the small size of the enhancing mass.

effect from the focal metastatic tumor and (2) increased intracranial pressure. The symptoms and signs of local tumor(s) depend on the anatomic location(s) of the metastases. The presentation is not specific for brain metastases but can be seen with any brain mass lesion. The symptoms of increased intracranial pressure are headache, nausea, vomiting, and mental confusion. The neurological signs of increased intracranial pressure include papilledema (not always present), and later, the signs of uncal or central herniation. Symptom development is usually subacute, over days to weeks, but can be more acute, particularly if there is hemorrhage into the metastases. Melanoma, testicular carcinoma, and choriocarcinoma are tumors that frequently hemorrhage.[1,26]

The most common symptom at diagnosis of brain metastases is headache in 26% to 57% of cases (Table 15–2).[27–33] Focal weakness is present in 26% to 75%, mental and behavioral symptoms in 22% to

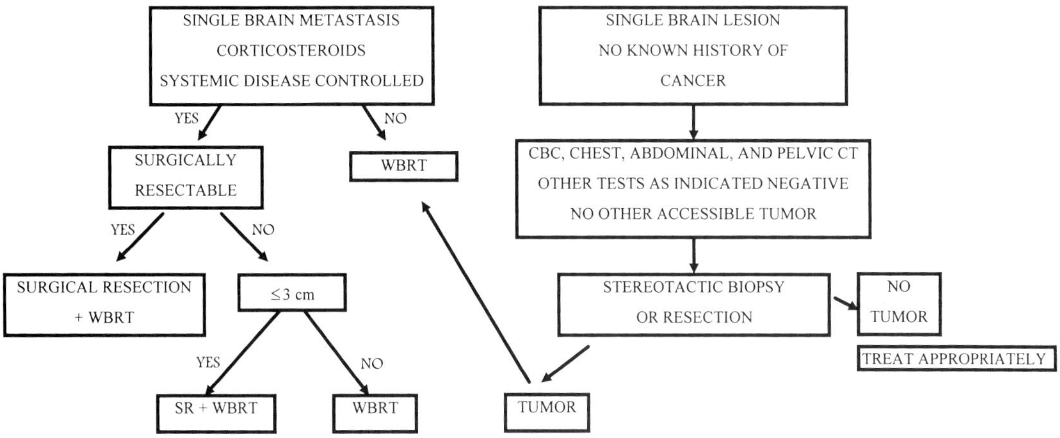

Figure 15–2. Single brain metastasis treatment pathways. SR = stereotactic radiosurgery; WBRT = whole brain radiation therapy.

77%, and seizures in 6% to 21%.[27–33] Headache and the cognitive symptoms can be caused by either local tumor mass or increased intracranial pressure.

In a patient with known cancer and signs or symptoms of a local mass or increased intracranial pressure, brain metastases should be the first consideration and an MRI or CT scan should be ordered. However, only 21% of patients with cancer and undiagnosed headache are ultimately found to have brain metastases. The differential diagnosis of headache in the cancer patient is shown in Table 15–3.[34] The most common cause of altered mental status in the patient with cancer is metabolic encephalopathy in 61%, with only 15% having metastases. The differential diagnosis of mental status change is in Table 15–4.[34]

DIFFERENTIAL DIAGNOSIS

The differential diagnosis of a single contrast-enhancing lesion includes metastatic brain tumor, primary brain tumor, cerebral infarct and hemorrhage, demyelinating disease, and brain abscess (see Table 15–5). In the setting of known systemic malignancy and a contrast-enhancing lesion, Patchell and colleagues[35] found that

Table 15–3. **Cancer: Differential Diagnosis of Headache**

Sign or Symptom	Incidence (%)
Fever or unclassified	38
Intracranial metastases	21
Migraine	13
Base of skull metastases	9
Intracranial bleed	6
Other nonstructural diagnoses	9
Other structural diagnoses	3
Total	99

Adapted from Clouston et al.,[34] p 270, with permission.

Table 15–4. **Differential Diagnosis of Altered Mental Status in the Cancer Patient**

Sign or Symptom	Incidence (%)
Metabolic encephalopathy	61
Intracranial metastases	15
Intracranial bleed	5
Other	16
Unknown	3
Total	100

Adapted from Clouston et al.,[34] p 270, with permission.

Table 15–5. **Single Brain Metastasis: Differential Diagnosis**

Primary brain tumor
Cerebral infarct
Cerebral hemorrhage
Brain abscess
Demyelinating disease

six patients (11%) had lesions other than brain metastases at biopsy. The six nonmetastatic brain lesions were two glioblastoma multiforme, one LGA, two brain abscesses, and one nonspecific inflammatory lesion. In a second study in which presumed metastases were biopsied, only one patient (3.1%) had a nonmetastatic lesion, glioblastoma multiforme.[36]

Cerebral infarcts may enhance on MRI images in the days following a stroke and be confused with metastases, but the enhancement in the infarct is usually serpiginous and heterogeneous, not spherical and homogeneous. A vascular history is usually acute, and the enhancing abnormality usually resolves in 6 to 8 weeks with vascular disease and progresses with metastatic disease. Occasionally, small metastatic lesions hemorrhage into brain, the hemorrhage obscuring the enhancing tumor. The diagnosis of multiple sclerosis (MS) might be confused with that of metastatic tumor, but is more easily confused with primary brain tumor. MS lesions are most often periependymal in location, and they enhance serpiginously and heterogeneously. Surgical resection of a single contrast-enhancing lesion is the procedure of choice in the patient with cancer and systemic disease in order to rule out treatable nonmetastatic disease and improve survival.[35,36]

In patients who present with a single contrast-enhancing lesion and no history of cancer, the differential diagnosis of the lesion is similar to that in the patient with cancer. However, only 15% of these patients have metastatic cancer.[37] A patient presenting with a brain metastatic neoplasm that pathologically cannot be characterized more fully has a lung primary tumor in 68% of cases and a gastrointestinal malignancy in 9%. Thyroid, melanoma, bladder, and lymphoma tumors each account for an additional 2% of the primary tumors.[25] The diagnostic workup for the unknown primary should include chest and abdominal CT scans, sputum cytology, stool guaiac, liver function tests, and carcinoembryonic antigen levels.[25]

The differential diagnosis of multiple contrast-enhancing lesions is multiple embolic infarcts, multiple brain abscesses, multifocal glioblastoma, and multifocal demyelinating disease.[38] All of these entities, except demyelinating disease, are considerably more common as a single lesion than multifocal disease. The likelihood of multiple contrast-enhancing lesions' being something other than metastatic disease is less than with a single metastatic lesion.

DIAGNOSTIC WORKUP

Contrast-enhanced MRI is the diagnostic procedure of choice for patients with suspected brain metastases.[14,39,40] CT is a good alternative, but not even delayed double-dose CT is as sensitive as contrast-enhanced MRI in determining the presence of multiple lesions, their location in space, and their exact number.[14,40] Radiological findings of a single contrast-enhancing lesion that point to a metastatic tumor include: (1) spherical shape with regular margin, (2) gray-white junction or watershed zone location, (3) homogeneous contrast enhancement in small lesions (larger lesions may have rim enhancement with central necrosis), and (4) a large amount of vasogenic edema surrounding a small lesion (see Fig. 15–1). The greater the number of radiologic findings, the more likely the enhancing abnormality is a single metastasis. A lumbar puncture has an extremely low diagnostic yield unless the patient has concurrent leptomeningeal metastases. At autopsy, approximately 29% of patients with parenchymal brain metastases have pathological evidence of leptomeningeal disease.[7] This figure is likely to be much lower during life, particularly if the patient does not have widely disseminated disease.

TREATMENT

Symptomatic

CORTICOSTEROIDS

Stable patients with brain metastases should be started on corticosteroid treatment at the time of diagnosis (Table 15–6). Corticosteroids rapidly reduce cerebral edema in the majority of patients (70% to 80%), with symptomatic improvement.[1,2,38] Dexamethasone is usually used in dosages of 4 mg, four times a day. The symptomatic improvement may occur as early as 8 hours after the first dose of dexamethasone. If no improvement occurs within 48 hours, the dexamethasone dose should be doubled.[1] Dosages up to 100 mg/d may be required. Patients should be maintained on as low a dose of dexamethasone as possible. Steroids are believed to decrease complications associated with whole-brain radiation therapy (WBRT), although proof is lacking. If a patient has markedly increased intracranial pressure, steroids are given for 48 to 72 hours before WBRT is started. Steroids are tapered, often during RT, with continuation of the taper after RT is complete, as permitted by symptomatology.

Table 15–6. **Brain Metastases: Treatment Considerations**

Symptomatic
Steroids
Anticonvulsants
Unstable patients (see Table 15–7)
Surgery
For single metastases (see Fig. 15–2)
For multiple metastases (see Fig. 15–3)
Reoperation
Radiation Therapy
Postoperative whole brain radiation therapy
Whole brain radiation therapy
Re-irradiation
Stereotactic radiosurgery
Chemotherapy

SEIZURES

Seizures occur in approximately 25% of patients with brain metastases at some time during their clinical course.[1] In 10% to 18% of patients with brain metastases, seizures are the presenting sign.[1,41] These patients should be treated with anticonvulsants. An additional 7% to 15% of patients develop seizures during their course. In a retrospective review of prophylactic anticonvulsant use in patients with brain metastases, the rate of seizure development (10%) was identical in both the prophylactic anticonvulsant group and those who received no treatment.[41] A double-blind, randomized, control trial of valproic acid versus placebo found no evidence that valproic acid prophylaxis decreased the incidence of seizures.[42] Therefore, prophylactic anticonvulsants are not routinely administered. In melanoma, which has a high incidence of hemorrhage and often invades the brain, prophylactic anticonvulsants are recommended.

UNSTABLE PATIENTS

In unstable patients (Table 15–7) with either increased or markedly increased intracranial pressure or herniation, the patient should be intubated and hyperventi-

Table 15–7. **Brain Metastases: Treatment of the Unstable Patient**

Intubation and hyperventilation to $Pa{CO_2}$ of 20–25 mm Hg
IV hyperosmolar mannitol 1.5–2.0 gm/kg over 20 min
Diuretics furosemide 80 mg IV stat
Dexamethasone 100 g IV push and then 1 mg–100 mg/dy
Emergency CT or MRI
Hydrocephalus consider ventricular drainage
When stable, treat according to Figure 15–2 or 15–3

CT = computed tomography.
IV = intravenous.
MRI = magnetic resonance imaging.

lated to a Pa_{CO_2} level of 20 to 25 mm Hg.[1] Hyperosmolar mannitol should be used in a dose of 1.5 to 2.0 mg/kg, given intravenously over 10 to 20 minutes. Furosemide prolongs and enhances the mannitol effect and is usually given in a dose of 80 mg.[1] Corticosteroids are begun acutely, usually dexamethasone in a dose of 100 mg intravenous bolus followed by 16 to 100 mg/d. Patients often improve in a few days, and then definitive treatment can begin.

Surgery

SINGLE BRAIN METASTASES

Patchell and colleagues[35] have shown that surgical resection followed by WBRT is the treatment of choice for single brain metastasis when the systemic disease is controlled. Patients were randomized to biopsy plus WBRT or surgical resection plus WBRT. WBRT was given in 12 total-dose daily fractions of 300 cGy or 3600 cGy. The median survival in the resection group was 40 weeks compared with 15 weeks in the biopsy group ($p<0.01$). In addition, recurrence at the original site was less in the resection group (20%) versus 52% in the biopsy group ($p<0.02$). Functional independence was significantly better in the resection group, and there was no difference in the 1-month mortality (4%) in the two groups.

Vecht and associates[36] performed a second similar study with randomization to surgery plus WBRT or WBRT alone, with no biopsy in the WBRT-only group. WBRT was delivered in a dosage of 200 cGy twice a day for 10 days for a total dose of 4000 cGy. Patients were stratified into lung cancer versus nonlung cancer. Surgical resection followed by WBRT led to a longer survival ($p=0.04$) and functionally independent status ($p=0.06$). Survival differences were most pronounced in patients with stable extracranial disease (12 versus 7 months). Patients with progressive systemic cancer had the same 5-month survival regardless of treatment. Surgical resection of brain metastases followed by WBRT cannot be expected to treat progressive systemic disease. The combined treatment resulted in better survival in both the lung and nonlung cancer stratification; however, the sample size was not adequate for statistical significance. The 1-month mortality rate was 9% in the surgery group and 0% in the WBRT group.

Surgical resection followed by WBRT is currently the treatment of choice when the patient has a single brain metastasis and stable systemic disease (see Fig. 15–2). Surgical resection offers a chance for a cure for the patients with a solitary brain metastasis. In a retrospective series of patients with solitary brain metastases or brain and systemic lung metastases, patients treated with combined surgery and WBRT had a median survival of 26 months compared with 14 months for the WBRT group.[43] A total of 22% of the patients treated with surgery lived 4 years.

Burt and coworkers[44] reported on resection of single brain metastases, in non–small cell lung cancer. They found that patients who had a complete resection at the local site had a significantly longer median survival than those with incomplete lung resection.

In order to obtain a tissue diagnosis, surgery is indicated in patients who present with a solitary brain lesion and no obvious systemic cancer. Surgery may rarely be indicated for patients with progressive brainstem compression from a large supratentorial mass. Patients can almost always be treated medically with intubation hyperventilation and hyperosmolar mannitol, furosemide, and high-dose dexamethasone, with clinical stabilization.[1]

Patients with single brain metastases and progressive systemic disease or surgically inaccessible metastases should be treated with WBRT. Single brain metastases are not operable in approximately 50% of patients.[43] Patients with inaccessible single brain metastases and stable systemic disease, should be considered for SR.

MULTIPLE METASTASES

Standard therapy for multiple brain metastases most often does not include surgery.[1,38] The standard treatment is WBRT (Fig. 15–3). Occasionally, neurosurgeons advocate removal of two or three small closely spaced metastases. Wronski and colleagues[45] found the median survival of patients with non–small cell lung cancer with resection of multiple metastases to be 8.5 months compared with 11 months with resection of a single brain metastasis (p=0.02 log-rank test). At times, a life-threatening large metastatic lesion will be removed, but the other metastatic lesions are not. These are individual physician clinical decisions; they have no definitive study to support or refute the practice.

Bindal and colleagues[46] conducted a retrospective review of 56 patients who underwent surgical resection for multiple metastases and compared the results with those of a group with single metastases who underwent resection. Twenty-one patients required multiple craniotomies. WBRT timing was variable at times before surgery and at other times after surgery. The WBRT was in fractions of 300 cGy each, for a total dose of 3000 cGy. At data analysis, patients with multiple metastases were divided into two groups: those with postoperative imaging documentation of complete resection and those who had incomplete resection. The group with complete resection of multiple metastases had a survival of 14 months, identical to that of the single-metastases comparison group. The incomplete resection group had a median survival of 6 months. The 30-day postoperative mortality rate was 3.5%. The authors concluded that complete surgical removal of multiple metastases results in a survival time similar to that for surgical resection of single metastases. They advocate surgical removal for multiple metastases, if the patient's primary disease is well controlled and all tumor is thought to be surgically resectable.

Hazuka and colleagues[47] retrospectively reviewed 28 patients with resection of single metastases and 18 patients with resection of multiple metastases. All but two patients were treated with WBRT to a median total dose of 30 Gy. Patients with single metastases had a median survival of 12 months compared with 5 months for the multiple-metastases group. The multi-

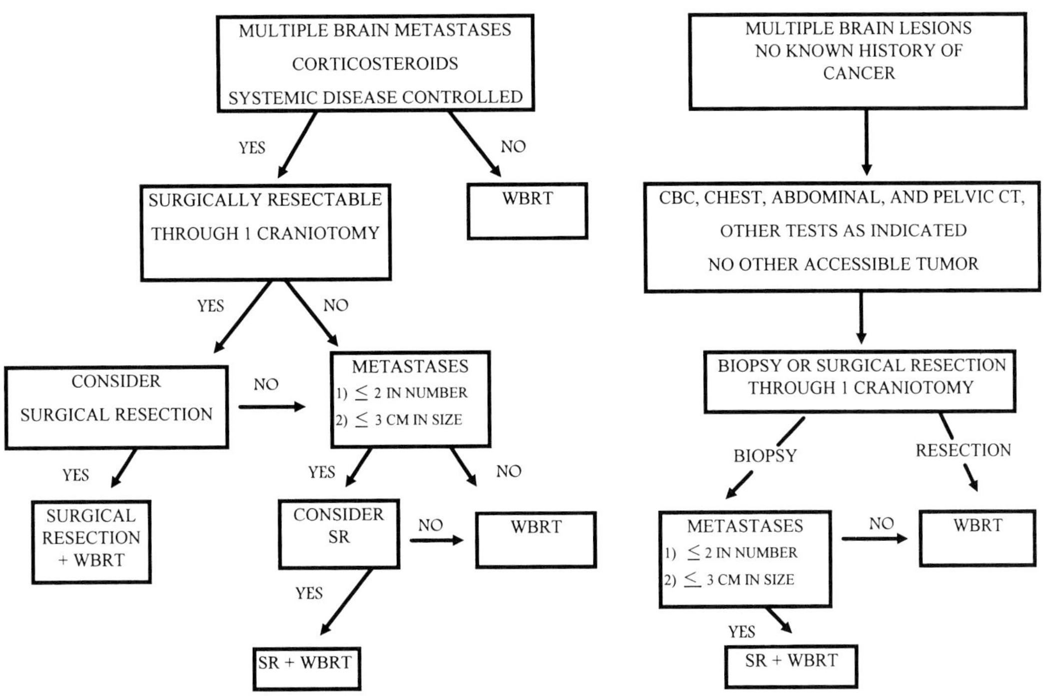

Figure 15–3. Multiple brain metastases treatment pathways. SR = stereotactic radiosurgery; WBRT = whole brain radiation therapy.

ple-metastases group had a disproportionate number of patients with infratentorial disease, an unfavorable prognostic indicator. However, on secondary analysis with exclusion of these patients, median survival of the remaining supratentorial patients was only 6 months. The 30-day postoperative mortality was 0%. The authors conclude that surgical resection of multiple metastases is not indicated, the opposite conclusion to that of the study by Bindal[46] and coworkers.

To restate, the standard of care for multiple brain metastases is WBRT. Three uncontrolled retrospective studies of the role of surgery in the management of multiple metastases have not reached similar or definitive conclusions. A controlled study is needed but will require a larger number of patients than the number used in the single-metastases study because when benefit is seen, it is only in the subset of those undergoing operation who have a complete resection.

REOPERATION FOR BRAIN METASTASES

Reoperation is an option for patients with a single brain metastasis and controlled systemic disease. Two retrospective series evaluating patients reoperated for recurrent brain metastases have been reported.[48,49] Bindal and colleagues[49] found the median time to local or distant first recurrence and a second operation was 10.4 months. The median time to a second recurrence after reoperation was 7.7 months. The 30-day operative mortality rate was 0% in both series. The median survival time after reoperation in the two series was 9 months[48] and 11 months, respectively.[49] Favorable prognostic factors in a univariate analysis were no systemic disease, time to recurrence of less than 4 months, and preoperative Karnofsky performance status greater than 70. In a multivariate analysis, age younger than 40 years and tumor type other than melanoma or breast were favorable prognostic indicators in addition to the prognostic factors in the univariate analysis.[49] A total of 26 patients developed a second recurrence in brain, and 17 of these underwent reoperation. Patients who underwent a second reoperation survived an additional 8.6 months compared with 2.8 months for patients not reoperated a second time.[49]

Radiation Therapy

POSTOPERATIVE WHOLE-BRAIN RADIATION THERAPY

Postoperative WBRT is administered to destroy cancer cells remaining at the resection site or elsewhere in the brain. The role of immediate postoperative WBRT after surgical resection of a single metastasis has been evaluated in a multigroup cooperative study that randomizes patients with single brain metastases to surgical resection followed by immediate WBRT or delayed WBRT on recurrence after surgical resection.[2] Recurrence of tumor anywhere in the brain was less frequent in the immediate radiotherapy group (18% versus 70%, $p < .001$). Postoperative radiotherapy prevented brain recurrence at the original metastatic site (10% versus 46%, $p < .001$), and at other brain sites (14% versus 37%, $p < .01$). Patients in the immediate WBRT group were less likely to die a neurologic death (14% versus 44%, $p < .003$). However, there was no significant difference in the two groups in length of survival or functional independence. This study supports the use of postoperative WBRT to prevent tumor recurrence and decrease the incidence of neurologic death.

Most other published evidence indicates that postoperative WBRT increases survival and decreases local and distant tumor recurrence.[50–52] In the first published study of postoperative WBRT, Dosoretz and associates[50] found no survival advantage for WBRT. DeAngelis and coworkers[51] reported a retrospective review of postoperative brain metastases. The median survival with postoperative WBRT was 20.6 months and 14.4 months with no RT (not statistically different). The time to local recurrence was significantly prolonged in the WBRT group. Smalley and colleagues[52] found the median survival was longer for the adjuvant WBRT group (21 versus 11.5 months, $p=0.02$) than for the observation group. After covariate analysis, the effect of WBRT was significant. In addition, pattern of failure analysis revealed local failure in 21% of the adjuvant WBRT group and 85% of the observation group. In patients in the adjuvant WBRT group who received more than 39 GY, the incidence of local recurrence was only 11%. Ultimately, 60% of patients in the observation group received RT because of brain relapse. At the present time, we would recommend postoperative WBRT (see Fig. 15–2) because of what appears to be improved survival and decreased local recurrence. WBRT on recurrence had a less-positive response in the study by Smalley[52] and coworkers. The WBRT dose should be conservative to minimize CNS complications.

WHOLE BRAIN RADIATION THERAPY

WBRT was first used for the treatment of brain metastases by Chao and colleagues[4] in 1954. It is the best alternative for patients with single metastases who are not surgical or radiosurgical candidates, and it is usually delivered after surgery or SR. WBRT is the standard of care for patients with multiple metastases. There are many studies on the treatment of brain metastases with WBRT. The median survival of patients with brain metastases treated with WBRT is generally 3 to 6 months, with a 10% to 15% 1-year survival rate.[1,9,11,32,38,43] Most studies report clinical response rates of between 50% and 75%. Response determination is subjective in most studies and is confounded by the administration of dexamethasone.

The optimal dose and fractionation for WBRT is unknown. Most patients receive a dose of between 3000 and 5000 cGy. In a series of studies, the Radiation Therapy Oncology Group (RTOG) has evaluated the following dose fractionation schemes: (1) 2000 cGy for 1 week, (2) 3000 cGy for 2 weeks, (3) 3000 cGy for 3 weeks, (4) 4000 cGy for 3 weeks, (5) 4000 cGy for 4 weeks, (6) 5000 cGy for 4 weeks, and (7) misonidazole radiosensitization with 3000 cGy for 2 weeks. There was no difference in survival between any of these treatments arms, with a median survival of between 13 and 20 weeks.[53–56] Young and colleagues[57] treated 83 patients with a rapid course of WBRT of 1500 cGy in two equal fractions. They compared outcomes to 79 patients treated with 3000 cGy in 15 treatments and found significantly more serious complications, with six cerebral herniations in the rapid course WBRT group versus three in the conventionally treated group. They noted that herniation occurred more often with evidence of increased intracranial pressure and cautioned against the use of rapid-course RT in this setting.

Sause and colleagues[58] reported an accelerated fractionation scheme for the treatment of brain metastases; WBRT delivered in doses of 1.6 Gy twice daily to 32 Gy, and a focal-boost dose of 16 to 42 Gy. The median survival was 4.2 months at 48 Gy, 5.2 months at 54 Gy, 4.8 months at 64 Gy, and 6.4 months at 74 Gy. In conclusion, a more effective WBRT regimen has not been found.

PROPHYLACTIC WHOLE BRAIN RADIATION THERAPY

The use of prophylactic whole brain radiation therapy (PWBRT) in patients with small cell carcinoma of the lung is based on the experience with acute lymphoblastic leukemia (ALL). In ALL, the use of prophylactic craniospinal RT with intrathecal methotrexate (MTX) chemotherapy decreased the incidence of brain relapse. Small cell carcinoma metastasizes to brain frequently, and WBRT was evaluated to prevent the development of brain metastases. PWBRT was found to decrease the incidence and delay the development of brain metastases but had no effect on median survival.[59,60] PWBRT timing was also critical: patients receiving the PWBRT after two to three courses of chemotherapy had a lower incidence of metastases, 13% versus 21%, in those treated after six courses of chemotherapy.[61] Rosenstein and coworkers[62] found PWBRT to be effective in prolonging survival for patients who achieved durable thoracic control. The results of this study are similar to those found by Burt and associates,[44] in which patients with non–small cell carcinoma who had surgical resection of their single brain metastases had the best outcome when their thoracic disease was controlled. However, PWBRT carries significant CNS neurotoxicity,[63–65] which is potentiated by the concurrent use of systemic chemotherapy.[GG]

RE-IRRADIATION FOR BRAIN METASTASES

Patients who were initially treated with surgery and WBRT or WBRT alone with a durable response (≥6 months) and who are not surgical candidates should be considered for re-irradiation.[1] The median survival in four series after re-irradiation was 8, 14, 17, and 22 weeks,[67–70] respectively, with at least 11 of 236 patients living more than 1 year. The incidence of radiation CNS toxicity increases with re-irradiation. If the intent of re-irradiation is palliation, radiation necrosis is predominantly a theoretical problem. If the development of radiation necrosis is delayed, and with a median survival of 8 to 22 weeks following reirradiation, most patients do not live long enough to develop radiation necrosis.

INTERSTITIAL BRACHYTHERAPY

Fourteen patients were treated with temporary interstitial Iodine-125 (^{125}I) radioactive implants: four adjuvantly after WBRT and 10 on recurrence 4 to 16 months after WBRT.[71] Six patients had lung primaries (non–small cell), four had breast carcinoma, three had melanoma, and one had uterine carcinoma. The median survival for the entire group was 80 weeks, with six deaths and eight patients alive. Two of the deaths were systemic, one CNS, and three a combination of both. Two patients were reoperated for radiation necrosis. In a second series of 10 patients (nine lung adenocarcinoma, one breast) with recurrent single brain metastasis after surgery and WBRT failure, Bernstein and colleagues[72] treated patients with a minimum of 70 Gy to the periphery of tumor, with a median survival of 46 weeks. Four patients lived 2 years or more, with two patients alive 183 and 324 weeks post-implant. Five of the deaths were due to brain recurrence at intervals of 20 to 143 weeks post-implant. Three patients underwent reoperation after implant; radiation necrosis was found in two. These three patients were among the four long-term survivors. Interstitial brachytherapy appcars to provide benefit to selected cases of single brain metastases, usually after treatment failure, with a median survival of 46 to 80 weeks after implant and 20% or more 2-year survival. Interstitial brachytherapy requires a second operation for removal of radiation necrosis in at least 25% of patients. It has largely been replaced by SR for the treatment of brain metastases.

STEREOTACTIC RADIOSURGERY

The potential advantages of SR for brain metastases are: (l) it can treat single deep lesions locally that are not amenable to surgery or interstitial brachytherapy (i.e., periventricular, deep gray or white matter, cerebellum, brainstem) (see Fig. 15–2); (2) it may be able to treat single lesions with high, focused, collimated doses of radiation and potentially obviate the need for craniotomy and its attendant hospital stay; and 3) it may be able to ablate multiple small lesions without surgery and with or without WBRT (see Fig. 15–3). Potential disadvantages are: (1) it cannot treat small microscopic foci of metastases that are not imaged unless combined with WBRT and (2) single high doses of SR may produce radiation necrosis requiring surgical resection. Therefore, SR is not likely to replace WBRT but may substitute for surgical resection.

Brain metastases are an ideal target for SR because they are often small and spherical, displace brain, and are well demarcated from normal brain with little invasion.[73,74] There are multiple uncontrolled series of SR treatment of brain metastases.[75–83] The great majority of patients have single metastases and have been treated with the combination of WBRT and an SR adjuvant boost (Table 15–8).[75–79] Outcome was reported in these series in terms of local control and median survival, with local control defined as lack of progression. The local control rate in the five cited series is high, varying between 79%[75] and 97%.[78] The local control rate does not include patients who have recurrence in brain regions untreated with SR. Median survival was 6 months in one series[77] and 9 or 10 months in the

Table 15–8. **Brain Metastases: Stereotactic Radiosurgery**

Study	Patient	Metastases #	Gamma Knife/Linac	WBRT + SR	Tumor Type	Dose	Local Control (%)	Median Survival (Months)
Coffey et al[75]	24	24	Gamma knife	20/24	All	15–20 Gy tm	94	10
Adler et al[76]	33	52	Linac	27/33	All	25 Gy i. 80%	90	NR
Engenhart et al[77]	69	102	Linac	10/69	All	21.5 Gy mean i. center (range 15–50 Gy)	95	6
Somaza et al[78]	23	32	Gamma knife	All	Melanoma	16 Gy tm	97	9
Alexander et al[79]	248	421	Linac	60/248	All	15 Gy	89	9.4
Laing et al[80]	22	26	Linac	11/22	All	10–20 Gy (two fractions)	70	18
Kihlström et al[81]	39	54	Linac	0	All	18 Gy mean (range 10–22 Gy)	93	NR
Voges et al[82]	200	300	Gamma knife	0	All	29 Gy	94	NR
Joseph et al[83]	120	194	Linac	100/120	All	26.6 Gy mean (range, 10–35 Gy)	94	8

i. = isodose.
NR = not reported.
tm = tumor margin.
WBRT + SR = whole-brain radiation therapy with stereotactic radiosurgery sequentially.

other four.[75,76,78,79] A total of 23 patients with radioresistant malignant melanoma were treated with WBRT plus SR, with a 97% local control rate and a median survival of 9 months.[78] Laing[80] reported the use of two fractionated SR treatments of 5 to 10 Gy, both in combination with WBRT and alone. A total of 24 patients with 28 brain metastases were treated with a median progression-free survival in the 22 evaluable patients of 18 months and median survival of l8 months. In the five patients treated with fractionated SR alone, all eight metastases had a radiological partial response (PR) or complete response (CR), and no patient had relapsed at 9 months.[80] Two series reported the use of SR alone for large numbers of patients.[81,82] The two series treated 239 patients with 354 metastatic tumors. Treatment dose was 29-Gy cobalt in one study[81] and a mean of 18-Gy photons[82] in the other. Local control was achieved in approximately 94%. Joseph and colleagues[83] found median survival equivalent for patients with one (33 weeks) or two (38 weeks) brain metastases treated with SR and significantly more than patients treated with three or four metastases (14 weeks). A total of 25% of patients developed additional brain metastases after SR.[83]

The acute complications of SR are nausea and vomiting, predominantly in metastases located in the area postrema near the fourth ventricle. Patients with a previous seizure history may have an increased frequency of seizures. Alopecia occurred in patients with superficial cortical metastases. Patients may develop a ring-enhancing lesion after steroids are tapered and may require steroids temporarily for symptomatic relief.[74] The most feared complication of SR is delayed radiation necrosis, occurring 7 or 8 months after SR. Two types of radiation necrosis occur, symptomatic radiation necrosis and a delayed cranial neuropathy.[74] The rate of symptomatic radiation necrosis is increased when lesions larger than 3 cm are treated and when SR in excess of 40 Gy is given.[74,76,83] The probability of radiation necrosis was also increased by prior or concurrent of delivery of WBRT.[83]

The exact role of SR in the treatment of single and multiple brain metastases is yet to be defined. Some of the questions that need to be answered are: (1) Will it replace surgery in the treatment of single brain metastases? (A multicenter, randomized trial is in progress for the treatment of single brain metastases that are 3 cm or less in size comparing biopsy followed by SR with surgical resection, both followed by WBRT.[74,79]) (2) Will WBRT be needed after SR for the treatment of single metastases? (3) Will SR be used as an adjuvant boost with WBRT in the treatment of multiple metastases? (4) Will SR replace WBRT in the treatment of multiple metastases? None of these questions has yet been answered in a controlled study. The optimal dose or fractionation of SR is also to be determined.

Chemotherapy

Surgery and WBRT are usually the first treatments for brain metastases. They are usually ineffective in producing a durable response; patients have either local or distant brain recurrence. The majority of brain metastases present clinically in the late stages of the systemic disease, and patients may have already failed several chemotherapy regimens.[84,85] Effective chemotherapy to treat brain metastases and extraneural disease would be significant progress in disease treatment.[84] The BBB is at least partially open in virtually all patients with brain metastases, yet water-soluble drugs still have difficulty passing an incompletely open BBB. The mode of action, route, dose, and complications of the common chemotherapeutic agents are shown in Table 7–7.

One hundred breast cancer patients with brain metastases were treated with chemotherapy.[86] The majority of patients were treated with one of two regimens, (1) cyclophosphamide, 5-fluorouracil (5-FU), and prednisone (n=52), or (2) cyclophosphamide, MTX, and vincrisitine (n=35). Fifty patients responded (CR 10 and PR 40) even though these drugs poorly cross an intact BBB. The median survival was 39.5 months for patients with a CR, 10.5

months for those with a PR, and 1.5 months for the nonresponders. Tamoxifen produced a prolonged PR in two patients with breast cancer and brain metastases.[87,88]

The chemotherapeutic treatment of brain metastases from small cell lung carcinoma was reviewed in 12 series, with 116 patients treated at diagnosis and relapse.[89] Eleven of the 12 treatment regimens contained a podophyllotoxin, and five had a combination of a podophyllotoxin and a platinum compound. Only three regimens contained lipophilic drugs. A total of 76% of 55 patients treated at diagnosis with chemotherapy had a CR or PR, with a median response duration of 5 to 6 months. A total of 45% of 40 patients treated on recurrence had a CR or PR, with a median response of 3 months. There were 12 toxic deaths secondary to the chemotherapy. In the two series in which it was reported, 50% of patients' tumor recurred in brain.[89]

Ushio and colleagues[90] conducted a controlled randomized study of 100 patients with lung carcinoma metastatic to the brain. There were three treatment groups: (A) WBRT alone, (B) WBRT and chloroethylnitrosoureas, and (C) WBRT with chloroethylnitrosoureas and tegafur. Complete resolution of tumor was noted in 29%, 69%, and 63% of the patients in groups A, B, and C, respectively. Tumor regression of 50% or greater was seen in 36%, 69%, and 74%, in groups A, B, and C, respectively. The difference between groups A and C was significant ($p<0.05$); however, the median survival rates weeks after treatment was similar in A (27), B (30.5), and C (29).

The treatment of testicular cancer with brain metastases was reviewed, and the the only long-term survivors were those treated with WBRT and multiagent chemotherapy.[91] Rodriguez and associates[92] reviewed the treatment of brain metastases secondary to ovarian carcinoma and noted that patients treated with a combination of surgery, WBRT, and multiagent chemotherapy did better than either those treated with WBRT or surgery plus WBRT. Choriocarcinoma brain metastases also responded to chemotherapy.[93]

In summary, well-documented responses to chemotherapy have been seen with breast, testicular, and ovarian cancer; small cell and other lung tumors; and choriocarcinoma.

PROGNOSIS

Brain metastases have a poor prognosis, regardless of treatment. The median survival for untreated patients with brain metastases is 4 to 7.5 weeks,[9,94] with all untreated patients dying a CNS death. Treatment clearly produces an increase in survival and an improvement in clinical symptomatology. Corticosteroid therapy improves symptoms in 70% to 80% of patients and increases median survival to 8 weeks.[95]

Patients with single brain metastases have a better prognosis than those with multiple metastases.[32] In randomized controlled studies, Patchell[35] and Vecht[36] and their coworkers reported that patients treated with surgical excision of the brain metastases and WBRT lived significantly longer, had fewer brain recurrences, and had better quality of life than patients treated with WBRT alone. In both studies, the median survival in the surgery-plus-WBRT group was significantly better (10 months) than in the control WBRT group (4 and 6 months). In the study by Vecht and associates[36], there was no difference in survival between the two treatment groups when patients had progressive extracranial disease. Patients older than age 60 years had a hazard ratio of dying of 2.7 times greater than those less than age 60 years but still did better with combined treatment.[37] Patchell and colleagues[35] performed biopsies or resected single-mass lesions in 54 patients thought to have brain metastases, and six were not brain metastases. Three biopsies revealed nonmalignant conditions: two were brain abscesses and one was a nonspecific inflammatory condition. The other three patients had astrocytomas, and two were malignant. Surgical biopsy, which provided the correct diagnosis, clearly improved the prognosis in three patients and guided appropriate treatment. SR with WBRT appears to produce a 6- to 10-month survival in selected patients with single metastases.[74–79] Its most obvious role is for patients with deep, non–surgically accessible, single lesions. SR alone achieves good local control, but its effect on survival is to be defined.[81,82]

In patients with multiple metastases, the median survival is approximately 4 months when they are treated with WBRT.[32] The role of SR with WBRT at diagnosis, or alone on recurrence, is not defined. Alexander and coworkers[79] treated 248 patients with 421 metastatic lesions, all with a Karnofsky of 70 or greater, with WBRT and adjuvant SR (15%) or with SR alone on recurrence (85%). The median survival for all patients from the date of SR was 40 weeks, with single metastases having a median survival of 44 weeks. A total of 69% of patients had single metastases, 21% had two metastases, and 10% had three or more metastases. Patients with three or more metastases had worse outcome. SR may have a role in the treatment of patients with two metastases.

In a large series of patients with single and multiple metastases, good prognostic factors (Table 15–9) were solitary brain metastases, ambulation at diagnosis, and onset with headache or visual symptoms. Additional favorable prognostic factors were a long time interval from diagnosis of primary tumor to brain metastases and positive estrogen receptors. Poor prognostic factors were advanced age, symptoms lasting less than 1 week, and impaired consciousness.[33]

Table 15–9. **Brain Metastases: Prognostic Variables**

Favorable
Headache symptoms
Visual symptoms
Ambulatory
Solitary brain metastasis
Single brain metastasis
Unfavorable
Advanced age
Symptoms lasting less than 1 week
Impaired consciousness

CHAPTER SUMMARY

Brain metastases are an important cause of morbidity and mortality for patients with cancer. Timely diagnosis and treatment lead to symptomatic neurological improvement and improvement in survival and quality of life in most patients. Systemic disease is the mode of death in the majority of patients. This is demonstrated in the PWBRT trials for small cell carcinoma in which the incidence of brain metastases is reduced in patients treated with WBRT, but the median survival is identical in both PWBRT and untreated patients.

Patients with single brain metastases and stable systemic disease should be treated with surgical resection followed by WBRT. Patients with single, surgically inaccessible lesions and stable systemic disease should be considered for SR (if available) followed by WBRT. Patients with single metastases and progressive systemic disease should be treated with WBRT. Rarely, brain metastases are cured with WBRT.

WBRT is the standard of care for patients with multiple metastases. The role of surgery or SR in the treatment of multiple metastases is yet to be determined. Chemotherapy has been shown to produce a response in breast, lung, testicular, and ovarian cancer and in choriocarcinoma. The development of more effective chemotherapeutic agents to treat brain and systemic disease simultaneously would be a tremendous advance.

REFERENCES

1. Posner, JB: Management of brain metastases. Rev Neurol (Paris) 148(6–7):477–487, 1992.
2. Patchell, RA: Single brain metastases. In: Gilman, S, Goldstein, G, and Waxman, S (eds). Neurobase. Arbor Publishing Corporation, San Diego, 1998.
3. Grant, FC: Concerning intracranial malignant metastases: Their frequency and the value of surgery in their treatment. Ann Surg 84:635–646, 1926.
4. Chao, J-H, Phillips, R, and Nickson, JJ: Roentgen-ray therapy of cerebral metastases. Cancer 7:682–689, 1954.
5. DeAngelis, LM: Management of brain metastases. Cancer Invest 12(2):156–165, 1994.

6. Cairncross, JG, Chernik, NL, Kim, J-H, and Posner, JB: Sterilization of cerebral metastases by radiation therapy. Neurology 29:1195–1202, 1979.
7. Posner, JB, Chernik, NL: Intracranial metastases from systemic cancer. In: Schoenberg, BS (ed): Advances in Neurology, Vol. 19. Raven Press, New York, 1978, pp 579–592.
8. Delattre, JY, Krol, G, Thaler ,HT, and Posner, JB: Distribution of brain metastases. Arch Neurol 45:741–744, 1988.
9. Cairncross, JG, and Posner, JB: The management of brain metastases. In: Walker, MD (ed): Oncology of the Nervous System. Martinus Nijhoff Publishers, Boston, 1983, pp 341–377.
10. Cox, J, and Komak, R: Prophylactic cranial irradiation for squamous cell carcinoma, large cell carcinoma, and adenocarcinoms of the lung: indications and techniques. Annual Clinical Conference on Cancer 28, The University of Texas System Cancer Center, Houston, pp 233–237, 1986.
11. Sawaya, R, and Bindal, RK: Metastatic brain tumors. In Kaye AH, Laws ER Jr (eds). Brain Tumors. An Encyclopedic Approach. Churchill Livingstone, New York, 1995, pp 923–946.
12. Graus, F, Walker, RW, and Allen, JC: Brain metastases in children. J Pediatr 103:558–561, 1983.
13. Vannucci, RC, and Baten, M: Cerebral metastatic disease in childhood. Neurology 24:981–985, 1974.
14. Sze, G, Milano, E, Johnson, C, and Heier, L: Detection of brain metastases: comparison of contrast-enhanced MR with unenhanced MR and enhanced CT. Am J Neuroradiol 11:785–791, 1990.
15. Ask-Upmark, E: Metastatic tumors of the brain and their localization. Acta Med Scand 154:1–9, 1956.
16. Chason, JL, Walker, FB, and Landers, JW: Metastatic carcinoma in the central nervous system and dorsal root ganglia: A prospective autopsy study. Cancer 16:781–787, 1963.
17. Graf, AH, Buchberger, W, Langmayr, H, and Schmid, KW: Site preference of metastatic tumors of the brain. Virchows Archives Pathol Anatomy and Histopathology 412:493–498, 1988.
18. Fidler, IJ: Critical factors in the biology of human cancer metastasis: Twenty-eighth G. H. A. Clowes Memorial Award Lecture. Cancer Res 50:6130–6138, 1990.
19. Fidler, IJ: Selection of successive tumor lines for metastasis. Nature New Biol 242:148–149, 1973.
20. Fidler, IJ: Metastasis: quantitative analysis of distribution and fate of tumor cell emboli labeled with ^{125}I-5-iodo-2'-deoxyuridine. J Natl Cancer Inst 45:773–782, 1970.
21. Liotta, LA, Steeg, PS, and Stetler-Stevenson, WG: Cancer metastasis and angiogenesis: an imbalance of positive and negative regulation. Cell 64:327–336, 1991.
22. Cho, KG, Hoshino, T, Pitts, LH, et al: Proliferative potential of brain metastases. Cancer 62:512–515, 1988.
23. Sundaresan, N, and Galicich, JH: Surgical treatment of brain metastases: Clinical and computerized tomography evaluation of the results of treatment. Cancer 55:1382–1388, 1985.
24. McKeever, PE, and Blaivas, M: The brain, spinal cord, and meninges. In: Sternberg, SS (ed): Diagnostic Surgical Pathology (Second Edition). Raven Press, Ltd., New York, 1994, pp 409–492.
25. Merchut, MP: Brain metastases from undiagnosed systemic neoplasms. Arch Intern Med 149: 1076–1080, 1989.
26. Nutt, SH, and Patchell, RA: Intracranial hemorrhage associated with primary and secondary tumors. Neurosurg Clin N Am 3:591–599, 1992.
27. Paillas, JE, and Pellet, W: Brain metastases. In: Vinken, PJ, and Bruyn, GW (eds). Handbook of Clinical Neurology. Tumours of the Brain and Skull. Part III, Vol 18. North-Holland Publishing Company, Amsterdam, 1975, pp 201–232.
28. Hildebrand, J: Early diagnosis of brain metastases in an unselected population of cancer patients. Eur J Cancer 9:621–626, 1973.
29. Posner, JB: Diagnosis and treatment of metastases to the brain. Clinical Bulletins 4:47–57, 1974.
30. Young, B, and Patchell, RA: Brain metastases. In: Youmans, J (ed): Neurological Surgery, 4th Edition. W. B. Saunders, Philadelphia, 1996, pp 2748–2760.
31. Takakura, K, Sano, K, Hojo, S, et al: Metastatic Tumors of the Central Nervous System. Igaku-Shoin Ltd, 1982.
32. Zimm, S, Wampler, GL, Stablein, D, et al: Intracerebral metastases in solid-tumor patients: Natural history and results of treatment. Cancer 48: 384–394, 1981.
33. Nisce, LZ, Hilaris, BS, and Chu, FC: A review of experience with irradiation of brain metastasis. Am J Roentgenol Radium Ther Nucl Med 111: 329–333, 1971.
34. Clouston, PD, DeAngelis, LM, and Posner, JB: The spectrum of neurological disease in patients with systemic cancer. Ann Neurol 31:268–273, 1992.
35. Patchell, RA, Tibbs, PA, Walsh, JW, et al: A randomized trial of surgery in the treatment of single metastases to the brain. N Engl J Med 322: 494–500, 1990.
36. Vecht, CJ, Haaxma-Reiche, H, Noordijk, EM, et al: Treatment of single brain metastasis: radiotherapy alone or combined with neurosurgery? Ann Neurol 33:583–590, 1993.
37. Voorhies, RM, Sundaresan, N, and Thaler, HT: The single supratentorial lesion. An evaluation of preoperative diagnostic tests. J Neurosurg 53: 364–368, 1980.
38. Patchell, RA: Multiple brain metastases. In: Gilman, S, Goldstein, G, and Waxman, S (eds). Neurobase. Arbor Publishing Corporation, San Diego, 1995.
39. Russell, EJ, Geremia, GK, and Johnson, CE: Multiple cerebral metastases: detectability with Gd-DTPA-enhanced MR imaging. Radiology 165:609–617, 1987.
40. Davis, PC, Hudgins, PA, Peterman, SB, and Hoffman, JC: Diagnosis of cerebral metastases: double-dose delayed CT vs contrast-enhanced

MR imaging. Am J Neuroradiol 12:293–300, 1991.
41. Cohen, N, Strauss, G, Lew, R, et al: Should prophylactic anticonvulsants be administered to patients with newly-diagnosed cerebral metastases? A restrospective analysis. J Clin Oncol 6:1621–1624, 1988.
42. Glantz, M, Friedberg, M, Cole, B, et al: Double-blind, randomized, placebo-controlled trial of anticonvulsant prophylaxis in adults with newly diagnosed brain metastases. Proc Amer Soc Clin Oncol 13:176, 1994.
43. Patchell, RA, Cirrincione, C, Thaler, HT, et al: Single brain metastases: Surgery plus radiation or radiation alone. Neurology 36:447–453, 1986.
44. Burt, M, Wronski, M, Arbit, E, Galicich, JH, and The Memorial Sloan-Kettering Cancer Center Thoracic Surgical Staff: Resection of brain metastases from non-small-cell lung carcinoma. J Thorac Cardiovasc Surg 103:399–411, 1992.
45. Wronski, M, Arbit, E, Burt, M, and Galicich, JH: Survival after surgical treatment of brain metastases from lung cancer: a follow-up study of 231 patients treated between 1976 and 1991. J Neurosurg 83:605–616, 1995.
46. Bindal, RK, Sawaya, R, Leavens, ME, and Lee, JJ: Surgical treatment of multiple brain metastases. J Neurosurg 79:210–216, 1993.
47. Hazuka, MB, Burleson, WD, Stroud, DN, et al: Multiple brain metastases are associated with poor survival in patients treated with surgery and radiotherapy. J Clin Oncol 11:369–373, 1993.
48. Sundaresan, N, Sachdev, VP, DiGiancinto, GV, and Hughes, JEO: Reoperation for brain metastases. J Clin Oncol 6:1625–1629, 1988.
49. Bindal, RK, Sawaya, R, Leavens, ME, et al: Reoperation for recurrent metastatic brain tumors. J Neurosurg 83:600–604, 1995.
50. Dosoretz, DE, Blitzer, PH, Russell, AH, and Wang, CC: Management of solitary metastasis to the brain: The role of elective brain irradiation following complete surgical resection. Int J Radiat Oncol Biol Phys 6:1727–1730, 1980.
51. DeAngelis, LM, Mandell, LR, Thaler, HT, et al: The role of postoperative radiotherapy after resection of single brain metastases. Neurosurgery 24:798–805, 1989.
52. Smalley, SR, Schray, MF, Law,s ER, and O'Fallon, JR: Adjuvant radiation therapy after surgical resection of solitary brain metastasis: Association with pattern of failure and survival. Int J Radiat Oncol Biol Phys 13:1611–1616, 1987.
53. Gelber, RD, Larson, M, Borgelt ,BB, and Kramer, S: Equivalence of radiation schedules for the palliative treatment of brain metastases in patients with favorable prognosis. Cancer 48: 1749–1753, 1981.
54. Kurtz, JM, Gelber, R, Brady, LW, et al: The palliation of brain metastases in a favorable patient population: A randomized clinical trial by the Radiation Therapy Oncology Group. Int J Radiat Oncol Biol Phys 7:891–895, 1981.
55. Borgelt, B, Gelber, R, Kramer, S, et al: The palliation of brain metastases: Final results of the first two studies by the Radiation Therapy Oncology Group. Int J Radiat Oncol Biol Phys 6:1–9, 1980.
56. Komarnicky, LT, Phillips, TL, Martz, K, et al: A randomized phase III protocol for the evaluation of misonidazole combined with radiation in the treatment of patients with brain metastases (RTOG-7916). Int J Radiat Oncol Biol Phys 20: 53–58, 1991.
57. Young, DF, Posner, JB, Chu, F, and Nisce, L: Rapid-course radiation therapy of cerebral metastases: results and complications. Cancer 34: 1069–1076, 1974.
58. Sause, WT, Scott, C, Krisch, R, et al: Phase I/II trial of accelerated fractionation in brain metastases RTOG 85–28. Int J Radiat Oncol Biol Phys 26:653–657, 1993.
59. Umsawasdi, T, Barkley, HT Jr, Booser, DJ, et al: Role of prophylactic brain irradiation (PBI) during combined chemoradiotherapy (CCRT) for inoperable adeno & squamous cell lung cancer (AS-CLC). Proc Am Soc Clin Oncol 1:148(C574), 1982.
60. Aroney, RS, Aisner, J, Wesley, MN, et al: Value prophylactic cranial irradiation given at complete remission in small cell lung carcinoma. Cancer Treat Rep 67:675–682, 1983.
61. Lee, JS, Umsawasdi, T, Barkley, HT, et al: Timing of elective brain irradiation: A critical factor for brain metastasis-free survival in small cell lung cancer. Int J Radiat Oncol Biol Phys 13: 697–704, 1987.
62. Rosenstein, M, Armstrong, J, Kris, M, et al: A reappraisal of the role of prophylactic cranial irradiation in limited small cell lung cancer. Int J Radiat Oncol Biol Phys 24:43–48, 1992.
63. Laukkanen, E, Klonoff, H, Allan, B, et al: The role of prophylactic brain irradiation in limited stage small cell lung cancer: Clinical, neuropsychologic and CT sequelae. Int J Radiat Oncol Biol Phys 14:1109–1117, 1989.
64. Pedersen, AG, Bishop, JF, Bleehen, NM, et al: Management of CNS metastases in small cell lung cancer: A consensus report. Lung Cancer 5: 140–142, 1989.
65. Johnson, BE, Patronas, N, and Hayes, W: Neurologic, computed cranial tomographic, and magnetic resonance imaging abnormalities in patients with small-cell lung cancer: further follow-up of 6- to 13-year survivors. J Clin Oncol 8: 48–56, 1990.
66. Turrisi, A: Brain irradiation and systemic chemotherapy for small-cell lung cancer: Dangerous liasons? J Clin Oncol 8:196–199, 1990.
67. Hazuka, MB, and Kinzie, JJ: Brain metastases: results and effects of re-irradiation. Int J Radiat Oncol Biol Phys 15:433–437, 1988.
68. Kurup, P, Reddy, S, and Hendrickson, FR: Results of re-irradiation for cerebral metastases. Cancer 46:2587–2589, 1980.
69. Cooper, JS, Steinfeld, AD, and Lerch, IA: Cerebral metastases: value of reirradiation in selected patients. Radiology 174:883–885, 1990.
70. Wong, WW, Schild, SE, Sawyer, TE, and Shaw, EG: Analysis of outcome in patients reirradiated for brain metastases. Int J Radiat Oncol Biol Phys 34:585–590, 1996.

71. Prados, M, Leibel, S, Barnett, CM, and Gutin, P: Interstitial brachytherapy for metastatic brain tumors. Cancer 63:657–660, 1989.
72. Bernstein, M, Cabantog, A, Laperriere, N, et al: Brachytherapy for recurrent single brain metastasis. Can J Neurol Sci 22:13–16, 1995.
73. Leksell, L: The stereotactic method and radiosurgery of the brain. Acta Chir Scand 102:316–319, 1951.
74. Loeffler, JS, Alexander, E III, Kooy, HM, et al: Radiosurgery for brain metastases. In: Devita, VT, Hellman, S, and Rosenberg, SA (eds). PPO Updates: Cancer. Principles & Practice of Oncology, Volume 5(2). Philadelphia, JB Lippincott, pp 1–12, 1991.
75. Coffey, RJ, Flickinger, JC, Bissonette, DJ, and Lunsford, LD: Radiosurgery for solitary brain metastases using the cobalt-60 gamma unit: methods and results in 24 patients. Int J Radiat Oncol Biol Phys 20:1287–1295, 1991.
76. Adler, JR, Cox, RS, Kaplan, I, and Martin, DP: Stereotactic radiosurgical treatment of brain metastases. J Neurosurg 76:444–449, 1992.
77. Engenhart, R, Kimmig, BN, Höver, K-H, et al: Long-term follow-up for brain metastases treated by percutaneous stereotactic single high-dose irradiation. Cancer 71:1353–1361, 1993.
78. Somaza, S, Kondziolka, D, Lunsford, LD, et al: Stereotactic radiosurgery for cerebral metastatic melanoma. J Neurosurg 79:661–666, 1993.
79. Alexander, E III, Moriarty, TM, Davis, RB, et al: Stereotactic radiosurgery for the definitive, noninvasive treatment of brain metastases. J Natl Cancer Inst 87:34–40, 1995.
80. Laing, RW, Warrington, AP, Hines, F, et al: Fractionated stereotactic external beam radiotherapy in the management of brain metastases. Eur J Cancer 29A(10):1387–1391, 1993.
81. Kihlström, L, Karlsson, B, and Lindquist, C: Stereotactic radiosurgery for single and multiple cerebral metastases. Acta Neurochir 122:158, 1993.
82. Voges, J, Treuer, H, Schlegel, W, et al: Linac-radiosurgery in brain metastases. Acta Neurochir 122:158, 1993.
83. Joseph, J, Adler, JR, Cox, RS, and Hancock, SL: Linear accelerator-based stereotaxic radiosurgery for brain metastases: The influence of number of lesions on survival. J Clin Oncol 14: 1085–1092, 1996.
84. Hildebrand, J: Chemotherapy of brain metastases. Eur J Cancer Clin Oncol 24:629–631, 1988.
85. Siegers, HP: Chemotherapy for brain metastases: recent developments and clinical considerations. Cancer Treatment Reviews 17:63–76, 1990.
86. Rosner, D, Nemoto, T, and Lane, WW: Chemotherapy induces regression of brain metastases in breast carcinoma. Cancer 58:832–839, 1986.
87. Carey, RW, Davis, JM, and Zervas, NJ: Tamoxifen-induced regression of cerebral metastases in breast carcinoma. Cancer Treat Rep 65:793–795, 1981.
88. Hansen, SB, Galsgård, H, von Eyben, FE, et al: Tamoxifen for brain metastases from breast cancer. Ann Neurol 20:544, 1986.
89. Kristensen, CA, Kristjansen, PEG, and Hansen, HH: Systemic chemotherapy of brain metastases from small-cell lung cancer: a review. J Clin Oncol 10:1498–1502, 1992.
90. Ushio, Y, Arita, N, Hayakawa, T, et al: Chemotherapy of brain metastases from lung carcinoma: a controlled randomized study. Neurosurgery 28:201–205, 1991.
91. Spears, WT, Morphis, JG II, Lester, SG, et al: Brain metastases and testicular tumors: long-term survival. Int J Radiat Oncol Biol Phys 22:17–22, 1991.
92. Rodriguez, GC, Soper, JT, Berchuck, A, et al: Improved palliation of cerebral metastases in epithelial ovarian cancer using a combined modality approach including radiation therapy, chemotherapy, and surgery. J Clin Oncol 10: 1553–1560, 1992.
93. Rustin, GJS, Newlands, ES, Begent, RHJ, et al: Weekly alternating etoposide, methotrexate, and actinomycin/vincristine and cyclophosphamide chemotherapy for the treatment of CNS metastases of choriocarcinoma. J Clin Oncol 7:900–903, 1989.
94. Markesbery, WR, Brooks, WH, Gupta, GD, and Young, AB: Treatment for patients with cerebral metastases. Arch Neurol 35:754–756, 1978.
95. Chang, D-B, Yang, P-C, Luh, K-T, et al: Late survival of non-small cell lung cancer patients with brain metastases. Chest 101:1293–1297, 1992.

INDEX